THE RECOVERY ROOM

A Critical Care Approach to Post Anesthesia Nursing

Second Edition

CECIL B. DRAIN

R.N., C.R.N.A., Ph.D.
Lieutenant Colonel, U.S. Army Nurse Corps
Brooke Army Medical Center
Fort Sam Houston, Texas

SUSAN SHIPLEY CHRISTOPH

R.N., D.N.Sc., C.C.R.N.
Lieutenant Colonel, U.S. Army Nurse Corps
Chief Nurse
United States Army Medical
    Research and Development Command
Fort Detrick
Frederick, Maryland

1987
W.B. SAUNDERS COMPANY

Philadelphia   London   Toronto
Sydney   Tokyo   Hong Kong

W. B. Saunders Company: West Washington Square
                          Philadelphia, PA 19105

Library of Congress Cataloging-in-Publication Data

Drain, Cecil B.

The recovery room.

Includes bibliographies and index.
1. Recovery room (Surgery).   2. Postoperative care.   3. Intensive
   care nursing.   I. Christoph, Susan Shipley.   II. Title.
   [DNLM: 1. Nursing Care. 2. Postoperative Care—nurses' instruction. 3. Post-operative Period—nurses' instruction. 4. Recovery
   Room—nurses' instruction. WY 154 D759r]

RD51.D7 1987   617'.919   86–17858

ISBN   0–7216–1065–X

Listed here are the latest translated editions of this book together
with the language of the translation and the publisher.

Portuguese (*1st Edition*)—Editora Guanabara Koogan S.A., Travessa do Ouvidor—
                          1, ZC 00 Rio de Janeiro, Brazil

Editor: Michael Brown
Designer: Dorothy Chattin
Production Manager: Bill Preston
Manuscript Editor: Diane Zuckerman
Illustration Coordinator: Peg Shaw
Indexer: David Prout

The Recovery Room   ISBN   0–7216–1065–X

Last digit is the print number: 9   8   7   6   5   4   3   2

To my parents, my wife Cindy, our sons Tim and Steve, and our daughter Kathryn, for their love and support; to O. M. "Sandy" Gammon, for a fine introduction into the world of professional nursing; to Mary Shofner, for teaching me the foundations of PACU nursing; to Jim Hunn, for making physiology exciting and enjoyable; to Arlene M. "Pam" Putt, for her splendid introduction into the world of graduate nursing education; to Glenn Ross Johnson, for his intellectual guidance during my doctoral education; and, finally to my recently departed friend, educator, and mentor, Hershal Wayne Bradshaw—the man who helped me "to be all that I can be."

CECIL B. DRAIN

This manuscript is lovingly dedicated to the young fast food experts of my family: Skip, my computer programmer; Gail, my typist; Bobby, my printer; and Hunter, my handyman; and to PACU nurses everywhere who have become not only helpful critics, but friends.

SUE CHRISTOPH

Contributors

MARIE H. DUTTON, R.N., M.S.N.
United States Army Nurse Corps (Retired)

BRYAN S. JORDAN, CAPTAIN, A.N.C.
United States Army Institute of Surgical Research
Fort Sam Houston
San Antonio, Texas

STEVEN SCHMIDT, MAJOR, M.C.
United States Army Institute of Surgical Research
Fort Sam Houston
San Antonio, Texas

ALAN SEYFER, COLONEL, M.C.
Chief, Plastic and Reconstructive Surgery
Walter Reed Army Medical Center
Washington, D.C.

KAREN D. SPADACCIA, R.N., B.S.N., C.C.R.N., C.E.N.
Staff Development/Critical Care Instructor
North Westchester Hospital Center
Mt. Kisco, New York

GAYLE WHITMAN, R.N. M.S.N., C.C.R.N.
Department Chairperson, Cardiac Nursing
Department of Hospital Nursing
Cleveland Clinic Foundation
Cleveland, Ohio

Preface to the Second Edition

Since the introduction of this book, post anesthesia nursing has become more firmly established as a specialty within critical care nursing, including the establishment of its own professional society. The authors hope that the first edition of this book helped support this development.

Historically, the special areas of a hospital designated for the close monitoring and intensive care of patients who have undergone anesthesia and surgery have been called "recovery rooms" or "recovery wards". In 1983, the American Society of Post Anesthesia Nurses (ASPAN) chose the term *post anesthesia care unit* (PACU) to apply to the work area and *post anesthesia nurse* (PAN) to designate the nurse specializing in that area of patient care. We have renamed the second edition to reflect the fact that post anesthesia nursing is a critical care specialty, and we have used the term post anesthesia care unit (PACU) to demonstrate our support of ASPAN, while maintaining continuity with the first edition by retaining *The Recovery Room* as part of the title.

The first edition gained remarkable acceptance in the nursing and medical communities; therefore, the second edition adheres to the original philosophy of providing a succinct discussion of the impact of physiologic, pharmacologic, and psychosocial considerations on the nursing care of the patient during this vulnerable period. We hope that the information provided will facilitate the implementation of sound nursing interventions in the PACU setting.

The first section of the book is an overview of the specialty of post anesthesia nursing. Specifically, Chapters One through Three reflect the most recent information on physical setup, specialization, management, and policies.

Section Two discusses the physiologic considerations in the nursing care of the patient in the post anesthesia care unit. Three new chapters are presented: Central Nervous System Anatomy and Physiology, Endocrine Physiology, and Immune System Physiology. Furthermore, the chapters in Section Two have been updated and expanded to reflect current physiological and clinical information, including that relating to the acquired immunodeficiency syndrome (AIDS).

Section Three, covering the basic concepts pertaining to anesthetic agents, has been largely rewritten to update the content, improve the organization, and delete discussions on outdated agents and techniques.

Section Four provides selected, in-depth discussions of the nursing care considerations following surgery to specific body systems. The important new information on the stir-up regimen in Chapter 18 is the result of ongoing nursing research. It is believed that the incorporation into nursing practice of this revised stir-up regimen (including the sustained maximal inspiration (SMI) maneuver, cascade cough, and repositioning) will enhance outcomes in the surgical patient. All chapters in this section have been updated, and three new chapters have been added. Chapter 19 deals with the management of postoperative pain. Because of the highly specialized postoperative nursing care required by the burn patient, Chapter 33 presents the current concepts in the care of the burn patient in the immediate postoperative period. Since many medical treatment facilities are now providing ambulatory surgery units, Chapter 34 is devoted to the postoperative care of the ambulatory surgical patient.

Section V is devoted to frequently encountered medical conditions and physical states that require specialized knowledge and skills. All the chapters in this final section have been revised, and two new chapters have been added. Chapter 39 provides a basic understanding of the nursing care required by the pregnant patient. Because of the strong interest in malignant hyperthermia, Chapter 42 presents the physiology, pharmacology, and nursing interventions for the patient who is suffering from this syndrome.

The authors believe that this book will continue to be a valuable aid to the beginning post anesthesia nurse. It will also serve as an informative review for the experienced critical care nurse and provide a comprehensive text for students.

Acknowledgments

LTC Cecil B. Drain would like to thank Dr. Glenn Ross Johnson, Ed.D.; Elizabeth Gardner, Ph.D.; LTC(Ret.) Keith L. Campman, C.R.N.A., B.S.; LTC(Ret.) Hershal W. Bradshaw, C.R.N.A., M.Ed.; Katherine Pitcoff, CPT(Ret.); Marie Dutton, R.N., M.S.; Cynthia M. Drain; and Robert O. Barney for their help and assistance.

LTC Susan B. Shipley Christoph would like to acknowledge that a number of persons have assisted with the review and preparation of this second edition of *The Recovery Room*. Some of these contributors have been acknowledged directly along with the chapter in which they made significant revisions.

In addition, I would like to thank Colonel William Rimm, MC, for assistance with the chapter on ophthalmic surgery, and Major Richard De Angeleis, ANC, for review of the thoracic and cardiac surgery chapters.

I extend my gratitude to Debbie Stover, R.N.; Pamela Williams, R.N.; and Joyce Staubs, R.N., PACU nurses at Prince George's General Hospital and Medical Center, Cheverly, Maryland, for their review of all the chapters on postoperative care.

And, finally, a note of appreciation to my family and friends for their continued support and encouragement despite my procrastination.

The authors appreciate the assistance and cooperation received from the staff of Academy of Health Sciences and Brooke Army Medical Center, San Antonio, Texas; Arizona Health Sciences Center and the College of Nursing, Tucson, Arixona; U.S. Texas A&M University, College of Medicine Library; Army Research and Development Command, Fort Detrick, Maryland; and from our many friends and educators.

The authors wish to thank the following individuals for reviewing the manuscript and for their helpful suggestions: Mary Lou Barnett, University of Minnesota, Member, ASPAN, American Society of Post-Anesthesia Nurses, Edina, Minnesota; Linda H. Bolton, R.N., Head Nurse, Post Anesthesia Recovery Unit, Grady Memorial Hospital, Atlanta, Georgia; Nancy Burden, R.N., AMI Single Day

Surgery, Clearwater, Florida; Lila Coates, B.S.N., M.S.N., Manager, Surgical Department, Health Center West, Kaiser Foundation, Portland, Oregon; Madelyn Dalton, B.S.N., B.S.Ed., Post Anesthesia Recovery, St. Francis Hospital, Tulsa, Oklahoma; Ernestine B. Davis, Ed.D., B.S., M.S., Nursing Administration, School of Nursing, University of North Alabama, Florence, Alabama; Dr. Dennis Johnson, Ph.D., Department of Pharmacology, College of Medicine, University of Saskatchewan, Saskatoon, Canada; Jeanne Maher, R.N., Nursing Coordinator, Post Anesthesia Care Unit, Galesburg Cottage Hospital, Galesburg, Illinois; Janice Silinsky, R.N., B.S., M.T.(A.S.C.P.), Clinical Coordinator, Recovery Room, Hahnemann University, Philadelphia, Pennsylvania; Katherine Stefos, Ph.D., R.Ph., University of Texas, School of Nursing, Houston, Texas; Jean Sutton, R.N., Sacred Heart Medical Center, Spokane, Washington.

We would also like to thank the authors, publishers, and companies who have granted us permission to use their material in this book.

Special thanks goes to the staff of W. B. Saunders Company, especially Mr. Michael J. Brown, Patricia Conway, and Diane Zuckerman.

Contents

SECTION V
Special Considerations

The Post Anesthesia Care Unit

1

The Physical Structure and Required Equipment

The recovery room or post anesthesia care unit (PACU) is one of the most important yet frequently undervalued facilities in the hospital. It should be designed to afford maximum safety to postoperative patients and to contribute to their comfort. Most importantly, the physical structure of the PACU must allow for close observation, prevention of complications, and ease of providing emergency care to control problems that may arise, such as airway obstruction, vomiting and aspiration, hypovolemia, shock, cardiac arrhythmias, and respiratory or cardiac arrest. This unit should be as self-sufficient as possible (Fig. 1–1).

Achieving the ideal physical design for a PACU is not always possible, especially when trying to establish it in a fixed structure or when working with a limited budget. Every effort should be made to provide an optimal working area. The following suggestions are offered as guidelines to that goal. Individual modifications must certainly be made according to the number and type of patients served and the availability of staff.

LOCATION

The PACU must be located as close to the operating suite as possible to allow unimpeded transfer of patients and ready access to the services of surgeons, anesthetists, and operating room nurses.

When the construction of a new hospital is planned, consideration should be given to locating the PACU, along with the other critical care areas, so that essential laboratory, radiology, and surgical resources are readily available to all areas, and duplication of common requirements is avoided. Clustering these areas is also advantageous in that special equipment can be used interchangeably as back-up in case of equipment failure or multiple emergencies, and additional nurses and physicians with special skills will be in the vicinity. In any case, the laboratory resources, including blood gas analysis capability and radiology facilities, must be readily accessible to the post anesthesia unit.

SIZE

The size of the PACU needed in each hospital must be based on the volume and the types of surgery performed. Useful guidelines are available from the Division of Hospital Facilities, United States Public Health Service; from the Joint Commission on Hospital Accreditation; and from individual health departments. A rule of thumb for general surgical procedures is that two

3

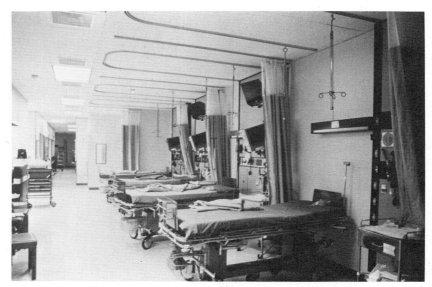

Figure 1–1. Typical PACU setup.

recovery beds will be required for every four to five procedures performed in 24 hours. In the planning of a new recovery facility, a survey of patient load and procedures performed over the past two years yields invaluable information about the size of the unit and the number of beds that will be required to provide the necessary services.

Once the required number of beds is established, the size of the unit can be planned. There should be enough room for at least 4 feet of maneuvering space on both sides of each bed (8 foot width per bed) and a stretcher radius of at least 38.5 square feet in the open areas. Additional space must be allocated for all special equipment. Wall-mounted oxygen and vacuum apparatuses conserve floor space and are convenient (Fig. 1–2). A means for hanging IV

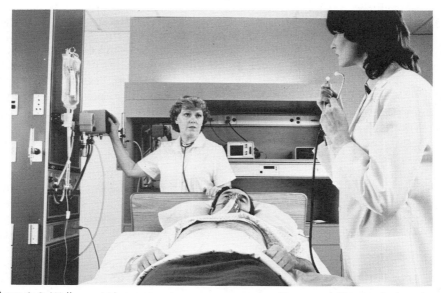

Figure 1–2. Wall-mounted oxygen and vacuum apparatuses. (Courtesy of Ohio Medical Products.)

fluids or other gravity-dependent fluids must be available at each patient space. This can be conveniently accomplished with ceiling suspensions.

There should be adequate space for a complete nurses' station. The nurses' station should include room for a medication storage area as well as a medication refrigerator. The increasing number of computer applications in health care makes allowance of room for computer terminals and perhaps a printer, a mandatory consideration. The number of terminals and the room needed, as well as location of the terminals, will depend upon their intended use. In order to maximize personnel efficiency, it seems wisest to plan terminal placement within the nursing station.

Commonly overlooked in the planning of a unit is the provision of adequate storage space. In order to plan for storage space, policies must be reviewed to determine what equipment will be kept in the recovery area. This includes additional stretchers, respiratory equipment, ventilators, and monitors, as well as daily supplies. A central area should be planned for placement of an emergency/cardiac arrest "crash" cart.

At least one private room should be set aside as an isolation room, and the recovery area should include an adjacent room for visiting family members. A conference room/office is essential. Allowance must also be made for utility rooms, both clean and contaminated.

THE FLOOR PLAN

The floor plan should be individualized to suit the needs of the particular institution. However, several considerations must be kept in mind. The floor plan should allow ease in transferring patients from the operating suite to the unit and from the unit to the parent wards; therefore, the placement of doors becomes critical. In order to provide for smooth traffic flow, recovered patients should leave the unit via doors separate from the ones through which anesthetized patients arrive from the operating room.

The floor plan should permit simultaneous observation of all patients present on the unit. One large main room with an open design is preferred. Postoperative patients are usually not acutely aware of the activities surrounding them because of the residual effects of anesthesia, the stress of the surgical procedure itself, or the sedative effects of analgesics; separation of patients can be provided, if necessary, by moveable, washable curtain partitions. The advantage of increased safety for patients (because of the constant surveillance capability provided by the open design) compensates for its disadvantages. Open design does have disadvantages: The noise level is higher, general activity is greater, privacy is minimal, and the risk of cross-contamination is greater than with separate rooms. Some institutions, therefore, prefer a multiple-room design to allow segregation of patients. Separate rooms or separate recovery units should be considered for ambulatory and pediatric patients, and for women who have had cesarean sections, since the needs of these patients are unique.

Staffing patterns must be carefully scrutinized: Multiple rooms require a greater number of professional staff than is required for the same number of beds included in the open design. If the multiple-room design is chosen, detailed planning must be accomplished to ensure that observation requirements are met and to provide ready access and easy communication between rooms. If several rooms are used, glass panels should form the walls to allow visual surveillance from all areas.

ESSENTIAL ARCHITECTURAL REQUIREMENTS

Several structural factors must be kept in mind when planning the post anesthesia care unit.

Doors

Doors must be wide enough and high enough to allow free passage of the postoperative bed, along with any additional apparatus and personnel accompanying the patient during the transfer process. Electronic doors are more than just a convenience and should be seriously considered.

Floors

Floors should be easy to maintain, have a smooth surface for ease of movement of beds and equipment, and be resilient for the comfort of personnel. Consideration must be given to acoustics; the ideal flooring material will dramatically reduce the noise level. However, this is definitely not an area for carpeting.

Electrical Considerations

Power Outlets

A sufficient number of electrical outlets should be located at each bedside. Recommended is a minimum of eight outlets, arranged in pairs, one pair on either side of the bed and the others about 3 feet from the bed. This allows easy access and additional outlets if necessary when other electrical equipment is already utilizing the bedside outlets. All outlets must be properly grounded to minimize electrical hazards, and separate circuit breakers must be supplied for every two beds. At least one pair of outlets at each bedside must be connected to the emergency power system of the hospital. At least one 220-volt outlet should be conveniently located on the unit for portable x-ray equipment.

Lighting

Good general illumination is essential in the recovery room. Adequate lighting must be provided, not only for observation of patients but also for minor surgical procedures, such as arterial line or Swan-Ganz catheter placement. High intensity lights, such as iodine-vapor lights, must be provided to illuminate the area when necessary. These are most convenient when ceiling-mounted.

Air Conditioning

Adequate heating, cooling, and humidification are essential in the recovery room for patient welfare and safety, staff comfort, and equipment functioning. The system should keep the air fresh (complete air exchange at least 12 to 15 times per hour), the temperature moderate (75°F ± 2°), and relative humidity at 50 percent ± 10 percent. Controls for the air conditioning system should be located within the nurses' station so that changes dictated by specific patient conditions can be met.

Plumbing

A staff toilet is a necessity. It should be located within the working area to maintain staff availability to the patients. Hand sinks with foot or elbow controls should be available in the work area in sufficient number, i.e., at least one for every four beds. Disposable towels should be available at each sink. In addition, at least two large sinks must be available in the utility rooms for the cleaning of equipment.

Additional Required Bedside Facilities

At least three vacuum outlets should be provided at each bedside: one for nasotracheal suction, one for gastrointestinal suction, and one for chest suction. At least two oxygen outlets should be provided at each bedside. An additional outlet for compressed air should also be available. Suspended tracts with moveable hooks for hanging intravenous solutions should be above each bed. Wall-mounted shelves at the head of each bed are convenient for storage of necessary bedside supplies and equipment. All these facilities allow appropriate and necessary supplies and equipment to be readily available without using valuable floor space, impeding traffic flow, or limiting access to the patient. At least one large-faced, wall-mounted clock with bold numerals should be provided on each wall. These clocks should ideally have elapsed-time mechanisms that can be started and stopped without interfering with the time mechanism. Many of these necessities have been incorporated into wall panels suitable for use in the PACU.

REQUIRED EQUIPMENT

No standardized list of equipment or supplies can be complete and appropriate for every situation. Each unit will have to incorporate in its list of equipment those linens, dressings, and other patient-care items necessary in the specific situation to supplement the suggested lists that follow.

EQUIPMENT THAT SHOULD BE IMMEDIATELY AVAILABLE WITHIN THE POST ANESTHESIA CARE UNIT

Bedside cardiac monitors
Bedside arterial pressure monitors
Defibrillator (with both adult and pediatric defibrillator paddles)
EKG machine
Pacemakers
Hypothermia machines
Bronchoscope cart
Respirometers
Ventilators (both IPPB and volume-controlled)
Chest tube cart
Tracheostomy tray
Post-tonsillectomy tray
Cutdown infusion tray
Ice machine
Blanket warmer
Fluid warmers
Heat lamps
Crash cart, including defibrillator, endotracheal tray, and emergency drugs. A separate pediatric crash cart (with dosage-by-weight charts for emergency drugs) should be kept in the pediatric area.
Equipment and drugs for malignant hyperthermia crisis
Endotracheal tray, including a complete assortment of laryngoscopes, tubes of various sizes, and connectors and an assortment of oropharyngeal airways stocked and readily accessible
Equipment for drawing blood samples, both venous and arterial, should be stocked on the unit.

DRUGS

Most hospitals now employ the unit-dose system and have intravenous sections in the pharmacy. Accessibility of the pharmacy and response time will, in part, dictate which intravenous solutions and parenteral medications must be stocked within the unit.

A full line of intravenous fluids and the required sets for their administration should be kept in the PACU. A refrigerator for drug storage and a separate blood refrigeration unit are required equipment. An adequate supply of various needles for drug administration and venipuncture and a variety of disposable syringes should be stocked.

A certain number of emergency drugs must be kept immediately available on the unit. At a minimum, the following drugs should be readily accessible. Our preference is to have them on an emergency cart that can be easily wheeled to the bedside if necessary, with back-up stock in the medication area.

EMERGENCY DRUGS

aminophylline
physostigmine salicylate (Antilirium)
metaraminol (Aramine)
atropine
diphenhydramine hydrochloride (Benadryl)
bretylium tosylate (Bretylol)
calcium chloride
calcium gluconate
dantrolene sodium (Dantrium)
dexamethasone (Decadron)
dextrose 50 percent
digoxin
phenytoin sodium (Dilantin)
epinephrine (Adrenalin)
ephedrine
furosemide (Lasix)

heparin sodium
diazoxide (Hyperstat)
propranolol hydrochloride (Inderal)
dopamine hydrochloride (Intropin)
isoproterenol hydrochloride (Isuprel)
levarterenol bitartrate (Levophed)
lidocaine hydrochloride (Xylocaine)
naloxone hydrochloride (Narcan)
pancuronium bromide (Pavulon)
phenylephrine hydrochloride (Neo-Synephrine)
phenobarbital (Luminal)
procainamide hydrochloride (Pronestyl)
sodium bicarbonate
hydrocortisone sodium succinate (Solu-Cortef)
edrophonium chloride (Tensilon)
diazepam (Valium)
succinylcholine chloride (Anectine)
tubocurarine chloride (Tubarine)

Other drugs that might be needed quickly include:
propantheline (Pro-Banthine)
oxytocin (Pitocin)
dobutamine hydrochloride (Dobutrex)
nitroglycerine IV (Tridil)
hydralazine HCl (Apresoline)
verapamil HCl (Isoptin)
sodium nitroprusside (Nipride)
regular insulin
glycopyrrolate (Robinul)
vasopressin (Pitressin)
prochlorperazine (Compazine)
chlorpromazine (Thorazine)
promethazine hydrochloride (Phenergan)
vitamin K
carbazochrome salicylate (Adrenosem)

A variety of both parenteral and oral analgesics should be available. These should include standard drugs as well as the preferred analgesics of the surgeons utilizing this facility. A suggested list includes:
meperidine hydrochloride (Demerol)
morphine sulfate
hydromorphone hydrochloride (Dilaudid)
codeine (parenteral and oral)
pentazocine lactate (Talwin) (parenteral and oral)
aspirin
acetaminophen (Tylenol)

Additions or deletions to these lists must be made according to the common practices within the institution. If there is no intravenous additive section in the pharmacy, a range of antibiotics, potassium chloride, and vitamin preparations must be added to the list of drugs stocked.

BEDSIDE SUPPLIES

Each bedside should be stocked with at least the following patient-care supplies, either in a bedside stand or on wall-mounted shelves at the head of the bed:
stethoscope
scissors
Kelly clamp
oxygen tubing
oxygen mask (clear)
nasal prongs
suction catheters
sterile gloves
sterile normal saline and water
alcohol prep swabs
sterile 4 × 4's
sterile 2 × 2's
paper and adhesive tape
safety pins
paper tissues
disposable emesis basin
bed linen protectors
oral airways
petrolatum ointment
water-soluble lubricant (K-Y Jelly or Surgilube)
tonsil sucker

REFERENCES

1. Brody, D. C.: Criteria for patient care. Curr. Rev. Recovery Room Nurses, 5(19):155–160, 1983.
2. Ennis, H. J.: Staffing of the recovery room: A view of systems. Curr. Rev. Recovery Room Nurses, 5(1):113–120, 1979.
3. Israel, J. S., and DeKornfeld, T. J. (eds.): Recovery Room Care. Springfield, Illinois, Charles C Thomas, publisher, 1982.
4. Schneider, M.: Planning the physical structure of a recovery room. Breathline, 1(3):11–13, 1981.
5. Willock, M. M.: Design and equipment of a modern recovery room. Curr. Rev. Recovery Room Nurses, 6(14):107–111, 1984.

2

Post Anesthesia Nursing as a Specialty

The provision of quality care in the post anesthesia unit requires strong, knowledgeable leadership and excellent management. Particular attention must be paid to developing the organizational structure of the unit and maintaining the best possible nursing staff.

ORGANIZATIONAL STRUCTURE

The recovery room should be under the immediate supervision, and be the responsibility of, the anesthesia department. The chief of anesthesiology should be the medical director of the unit. If the hospital and the unit are large, the chief of anesthesiology may wish to appoint an assistant director. The medical director of the unit is responsible for coordinating the medical care provided in the unit. Anesthesiologists are readily available, are constantly in the operating room, and by virtue of their specialized training are best equipped to handle the problems of respiration and circulation that may arise in the immediate postoperative period. Other problems that may arise related to the surgery performed may be handled by the anesthesiologist on an emergency basis with consultation with the surgeon as soon as possible.

The medical director also works closely with the head nurse in developing policies and procedures, assisting with continuing education for the nursing staff, and coordinating the quality assurance program for the unit.

Administrative control of the nursing staff should come from the department of nursing through the head nurse of the unit. Nurses must be directly responsible to the anesthesiologists and follow their orders; thus, the nurse is in a dual chain of command. The supervisor and head nurse positions must be filled with mature, cooperative, and experienced nurses who can form good working relationships with the anesthesiologists, yet are assertive enough to "hold their ground" when necessary, and back the nurses when unforeseen problems arise. Freedom for independent decisions, which may mean an occasional setting aside of some of the hospital's rules and regulations, must be afforded these persons to allow the exercise of nursing judgment specific to the clinical situation. This is essential in fulfilling the purpose of the PACU.

Staffing

Selection of Nurses

The most important ingredient in a successful PACU is a well educated, highly skilled nursing staff. The post anesthesia

9

nurse must be a "jack of all trades." Not only must he or she have a solid background in physiology, pathophysiology, and surgical procedures but also an understanding of medicine, pediatrics, and geriatrics. In addition, nurses must be thoroughly versed in the pharmacodynamics of anesthesia and analgesia.

Careful selection of nursing personnel for the PACU is of the utmost importance. Qualifications for such nursing positions should be established by the head nurse of the area in conjunction with the director of the unit. These should be written and utilized in all employment or assignment proceedings. This practice tends to preclude, or at least minimize, subsequent problems, such as job dissatisfaction, unsatisfactory work performance, and undue turnover of personnel, and helps ensure a smoothly functioning PACU. The following characteristics should be considered for inclusion in the selection criteria, but this list is not necessarily complete.

Personal Qualifications

1. A sincere interest in the specialized role of post anesthesia nursing.
2. Commitment to providing high-quality, individualized patient care.
3. Stability and maturity.
4. Ability to form good working relationships with a variety of health care team members.
5. Capacity for making intelligent, independent decisions, and initiating appropriate action, as well as a willingness to accept responsibility.
6. Interest and ability in learning the scientific principles and theory underlying patient care as well as the technologic aspects of post anesthesia nursing.
7. Motivation for continuing education.

8. Excellent health.
9. Dependability (previous evidence of good work attendance).
10. Intention of spending at least a year in service on the unit.

The orientation and training of a recovery room nurse takes significant time, energy, and budget, and temporary assignment to the recovery room is not worthwhile except as a student learning experience.

Professional Qualifications

1. Educationally prepared at the baccalaureate level.
2. At least one year of general nursing experience.
3. A demonstrated ability to coordinate care being rendered by a variety of health team members.
4. A demonstrated ability to function effectively in crisis situations.

Certification by one of the professional nursing associations (Table 2–1) demonstrates commitment to professional excellence and should be considered very positively when selecting PACU nurses. Commitments to professional organizations should also help the candidate to be considered in a positive light.

Nursing personnel assigned to the PACU should be permanent and should not be given any other assignments. At least one registered professional nurse should be assigned for every 2.5 beds. Higher nurse-to-patient ratios are necessary if the unit cares for patients with particularly demanding requirements, such as those undergoing open heart surgery, thoracic surgery, or very radical procedures. A head nurse should be assigned and not included in the number of nurses required to provide optimal direct patient care. Optimal patient care is the goal of the unit, and continuous

TABLE 2–1. Certification by Professional Nursing Associations

Professional Association	Credential
American Nurses' Association	Medical-Surgical Certification
American Association of Critical Care Nurses	CCRN
Association of Post Anesthesia Nurses	CPAN
Association of Operating Room Nurses	CNOR
Emergency Nurses' Association	CEN

professional nursing judgment is required in this area. Therefore, ideally, only professional nurses are assigned patient care. Minimal numbers of ancillary personnel should be assigned to the unit. Auxiliary personnel, such as licensed vocational or practical nurses, may be assigned to the unit to assist professional nurses with technical functions and duties, such as restocking supplies, the transfer of patients, preparation of postoperative beds, errands to the laboratory, central supply, and other locations, and so forth. It is obvious that such work will not permit use of licensed vocational nurses in their fullest capacity. Orderlies or nurse's aides could be assigned to the unit to perform some of these tasks but would not be as technically helpful to the nurses. A well-chosen secretary/clerk is a definite asset to the PACU. The clerk should be assigned to clerical duties, restocking paper supplies and answering the never-ending telephone calls.

Head Nurse. The head nurse of the PACU must be most carefully selected by the same criteria used for selection of the staff nurses. The head nurse must have at minimum a baccalaureate degree in nursing. In addition, the head nurse must be exceptionally well prepared in all aspects of PACU nursing in order to provide expert supervision, guidance, and training of the PACU staff. The head nurse is responsible for the quality of care rendered within this critical care unit.

BASIC ORIENTATION OF STAFF

Before starting in the PACU, the nurse should attend a basic orientation program. Nurses should be thoroughly familiar with hospital and post anesthesia unit policies and procedures.

The basic PACU orientation program should include formal lectures and discussion as well as informal demonstrations and supervised practice. Anesthesiologists, surgeons, and the PACU nursing staff should develop and coordinate this program using all available resources. A list of basic classes geared to providing the beginning PACU practitioner with the required knowledge and skills is listed here. The topics may be varied according to the needs of the class or individuals.

Recovery Room Classes

I. Review of the Anatomy and Physiology of the Cardiorespiratory System
   1. Pathophysiologic processes of the cardiorespiratory system
   2. Factors altering circulatory or respiratory function following surgery and anesthesia:
      a. Position of patient
      b. Type of incision
      c. Medication
      d. Blood loss and replacement
      e. Anesthetic agent
      f. Type of operative procedure
   3. Monitoring techniques
   4. Cardiac arrhythmias
   5. Airway maintenance, equipment, and procedures
   6. Ventilatory support, equipment, and procedures
   7. Cardiorespiratory arrest and its management

II. Review of Other Physiologic Considerations in PACU
   1. Neurologic system
   2. Musculoskeletal system
   3. Genitourinary system—fluid and electrolyte balance
   4. Gastrointestinal system
   5. Integumentary system
   6. Pediatric physiology
   7. Geriatric physiology
   8. Physiology of pregnancy

III. Anesthesia
   1. General concepts—induction and emergence
   2. Administration and properties of selected agents (must include all agents routinely used in the institution)
      a. Gaseous agents
      b. Intravenous agents
      c. Muscle relaxants
      d. Conduction anesthesia

IV. Care of the PACU Patient
   1. Physical assessment of the postoperative patient

2. General PACU care
   a. Psychologic considerations
   b. The stir-up regimen
   c. IV therapy and blood transfusion
   d. Infection control
   e. General comfort and safety measures
3. Specific care required following surgical procedures
   a. ENT surgery
   b. Ocular surgery
   c. Cardiothoracic surgery
   d. Neurosurgery
   e. Orthopedic surgery
   f. Genitourinary surgery
   g. Gastrointestinal surgery
   h. Gynecologic and obstetric surgery
   i. Plastic surgery

Once nurses finish formal classes they should work continuously on improving their background theory and skills. This may be accomplished by active participation in on-the-job training, nursing in-services provided on the unit, outside reading, and attendance at both in-house and outside-sponsored seminars. Constant review of basic knowledge and procedures is essential. Keeping abreast of new scientific information and innovations is necessary to ensure quality care. It is important that the budget for the unit include funds to send nurses to important information-sharing meetings. An investment made to stimulate professional development of the nursing staff will be directly reflected in the level of care provided to the patient.

Stress and Burnout for the Post Anesthesia Nurse

Emotional exhaustion, commonly referred to as "burnout" in the recent literature, is a concern in the PACU because the nursing profession seems to be particularly vulnerable to this syndrome. Burnout may be reflected in increased tardiness and absenteeism, physical complaints, conflicts with fellow workers, and "dropout" (Table 2–2).

The contributors to burnout include the physical and emotional demands of patient

TABLE 2–2. Signs and Symptoms of Nursing Burnout

Increased absenteeism
Increased tardiness
Somatic complaints
Headaches
Fatigue
Upset stomach
Itches and rashes
Depression
Irritability
Intrastaff conflicts
Dropout
Request for transfer
Change of profession

care responsibilities and the frequent frustrations involved with the dual chain of command. One of the significant factors identified as causing burnout for nurses is the lack of respect shown for nurses and nursing by physician colleagues. Shift rotation, overtime, interactions with a diverse population, and demanding supervisors can also lead to burnout. For PACU nurses, burnout could result from the lack of positive feedback received from patients who do not remember them. The PACU nurse rarely has the opportunity to see the results of care unless postoperative visiting is included in the PACU routine. Vulnerability to burnout may be assessed by reviewing the factors identified as putting individuals at risk for burnout (Table 2–3).

While PACU nurses may be susceptible to burnout because they experience many of the same frustrations as other nurses, the actual incidence of burnout for PACU nurses seems to be relatively low. The reasons for this have not been explicated, but it would seem that the regular hours as well as the social support gleaned from the close relationships developed with the surgical team assist in prevention.

TABLE 2–3. Burnout Risk Factors

Single
Female
New and inexperienced
Large institution
Shift rotation
Overtime (on duty more than 40 hours/week)
Unrealistic demands by supervisors and physicians
Complex patient situations
Role conflict

TABLE 2–4. Measures for Alleviation of Burnout

Social Support
Within the work environment
  Support groups
  Team spirit
  Supervisory support
Outside of work

Changes in Work Climate
  Improved working environment
  Improved policies and procedures
  Interdisciplinary committees

Vacation Time

Even though the incidence of burnout appears to be low, the head nurse as well as colleagues in the post anesthesia unit should remain alert to the signs and symptoms of burnout for the nurse so that measures for its alleviation can be instituted (Table 2–4).

REFERENCES

1. Brody, D. C.: Criteria for patient care. Curr. Rev. Recovery Room Nurses, 5(19):155–159, 1983.
2. Constable, J. F.: The effects of social support and the work environment upon burnout among nurses. Unpublished doctoral dissertation. Ames, University of Iowa, 1983.
3. DeKornfeld, T. J.: Medico-legal implications of recovery room care. Curr. Rev. Recovery Room Nurses, 4(1):27–31, 1979.
4. Ennis, H. J.: Staffing of the recovery room: A view of systems. Curr. Rev. Recovery Room Nurses, 5(1):113–120, 1979.
5. Guidelines for Management Standards in the Post-Anesthesia Care Unit. Richmond, Va., The American Society of Post Anesthesia Nurses, 1984.
6. Guidelines for Standards of Care in the Post-Anesthesia Care Unit. Richmond, Va., The American Society of Post Anesthesia Nurses, 1984.
7. Jones, J. W.: The Burnout Syndrome. Park Ridge, Ill., London House Press, 1981.
8. Maslach, C.: Burnout—The Cost of Caring. Englewood Cliffs, N. J., Prentice-Hall, 1982.
9. Selvin, B. L.: Recovery room policy manual: A model. Md. State Med. J., 30(19):56–59, 1981.
10. Willock, M. M.: Management and staffing in the recovery room. Curr. Rev. Recovery Room Nurses, 6(11):83–87, 1984.
11. Wilson, E. A.: The recovery room staff: Planning, selection, development and management. ASPAN Newsletter, 1(2):11–15, 1981.

3

Post Anesthesia Care Unit Management and Policies

All management procedures and policies for the PACU should be established through joint efforts of the directors of the unit and the head nurse. These must be written and readily available to all staff working in the PACU and all physicians who utilize the area for recovery of their patients following surgery. Policies and procedures are developed to provide a basis for smooth functioning of the unit, and, once established, the policies should be soundly backed by the director and head nurse. However, policies and procedures are not fixed in cement, and they should be reviewed frequently, with enough flexibility maintained so that appropriate changes can be made when deemed necessary.

Changes in the clinical situation of the hospital and advances in science and technology make revision of policies and procedures a continuous challenge. Some suggested areas that most often require written policy for the unit per se in addition to hospital regulations are noted in Table 3–1. The opinions of the authors reflect experience in a variety of institutions; however, as with the development of other facets of the unit, the policies and procedures must be tailored to meet the individual unit's needs.

PURPOSE OF THE PACU

The post anesthesia care unit is designed and staffed to provide intensive observation and care of patients following an operative procedure for which an anesthetic agent has been required. Criteria for admission to the PACU should be clearly outlined. Particular attention should be directed toward delineation of any exceptions to the policy as written. Of special concern, owing to the effects on staffing and utilization of post anesthesia beds, is use of the recovery area as a place to perform special procedures or to observe patients who have undergone special procedures, such as cardiac catheterization, arteriography or other specialized radiologic tests, and electroshock therapy.

Each patient admitted to the unit should be retained until the effects or possible complications of anesthesia have been eliminated. Patients who have major surgical or medical problems and who cannot be transferred to the parent ward should be transferred to the appropriate intensive care area or ward with special nursing attention.

Some institutions, especially smaller hospitals (under 200 beds), have found it impossible to staff or to provide the budget for separate units and have combined the

TABLE 3–1. Suggested Policies and Procedures for the PACU

Purpose of the Unit
Philosophy of nursing
Admission and discharge criteria
Admission and discharge procedures
Job Descriptions
Lines of authority
Medical director
Head nurse
Staff nurses
Unit clerk
Nursing Procedures
All specific procedures
Nursing orders
Documentation of care
Special Procedures, Equipment, and Supplies
Maintenance and Safety
Electrical safety
Control of radioactive materials
Role of biomedical engineers
Respiratory Care
Infection Control
Isolation
  Protective
  Isolation of infectious disease
Review of antibiotic use
Traffic control
Visitors
Laboratory Procedures
Physicians' Orders
Standing orders
Intravenous medications
Intravenous fluids
Blood or blood component transfusions
Staff Education
Orientation
Continuing education
Basic life-support programs and certification
Advanced life-support programs and certification
Quality Assurance
Audits
Morbidity and mortality reviews
Infection control statistics
Multidisciplinary surgical team conferences

surgical intensive care unit with the PACU. When this is the case, it is imperative that a separate area within the unit be designated as the recovery area. Grouping the post anesthesia patients together and separating them from the surgical intensive care patients assist in ensuring that the intense observation for the effects and complications of anesthesia is carried out. There is a tendency for the staff to neglect specific observations when all patients are randomly grouped together. There is also a tendency to provide more intensive care for surgical patients because they are so sick or because there are so many tasks to be ac-

complished. Consequently, PACU staff may fail to notice subtle changes in the patient who is emerging from anesthesia following minor surgery. This is a hazard that must be eliminated with the combined type of unit.

STAFF

Nursing staff should consist of registered professional nurses to provide direct patient care. Licensed vocational nurses may be utilized in the area to assist the professional nurse. Nursing staff should be permanent and should not be rotated through other assignments in the hospital. Student nurses should not be utilized to staff the PACU. Students serve primarily as observers, and any patient care given by student nurses should be accomplished only under the direct supervision of a permanent staff nurse. No private duty nurses or "float pool" nurses should be used to staff the post anesthesia unit.

VISITORS

Visitors are not permitted in the PACU at any time. Exceptions to this policy may be valid, if staffing and the physical structure of the unit permit, in the following clinical situations:

1. Immediate family members may visit for a short time when the patient is in extremis and death may be imminent.

2. Immediate family members may visit for a short time when the patient must return to surgery.

3. Immediate family members may visit when an extended PACU stay is planned.

4. It may be permissible to allow a parent to stay with a child whose physical well-being may depend upon the calming effect of the parent's presence.

5. A significant other may be allowed in the recovery room when the patient's well-being depends upon that person's presence. Patients who may fall into this category include the mentally retarded, the mentally ill, or persons with profound sensory deficits.

These exceptions to policy must not be

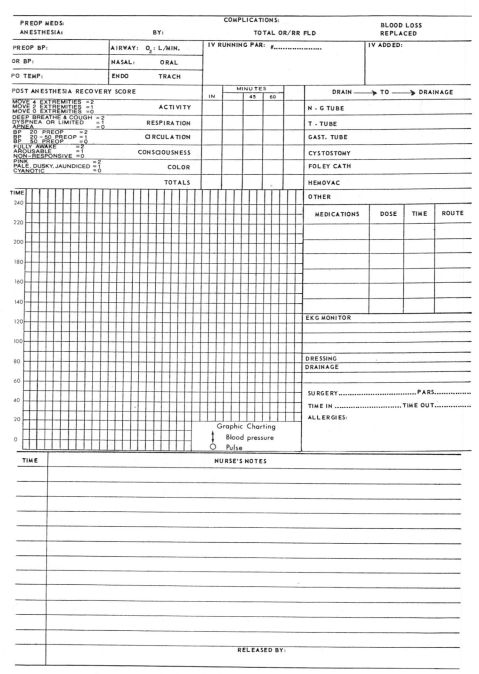

Figure 3–1. PACU clinical record.

abused and require the exercise of good nursing judgment. Whether or not these exceptions to policy are permitted may also be determined, at least in part, by whether the unit is a combined surgical intensive care unit and PACU.

PATIENT RECORDS

All physicians' orders should be written and signed. Some units have standing physicians' orders for routine uncomplicated procedures; however, these should be reviewed and individualized as necessary for each patient.

A post anesthesia record should be kept on every patient admitted to the unit. A suggested format is included that may be modified to meet the needs dictated by specific procedures (Fig. 3–1). Anecdotal notes should detail an admission note, the assessment, planning, and implementation phases of the nursing process in the PACU, as well as an evaluation of how the patient responded to the care provided, and a discharge summary. A discharge note by the anesthetist must be included in the record prior to transfer of the patient from the recovery unit.

DISCHARGING THE PATIENT FROM THE PACU

Criteria for discharge of the patient from the PACU must be set and should include: (1) when the patient has regained consciousness and is oriented to time and place (provided he was oriented to time and place preoperatively); (2) when the airway is clear and danger of vomiting and aspiration is past; and (3) when circulatory and respiratory vital signs are stabilized. Many institutions have incorporated the Post Anesthesia Recovery Score (PARS) in their criteria for discharge (Table 3–2). Our interpretation of this system follows. It consists of five assessments of the patient's physical condition. When the patient scores 10 points he may be discharged from the PACU to the parent ward. If the patient does not score 10 points, he must be further evaluated by the anesthetist or surgeon or both and appropriate disposition made either to the surgical intensive care unit or to a ward with special nursing care.

Color is probably the most difficult entity to assess with any reliability, and many PACUs have elected to eliminate this parameter from the score. In that case, the required number of points on the score for discharge would be eight. This scoring system does not include detailed observations, such as urinary output, bleeding or other drainage, or temperature trends that should be considered when determining readiness for discharge, but it does provide a gross scoring system. No specific time required for the PACU stay can be stated, since patient conditions vary with surgical procedure, anesthesia used, use of analgesics,

TABLE 3–2. Postanesthesia Recovery Score (PARS)

Activity
0 = Unable to lift head or move extremities voluntarily or on command
1 = Moves two extremities voluntarily or on command and can lift head
2 = Able to move four extremities voluntarily or on command. Can lift head and has controlled movement.
   Exception: Patients with a prolonged IV block such as marcaine may not move affected extremity for as long as 18 hours. *Exception:* Patients who were immobile preoperatively

Respiration
0 = Apneic. Condition necessitates ventilator or assisted respiration
1 = Labored or limited respirations. Breathes by self but has shallow slow respirations. May have an oral airway
2 = Can take a deep breath and cough well, has normal respiratory rate and depth

Circulation
0 = Has abnormally high or low blood pressure: BP—50 of preanesthetic level
1 = BP—20–50 of preanesthetic level
2 = Stable BP and pulse. BP—20 of preanesthetic level (minimum 90 mm Hg systolic). *Exception:* Patient may be released by anesthetist after drug therapy

Neurologic Status
0 = Not responding or responding only to painful stimuli
1 = Responds to verbal stimuli but drifts off to sleep easily
2 = Awake and alert, oriented to time, place, and person. *Note:* After ketamine anesthesia the patient must have no nystagmus when released

Color
0 = Cyanotic, dusky
1 = Pale, blotchy
2 = Pink

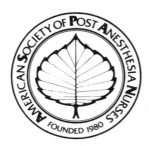

Guidelines for Standards of Care in the Post Anesthesia Care Unit

I. Assessment

Health status data is collected. This data is recorded, retrievable, continuous and communicated. Data is obtained by physical exam, review of records and consultation.

1. Assessment factors include but are not limited to:
   a. relevant preoperative status, including: electrocardiogram, vital signs, radiology findings, laboratory values, allergies, disabilities, drug use, physical or mental impairments, mobility limitations, prostheses (including hearing aids)
   b. anesthesia technique (general, regional, local), effect of pre-op medications
   c. anesthestic agents, muscle relaxants, narcotics and reversal agents used
   d. length of time anesthesia administered
   e. type of surgical procedure
   f. estimated fluid/blood loss and replacement
   g. complications occurring during anesthetic course, treatment initiated, response
2. Initial physical assessment to include the documentation of:
   a. vital signs
      1. respiratory rate and competency, airway patency, type of artificial airway, mechanical ventilator and settings
      2. blood pressure — cuff or arterial line
      3. pulse — apical — peripheral — cardiac monitor pattern
      4. temperature — oral — rectal — axillary — digital through dermal sensors
   b. pressure readings — central venous — arterial blood — pulmonary artery wedge
   c. position of patient
   d. condition and color of skin
   e. circulation — peripheral pulses and sensation of extremity(ies) as applicable
   f. condition of dressings
   g. condition of suture line, if dressings are absent
   h. type and patency of drainage tubes, catheters and receptacle
   i. amount and type of drainage
   j. muscular response and strength
   k. fluid therapy, location of lines, type and amount of solution infusing (including blood)
   l. level of consciousness
   m. level of comfort
3. Numerical score if used

II. Nursing Diagnosis

Nursing diagnosis is a concise statement and represents a decision based upon analysis of the data collected during the assessment phase.

1. Nursing diagnosis is consistent with current scientific knowledge
2. Nursing diagnoses are based on identifiable data as compared to established norms or previous conditions
3. Nursing diagnoses include but are not limited to:
   a. altered level of consciousness
   b. alterations in comfort
   c. anxiety
   d. alterations in cardiac output
   e. alterations in fluid volume (both excess and deficit)
   f. impairment of mobility (including decrease in muscle strength)

g. potential for physical injury
h. respiratory dysfunction
i. impairment in skin integrity
j. abnormal tissue perfusion
k. alterations in urinary elimination

III. Care Plan

The plan for nursing care describes a systematic method for achieving the goal of post anesthesia nursing care—to assist the patient in returning to a safe physiological level after an anesthetic.

1. The plan includes setting priorities for appropriate nursing actions
2. The plan is based on current scientific knowledge
3. The plan is developed with and communicated to the patient, family and/or significant others and appropriate health care team personnel
4. The plan is formulated in conjunction with preoperative, intraoperative, and current post anesthetic health status assessments
5. The plan includes but is not limited to the following nursing actions:
   a. identification of the patient
   b. monitor, maintain, and/or improve respiratory function
   c. monitor, maintain, and/or improve circulatory function
   d. promote and maintain physical and emotional comfort
   e. receive report from operating room nurse, anesthesiologist, and/or anesthetist
   f. monitor surgical site
   g. interpretation and documentation of data obtained during assessment
   h. documentation of nursing plan, action, and/or interventions with outcome
   i. notify family and/or significant others of patient's arrival and discharge from PACU
   j. notify patient care unit of any needed equipment
   k. notify patient care unit when patient is ready for discharge from PACU
   l. out-patient surgicals — discharge planning with patient and family

IV. Implementation

The plan for nursing care is implemented to achieve the goal as stated under care plan.

1. Nursing actions remain consistent with the written plan to provide continuity of care in accordance with established policy and procedure
2. Comfort, safety, efficiency, skill, and effectiveness are reflected in nursing actions
3. Nursing decisions and actions regarding patient care reflect upholding the dignity of the patient and family
4. The plan may be altered to meet the changing needs of the patient

V. Evaluation

The plan for nursing care is evaluated

1. Current assessment data are collected and recorded to evaluate the patient's status for discharge:
   a. airway patency and respiratory function
   b. stability of vital signs, including temperature
   c. level of consciousness and muscular strength
   d. mobility
   e. patency of tubes, catheters, drains, intravenous lines
   f. skin color and condition
   g. intake and output
   h. comfort
2. The nurse informs the family and/or significant others and health care team personnel of the patient's status

VI. Discharge

The post anesthesia nurse shall discharge the patient in accordance with written policies set forth by the Department of Anesthesia and also in accordance with the criteria and data collected through use of the nursing process. A final nursing assessment and evaluation of the patient's condition will be performed and documented. If a numerical scoring system is used, the discharge score will be recorded to reflect the patient's status. The post anesthesia nurse arranges for the safe transport of the patient from the PACU to his or her room.

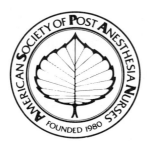

Guidelines for Management Standards in the Post Anesthesia Care Unit

I. Personnel

A. Head Nurse

The Head Nurse must be a Registered Nurse with appropriate education, experience and ability to demonstrate proficiency in nursing practice and management. Plans, coordinates, directs, evaluates, and delegates nursing activities for the PACU, twenty-four hours a day.

The Head Nurse is administratively responsible to a designee of the Department of Nursing and medically responsible to the Chairperson of the Department of Anesthesia. The Head Nurse has the responsibility and authority to take those actions needed to assure that optimal care is given in the PACU.

B. Staff Nurse

The Staff Nurse must be currently registered and complete a formal orientation program that is specific to the PACU. The Staff Nurse must be able to function in emergency situations and possess the skills required for the use of the Nursing Process.

C. Ancillary Staff

Ancillary staff shall meet requirements set by hospital policy, position descriptions and be familiar with PACU procedure.

II. Education

Educational preparation for the RN in the PACU will include but is not limited to:
1. airway management
2. management of the patient during altered states of consciousness
3. management of monitoring and respiratory equipment
4. management of fluid lines
5. management of tubes, drains, and catheters
6. cardiopulmonary resuscitation
7. administration of drugs and drug related problems
8. knowledge of anesthetic agents, techniques, actions, and interactions
9. arrhythmia recognition and treatment

An educational curriculum will be developed to promote clinical experience and professional growth. Programs will be on-going to reflect new developments in patient care and offer continued opportunity for self-fulfillment. Individual educational records will be maintained with documentation of participation in educational programs.

III. Patient-Staff Ratio

Will vary according to patient classification and is recommended as follows:
1. 1:1 — One nurse to one patient at the time of admission to the PACU for any patient requiring life support care. A second nurse must be available to assist as needed.
2. 1:2 — One nurse to two patients: (a) patients who have undergone major surgery and whose systems have stabilized, (b) any stable, unconscious patient, (c) any uncomplicated pediatric patient.
3. 1:3 — One nurse to three patients, uncomplicated patients.

It is recommended that two licensed staff nurses, one of whom is an RN, be in the PACU whenever one patient is recovering from anesthesia.

IV. Physical Aspects

A. The Post-Anesthesia Care Unit will be in close proximity to the area in which anesthesia is to be administered.

B. One and one half beds will be available in the PACU for every one operating room.

C. Each patient care unit will be equipped to provide various means of oxygen delivery, constant and intermittent suction, a means to monitor blood pressure, adjustable lighting and the capacity to ensure patient privacy.

D. There will be one EKG monitor for every two patient care units. Monitors for arterial, central venous, and/or pulmonary arterial pressures, for those patients requiring these measurements, will be available.

E. One ventilator will be maintained in the PACU at all times. A sufficient number of ventilators will be available to care for any post-anesthesia patient who requires one.

F. Portable oxygen, suction, and cardiac monitoring equipment will be available for those patients requiring such equipment during transport.

G. Patients requiring isolation (as detailed by the Infection Control Committee or Department) will be cared for in a designated area in the PACU, (preferably a separate room), apart from other patients. If such an area is not available, continuous nursing care will be provided elsewhere in the hospital. The quality of care in this situation will be equal to that available in the PACU.

H. Those patients requiring strict or respiratory isolation must be housed in a private room.

I. A method of calling for assistance in emergency situations shall be provided.

and patient response. Professional judgment is required to determine when the patient is ready for discharge from the post anesthesia unit.

Patients should receive a follow-up visit in the PACU by the anesthesiologist or anesthetist and be released to the parent ward. In instances in which the nursing staff of the PACU is appropriately trained, the anesthetist may write the post anesthesia order at the post anesthesia visit: "Release when PARS is 10." This policy must remain flexible enough to allow the nurse in charge to release the patient who meets the criteria when space must be made available for the admission of patients in certain clinical situations, e.g., when a rapid influx of emergency surgical procedures ties up the anesthesiologists in the operating room.

QUALITY ASSURANCE

Each PACU should have a planned quality assurance program. The goal of the quality assurance program is professional self-evaluation and regulation to ensure that each patient receives a specified level of care. The program should involve input from a variety of sources and include mechanisms to identify and address problems as they arise.

The American Society of Post Anesthesia Nurses has developed guidelines for standards to be used in the PACU. These are reprinted here with their permission.

These guidelines should provide sound direction for the development of policies for the post anesthesia unit. They may also be used as the basis for development of a quality assurance program.

REFERENCES

1. Aldrete, J. A., and Kroulik, D.: A postanesthetic recovery score. Anesth. Analg., *49:*924–933, 1970.
2. Brody, D. C.: Criteria for patient care. Curr. Rev. Recovery Room Nurses, *19*(5):155–159, 1983.
3. Cramer, C.: The postanesthetic record. Curr. Rev. Recovery Room Nurses, *21*(6):166–171, 1984.
4. DeKornfeld, T. J.: Medico-legal implications of recovery room care. Curr. Rev. Recovery Room Nurses, *1*(4):27–31, 1979.
5. Diniaco, M. J., and Ingoldsby, B. B.: Parental presence in the recovery room. AORN J., *38*(4):685–693, 1983.
6. Fraulini, K. E.: Policies, procedures, and chart forms. Curr. Rev. Recovery Room Nurses, *6*(6):43–46, 1984.
7. Selvin, B. L.: Recovery room policy manual: A model. Md. State Med. J., *30*(19):56–59, 1981.
8. Willock, M. M.: Management and staffing in the recovery room. Curr. Rev. Recovery Room Nurses, *6*(11):83–87, 1984.
9. Wilson, E. A.: The recovery room staff: Planning, selection, development and management. ASPAN Newsletter, *1*(2):11–15, 1981.

Physiologic Considerations in the Post Anesthesia Care Unit

4

Respiratory Anatomy and Physiology

The inhalational anesthetic agents depress respiratory function. They also depend largely upon the respiratory system for their removal during emergence from anesthesia. The other anesthetic agents, such as intravenous agents, also depress respiration. Much of the morbidity and mortality that occur in the post anesthesia care unit (PACU) can be attributed to an alteration in lung mechanics and dysfunctions in airway dynamics. In fact, it is postulated that 70 to 80 percent of the morbidity and mortality occurring in the PACU is associated with some form of respiratory dysfunction. Consequently, a detailed discussion of the many facets of respiratory anatomy and physiology will be presented in this chapter. If the PACU nurse incorporates this information into nursing practice, the recovery of the surgical patient will be enhanced.

Definitions

Acidemia: lower than normal blood pH (increased hydrogen ion concentration).

Acidosis: the process leading to an increase in hydrogen ion concentration in the blood.

Adventitious Sounds: abnormal noises that can be heard superimposed on the patient's breath sounds.

Alkalemia: higher than normal blood pH (decreased hydrogen ion concentration).

Alkalosis: the process leading to a decrease in hydrogen ion concentration in the blood.

Apnea: absence of breathing.

Apneustic Breathing: prolonged inspiratory efforts interrupted by occasional expirations.

Atelectasis: collapse of the alveoli.

Bradypnea: respiratory rate in the adult that is lower than 8/minute.

Bronchiectasis: dilatation of the bronchi.

Bronchospasm: constriction of the bronchial airways due to an increase in smooth muscle tone in the airways.

Cheyne-Stokes Respirations: periods of apnea alternating with rhythmic shallow, progressively deeper and then shallower respirations that are associated with brain damage, heart or kindey failure, or drug overdose.

Compliance (lung compliance): a measure of distensibility of the lung— the amount of change in volume per change in pressure across the lung.

Cyanosis: a sign of poor oxygen transport, characterized by a bluish discoloration of the skin produced when more than 5 grams of hemoglobin per dl of arterial blood are in the deoxy or reduced state.

Dyspnea: a feeling of shortness of breath, as perceived by the patient.

Epistaxis: hemorrhage from the nose.

Fio$_2$: fractional inspired concentration of oxygen.

Hypercapnia: increased carbon dioxide tension in the blood.

Hyperpnea: increased rate of respirations.

Hyperoxemia: increased oxygen tension in the blood.

Hyperventilation: overventilation of the alveoli in relation to the amount of carbon dioxide being produced by the body.

Hypocapnia: decreased carbon dioxide tension in the blood.

Hypoventilation: underventilation of the alveoli in relation to the amount of carbon dioxide being produced by the body.

Hypoxemia: decreased oxygen tension in the blood.

Hypoxia: inadequate tissue oxygen levels.

Kussmaul Respirations: rapid, deep respirations associated with diabetic ketoacidosis.

Methemoglobin: hemoglobin that has the iron atom in the ferric state.

Minute Ventilation ($\dot{V}_E$): the volume of air expired over a period of one minute.

Orthopnea: severe dyspnea that is relieved by the patient when he elevates his head and chest.

Oxyhemoglobin: hemoglobin that is fully oxygenated.

Paroxysmal Noctural Dyspnea (PND): sudden onset of severe dyspnea when the patient is lying down.

Partial Pressure: the pressure exerted by each individual gas when mixed in a container with other gases.

PEEP: positive end-expiratory pressure.

Polycythemia: increased number of red blood cells in the blood.

Rales: Short, discontinuous, explosive adventitious sounds (usually called crackles).

Reduced Hemoglobin: hemoglobin in the deoxy state (not fully saturated with oxygen).

Respiration: the process by which oxygen and carbon dioxide are exchanged between the outside atmosphere and the cells in the body.

Ronchi: continuous musical adventitious sounds.

Torr: units of the Torricelli scale, the classic mercury scale, which is used to express the same value as mm Hg.

Wheeze: a high-pitched sibilant rhonchus usually produced on expiration.

RESPIRATORY ANATOMY

The Nose

The nose is the first area in which inhaled air is filtered (Fig. 4–1). It is lined with ciliated epithelium: The cilia move mucus and particles of foreign matter to the pharynx to be expectorated or swallowed (Fig. 4–2). Other functions of the nose include humidification and warming of the inhaled air, and the olfactory function of smell.

It is important to remember that the administration of dry gases during anesthesia and in the post anesthesia care unit will dry the mucous membrane and slow the action of the cilia. The administration of moist gases by various humidification and mist therapy devices will keep this physiologic filter system viable.

A tracheostomy will preclude the functions of the nose, and it is very important that proper tracheostomy care, including the administration of humidified oxygen, be instituted.

The blood supply to the nose is provided by the internal and external maxillary arteries, which are derived from the external carotid, and by branches of the internal carotid arteries. The venous plexus of the nasal mucosa is drained into the common facial vein, anterior facial vein, the exterior jugular vein, or the ophthalmic vein. There is a highly vascular plexus of vessels located in the mucosa of the anterior nasal septum. They are referred to as Kiesselbach's plexus or Little's area. In a majority of instances, this area is the source of epistaxis.

Epistaxis may occur in the post anesthesia care unit owing to trauma to the nasal veins from nasotracheal tubes or to nasal airways during anesthesia. If epistaxis occurs, prompt action should be taken to prevent aspiration of blood into the lungs. The pa-

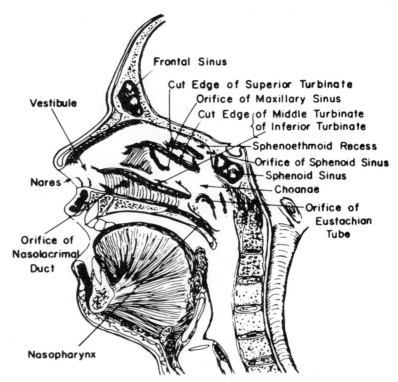

Figure 4–1. Sagittal section through the nose. (From Lough, M., Boat, T., and Doershuk, C. F.: The nose. Resp. Care, *20*[9]:844, 1975.)

tient should be positioned with his head up and flexed forward toward the chest. The application of cold to the bridge of the nose and neck may be effective in slowing or stopping the bleeding. If the bleeding is profuse, the oral cavity should be suctioned carefully and the attending physician should then be notified. A nasal pack or cautery with silver nitrate or electrical current may be necessary to stop the bleeding.

The Pharynx

The pharynx originates at the posterior aspect of the nasal cavities. It is called the nasopharynx until it reaches the soft palate, where it becomes the oropharynx. The oropharynx extends to the level of the hyoid bone, where it becomes the laryngeal pharynx, which extends caudally to below the hyoid bone.

The Larynx

The larynx, or voice box (Fig. 4–3), is situated anterior to the third, fourth, and fifth cervical spine in the adult male. It is higher in females and children. It is composed of nine cartilages, which are held together by ligaments and intertwined with

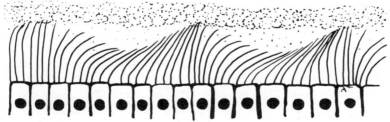

Figure 4–2. Mucus blanket of the nasal airways. The outer (gel-like) layer rests on the tips of the beating cilia, and the inner (water) layer bathes the cilia. Particles are trapped on the sticky outer blanket and carried posteriorly into the nasopharynx by the organized beating of cilia. (From Lough, M., Boat, T., and Doershuk, C. F.: The nose. Resp. Care, *20*[9]:845, 1975.)

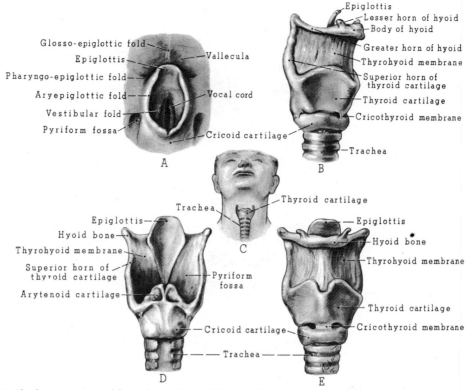

Figure 4–3. The larynx as viewed from above (A), and the side (B), in relation to the head and neck (C), from behind (D), and from the front (E). (From Jacob, S. W., Francone, C. A., and Lossow, W. J.: Structure and Function in Man. 4th ed. Philadelphia, W. B. Saunders Co., 1978, p. 425.)

many small muscles. The thyroid cartilage, which is the largest, is V-shaped, and its protruding prominence is commonly referred to as the Adam's apple. It is attached to the hyoid bone by the hyothyroid membrane and to the cricoid cartilage. The cricoid cartilage is situated below the thyroid cartilage and forms a ring anteriorly. It is in the shape of a signet ring. The "signet" lies posteriorly as a quadrilateral lamina joined in front by a thin arch. The inner surface of the cricoid cartilage is lined with a mucous membrane. In children up to age 10, the cricoid cartilage is the smallest opening down to the bronchi of the lungs.

The epiglottis is a cartilage of the larynx. It is an important landmark for tracheal intubation and serves to deflect foreign objects away from the trachea. It is leaf-shaped and projects outward above the thyroid cartilage over the entrance to the trachea. The lower portion is attached to the thyroid

lamina, and the anterior surface is attached to the hyoid bone and thereby to the base of the tongue. The valleys on either side of the glossoepiglottic fold are termed the valleculae.

The arytenoid cartilages are paired and articulate with the lamina of the cricoid through the articular surface on the base of the arytenoid. The anterior angle of the arytenoid cartilage projects forward at a point to form the vocal process. The medial surface of the cartilage is covered by mucous membrane to form the lateral portion of the rima glottidis (split between the vocal cords), which is completed anteriorly by the thyroid cartilage and posteriorly by the cricoid cartilage.

The corniculate cartilages are two small nodules lying at the apex of the arytenoid. The cuneiform cartilage is a flake of cartilage within the margin of the aryepiglottic folds. It probably serves to stiffen the folds.

There are nine membranes and ligaments, the latter being either extrinsic or intrinsic. The extrinsic ligaments connect the thyroid cartilage and the epiglottis with the hyoid bone, and the cricoid cartilage with the trachea. The intrinsic ligaments connect the cartilages of the larynx with each other.

The fissure between the vocal folds, or true cords, is termed the rima glottidis or glottis. In the adult, this opening between the vocal cords is the narrowest part of the laryngeal cavity, and any obstruction in this area will lead to death by suffocation if not promptly relieved. The rima glottidis divides the laryngeal cavity into two main compartments. The upper portion is the vestibule, which extends from the laryngeal outlet to the vocal cords. It includes the laryngeal sinus, which is sometimes referred to as the middle compartment. The lower compartment extends from the vocal cords to the lower border of the cricoid cartilage and thereafter is continuous with the trachea.

The muscles of the larynx are also either intrinsic or extrinsic. The intrinsic muscles control the movements of the laryngeal framework. They open the cords on inspiration, close the cords and the laryngeal inlet during swallowing, and alter the tension of the cords during speech. The extrinsic muscles are involved in the movements of the larynx as a whole, such as in swallowing.

The nerve supply to the larynx is from the vagus (tenth cranial nerve) via its superior and recurrent laryngeal nerves. The superior laryngeal nerve passes deep to both the internal and the external carotid and divides into a small external branch that supplies the cricothyroid muscles that tense the vocal ligaments. The larger internal branch pierces the thyrohyoid membrane to provide sensory fibers to the mucosa of both sides of the epiglottis and the larynx above the cords.

The recurrent laryngeal nerve on the right side exits from the vagus as it crosses the right subclavian artery and ascends to the larynx in the groove between the trachea and esophagus (Fig. 4–4). Once it reaches the neck, it assumes the same relationships as on the right. This nerve provides the motor function to the intrinsic muscles of the larynx, with the exception of the cricothyroid. It also provides sensory function to the laryngeal mucosa below the vocal cords.

Laryngospasm, which is spasm of the laryngeal muscle tissue, may be complete, when there is complete closure of the vocal cords, or incomplete, when the vocal cords are partially closed. Patients experiencing partial or complete airway obstruction, such as laryngospasm, will usually have a paradoxical, rocking motion of the chest wall. This motion can be misinterpreted as normal abdominal breathing. Hence, the PACU nurse should *always* auscultate the patient's lungs to determine the degree of ventilation, and not rely upon just a visual assessment of the motion of the chest.

If a laryngospasm occurs in the post anesthesia care unit, prompt emergency treatment is necessary to save the patient's life. The PACU nurse should have someone on the PACU staff summon the anesthetist when a laryngospasm is suspected. Treatment consists of mask ventilation using *sustained moderate pressure* on the reservoir bag. This usually will help to overcome the partial laryngeal spasm. If the laryngeal spasm is of the complete closure type and is not relieved by positive pressure within at least one minute, more aggressive treatment should be instituted. Intravenous (0.5 mg/kg) or intramuscular (1 mg/kg) succinylcholine should be administered to relax the smooth muscle of the larynx. Endotracheal intubation may be necessary. The nurse must remember that ventilation of the patient should be continued until *complete* respiratory functioning has returned.

The Trachea

The *trachea* is a musculomembranous tube surrounded by 16 to 20 incomplete cartilaginous rings. These C-shaped rings prevent the collapse of the trachea, thereby maintaining free passage of air. The trachea is lined by ciliated columnar epithelium,

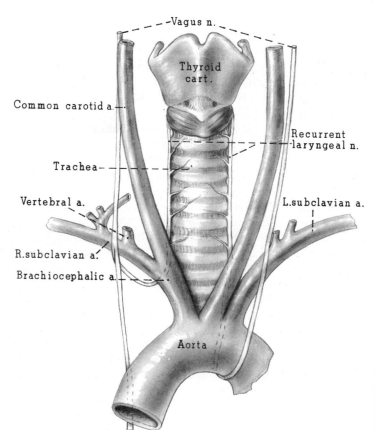

Figure 4–4. Course of recurrent laryngeal nerve. (From Jacob, S. W., Francone, C. A., and Lossow, W. J.: Structure and Function in Man. 4th ed. Philadelphia, W. B. Saunders Co., 1978, p. 273.)

which aids in the removal of foreign material.

The area at the distal end of the trachea at the point of bifurcation into the right and left mainstem bronchi is called the *carina* (Fig. 4–5). The carina appears to contain sensitive pressoreceptors, which upon stimulation, such as by an endotracheal tube, will cause the patient to cough and "buck." The angle created at the point of bifurcation into the right and left mainstem bronchi is of clinical significance to the PACU nurse. The angle at which the bronchi bifurcate from the trachea varies according to the age of the individual (Table 4–1). The significance of the lesser angle of the right mainstem bronchus as compared with the left mainstem bronchus is that foreign material will usually go down the right mainstem bronchus rather than the left. This is also important in regard to endotracheal tubes, which, if advanced too far, will usually enter the right mainstem bronchus and oc-

clude the left mainstem bronchus; thus, the left lung cannot be ventilated. Signs of this complication are decreased or absent breath sounds in the left side of the chest, tachycardia, and uneven expansion of the chest on inspiration and expiration.

Intubation of the Trachea

Intubation of the trachea is a skill that should be reserved for medical personnel who are specifically trained to perform this maneuver. The PACU nurse should be familiar with the technique and capable of performing intubation quickly and efficiently. The technique of orotracheal intubation is presented in detail in Chapter 44.

Endotracheal intubation and *intratracheal intubation* are synonymous terms indicating the placement of a tube directly into the trachea. When the endotracheal tube is placed through the mouth, the method is referred to as *orotracheal intubation*. When the tube is inserted through the nose, the

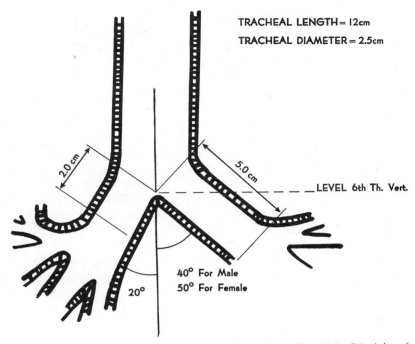

TRACHEAL LENGTH = 12cm

TRACHEAL DIAMETER = 2.5cm

2.0 cm

5.0 cm

_____ LEVEL 6th Th. Vert.

40° For Male
50° For Female

20°

Figure 4–5. Bifurcation of the trachea into the main stem bronchi. (From Collins, V. J.: Principles of Anesthesiology. 2nd ed. Philadelphia, Lea & Febiger, 1976, p. 351.)

method is referred to as *nasotracheal intubation*. Nasotracheal intubation is sometimes done without the use of a laryngoscope; then the method is referred to as a *blind nasotracheal intubation*. *Direct vision intubation* is the insertion of an endotracheal tube with the aid of a laryngoscope. When using the direct vision method to perform a nasotracheal intubation, the nurse may use Magill forceps (Fig. 4–6). A description of the nasal intubation technique can be found in many anesthesia textbooks.

Intubation has many advantages. It provides a route for mechanical ventilation, reduces the amount of anatomic dead space, and protects the patient from aspiration of blood, mucus, or foreign material into the tracheobronchial tree. It also relieves upper airway obstruction and pro-

vides an access route for removing excess secretions in the airways.

The disadvantage of intubation is that it may produce trauma to the teeth, lips, soft palate, epiglottis, vocal cords, and other tissues in that region.

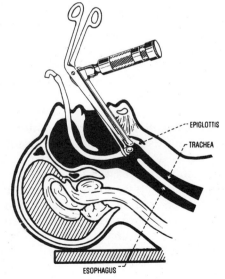

EPIGLOTTIS

TRACHEA

ESOPHAGUS

Figure 4–6. Use of Magill's forceps for nasal intubation. (From Collins, V. J.: Principles of Anesthesiology. 2nd ed. Philadelphia, Lea & Febiger, 1976, p. 334.)

TABLE 4–1. Variations of Bronchial Bifurcation Angles in Adults and Children

	Right Bronchus (degrees)	Left Bronchus (degrees)
Newborn	10–35	30–65
Adult Male	20	40
Adult Female	19	51

PACU Care of the Intubated Patient. Nursing care of the intubated patient involves (1) frequent auscultation of the chest for bilateral breath sounds to ensure correct placement of the endotracheal tube; (2) frequent suctioning of the oral cavity and, if clinically required, suctioning down the inside of the endotracheal tube to remove secretions; and (3) maintenance of verbal communication with the intubated patient to reduce anxiety. The PACU nurse must reassure the patient that the attendants are constantly observing him or her, and the nurse should provide the patient with a means of communication. **Warning:** When suctioning down an endotracheal tube, *always* administer at least five maximal ventilations of 100 percent oxygen before performing the suctioning procedure.

Postoperative Sore Throat. Upon emergence from anesthesia, some patients who have been intubated intraoperatively will complain of a very sore throat. Although the incidence of a sore throat after intubation is low, it is a significant discomfort to the patient. The incidence of sore throat increases dramatically when the patient's head is turned frequently or when the head is in an abnormal position intraoperatively.

Assessment of the patient complaining of sore throat should include visual assessment of the oropharynx and auscultation of the chest. Abnormal findings should be reported to the anesthesiologist. Counseling the patient is probably the most important nursing intervention. The nurse should review the anesthesia record to determine if the patient was intubated and if the procedure was traumatic (i.e., multiple attempts, difficult intubation, and the like). Sore throats usually result from traumatic intubations.

Interventions consist of telling the patient that he had a tube in his throat during surgery to help him breathe and that he may experience throat discomfort for one to three days. Many times, when the patient understands the reason for the discomfort and learns that it is not life-threatening, the discomfort will become less severe. If treatment is required, dexamethasone (Decadron) may be given to reduce the inflammation; also, an ice bag or chips of ice may be given to the patient to help relieve the symptoms.

The Bronchi and Lungs

Within the lungs each primary bronchus supplies a number of lobar bronchi (Fig. 4–7). In humans there are, on the right, an upper, middle, and lower lobe bronchus, and on the left. an upper and lower lobe bronchus. Within each pulmonary lobe a lobar (secondary) bronchus soon divides into tertiary branches remarkably constant as to their number and distribution within the lobe. The segment of a lobe aerated by a tertiary bronchus is usually well delineated from adjoining segments by more or less complete planes of connective tissue. The fact that these areas of the lung are rather well defined explains why pulmonary diseases may be limited to a particular segment or segments of a lobe.

The bronchi bifurcate 22 to 23 times from the mainstem bronchus to the terminal bronchus. These bronchi have connective tissue support and have cartilaginous support. The terminal bronchus gives rise to the bronchioles. They are said to have a diameter of 1 mm or less and tend to be devoid of cartilaginous support. They have thin, highly elastic walls composed of smooth muscle, which is arranged circularly. When this circular smooth muscle is contracted, the bronchiolar lumen is constricted. This circular smooth muscle is innervated by the vagus (parasympathetic nervous system), which causes constriction, and the sympathetic nervous system, which is dilative in action. The patency of the terminal bronchioles, therefore, is determined by the amount of tonus of the muscle produced by a balance between the two components of the nervous system. Bronchospasm occurs when the smooth muscles constrict or go into spasm, which causes airway obstruction.

The terminal bronchiole usually divides into the respiratory bronchioles in which actual gas exchange first occurs. The respi-

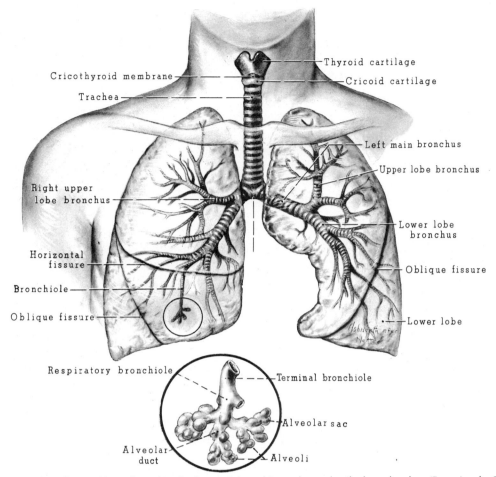

Thyroid cartilage

Cricothyroid membrane

Cricoid cartilage

Trachea

Left main bronchus

Upper lobe bronchus

Right upper lobe bronchus

Lower lobe bronchus

Horizontal fissure

Oblique fissure

Bronchiole

Oblique fissure

Lower lobe

Respiratory bronchiole

Terminal bronchiole

Alveolar sac

Alveolar duct

Alveoli

Figure 4–7. Distribution of bronchi within the lungs. Enlarged inset shows detail of an alveolus. (From Jacob, S. W., Francone, C. A., and Lossow, W. J.: Structure and Function in Man. 4th ed. Philadelphia, W. B. Saunders Co., 1978, p. 432.)

ratory bronchioles usually bifurcate to form alveolar ducts, and these, in turn, terminate in a spherical enclosure called the alveolar sac. The sacs bear a small but variable number of terminal alveoli.

The number of alveoli in an average adult's lungs is estimated at about 750 million. The surface area available for gas exchange is approximately 125 square meters. The alveoli are shaped like soap bubbles in a glass. The interalveolar septum has a supporting latticework composed of elastic collagenous and reticular fibers. The capillaries are incorporated into and supported by the fibrous lattice. The capillary networks in the lungs are the richest in the body.

Unoxygenated blood to the lungs arises from the left and right pulmonary arteries, which originate from the right ventricle of the heart. The divisions of the pulmonary arteries tend to follow the bifurcations of the airway. There are typically two pulmonary veins exiting from each lung, all four emptying separately into the left atrium. Although the blood arriving in the rich pulmonary capillary network from the pulmonary arteries provides for the metabolic needs of the pulmonary parenchyma, the other portions of the lungs, such as the conducting vessels and airways, require their own private circulation. The bronchial arteries, which arise from the aorta, provide the oxygenated blood to the lung tissue.

The blood of the bronchial arteries returns to the heart by way of the pulmonary veins.

Each lung is contained in a thin, elastic membranous sac, called the visceral pleura, which is adherent to the external surface of the lung. Another membrane, the parietal pleura, lines the chest wall. These two membranes normally are very close to each other. A few milliters of viscous fluid are secreted between them to provide lubrication. The visceral pleura continuously absorbs this fluid.

PULMONARY PHYSIOLOGY

Lung Volumes and Capacities

The care of the PACU patient is based largely on knowledge of the physiology and pathophysiology of the lung volumes and capacities. In fact, the dysfunction of lung volumes and capacities that occurs in the postoperative patient is the compelling reason for instituting the stir-up regimen in the post anesthesia care unit. Accordingly, the physiology of the lung volumes and capacities as well as lung mechanics will be described in detail. Table 4–2 provides the definition and normal value for each lung volume and capacity. As shown in Table 4–2 and Figure 4–8, the lung capacities comprise two or more lung volumes.

The Lung Volumes

The *tidal volume* (V_T) represents the amount of air moved into or out of the lungs during a normal ventilatory excursion. It is an important lung volume to monitor when the patient is receiving ventilatory support. However, the measurement of the tidal volume is highly variable and therefore not an extremely helpful parameter on pulmonary function tests. Clinically, the tidal volume can be estimated at 7 ml per kg. For example, a 70 kg man will have a tidal volume of approximately 490 ml (7 × 70 = 490).

The *expiratory reserve volume (ERV)* reflects muscle strength, thoracic mobility, and balance of forces that determine the resting position of the lungs and chest wall following a normal expiration. The ERV is the maximum amount of air that can be expired from the resting position following a normal spontaneous expiration. The ERV is a lung volume that is usually decreased in patients who are morbidly obese (see Chapter 36). This is also a lung volume that is decreased immediately postoperatively in patients who have had upper abdominal or thoracic operations.

The *residual volume (RV)* is the volume of air that remains in the lungs at the end of a maximum expiration. This lung volume represents the balance of forces of the lung

TABLE 4–2. Lung Volumes and Capacities*

Terminology	Definition	Normal Male†	Normal Female†
Tidal volume	Volume of air inspired or expired at each breath	660 (230)	550 (160)
Inspiratory reserve volume	Maximum volume of air that can be inspired after a normal inspiration	2240	1480
Expiratory reserve volume	Maximum volume of air that can be expired after a normal expiration	1240 (410)	730 (300)
Residual volume	Volume of air remaining in the lungs after a maximum expiration	2100 (520)	1570 (380)
Vital capacity	Maximum volume of air that can be expired after a maximum inspiration	4130 (750)	2760 (540)
Total lung capacity	The total volume of air contained in the lungs at maximum inspiration	6230 (830)	4330 (620)
Inspiratory capacity	The maximum volume of air that can be inspired after a normal expiration	2900	2030
Functional residual capacity	The volume of gas remaining in the lungs after a normal expiration	3330 (680)	2300 (490)

*From Wylie, W. B., and Churchill-Davidson, H.C., eds.: A Practice of Anesthesia. 4th ed. London, Lloyd-Luke (Medical Books), 1978. Reproduced by permission of the publisher and the authors.
†The figures given are mean values, with the standard deviation in parenthesis.

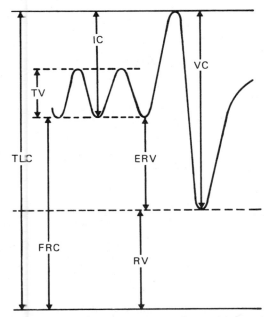

Figure 4—8. Graphic representation of normal lung volumes and capacities. TLC = total lung capacity; TV = tidal volume; FRC = functional residual capacity; IC = inspiratory capacity; ERV = expiratory reserve volume; RV = residual volume; VC = vital capacity. (From Drain, C.: The anesthetic management of the patient: A broad view of the anesthetic considerations necessary regarding the respiratory system. AANA J, 50[2]:192–201, 1982.)

elastic forces and thoracic muscle strength. Patients who did not have their skeletal muscle relaxant adequately reversed at the end of the anesthetic may experience an elevated RV because they are unable to generate enough muscle strength to force all the air out of their lungs. As the RV increases, more air will remain in the lungs, so that it will not participate adequately in gas exchange and will become dead-space air. As the dead-space volume of air increases it can impinge on the tidal volume, and hypoxemia can ensue. The importance of the residual volume is that it allows for continuous gas exchange throughout the entire breathing cycle by providing air to most of the alveoli and aerates the blood between breaths. Consequently, the residual volume prevents wide fluctuations in oxygen and carbon dioxide concentrations during inspiration and expiration.

The *inspiratory reserve volume (IRV)* reflects a balance of the lung elastic forces, muscle strength, and thoracic mobility. It is the maximal volume of air that can be inspired at the end of a normal spontaneous inspiration. Physiologically, the IRV is available to meet increased metabolic demand at a time of excess physical exertion. It assists in moving a larger volume of air into the alveoli through each ventilatory cycle to increase the overall performance and efficiency of the respiratory system.

The Lung Capacities

The *inspiratory capacity (IC)* is the maximum volume of air that can be inspired from the resting expiratory position. The IC is the sum of the tidal volume and the inspiratory reserve volume.

The *functional residual capacity (FRC)* represents the previously mentioned resting position. The FRC is the volume of air remaining in the lungs at the end of a normal expiration when no respiratory muscle forces are applied. At FRC the mechanical forces of the lung and thorax are at rest and no air flow is present. This particular lung capacity is of great importance to the PACU nurse when rendering intensive nursing care to the patient recovering from anesthesia. This is because the functional residual capacity is usually reduced in patients recovering from anesthesia. That is why breathing maneuvers such as the sustained maximal inspiration (SMI) are instituted in the PACU—to raise the FRC (see Lung Mechanics). The FRC represents the sum of the expiratory reserve volume and the residual volume. A severe increase in the FRC is often associated with pulmonary distention, which is technically a state of hyperinflation of the lung. This state of hyperinflation can be caused by two abnormal conditions: airways obstruction and loss of elasticity. Airways obstruction could be exemplified by an attack of acute bronchial asthma; a loss of lung elasticity is usually associated with emphysema. A severe decrease in FRC is associated with the disease pulmonary fibrosis and can be the sequela of postoperative atelectasis.

The *vital capacity (VC)* is the amount of air that can be expired following the deepest possible inspiration. It is the sum of the tidal volume, the expiratory reserve volume, and the inspiratory reserve volume. The VC measures many factors that simultaneously affect the ventilation process, including activity of respiratory centers, motor nerves, and respiratory muscles, as well as thoracic compliance, airway and tissue resistance, and lung volume.

The *total lung capacity (TLC)* is simply the total amount of air in the lung at a maximal inspiration. The total lung capacity is the sum of the vital capacity and the residual volume.

The TLC, FRC, and RV are difficult to measure clinically because these measurements include a gas volume that cannot be exhaled. Therefore, performance of these measurements requires sophisticated pulmonary function testing equipment utilizing gas dilution techniques or plethysmography. As will be seen, measurements of lung volumes and capacities are very useful in the evaluation of lung function.

Lung Mechanics

Mechanical Features of the Lungs

To understand how these lung volumes and capacities are determined and how they are affected by anesthesia and surgery, the PACU nurse should become familiar with the "balance of forces" concept of the respiratory system. The mechanical forces of the respiratory system actually determine the previously described lung volumes and capacities. The PACU stir-up regimen is designed to enhance the postoperative patient's lung volumes and capacities by enhancing the mechanical forces of the respiratory system.

The lungs and chest wall are viscoelastic structures, one within the other. Because they are elastic, the lungs always want to collapse or to recoil to a smaller position. Therefore, as can be seen in the pressure-volume (P-V) curve of the lungs alone (Fig. 4–9), below residual volume the lungs are collapsed and no pressure is transmitted across the lungs (i.e., there is no transpulmonary pressure). When the lungs are in-

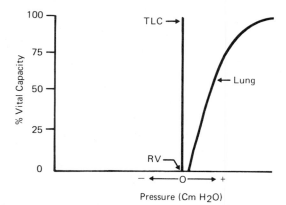

Figure 4–9. Static deflation pressure-volume (P-V) curve for the lung. The positive pressures represent pressures tending to decrease lung volume. (From Drain C.: The anesthetic management of the patient: A broad view of the anesthetic considerations necessary regarding the respiratory system. AANA J, *50*[2]:192–201, 1982.)

flated to a volume halfway between RV and TLC, the lungs seek to recoil or collapse back to the resting position at or actually below RV; this is reflected by an increase in transpulmonary pressure. When the lungs are fully inflated at TLC, a maximal transpulmonary pressure is also exhibited. To use an analogy, when a balloon is completely deflated, the pressure measured at the mouth of the ballon is zero. When the balloon is partially inflated, the pressure increases because the elastic forces of the balloon are trying to make the balloon recoil to its resting position. If the balloon were maximally inflated, the elastic recoil of the balloon would be greater, as would the pressure measured at the mouth of the balloon.

Pulmonary Hysteresis

As seen in Figure 4–10, the inflation and deflation paths of the pressure-volume (P-V) curve of the lung are not aligned on top of each other. More specifically, the path of deformation (inspiration) to total lung capacity is different from the path followed when the force is withdrawn (expiration) from TLC to RV. This phenomenon is known as *pulmonary hysteresis*. The factors that contribute to pulmonary hysteresis are (1) properties of the tissue elements (a minor factor); (2) recruitment of lung units;

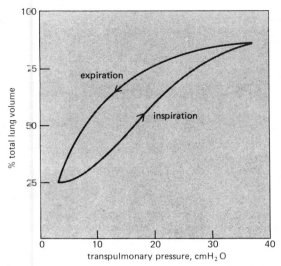

Figure 4–10. The inflation and deflation paths of the pressure-volume (P-V) curve of the lungs. (From Levitzky, M.: Pulmonary Physiology. New York, McGraw-Hill, Inc., 1982, p. 21.)

and (3) the surface tension phenomenon (surfactant).

Elastic Properties of the Lung. The elastic properties of the lung tissue contribute only a small part to the phenomenon of hysteresis.

Recruitment of Lung Units. Recruitment of lung units has an important part in pulmonary hysterersis. To understand recruitment of lung units, the nurse must be familiar with the concept of *airway closure*. In the lung, there is an apex-to-base gradient of alveolar size (Fig. 4–11). This is because of the weight of the lung, which tends to "pull" the lung down toward the base. As a result, the pleural pressure is more negative at the apex than at the base of the lung. Ultimately, at low lung volumes, the alveoli at the apex are *inflated*

more than the alveoli at the base. In fact, at the base of the lungs, some alveoli are closed to ventilation because the weight of the lungs in that area causes the pleural pressure to become positive. Airways open only when their critical opening pressure is achieved during inflation, and the lung units peripheral to them are recruited to participate in volume exchange. This is called *radial traction* or a *tethering* effect on airways. An analogy of a nylon stocking may aid in explaining this concept: When no traction is applied to the nylon stocking, the holes in the stocking are very small. As traction is applied to the stocking from all sides, each nylon filament pulls on the others, which will spread apart all the other filaments, and the holes in the stocking will enlarge. Similarly, as one airway opens, it produces radial traction on the next airway and pulls the next airway open; in other words, it recruits airways to open. The volume of air in the alveoli behind the closed airways is termed *closing volume (CV)*. The CV plus the residual volume is termed *closing capacity (CC)*. The CC normally occurs below the FRC (see Fig. 4–22). Patients in the PACU, during their early emergence phase, usually have low lung volumes, which can lead to airway closure. Consequently, a postoperative breathing maneuver having a maximal alveolar inflating pressure, a long alveolar inflating time, and high alveolar inflating volume, such as the *sustained maximal inspiration* or *yawn maneuver*, should facilitate the maximal recruitment of lung units. With the recruitment of lung units, the FRC could be raised out of the closing volume range, and ultimately there would be a reduction in hypoxemia.

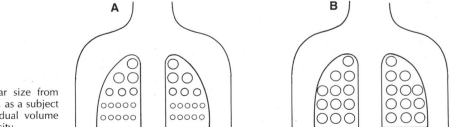

Figure 4–11. Alveolar size from apex to base of lungs, as a subject inhales from *(A)* residual volume to *(B)* total lung capacity.

Surface Tension Phenomenon. The surface tension phenomenon basically has to do with the action of surfactant on lung tissue. Surfactant is a phospholipid rich in lecithin that is produced by the type II alveolar cells. Surfactant lines the alveolus as a thin surface-active film. This film has a physiologic action of reducing the surface tension of the alveoli and terminal respiratory airways. If the surfactant were not present, the surface tension would be fixed and greater pressure would be required to keep the alveolus open. As a result, small alveoli would empty into larger ones, atelectasis would regularly occur at low lung volumes, and large expanding pressures would be required to reopen collapsed lung units. Surfactant is also an important factor in alveolar inflation because it provides uniformity in the inflation of lung units. In these ways, surfactant helps to impart stability to alveoli in the normal lung. Besides playing a major role in pulmonary hysteresis, surfactant also contributes to lung recoil and reduces the workload of breathing.

Lung Compliance

Several other terms relating to the P-V curve of the lung deserve attention. One is *lung compliance* (C-L), which is defined as the change in pressure over the change in volume.

$$C_L = \frac{\Delta V}{\Delta P}$$

Compliance is a measure of elasticity of the lung. According to convention, lung compliance means the slope of the static deflation portion of the P-V curve over the tidal volume range. So it can be said that C_L is the slope of the P-V curve, and may remain unchanged even if there are marked changes in lung elastic properties resulting in a shift of the P-V curve to the left or right. Hence, when the compliance of the lung is measured clinically, it is done over the tidal volume range, during deflation. Measuring the C_L over any other portion of the P-V curve may result in an inaccurate

reading as compared with normal. Lung elastic recoil, or Pst_L, is the pressure exerted by the lung (transpulmonary pressure) because of its tendency to recoil or collapse to a smaller resting state. At low lung volumes, the Pst_L will be low, and at high lung volumes, the Pst_L will be high. This elastic retractive force (Pst_L) is due to the overall structural elements of the lung combined with the lung surface tension forces. So it can be said that the C_L represents the slope of the P-V curve, and the Pst_L represents the points along the P-V curve. Changes in C_L and Pst_L have dramatic implications in the alteration of the lung volumes that occur in the immediate postoperative period (see p. 58).

Mechanical Features of the Chest Wall

Of next concern is the chest wall. The chest wall wants to spring out or recoil outward, seeking larger resting volume. The resting volume of the lungs alone is below RV and the resting volume of the chest wall is about 60 percent of the vital capacity. Action of the chest wall can be illustrated by using the analogy of a wire screen attached around a balloon. The wire screen tends to spring outward, so at lower balloon volumes the screen will pull the balloon open. Measuring the pressure at the mouth of the balloon would reflect a negative number. At a certain point, which is about 60 percent of the total capacity of the balloon, the screen will not tend to spring outward anymore. At that point, the addition of air causes the screen to push down on the balloon, reflecting a positive pressure at the mouth of the balloon. The screen around the balloon can be likened to the chest wall. Looking at Figure 4–12, it is clear that at lower lung volumes the chest wall is inclined to recoil outward, which creates a negative pressure, and at about 60 percent of the vital capacity the chest wall starts to push down on the lungs, creating a positive pressure. The result of the interplay of the chest wall's strong tendency to spring outward and the lung's strong tendency to recoil inward is the subatmos-

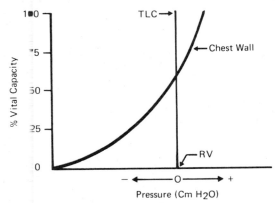

Figure 4–12. The pressure-volume (P-V) curve of the chest wall during deflation going from total lung capacity to residual volume. Positive pressures of the chest wall represent pressures tending to decrease lung size and the negative pressures represent the pressure tending to increase lung volume because of the outward recoil tendency of the chest wall at about 60 percent of the vital capacity, or less. (From Drain, C.: The anesthetic management of the patient: A broad view of the anesthetic considerations necessary regarding the respiratory system. AANA J, 50[2]:192–201, 1982, p. 194.)

pheric pleural pressure. The pleural pressure can become positive during a forced expiratory maneuver such as a cough. Pneumothorax can occur when the chest wall is opened or when air is injected into the pleural cavity. When this occurs, the lungs collapse because they naturally recoil to a smaller position. Also, when pneumothorax occurs, the ribs will flare outward, because of their natural inclination to recoil outward. Clinically, when a patient has a pneumothorax, inspection may reveal that the ribs on the affected side are protruding outward. There are two types of pneumothorax—open and closed. *Simple pneumothorax* occurs when there is airflow into the pleural space which results in a positive pleural pressure. The lungs collapse because their recoil pressure is not counterbalanced by the negative pleural pressure. Treatment for a pneumothorax can be conservative or more aggressive depending on the type and amount of pneumothorax. Aggressive treatment consists of the insertion of chest tubes into the pleural space to recreate the negative pleural pressure. This will reestablish normal ventilatory excursions. In most cases, the air leak between the lung and the pleural space will seal after

the chest tubes have been removed. If air continues to flow into the intrapleural space and cannot escape, a one-way valve mechanism can result, in which the intrapleural pressure continually increases with each succeeding inspiration. This one-way valve mechanism is known as a *tension pneumothorax*. It is a medical emergency because in a very short time, as the intrapleural pressure increases, it compresses the affected lung and puts a great amount of pressure on the mediastinum. Hypoxemia and a reduction of cardiac output result, and if treatment is not instituted immediately the patient can die. Treatment consists of immediate evacuation of the excess air from the intrapleural space, either by chest tubes or by a large-bore needle.

The Combined Mechanical Properties of the Lungs and Chest Wall

The combined pressure-volume (P-V) characteristics of the lung and the chest wall have many implications for the nurse in the post anesthesia care unit. The combined P-V curve is the algebraic sum of the individual P-V curves of the lung and chest wall. As shown in Figure 4–13, when no muscle forces are applied to the respiratory system, the functional residual capacity (FRC) is determined by a balance of elastic forces between the lung and the chest wall. Any pathophysiologic or pharmacologic process that affects the elasticity of either the lung or chest wall will affect the FRC.

Alterations in the Balance of Pulmonary Forces in the PACU Patient

It is suggested that during induction of anesthesia the shape of the P-V curve of the chest wall is altered. This agent-independent phenomenon is probably due to loss of elasticity of the chest wall. Thus, the P-V curve of the chest wall of a patient with normal lung function is shifted to the right, the balance of forces occurs sooner, and the FRC decreases (Fig. 4–14). This shift to the right has an impact on the P-V curve of the lung: it also shifts to the right, and secondary changes occur in the lung. More spe-

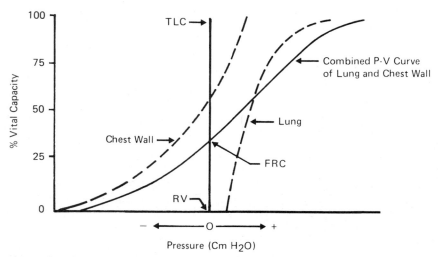

Figure 4–13. The combined pressure-volume (P-V) curves of the lungs and chest wall. The individual pressure-volume curves of the lungs and chest wall are represented by dashed lines. They are transposed from the static deflation P-V curves of the lungs (Fig. 4–9) and chest wall (Fig. 4–12). The combined P-V curve is the algebraic sum of the deflation curves of the lungs and chest wall. In the combined P-V curve it can be seen that the FRC is determined by the balance of elastic forces of the lungs and chest wall when no respiratory muscles are applied. (From Drain, C.: The anesthetic management of the patient: A broad view of the anesthetic considerations necessary regarding the respiratory system. AANA J, *50*[2]:192–201, 1982, p. 194.)

cifically, the changes consist of an increase in lung recoil ($\uparrow$ Pst_L) and a decrease in lung compliance ($\downarrow$ C_L). Ultimately, the lung becomes stiffer and the FRC decreases and may drop into the closing capacity range. Hence, during tidal ventilation, some airways are closed to ventilation, and ventilation-perfusion mismatching occurs ($\downarrow$ $\dot{V}/\dot{Q}$), which ultimately leads to hypoxemia. Research indicates that this phenom-

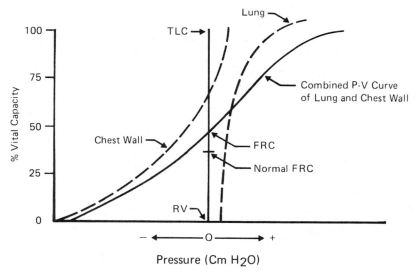

Figure 4–14. Pressure-volume (P-V) curve representing the lung mechanics of a patient in the immediate postoperative period who has undergone an upper abdominal or thoracic surgical procedure. This patient will have a loss of chest wall elastic recoil causing the lungs to become less compliant. Consequently, the combined P-V curve will shift to the right, leading to a decline in the functional residual capacity (FRC) because the balance of forces occur at lower lung volumes. (From Drain, C.: The anesthetic management of the patient: A broad view of the anesthetic considerations necessary regarding the respiratory system. AANA J, *50*[2]:192–201, 1982, p. 196.)

enon plus sighless breathing patterns in the post anesthesia care unit can cause patients to experience hypoxemia in the recovery phase of the anesthetic (see Postoperative Lung Volumes, p. 58).

Pulmonary Circulation

The basic functions of the pulmonary circulation are exchanging gas, providing a reservoir for the left ventricle, furnishing nutrition, and protecting the lungs.

Gas Exchange. The major aspects of gas exchange are discussed on page 44, but because of the implications for PACU nursing care, the concepts of transit time and pulmonary vascular resistance will be presented here.

Of the 5 liters of blood that flow through the lungs every minute, only 70 to 200 ml are active in gas exchange at any one time. The time it takes a red blood cell (RBC) to cross the pulmonary capillary bed is 0.75 second, yet it only takes the red blood cell 0.25 second to become saturated with oxygen, that is, until all the oxygen-bonding sites on the hemoglobin molecule are occupied. Because the transit time is 0.75 second and the saturation time is only 0.25 second, the body has a tremendous backup of one-half second for hemoglobin saturation with oxygen. If the RBCs move across the pulmonary capillary bed at an accelerated pace (decreased transit time), the amount of time available for O_2 to saturate the RBCs is decreased; but during stress or exercise, the complete saturation of the hemoglobin can still be accomplished because the transit time of a red blood cell rarely decreases below 0.25 second.

However, this is not true for patients with interstitial fibrosis who have a thickened respiratory exchange membrane. They may have a normal PaO_2 at rest, but exercise or exertion of surgery will increase the cardiac output, which will lower the red blood cell transit time, and the hemoglobin will not become completely saturated during its passage through the pulmonary capillary bed. This happens because more time is needed for oxygen to pass through the diseased membrane. For these patients, the lower limit for complete saturation may be 0.5 second, not 0.25 second. Hence, patients with disorders of the respiratory exchange membrane can demonstrate hypoxemia on blood gas analysis when they experience any exertion that could decrease red blood cell transit time. Clinically this phenomenon is sometimes called *desaturation on exercise*. Therefore, in the post anesthesia care unit, patients suspected of having this problem should be given low-flow oxygen and measures should be started to reduce the extrinsic factors, such as stress, elevated body temperature, and anxiety, which increase the cardiac output.

The pulmonary circulation and the systemic circulation have the same pump (the heart), so the pulmonary system receives the same cardiac output as the systemic circulation—approximately 5 liters per minute. The pulmonary circulation, compared with the systemic circulation, is a low-pressure system, with low resistance to flow, having very distensible vessels with very thin walls and a small amount of smooth muscle. Many stimuli affect pulmonary vascular resistance. Probably the most potent vasoconstrictor of the lung is alveolar hypoxia. Research indicates that *neuroendothelial bodies (NEBs)*, which respond to a low P_AO_2 may exist close to the pulmonary vascular bed. Also, the NEBs may liberate prostaglandins or histamine or both when alveolar hypoxia is present. In the postoperative period, if a patient experiences atelectasis in some portion of his lungs, the P_AO_2 in that particular area of the lungs will be reduced. As a result, the NEBs will be stimulated to produce an increased pulmonary vascular resistance in that area of the lungs. Eventually, the blood will be redirected or shunted to areas of the lungs that are adequately ventilated. Because of this, the first arterial blood gas value in a patient with atelectasis may indicate hypoxemia. Upon the second arterial blood gas determination, the hypoxemia may be slightly improved because of the increased pulmonary vascular resistance in the area of atelectasis. Therefore, the PACU nurse should continue to use an aggressive stir-up regimen on a patient with atelectasis, even though the patient's arterial blood gases indicate a slight improvement.

Reservoir for the Left Ventricle. In regard to their functioning as a reservoir for the left ventricle, the pulmonary veins are considered to be an extension of the left ventricle.

Nutrition. The pulmonary circulation can be divided into the bronchial circulation and the actual pulmonary circulation. The bronchial circulation carries nutrition and oxygen down to the respiratory bronchioles in the lungs. The bronchial circulation empties its deoxygenated blood via the pulmonary veins to the left heart. The pulmonary circulation carries nutrition to the respiratory bronchioles and the alveoli.

Protection. The role of the lungs in protection is vital for the preservation of the human organism. For example, on the surface of the pulmonary epithelium are invaginations called *caveoli*. Bradykinin and angiotensin I are handled on the surface of the caveoli. Ninety percent of the bradykinin is deactivated in the caveoli during each pass through the lungs, and angiotensin I is converted to angiotensin II via angiotensin-converting enzyme in the lungs. In the presence of hypoxia, the conversion of angiotensin I to angiotensin II is inhibited. Also, in the hypoxemic state, less than 10 percent of the bradykinin is deactivated by the lungs. In the hypoxemic state the liberated bradykinin then becomes prostaglandins. Interestingly, the inappropriate levels of prostaglandins due to hypoxemia in the chronic state are thought to produce the clubbing of the fingers in patients who suffer from long-standing chronic hypoxemia. Finally, the pulmonary epithelium also deactivates norepinephrine and serotonin. Serotonin plays an important part in platelet aggregation. Increased levels of serotonin due to decreased lung function caused by hypoxia or lung disease lead to a high risk of developing a venous thrombus. This can have ramifications in the post anesthesia care unit, therefore patients who are immobile and hypoxemic should be monitored for pulmonary and systemic thromboemboli.

Other lung reflexes associated with protection are presented later in this chapter under Regulation of Breathing.

Water Balance in the Lung

The alveoli stay dry by a combination of pressures and lymph flow (Fig. 4–15). The forces tending to push fluid out of the pulmonary capillaries are the *capillary hydrostatic pressure* (P_{cap}) minus the *interstitial fluid hydrostatic pressure* (P_{is}). The forces tending to pull fluid into the pulmonary capillaries are the *colloid osmotic pressure of the proteins in the plasma of the pulmonary capillaries* (π_{pl}) minus the *colloid osmotic pressure of the proteins in the interstitial fluid* (π_{is}). The Starling equation describes the movement of fluid across the capillary endothelium:

$$Q_f = K_f (P_{cap} - P_{is}) - \sigma_f (\pi_{pl} - \pi_{is})$$

where Q_f = net flow of fluid
K_f = capillary filtration coefficient. This describes the permeability characteristics of the membrane to fluids.
σ_f = reflection coefficient. This describes the ability of the membrane to prevent extravasation of solute particles. Thus the membrane is permeable to fluid, and in normal circumstances σ_f is equal to 1.0 in the equation.

Substituting normal values into the Starling equation,

$$Q_f = K_f [10 \text{ torr} - (-3)]$$
$$- \sigma_f [25 \text{ torr} - 19 \text{ torr}]$$

where K_f and σ_f are dropped out of the equation because they are considered normal and do not affect the outcome of the example; therefore

$$Q_f = 13 \text{ torr} - 6 \text{ torr}$$
$$Q_f = +7 \text{ torr}$$

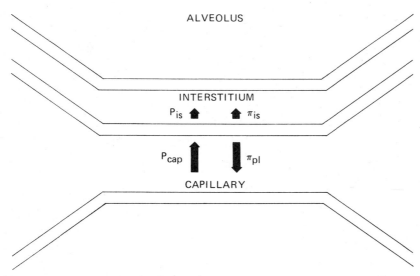

Figure 4–15. Illustration of the factors that affect the movement of fluid from the pulmonary capillaries. P_{cap} = capillary hydrostatic pressure; P_{is} = interstitial hydrostatic pressure (assumed to be negative); π_{pl} = plasma colloid pressure; π_{is} = interstitial colloid osmotic pressure. (From Levitzky, M.: Pulmonary Physiology. New York, McGraw-Hill, Inc., 1982, p. 101.)

Thus, the pressure is favoring flow out of the capillaries to the interstitium of the alveolar wall tracts through the interstitial space to the perivascular and peribronchial spaces to facilitate transport of the fluid to the lymph nodes. Hence, there is a net pressure of +7 pushing fluid to the interstitial space. The lymph flow draining the lungs is about 20 ml/hr in rate of flow. Thus, the lungs depend on a continuous net fluid flux to remain in a consistently "dry" state.

Pulmonary edema, defined as increased total lung water, is associated with dysfunction of any parameter of the Starling equation. Examples of conditions that produce an overwhelming amount of fluid to be drained by the lymphatic system are elevated pulmonary capillary pressure (due to left-sided heart failure), decreased capillary colloid osmotic pressure (due to hypoproteinemia or overadministration of intravenous solutions), and extravasation of fluid through the pulmonary capillary membrane (due to adult respiratory distress syndrome). It is notable that the earliest form of pulmonary edema is characterized by engorgement of the peribronchial and perivascular spaces and is known as *interstitial*

edema. This, in turn, if allowed to continue, leads to frank alveolar pulmonary edema.

Pulmonary edema is hard to assess in its early stages. As the fluid volume increases in the interstitium that surrounds the blood vessels and airways, reflex bronchospasm may occur. A chest x-ray at this time would reveal Kerley's B lines, which denote fluid in the interstitium. Once the lymphatics become completely overwhelmed, fluid will enter the alveoli. In the beginning of this pathophysiologic process, fine crackles will be heard upon auscultation. As the pulmonary edema progresses into the alveoli, coarse crackles will be heard, especially at the base of the lungs. Owing to the direct stimulation of the J receptors in the interstitium, the patient will have a tachypneic ventilatory pattern. Initial arterial blood gases will demonstrate a low PaO_2 and $PaCO_2$. As the pulmonary edema progresses, the $PaCO_2$ will increase because the hyperventilation (tachypnea) will not be able to counterbalance the rise in the carbon dioxide tension in the blood. Finally, when the pulmonary edema becomes fulminant, the sputum will become frothy and blood-tinged.

Treatment of pulmonary edema is based

upon the Starling equation. If the edema is cardiogenic, the focus of the treatment is to lower the hydrostatic pressures within the capillaries. Noncardiogenic pulmonary edema is usually treated with the infusion of albumin to increase the osmotic forces. Diuretics and dialysis also may be used in noncardiogenic edema in an effort to lower the vascular pressures. Positive end-expiratory pressure (PEEP) or continuous positive airway pressure (CPAP) are used with high oxygen concentrations to correct the hypoxemia.

Blood Gas Transport

Respiration is defined as the gas exchange between cellular levels in the body and the external environment. There are three phases of respiration: (1) ventilation, the phase of moving air in and out of the lungs; (2) transportation, which includes diffusion of gases in and out of the blood in both pulmonary and systemic capillaries, and the reactions of carbon dioxide and oxygen in the blood; also in this category is the circulation of blood between the lungs and the tissue cells; and (3) gas exchange, during all respiration, in which oxygen is utilized and carbon dioxide is produced as a waste product. Blood gas transport is the important link in carrying gas to or from the cell.

At sea level the barometric pressure is 760 torr. Air contains approximately 21 percent oxygen, which exerts a partial pressure of 159 torr. This is in accordance with Dalton's law of partial pressure, which states that the total pressure of a given volume of a gas mixture is equal to the sum of the separate or partial pressures that each gas would exert if that gas alone occupied the entire volume. Therefore, the total pressure is equal to the sum of the partial pressures of the major gases in the atmosphere. For example, the total atmospheric pressure (P_{total}) = partial pressure of nitrogen (P_{N_2}) + partial pressure of oxygen (P_{O_2}); therefore

$$P_{total} = P_{N_2} + P_{O_2}$$

If the actual numerical quantities are then substituted into the formula, 760 torr = 601 torr + 159 torr. Expressed in percentages: 100 percent (total atmospheric pressure) is equal to 79.03 percent (nitrogen) plus 20.93 percent (oxygen). Thus, nitrogen is 601 torr (0.7903×760) and oxygen is 159 torr (0.2093×760). In the lower airways, water vapor exerts a pressure that can be accounted for by Dalton's law. At the body temperature of 37°C the water vapor pressure in the lower airways is 47 torr. Because the water vapor pressure affects the partial pressures of both nitrogen and oxygen, it is subtracted from the atmospheric pressure of 760 torr, which results in a pressure of 713 torr (760 torr − 47 torr = 713 torr). To determine the partial pressure of oxygen in the lower airways, the percent oxygen (20.93) is multiplied by the 713 torr with a resultant oxygen partial pressure of 149.2 torr. The respiratory exchange ratio can be used to understand how the alveolar partial pressure of oxygen is determined. This ratio represents carbon dioxide production divided by oxygen consumption. The normal respiratory exchange ratio is 0.8. In theory then, *for every 10 torr of carbon dioxide that is added to the alveolus, 12 torr of oxygen is displaced.* Therefore, with no respiratory pathophysiology present, if the Pa_{CO_2} is 40 torr, then 48 torr of oxygen will be removed from the alveolus. Where

$$4 \times 10 = 40 \text{ torr (carbon dioxide)},$$
$$\text{so } 4 \times 12 = 48 \text{ torr (oxygen)}$$

This results in an alveolar partial pressure for oxygen of 101 torr (149 torr − 48 torr = 101 torr). This is called the *12–10 concept* and is very helpful in assessing arterial blood gas determinations in the PACU (see p. 51).

As the oxygen diffuses across the pulmonary membrane, the partial pressure of oxygen is further decreased to 95 torr by a venous admixture. This is because of vascular shunts that normally redirect 1 to 2 percent of the total cardiac output either to nonaerated areas in the lungs themselves or directly through the heart, bypassing the lungs.

Oxygen Transport

Oxygen is carried in the blood in two forms: in combination with hemoglobin or in simple solution. About 98 percent of the oxygen transported from the lungs to the cells is carried in combination with hemoglobin in the red blood cell. It is a reversible chemical combination. The remaining 2 percent is dissolved in the plasma and in the cytoplasm of the red blood cell. The amount of oxygen transported in both forms is directly proportional to the partial pressure of oxygen.

When the blood passes through the lungs, it does not normally become completely saturated with oxygen. Usually, the hemoglobin will become about 97 percent saturated. When hemoglobin is saturated with oxygen it is called *oxyhemoglobin*.

Normally, the oxygen content of the arterial blood is 19.8 ml/dl of blood. This total oxygen content in the arterial blood (CaO_2) is equal to the oxygen-carrying capacity of hemoglobin, which is 1.34 times the number of grams of hemoglobin. That number divided by 100 is the oxygen content carried by the hemoglobin. To determine the total amount of oxygen in the blood, the oxygen content that is dissolved in the plasma must be added to the oxygen content of the hemoglobin. The amount of oxygen dissolved in the plasma is determined by multiplying the PaO_2 times the solubility coefficient for oxygen in plasma, which is 0.003. Therefore, the equation for the total oxygen content in the blood is:

$$CaO_2 = \frac{(Hb \times 1.34 \times \% \ Hb \ saturation)}{100} + (PaO_2 \times 0.003)$$

If the normal values of Hb = 15 gm, percent Hb saturation = 97, and PaO_2 = 95 torr, are substituted into the equation:

$$CaO_2 = \frac{(15 \times 1.34 \times 97)}{100} + (95 \times 0.003)$$

$$CaO_2 = 19.497 + 0.285$$

$$CaO_2 = 19.782 \text{ ml oxygen/dl of blood.}$$

It must be remembered that oxygen content is different from oxygen partial pressures. Content refers only to the amount of oxygen carried by the blood, not to its partial pressure (PO_2).

At the lungs, venous blood is oxygenated or arterialized. The oxygen bond with hemoglobin is loose and reversible. The bond is also PO_2-dependent; that is to say, the higher the PaO_2, the more oxygen saturation of the hemoglobin. However, the hemoglobin cannot be supersaturated, because when all the bonding sites on the hemoglobin molecule are occupied by oxygen, no matter how much more oxygen is presented to the hemoglobin, it will not be able to bond to the hemoglobin.

The *oxygen-hemoglobin dissociation curve* relates the percentage of oxygen saturation of hemoglobin to the PaO_2 value. Note in Figure 4–16 that the curve is sigmoid in shape with a very steep portion between the 10 and 50 torr PaO_2 range, with a leveling off noted above the 70 torr level. The flat portion of the curve indicates the capacity to oxygenate most of the hemoglobin despite wide variations in the partial pressure of oxygen (70 to 98 torr). This flat portion of the curve can be referred to as the *association* portion of the curve, and it corresponds to the external respiration that is taking place in the lungs. The steep portion of the curve indicates the capacity to unload large amounts of oxygen in response to small tissue PO_2 changes. This part of the curve is called the *dissociation* portion of the oxygen-hemoglobin dissociation curve.

As discussed, the normal oxygen content at the association portion of the curve is about 19.8 ml of oxygen/dl of blood. At the venous dissociation portion of the curve, the content of oxygen is 15.2 ml of oxygen/dl of blood. The following formula is used to derive the content of oxygen in the venous blood (CvO_2):

$$CvO_2 = \frac{(Hb \times 1.34 \times \% \ Hb \ saturation)}{100} + (PvO_2 \times 0.003)$$

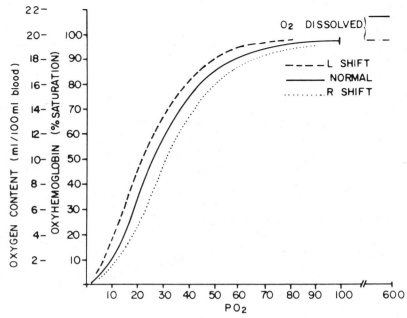

Figure 4–16. Oxyhemoglobin dissociation curve. (From Guenter, C., and Welch, M.: Pulmonary Medicine. Philadelphia, J. B. Lippincott Co., 1977, p. 151.)

Substituting normal values for venous blood of Hb = 15 gm, percent Hb saturation = 75, and the Pvo_2 = 40, into the formula:

$$Cvo_2 = \frac{(15 \times 1.34 \times 75)}{100} + (40 \times 0.003)$$

$Cvo_2 = 15.08 + 0.12$

$Cvo_2 = 15.20$ ml oxygen/dl blood.

Therefore, in this example the net delivery of oxygen to the tissues is 4.6 ml of oxygen/dl of blood (19.8 − 15.2 = 4.6).

Factors Affecting Oxygen Transport

The association portion of the oxygen-hemoglobin dissociation curve is not necessarily a fixed line determined solely by the Pao_2. The height of the curve and the slope of it are dependent upon many factors, such as pH and temperature. Generally, a decrease in the pH (H^+ increase) or an increase in body temperature will cause a shift of the curve to the right, which leads to a decrease in the height and slope of the curve. Ultimately, there will be less saturation (loading) of the hemoglobin for a given Pao_2. Hence, patients who have a low pH and/or high temperature will probably ben-

efit from a higher Fio_2 than normal to facilitate an appropriate level of saturation of their hemoglobin. However, before changes in the Fio_2 are made, arterial blood gases should be drawn and analyzed.

At the dissociation portion of the oxygen-hemoglobin dissociation curve, the same is true. It is not a fixed line, as it also changes position in response to physiologic processes. At the tissue level, metabolically active tissues will produce more carbon dioxide, more acid (↓ pH), and will have an elevated temperature. All these products of metabolism will shift the curve to the right. The curve shifts far more in response to physiologic processes in the dissociation portion than in the association part. Metabolically active tissues produce more carbon dioxide and need more oxygen. The effect of carbon dioxide on the curve is closely related to the fact that deoxyhemoglobin binds H^+ more actively than oxyhemoglobin. As a result, at the tissue level, increased carbon dioxide decreases the affinity of hemoglobin for oxygen. Thus, the dissociation portion of the curve is shifted to the right and more oxygen is given to the tissue. This effect of carbon dioxide on oxygen transport is called the *Bohr effect*.

2,3 Diphosphoglycerate (2,3 DPG) regulates the release of oxygen to the tissue. It is a glycolytic intermediary metabolite that is more concentrated in the red blood cell than anywhere else in the body. High concentrations of 2,3 DPG shift the curve to the right, making oxygen more available to the tissues. Lower concentrations of 2,3 DPG will cause a shift of the curve to the left, ultimately leading to the release of less oxygen to the tissues. The clinical implications here involve the administration of outdated whole blood. Whole blood stored longer than 21 days will have low levels of 2,3 DPG. This means that if the blood were administered to a patient, the tissues would not receive an appropriate amount of oxygen owing to the shift to the left of the oxygen-hemoglobin dissociation curve.

Carbon Dioxide Transport

The transport of carbon dioxide begins within each cell in the body. The carbon dioxide is mainly a byproduct of the energy-supplying mechanisms of the cell. Approximately 200 ml per minute of carbon dioxide are produced within the body at rest. Carbon dioxide is 20 times more soluble in water than oxygen, the therefore it traverses

the fluid compartments of the body very rapidly. The intracellular partial pressure of carbon dioxide is 46 torr. A 1 torr gradient exists between the cell and the interstitial fluid. Carbon dioxide will diffuse out of the cell to the interstitial fluid and have a new partial pressure of 45 torr. When the tissue capillary blood enters the venules, the partial pressure of the carbon dioxide is 45 torr.

Carbon dioxide is transported in the blood in three forms: (1) physically dissolved in solution, (2) as carbaminohemoglobin, and (3) as bicarbonate ions.

Carbon Dioxide in Simple Solution. About 10 percent of the total amount of carbon dioxide transported in the body is physically dissolved in solution.

Carbaminohemoglobin. Approximately 30 percent of carbon dioxide is transported as *carbaminohemoglobin*, a chemical combination of carbon dioxide and hemoglobin that is reversible because the binding point on the hemoglobin is on the amino groups and is a very loose bond. This chemical bonding of carbon dioxide with hemoglobin can be graphically described by the use of the *carbon dioxide dissociation curve*. There are two differences between the carbon dioxide dissociation curve (Fig. 4–17) and the oxygen-hemoglobin dissociation curve. First, over

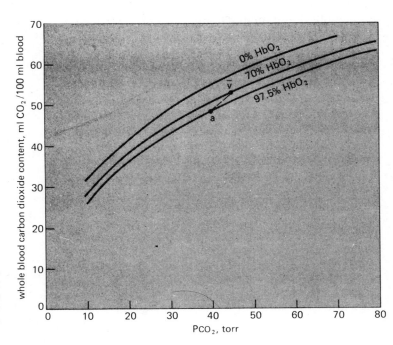

Figure 4–17. Carbon dioxide dissociation curves for whole blood at 37°C at different hemoglobin oxygen saturations. (From Levitzky, M.: Pulmonary Physiology. New York, McGraw-Hill, Inc., 1982, p. 146.)

the normal operating range of blood P_{CO_2} from 47 torr (venous) and 40 torr (arterial), the slope of the carbon dioxide dissociation curve is nearly linear and not sigmoid like the oxygen-hemoglobin dissociation curve. Second, the total carbon dioxide content is about twice the total oxygen content. Oxygen has a very definite effect on carbon dioxide transport. On the upper curve or venous portion of the carbon dioxide curve, note that the point for the P_{VCO_2} is 47 and the P_{VO_2} is 40. On the lower curve or arterial carbon dioxide curve, observe the points for the Pa_{CO_2} of 40 torr and the Pa_{O_2} of 100 torr. Notice how the venous carbon dioxide curve is shifted to the left and is above the arterial curve. This is the effect of oxygen on carbon dioxide transport or the *Haldane effect*. In terms of physiologic significance, the Haldane effect plays a more important role than the Bohr effect in gas transport. Specifically, at the lungs the binding of oxygen with hemoglobin tends to displace carbon dioxide from the hemoglobin (oxyhemoglobin is more acidic than deoxyhemoglobin). At the tissue level, oxygen is removed from the hemoglobin (owing to pressure gradient), reducing the acidity of the hemoglobin, and enabling it to bind more carbon dioxide. In fact, because the hemoglobin is in the reduced state (deoxyhemoglobin) the hemoglobin can carry 6 volumes percent more carbon dioxide than the amount of carbon dioxide that could be carried by oxyhemoglobin.

Bicarbonate. Sixty-five percent of carbon dioxide is transported in the form of bicarbonate, which is the product of the reaction of carbon dioxide with water. When the carbon dioxide and water join they form carbonic acid. Almost all the carbonic acid dissociates to bicarbonate and hydrogen ions, as seen in the following equation:

$$CO_2 + H_2O \xrightarrow{\text{carbonic anhydrase}} H_2CO_3^- \rightarrow H^+ + HCO_3^-$$

This reaction occurs mostly within the red blood cells as carbonic anhydrase accelerates the hydration of carbon dioxide to carbonic acid 220 to 300 times faster than if

carbon dioxide and water were joined without this enzymatic catalyst.

When the bicarbonate produced in this reaction in the red blood cells exceeds the bicarbonate ion level in the plasma, it will diffuse out of the cell. The positively charged hydrogen ion tends to remain within the red blood cell and is buffered by hemoglobin. Because of ionic imbalance, chloride, a negatively charged ion that is abundant in the plasma, diffuses into the red blood cell to maintain electrical balance. This movement is referred to as the *chloride shift*. Because of the increase of osmotically active particles within the cell, water from the plasma diffuses into the red blood cell. This is why the red blood cells in the venous edge of the circulation are slightly larger than the arterial red blood cells (Fig. 4–18).

As the venous blood enters the pulmonary capillaries, the carbon dioxide in simple solution freely diffuses to the alveoli. The carbaminohemoglobin reverses to free the carbon dioxide, which diffuses across the alveoli and is then expired. The hydrogen and the bicarbonate combine to form carbonic acid, which is rapidly broken down by carbonic anhydrase to form carbon dioxide and water. The carbon dioxide then diffuses through the alveoli and is expired.

Not all carbon dioxide is eliminated by pulmonary ventilation. Other buffer systems that remove excess carbon dioxide are acid-base buffers and urinary excretion by the kidneys. The respiratory system can adjust to rapid fluctuations in carbon dioxide, whereas the kidneys may require hours to restore a normal carbon dioxide tension.

Acid-Base Relationships

A buffer is a substance that causes a lesser change in hydrogen ion (H^+) concentration to occur in a solution, upon addition of acid or base, than would have occurred had the buffer not been present. The buffers can respond in seconds to fluctuations in carbon dioxide tension. Some buffers are the carbonic acid/bicarbonate system, the proteinate/protein system, and the hemoglobinate/hemoglobin system.

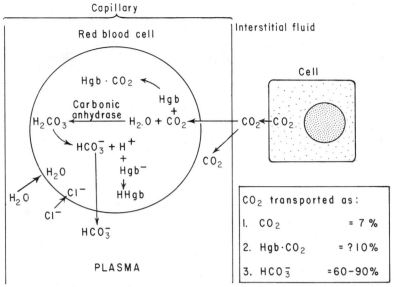

Figure 4–18. Transport of carbon dioxide in the blood. (From Jacob, S. W., and Francone C. A.: Structure and Function in Man. 3rd ed. Philadelphia, W. B. Saunders Co., 1974, p. 410.)

The pH is a measurement of alkalinity or acidity. It is dependent on the concentration of hydrogen ions. The more hydrogen ions, the more acidic the solution will be, and the fewer hydrogen ions, the more alkaline. pH is described in logarithmic form, and the greater the amount of hydrogen ions, the lower the pH (which would indicate acidity). If, on the other hand, the hydrogen ion concentration is low, then the pH is high, indicating alkalinity. The pH range is from 1 to 14, with 7 being equilibrium or pK. The normal pH in extracellular fluid is 7.35 to 7.45, which is slightly alkaline.

The normal bicarbonate level in the extracellular fluid is 24 mEq. Base excess is used to describe alkalosis or acidosis. If a plus base excess number is noted, this indicates more base in the extracellular fluid. If a minus number is reported, the base is being used to neutralize the acid to a point of encroaching on the amount of available base, which is demonstrated by a minus value for the base excess (acidosis).

Respiratory Acid-Base Imbalances

Respiratory acidosis is characterized by an increased $PaCO_2$ above the normal range of 36 to 44 torr. All other primary processes tending to cause acidosis are metabolic.

Some common causes of carbon dioxide retention and respiratory acidosis are summarized in Table 4–3.

Respiratory alkalosis is characterized by a lowering of the arterial carbon dioxide tension. Hyperventilation is a frequent clinical finding as the cause of this disorder. Some common causes of excessive carbon dioxide elimination and respiratory alkalosis are summarized in Table 4–4.

In respiratory alkalosis or acidosis, a lin-

TABLE 4–3. Common Causes of Carbon Dioxide Retention and Respiratory Acidosis (Hypoventilation)

Normal Lungs
Anesthesia
Sedative drugs (overdose)
Neuromuscular disease
  Poliomyelitis
  Myasthenia gravis
  Guillain-Barré syndrome
Obesity (Pickwickian syndrome)
Brain damage
Cardiac arrest
Pneumothorax
Pulmonary edema
Bronchospasm
Laryngospasm
Abnormal Lungs
Chronic obstructive pulmonary disease (chronic
  bronchitis, asthma, and emphysema)
  Diffuse infiltration pulmonary disease (advanced)
  Kyphoscoliosis (severe)

TABLE 4–4. Common Causes of Excessive Carbon Dioxide Elimination and Respiratory Alkalosis (Hyperventilation)

Normal Lungs
Anxiety
Fever
Drugs (aspirin)
Central nervous system lesions
Endotoxemia
Abnormal Lungs
Pneumonia
Diffuse infiltrative pulmonary disease (early)
Acute bronchial asthma (early)
Pulmonary vascular disease
Congestive heart failure (early)

ear exchange takes place between the carbon dioxide and bicarbonate concentrations, which are summarized as follows:

1. In acute respiratory acidosis bicarbonate concentration is approximately 1 mEq/L for each 10 torr change in $Paco_2$.

2. In chronic respiratory acidosis, the change in actual bicarbonate concentration is approximately 2 mEq/L for each 10 torr change in $Paco_2$.

3. The change in actual bicarbonate concentration with a chronic change in $Paco_2$ above the range of 40 torr change is approximately 4 mEq/L for each 10 torr change in $Paco_2$. This rule holds true for one or two days after onset of the disorder because of the slow renal buffer system.

Another rule of thumb to determine if the acid-base disorder is entirely respiratory in origin is: *An acute increase of $Paco_2$ by 10 torr produces a corresponding decrease in pH by 0.07 pH units. In chronic hypercapnia each increase of $Paco_2$ by 10 torr results in a corresponding decrease in pH by 0.03 pH units.* When the $Paco_2$ and pH changes are significantly outside these standards, this suggests that the acid-base disorder is not completely respiratory in origin. For example, if a patient recovering from a spinal anesthetic in the post anesthesia care unit has blood gases (room air) of Pao_2 = 92 torr, $Paco_2$ = 30 torr, and a pH of 7.47, as compared with his preoperative arterial blood gases (room air) of Pao_2 = 80 torr, $Paco_2$ = 40 torr, and a pH of 7.40, the rule of thumb can be applied. Because the $Paco_2$ decreased by 10 torr and the pH increased

by 0.07 pH units, it is clear that the patient is suffering from *respiratory* alkalosis, not from any metabolic disorder. Further, using the 12–10 concept, it can be determined that this patient is probably suffering from acute hyperventilation.

Metabolic Acid-Base Imbalances

Metabolic acidosis usually results when there is an increase in nonvolatile acids or a loss of bases from the body. The usual result is a deficit in buffer base, base excess, and bicarbonate. Because acidosis stimulates respiration, the $Paco_2$ will usually drop. The magnitude of the ventilatory response will usually serve to differentiate between acute and chronic metabolic acidosis. Some of the common causes of metabolic acidosis are summarized in Table 4–5.

Metabolic alkalosis is produced by an excessive elimination of nonvolatile acids (vomiting, gastric aspiration, hypokalemic alkalosis), or by increase in bases (alkali administration or hypochloremic alkalosis caused by some diuretics).

A summary of blood gas discrepancies in each condition is given in Table 4–6.

Matching of Ventilation to Perfusion

Distribution of Ventilation. There is a gravity-dependent gradient of pleural pressure in the upright lung at resting lung volumes. The weight of the lung tends to pull the lung tissue toward the base of the lung. As

TABLE 4–5. Common Causes of Metabolic Acidosis

Increased nonvolatile acids
Diabetes mellitus
Uremia
Severe exercise
Hypoxia
Shock
Idiopathic
Methyl alcohol ingestion (formic acid)
Aspirin ingestion (salicylic acid)
Excessive loss of bases (usually $NaCO_3$ from lower gastrointestinal tract)
Severe diarrhea (e.g., cholera, diarrhea in infants)
Fistulas (e.g., pancreatic, biliary)

TABLE 4–6. Summary of Blood Gas Discrepancies

Condition	HCO_3^-	Pco_2	pH
Metabolic acidosis	↓	↓	↓
Respiratory acidosis	↑	↑	↓
Metabolic alkalosis	↑	↑	↑
Respiratory alkalosis	↓	↓	↑

a result, the intrapleural pressure is more negative at the apex of the lung as compared to the intrapleural pressure at the base and over the tidal volume range, the alveoli at the apex being more fully inflated as compared with the alveoli at the base. Consequently, the alveoli at the base have a greater capacity for volume change during inspiration, whereas the alveoli at the apex are already "stretched" or distended. In a normal subject who breathes out to residual volume (RV) and then inspires in small steps, the initial inspired air (a small portion) goes to the apex and the base remains completely underventilated. After a certain lung volume is attained, the base of the lung will receive almost all of the air because of the capacity of the alveoli at the base of the lung for volume change. Therefore, because of the mechanical properties of the lung, during inspiration from RV to TLC the greatest volume change occurs near the base of the lungs.

Distribution of Perfusion. There is a gravity-dependent gradient for perfusion in the lungs, with approximately 80 to 90 percent of the blood flow occurring from the middle portion to an area near the base of the lungs. Therefore, the blood flow per unit lung volume increases down the lung from apex to base.

Matching. Matching of alveolar ventilation ($\dot{V}_A$) to perfusion ($\dot{Q}_C$) is defined in terms of a certain volume of alveolar gas that is required to arterialize a given volume of mixed venous blood. The normal alveolar ventilation ratio is:

$$\frac{\dot{V}_A}{\dot{Q}_C} = \frac{4,000 \text{ ml/min}}{5,000 \text{ ml/min}} = 0.8$$

If blood and gas were matched equally throughout the lung, the $\dot{V}_A/\dot{Q}_C$ ratio would

be 1.0. However, in the normal lung the matching of ventilation to perfusion is not proportional, which results in varying $\dot{V}_A/\dot{Q}_C$ ratios throughout the lung. More specifically, at the apex ventilation is high as opposed to perfusion, and perfusion is higher than ventilation at the base of the lung. Finally, if all the $\dot{V}_A/\dot{Q}_C$ relationships were summed up together, the mean ratio would be 0.8.

Causes of Hypoxemia

Hypoventilation

The Pao_2 and $Paco_2$ are determined by the balance between the addition of oxygen and the removal of carbon dioxide by the alveolar ventilation, and the removal of oxygen and the addition of carbon dioxide by the pulmonary capillary blood flow. If the alveolar ventilation is decreased (with no other lung pathology present), the Pao_2 will decrease and the $Paco_2$ will increase. In fact, the Pao_2 will fall almost proportionally to the rise in the $Paco_2$. Recall the calculations made in the 12–10 concept. At any specific inspired oxygen tension, a 10 torr rise in the $Paco_2$ will cause an approximate fall in the arterial oxygen tension of 12 torr. For example, if the normal $Paco_2$ is equal to 40 torr and the Pao_2 is equal to 95 torr and the patient's alveolar ventilation decreased owing to narcotics given in the post anesthesia care unit, the $Paco_2$ increases to 60 torr. The new Pao_2 should be 71 torr (change of 20 torr in the $Paco_2$, so 12 + 12 = 24 − 95 = 71). Therefore, when one is assessing blood gas data and the 12–10 relationship is determined to be present, hypoventilation should be suspected. Remember, the 12–10 relationship does not have to be exact, but if the numbers are close to the 12–10 relationship, hypoventilation is the probable cause. An increased inspired oxygen concentration will affect the 12–10 relationship. However, most patients in the post anesthesia care unit receive low-flow oxygen therapy and, therefore, the Fio_2 is usually 0.24 to 0.28. Consequently, if the values seem to change proportionally, hypoventilation can still be suspected. Hypoventilation is the most common cause of hypoxemia in the PACU. Nursing interventions should include administration of a higher FiO_2 via low-flow oxygen therapy, stimulation of the patient, use of an aggressive stir-up regimen, and possible pharmacologic reversal of narcotics or muscle relaxants.

Ventilation/Perfusion Mismatching

If the 12–10 relationship is not present during the analysis of the arterial blood gases, ventilation/perfusion ($\dot{V}_A/\dot{Q}_C$) mismatching is probably the cause. However, it is difficult to determine if the mismatching problem is due to increased or decreased $\dot{V}_A/\dot{Q}_C$. As seen in Figure 4–19, *normal* $\dot{V}_A/\dot{Q}_C$ exists when there is appropriate matching of ventilation to perfusion. *Decreased* $\dot{V}_A/\dot{Q}_C$ occurs when the matching ventilation is reduced as compared with perfusion of the alveoli, and *increased* $\dot{V}_A/\dot{Q}_C$ is caused by increased ventilation as compared to perfusion.

Decreased Ventilation to Perfusion ($\downarrow$ $\dot{V}_A/\dot{Q}_C$). The reduced ventilation as compared to perfusion may be due to excessive secretions or partial bronchospasm. When atelectasis or airway closure occurs, intrapulmonary shunting results. In these situations, oxygen cannot diffuse properly across to the pulmonary capillary blood. In decreased $\dot{V}_A/\dot{Q}_C$, some oxygen will diffuse across from the alveoli to the pulmonary capillary blood. Thus, the alveolar-arterial oxygen difference [(A-a)DO_2] will be slightly reduced. If there is a large gradient in the [(A-a)DO_2], intrapulmonary shunting is probably present. For a patient breathing room air, the normal [(A-a)DO_2] is between 5 and 15 torr. When a patient is breathing oxygen at a FiO_2 of 0.5 (50 percent), the alveolar-arterial oxygen gradient should be about 50 torr. A gradient greatly in excess of 50 torr suggests $\dot{V}_A/\dot{Q}_C$ mismatching. The focus of the nursing interventions to improve decreased $\dot{V}_A/\dot{Q}_C$ are airway clearance, reinflation of alveoli, and enhanced patency of the airways. The newly advocated stir-up regimen of turn, cascade cough, and sustained maximal inspiration

should improve the decreased $\dot{V}_A/\dot{Q}_C$. Percussion or vibration, or both, may also need to be instituted to facilitate secretion clearance. Also, if partial bronchospasm (expiratory wheeze) is suspected, the attending physician should be consulted about the institution of appropriate bronchodilator therapy.

At this point, a clarification of terms used to describe decreased $\dot{V}_A/\dot{Q}_C$ and shunt is in order. Basically, *intrapulmonary shunts* result in the mixing of venous blood that has not been properly oxygenated into the arterial blood (pulmonary vein). *Anatomic shunts*, which occur normally, are attributed to the two to three percent of the cardiac output that bypasses the lungs. The shunted, unoxygenated venous blood comes mainly from the bronchial circulation, which empties into the pulmonary veins, and from the thebesian vessels that drain the myocardium into the left heart. Intrapulmonary shunts occur when mixed venous blood does not become oxygenated when it passes by underventilated, unventilated, or collapsed alveoli. *Absolute intrapulmonary shunts*, sometimes called *true shunts*, are associated with totally unventilated or collapsed alveoli. *Shunt-like intrapulmonary shunts* are the areas of low $\dot{V}_A/\dot{Q}_C$ in which blood draining the partially obstructed alveoli has a lower arterial oxygen content in comparison with the alveolar capillary units that are well matched. As a result, the presence of anatomic shunts is normal. Abnormal shunts can be classified as physiologic shunts. *Physiologic shunts* are made up of the anatomic shunts plus *intrapulmonary shunts* (absolute and shunt-like intrapulmonary shunts).

Increased Ventilation to Perfusion. According to Figure 4–19, when the circulation to the individual alveolar-capillary unit is compromised, there is an excess of ventilation as compared with perfusion. If the flow of blood in the pulmonary capillary is partially obstructed, increased $\dot{V}_A/\dot{Q}_C$ results. If the flow of blood is completely obstructed, such as by a pulmonary embolus, only ventilation continues, producing wasted or dead space. Wasted ventilation is the total

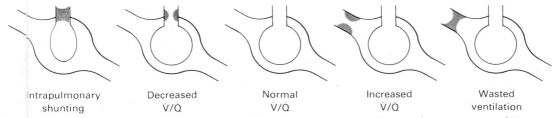

Intrapulmonary   Decreased   Normal   Increased   Wasted
shunting   V̇/Q̇   V̇/Q̇   V̇/Q̇   ventilation

Figure 4–19. Graphic representation of normal and abnormal matching of ventilation (V̇A) to perfusion (Q̇C). (From Harper, R.: A Guide to Respiratory Care: Physiology and Clinical Applications. Philadelphia, J. B. Lippincott Co., 1981, p. 98.)

amount of inspired gas that does not contribute to carbon dioxide removal; it is also known as physiologic dead space. *Physiologic dead space* (V_D physio) is that volume of each breath which is inhaled but does not reach functioning terminal respiratory units. Physiologic dead space has two components, alveolar and anatomic dead space. *Alveolar dead space* (V_D alv), as depicted in Figure 4–20, is that volume of air contributed by all those terminal respiratory units which are overventilated relative to their perfusion. *Anatomic dead space* (V_D anat) consists of the volume of air in the conducting airways that does not participate in gas exchange. This includes all air down to the respiratory bronchioles. The following formula depicts physiologic dead space:

$$V_D \text{ physio} = V_D \text{ alv} + V_D \text{ anat}$$

Normally, physiologic dead space consists mainly of anatomic dead space, with the alveolar dead space component being very small. That is why the normal physiologic dead space volume in milliliters is approximately equal to the weight of an individual in pounds. For example, a person weighing 150 pounds will have a physiologic dead space of 150 ml. When alveoli become overventilated as compared with perfused, the alveolar dead space increases, which in turn increases the physiologic dead space.

The amount of physiologic dead space can be determined by the Bohr equation. Clinically, the Bohr equation is commonly referred to as the V_D/V_T. The ratio of dead space (V_D) to tidal volume (V_T) can be used to determine whether the obstruction to pulmonary capillary blood flow is partial ($\dot{V}_A/\dot{Q}_C$) or complete (wasted ventilaton). The V_D/V_T can be derived from the following equation:

$$\frac{V_D}{V_T} = \frac{P_{aCO_2} - P_{E}CO_2}{P_{aCO_2}}$$

where the P_{aCO_2} is the arterial carbon dioxide partial pressure and the $P_{E}CO_2$ is the

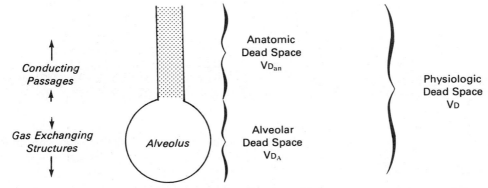

Conducting Passages

Gas Exchanging Structures

Alveolus

Anatomic
Dead Space
$V_{D_{an}}$

Alveolar
Dead Space
V_{D_A}

Physiologic
Dead Space
V_D

Figure 4–20. Graphic representation of dead space. The physiologic dead space represents the sum of the anatomic dead space in the conducting passages (shaded area) and alveolar dead space in the alveoli (circle). (From Harper, R.: A Guide to Respiratory Care: Physiology and Clinical Applications. Philadelphia, J. B. Lippincott Co., 1981, p. 48.)

partial pressure of the expired carbon dioxide. The V_D/V_T ratio is normally 0.3. If the V_D/V_T goes up to 0.6, more than half of the tidal volume is dead space. Most patients can double their minute ventilation ($\dot{V}_E$), but beyond that amount the effort is too exhausting, and a V_D/V_T ratio of > 0.6 usually mandates that the patient's ventilation be assisted mechanically.

REGULATION OF BREATHING

In the past, medullary control of breathing was thought to be a function of reciprocal inhibition between the inspiratory and expiratory centers. Research now indicates a more discrete regulatory process occurring at two levels—the sensors and the controllers. Patients with altered regulation and control of breathing present a significant challenge to the PACU nurse. Also, anesthesia, surgery, and medications administered in the post anesthesia care unit can have a profound impact on the patient's regulatory processes of breathing.

The Sensors

Peripheral Chemoreceptors. The carotid and aortic bodies are the peripheral chemoreceptors and are located at the bifurcation of the common carotid arteries and at the arch of the aorta, respectively. The carotid and aortic bodies are responsible for the immediate increase in ventilation due to lack of oxygen. These peripheral chemoreceptors are made up of very vascular tissue and glomus cells. The carotid and aortic bodies monitor only the partial pressure of oxygen (PaO_2), not the oxygen saturation (CaO_2) of the hemoglobin. Therefore, the receptors are not stimulated in conditions such as anemia and carbon monoxide and cyanide poisoning.

The carotid bodies are much more important physiologically than the aortic bodies. The carotid bodies respond, in order of degree of response, to low PaO_2, high $PaCO_2$, and low pH. The carotid bodies respond to a low PaO_2, and the response is augmented by a high $PaCO_2$ and/or low pH.

The physiologic responses to the stimulation of the carotid sinus are hyperpnea, bradycardia, and hypotension. The aortic bodies, on the other hand, respond to a low PaO_2 and high $PaCO_2$ but not to pH. The results of stimulation of the aortic bodies are hyperpnea, tachycardia, and hypertension.

The carotid and aortic bodies mainly respond to a low PaO_2. This response is commonly referred to as the *hypoxic drive* or *secondary drive*. The impulse activity in these chemoreceptors begins at a PaO_2 of about 500 torr. A rapid rise in impulses occurs at a PaO_2 below 100 torr. The impulses are *greatly increased* as the PaO_2 falls below 60 torr. Below 30 torr, the impulse activity from the chemoreceptors decreases owing to direct oxygen lack in the glomus cells. In addition, these peripheral arterial chemoreceptors are stimulated by a low arterial blood pressure and increased sympathetic activity.

Central Chemoreceptors. The central chemoreceptors lie near the ventral surface of the medulla. Specifically, these chemosensitive areas are near the choroid plexus (venous blood) and next to the cerebral spinal fluid. The central chemoreceptors respond *indirectly* to carbon dioxide. This is because the blood-brain barrier will allow lipid-soluble substances, such as carbon dioxide, oxygen, and water to cross the barrier, whereas water-soluble substances, such as sodium, potassium, hydrogen ion, and bicarbonate pass through the membrane at a *very slow rate*. Bicarbonate requires active transport to cross the barrier. Therefore, the carbon dioxide enters the cerebrospinal fluid (CSF) and is hydrated to form carbonic acid (H_2CO_3). The H_2CO_3 rapidly dissociates to form hydrogen ion (H^+) and bicarbonate (HCO_3^-). The hydrogen ion concentration in the CSF parallels the arterial PCO_2. Actually, it is the hydrogen ion concentration that stimulates ventilation via hydrogen receptors located in the central chemoreceptor area. In summary, carbon dioxide has very little direct effect on the stimulation of the receptors in the central chemoreceptor area but does have a *potent* *indirect effect*. This indirect effect is due to the inability of hydrogen ions to easily cross the blood-brain barrier. For this reason, changes in hydrogen ion concentration in the blood have considerably less effect in stimulating the chemoreceptor area than do changes in carbon dioxide. Consequently, the central chemoreceptor area precisely controls ventilation and therefore the $PaCO_2$. For that reason, *the index to the adequacy of ventilation is the $PaCO_2$*.

In the CSF, bicarbonate is the only major buffer. The pH of the CSF is a result of the ratio between bicarbonate and carbon dioxide in the CSF. As stated, carbon dioxide is freely diffusible in and out of the CSF via the blood-brain barrier. However, bicarbonate is not freely diffusible and requires active or passive transport to enter or to leave the CSF. Therefore, when an acute rise in the $PaCO_2$ occurs, the CO_2 enters the CSF, is hydrated, and hydrogen ions and bicarbonate are formed. The hydrogen ion stimulates the chemoreceptors, and the bicarbonate decreases the pH of the CSF. The resultant hyperpnea will lower the blood $PaCO_2$, creating a gradient favoring the diffusion of CO_2 out of the CSF. The blood $PaCO_2$ and pH will be corrected immediately, but the pH in the CSF will require some time to reestablish a normal carbon dioxide–bicarbonate level owing to the poor diffusibility of bicarbonate. This is usually not a problem for the person with normal respiratory function. However, for the patient with chronic carbon dioxide retention (chronic hypercapnia) who is hyperventilated to a "normal" $PaCO_2$ of 40 torr, serious deleterious effects can occur. Patients with a chronically elevated $PaCO_2$ will have a higher amount of carbon dioxide and bicarbonate in the CSF, but the ratio will be maintained in a chronic situation. In this case, the patient will be breathing at a higher *set point*. That is, instead of being maintained at 40 torr, the normal $PaCO_2$ for this patient might be maintained at 46 torr, and near-normal sensitivity to changes in the $PaCO_2$ would be present. If this patient were aggressively ventilated in the PACU with the goal of lowering his $PaCO_2$ to 40

torr, significant negative repercussions could occur. With a lower $PaCO_2$ the CO_2 in the CSF will diffuse out and the bicarbonate will remain, owing to its inability to diffuse out of the CSF. Thus, an excess of bicarbonate as compared with CO_2 ($\uparrow$ bicarbonate pool) will exist in the CSF causing the primary stimulus to ventilation to *cease*. Since the patient was hyperventilated, the $PaCO_2$ will fall and the alveolar PO_2 will rise (because of the 12–10 concept; see pg. 44). Therefore, the secondary (hypoxic) drive may also become extinguished so that this patient will have no effective drive for ventilation. If chronic hypercapnic patients are acutely hyperventilated, they must be monitored for apnea once the accelerated ventilation is discontinued. It would be more appropriate to maintain the $PaCO_2$ at the level that is normal for that patient to avoid an apneic situation,. Thus, for the patient with chronic carbon dioxide retention who is emerging from anesthesia, an overaggressive stir-up regimen (hyperventilation) should be avoided. The patient should perform the sustained maximal inspiration at normal intervals, and his or her arterial blood gases should be closely monitored.

In some patients with chronic carbon dioxide retention (chronic hypercapnia), the sensitivity to hydrogen ions via the carbon dioxide may be effectively decreased to the point at which the primary stimulus to ventilation becomes the low arterial partial pressure of oxygen at the carotid and aortic bodies. The low PaO_2 becomes an effective stimulus to ventilation, especially when the $PaCO_2$ is elevated. The high arterial carbon dioxide level will augment the response to the low PaO_2 by the peripheral chemoreceptors. For this reason, the patient is breathing via his or her hypoxic drive. Since the carotid bodies are the major peripheral chemoreceptors, patients using the hypoxic drive may also experience bradycardia and hypotension. For that reason, patients with abnormally high preoperative $PaCO_2$ values who have bradycardia and hypotension should be suspected of using the hypoxic drive as their primary drive to ventilation. In the post anesthesia care unit, patients suspected of primarily using this drive should be monitored closely and given oxygen to attain adequate oxygen content (a hemoglobin saturation of between 80 and 90 percent). The primary goal is to keep the patient oxygenated without extinguishing his or her main control of ventilation. Low-flow oxygen techniques using 1 to 2 liters per minute, or high-flow techniques using a mask that works on the Venturi principle to ensure precise FiO_2's (i.e., 24 to 28 percent) can be utilized with these patients.

The Response to Carbon Dixoide. Carbon dioxide is the primary stimulus to ventilation. The carbon dioxide response test is used to assess the ventilatory response to carbon dioxide. In this test, the subject inhales carbon dioxide mixtures (with the PaO_2 held constant) so that the inspired PCO_2 gradually rises. Normally, the minute ventilation increases linearly as the PCO_2 rises (Fig. 4–21). Some disease states and drugs cause the CO_2 response curve to shift to the left or the right. If the curve shifts to the left, the subject is more responsive to CO_2. Such factors as thyroid toxicosis, aggressive personality, salicylates, and ketosis will shift the curve to the left. A decreased ventilatory response to carbon dioxide occurs when the curve is shifted to the right. This is called a *blunted response.* Patients who have a blunted response to carbon dioxide require intense PACU nursing care. The ventilatory response to an increased concentration of inspired carbon dioxide is blunted by *hypothyroidism, mental depression,* *aging, general anesthetics, barbiturates,* and *narcotics.* Many patients in the PACU either have these conditions or have received these drugs intraoperatively. This blunted response to carbon dioxide is one of the main justifications for giving supplemental oxygen to all patients emerging from anesthesia in the PACU. It is also the rationale behind the need for critical PACU nursing care that includes frequent assessment and interventions such as the stir-up regimen to prevent respiratory depression.

Upper Airways Receptors. There are receptors that are sensitive to mechanical stimulation and chemical agents. Located in the nose, these receptors have afferent pathways via the trigeminal and olfactory nerves. Activation of these receptors can cause apnea, bradycardia, and, most commonly, a sneeze. The implications for the PACU nurse are related to the procedure of nasotracheal intubation. If a patient is to be intubated nasally, the PACU nurse should monitor for bradycardia and apnea and be prepared for necessary interventions. Drugs that may be required are atropine or glycopyrrolate (Robinul) for their vagolytic effect and succinylcholine to facilitate the intubation. Finally, a means of providing positive pressure ventilation (bag-valve-mask setup) should be immediately available in case apnea should occur.

Receptors located in the epipharynx are sensitive to mechanical stimulation. Their activation is associated with the *sniff* or *aspiration reflex.* Mechanical stimulation of these receptors will cause a deep inspiration, bronchodilation, and hypertension. This is a protective reflex allowing material in the epipharynx to be brought down to the pharynx, clearing the nasal airways. In the larynx are irritant receptors that respond both to mechanical and to chemical stimulation. Afferent pathways from these receptors travel along the internal branch of the superior laryngeal nerve. Stimulation of them invokes any of a number of responses, such as coughing, slow deep breathing, apnea, bronchoconstriction, and hypertension. In addition, the trachea possesses irritant receptors. Stimulation of these recep-

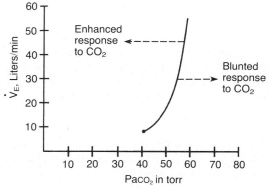

Figure 4–21. Carbon dioxide response curve (see text for details).

tors can cause responses such as coughing, bronchoconstriction, and hypertension. Again, during any procedure that involves the intubation of the trachea, the PACU nurse should be prepared to assess the appropriate cardiorespiratory parameters and implement nursing care as required.

Lung Receptors. *Pulmonary stretch receptors (PSR)* lie within the smooth muscle of the small airways. These receptors are activated by marked distention or deflation (atelectasis) of the lungs. Upon marked inflation of the lungs, the activation of the PSR will lead to a slowing of inspiratory frequency owing to an increase in expiratory time. Bronchodilation and tachycardia also may result from activation of these receptors. The PSRs are thought to be part of the *Hering-Breuer reflex*. The low threshold for the PSR is present for approximately the first three months of life; after that the threshold is high throughout adulthood. Hence, for the adult, the Hering-Breuer reflex is not important in the control of ventilation except in the anesthetized state. When an adult is under general anesthesia and ventilated with prolonged maximal lung inflations, a prolonged expiratory time can result owing to activation of the PSR.

Of great interest in regard to the pathogenesis of asthma are the *irritant receptors* that lie between the airway epithelial cells. These receptors respond to chemical irritants, such as histamine, and mechanical irritants, such as small particles and aerosols that irritate the pulmonary epithelium. The irritant receptors are mediated by vagal afferent fibers, and, upon receptor stimulation, bronchoconstriction and hyperpnea occur. It is suggested that the pathogenesis of asthma revolves around the sequence of histamine release, which stimulates the irritant receptors, which ultimately leads to bronchoconstriction mediated via the vagus nerve.

The *J receptors*, or *juxtapulmonary capillary receptors*, are located in the wall of the pulmonary capillaries. Like the irritant receptors, J receptors' afferent impulses are transmitted to the CNS by the vagus nerve. Normal stimuli of the J receptors include pneumonia, pulmonary congestion, and increased interstitial fluid pressure. Stimulation of these receptors by interstitial or pulmonary edema will result in tachypnea, bradycardia, and hypotension. Therefore, when assessing patients who are at risk for developing pulmonary edema, the nurse should always evaluate the rate of ventilation. Knowing that interstitial edema usually precedes pulmonary edema, and that increased interstitial congestion will stimulate the J receptors, the nurse should consider a rapid, shallow breathing pattern to be a danger signal and report it to the attending physician.

Located in the walls of the large systemic arteries, especially in the aortic and carotid sinuses, are *stretch receptors* called *baroreceptors*. These receptors help to control the systemic blood pressure. They also affect ventilation. When the systemic blood pressure increases, a reflex hypoventilation will occur owing to stimulation of the baroreceptors. On the other hand, a low systemic blood pressure will cause the baroreceptors to produce a reflex hyperventilation. Hence, if a patient in the PACU experiences a significant amount of hyper- or hypotension, a reflex ventilatory response will usually occur owing to the stimulation of the baroreceptors in the large systemic arteries.

The Controllers

The controllers of breathing are located in the central nervous system. They are composed of two functionally and anatomically separate components. Voluntary breathing is controlled in the cortex of the brain. Automatic breathing is controlled by structures within the brainstem. The spinal cord functions to integrate the output of the brainstem and cortex. The cortex can override the other controllers of breathing if voluntary control is desired. Examples of voluntary control include voluntary hyperventilation and breath-holding.

The Brainstem. Located bilaterally in the upper pons is the *pneumotaxic center (PNC)*. This center functions to fine-tune the respiratory pattern by modulating the activity of the apneustic center and regulating the respiratory system's response to such stimuli as hypercarbia, hypoxia, and lung inflation. Near the pontomedullary border lies the *apneustic center (APC)*. This center is probably the site of the inspiratory cutoff switch that terminates inspiration. In fact, apneusis, which consists of prolonged inspirations with occasional expirations, results when the apneustic center has been deactivated. Consequently, the apneustic center is also a fine-tuner of the rhythm of breathing.

Located in the medullary center, above the spinal cord, are two groups of neurons—the *dorsal respiratory group (DRG)* and the *ventral respiratory group (VRG)*. The dorsal respiratory group is composed of inspiratory neurons and is the initial intracranial processing site for many reflexes affecting breathing. It is probably the site of origin of the rhythmic respiratory drive. The DRG sends motor fibers via the phrenic nerve to the diaphragm. It sends inspiratory fibers to the ventral respiratory group (VRG), which is also part of the medullary center. However, the ventral respiratory group does not send fibers to the dorsal respiratory group; therefore, the reciprocal inhibition theory of the regulation of breathing seems unlikely. The ventral respiratory group is made up of both inspiratory and expiratory cells. The VRG neurons are driven by the cells of the DRG and, therefore, respiratory rhythmicity and the processing of sensory inputs do not occur initially within the VRG. The major function of the ventral respiratory group is to project impulses to distant sites and drive either spinal respiratory motor neurons (primary intercostal and abdominal) or the auxiliary muscles of breathing innervated by the vagus nerve.

The dorsal respiratory group (DRG) receives information from almost all the chemoreceptors, the baroreceptors, and the other sensors in the lung. In turn, the DRG generates a breathing rhythm that is fine-tuned by the APC (inspiratory cutoff switch) and the PNC. The inspiratory motor impulses are sent to the diaphragm and to the VRG. The VRG then drives spinal respiratory neurons (innervating the intercostal and abdominal muscles) or the auxiliary muscles of respiration innervated by the vagus nerve. Again, the cerebral cortex can override these centers if voluntary control of breathing is desired. Also, it should be stated that the vagus nerve has a profound effect on many aspects of the control of breathing. That is because the afferent pathways of the vagus nerve from the stretch, J, and irritant receptors serve to modulate the rhythm of breathing. Thus, any dysfunction that includes transection of the vagi will result in irregular breathing patterns, depending on the level of dysfunction (pons or medulla).

POSTOPERATIVE LUNG VOLUMES

Postoperative pulmonary complications are the greatest single cause of morbidity and mortality in the postoperative period. The reported incidence of postoperative pulmonary complications ranges from 4.5 to 76 percent.

Patients with Abnormal Pulmonary Function

When patients undergo anesthesia and surgery, certain risk factors predispose them to develop postoperative pulmonary complications. Patients at the highest risk are those with preexisting pulmonary problems with abnormal pulmonary function before surgery. The other major risk factors associated with postoperative pulmonary complications are chronic cigarette smoking, obesity, and advanced age.

Preexisting Pulmonary Disease. Patients with pre-existing pulmonary disease can have clinical or subclinical manifestations of their disease state. Consequently, preoperative pulmonary function tests are valuable in assessing the presence or absence of pulmonary pathophysiology as well as in determining operative risk. Obstructive lung disease, the most common category of lung disease, can be assessed by flow-volume measurements. Burrows suggests that a maximum voluntary ventilation (MVV) that is less than 50 percent of what is predicted, a maximum expiratory flow rate (MEFR) below 220 L/min, or a forced expiratory volume in one second (FEV$_1$) below 1.5 liters, indicates increased operative risk for pulmonary complications. These flow-volume measurements are valuable predictors of the patient's ability to generate an adequate cough, which is a pulmonary defense mechanism rendered ineffective in the immediate postoperative period by anesthesia and surgery. Consequently, these patients require vigorous, informed nursing care in the immediate postoperative period. Priorities of nursing care should include the frequent utilization of the stir-up regimen of turn, cascade cough, and sustained maximal inspiration, along with the use of appropriate nursing interventions designed to enhance secretion clearance, which will ensure airway patency.

Patients with restrictive lung disease represent a significant risk for postoperative pulmonary complications when their pulmonary function test reveals vital capacity (VC) or a diffusion capacity (D$_L$) of less than 50 percent of predicted values, or exercise arterial blood gases that demonstrate slight hypoxemia on exertion. In the PACU, these patients require a vigorous stir-up regimen with attention to tissue oxygenation via monitoring for hypoxemia. This is needed because during the surgical experience and in the post anesthesia care unit, physiologic stress can occur. One of the major products of physiologic stress is an increase in cardiovascular parameters. This will reduce the transit time of the red blood cells across the respiratory gas exchange membrane. Because of the pathologic changes in the respiratory membrane, patients with restrictive lung disease can desaturate upon exertion, such as in the stress reaction (see p. 41).

Chronic Cigarette Smoking. Chronic cigarette smoking has been shown to increase the incidence of postoperative pulmonary complications. Morton suggests that patients smoking only ten cigarettes a day have a sixfold increase in pulmonary morbidity in the postoperative period. The incidence of pulmonary embolism is higher in the smoker because of increased coagulability produced by chronic cigarette smoking. The ciliated epithelium of the lungs will be damaged by chronic cigarette smoking. This damage can cause some blockage of the mucociliary transport system, which will finally result in bronchiolar obstruction, infection, and atelectasis. Patients who smoke should be encouraged to stop smoking for *at least two weeks* before surgery. Two weeks of no smoking will allow the mucocillary transport system to return to a nearly normal level of function. The focus of nursing care for the active chronic cigarette smoker should be similar to the interventions discussed for the patient with obstructive lung disease.

Obesity. The markedly overweight patient has a very significant chance of developing postoperative pulmonary complications. This is due to the altered lung volumes and capacities caused by the excess adipose tissue. More specifically, the expansion of the lungs is hindered by an enlarged abdomen, which elevates the diaphragm, and by the weight on the chest wall, which hinders the outward recoil of the chest wall. This leads to a decreased thoracic wall and lung compliance and a reduced functional residual capacity (FRC). Finally, these complications result in hypoxemia from increased airway closure and $\dot{V}_A/\dot{Q}_C$ abnormalities (see Chapter 36). The focus of nursing interventions in the post anesthesia care unit is on preventing further airway closure. Thus, a vigorous stir-up regimen, including early ambulation, should help to prevent further reduction in the FRC. That will reduce the amount of airway closure, alleviate the hypoxemia, and ultimately improve the outcome of the patient.

Advanced Age. In patients of advanced age (>65 years old), there may be a slightly higher risk of developing postoperative pulmonary complications. A greater decrease in the functional residual capacity (FRC) following surgery in patients of advanced age has been demonstrated. Since the closing volume increases with age, significant airway closure can occur during tidal ventilation postoperatively. Although advanced age does not carry the same degree of risk as the factors previously discussed, it certainly can increase the danger of the other risk factors. However, patients of advanced age should receive a vigrous stir-up regimen in the post anesthesia care unit if only because of the alterations in their lung mechanics.

Patients with Normal Pulmonary Function

Because of the change in the mechanical properties of the lungs and chest wall, patients emerging from anesthesia will experience a decrease in their lung volumes and capacities (Fig. 4–22). This is especially true of the patient who has undergone a thoracic or upper abdominal surgical procedure. In the PACU, a further reduction in lung volumes and capacities may be seen. The major factor contributing to this reduction in lung volumes in the postoperative patient is a shallow, monotonous, *sighless* breathing

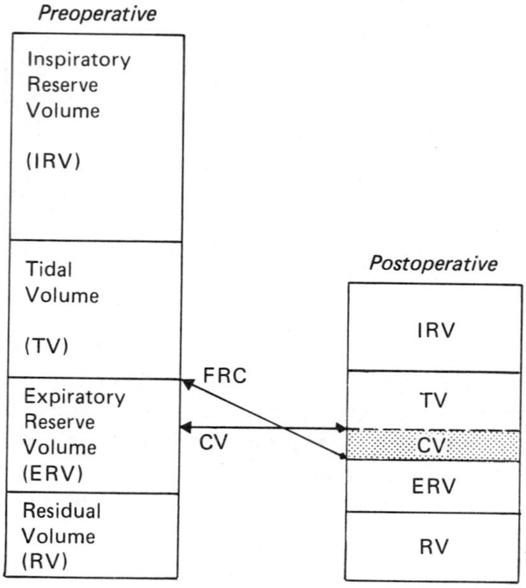

Figure 4–22. Graphic comparison of preoperative lung volumes to the probable lung volumes in the immediate postoperative period in a patient who has undergone an upper abdominal surgical procedure. (From Drain, C.: Postanesthesia Lung Volumes in Surgical Patients. AANA J, 49[3]:261–268, 1981, p. 263.)

pattern that is caused by general inhalational anesthesia, pain, and narcotics. Sighless ventilation may result in an uneven distribution of surfactant and a loss of stability of the small airways and alveoli, which can then lead to alveolar collapse and, ultimately, to atelectasis. Normally, adults breathe regularly and rhythmically, spontaneously performing a maximal inspiration that is held for about three seconds at the peak of inspiration. This physiologic process or sustained maximal inspiration is commonly referred to as a *sigh* or a *yawn*.

In normal lungs, the closing volume (CV) is less than the resting lung volume (i.e., FRC) and airways remain open during tidal breathing. In the immediate postoperative period, patients who have a sighless, monotonous, low tidal volume ventilatory pattern usually have a reduced FRC. When the FRC plus tidal volume is within the closing volume range, the airways leading to dependent lung zones may be effectively closed throughout tidal breathing (Fig. 4–22). Inspired gas is then distributed mainly to the upper or nondependent lung zones. Perfusion continues to follow the normal gradient, with higher flows to the dependent areas of the lung.

In the immediate postoperative period, as airway closure occurs, gas is trapped behind closed airways. This sequestered air can become absorbed and the alveoli will then become airless (atelectasis). The atelectasis, as it becomes more widespread, will lead to a decrease in ventilation as compared with perfusion (low $\dot{V}_A/\dot{Q}_C$), which results in a widening of the alveolar-oxygen gradient, and, ultimately, to hypoxemia. It should also be stated that atelectatic areas in the lung do provide an excellent culture medium in which pneumonia can develop.

Various investigators have demonstrated a decrease in lung volumes in the postoperative period. As can be seen in Figure 4–23, patients who have undergone an upper abdominal surgical procedure experience an immediate fall in the FRC from hour one to hour two postoperatively. The FRC then seems to return to near the baseline value by about the fourth postoperative hour. A second subsequent fall of the FRC is then

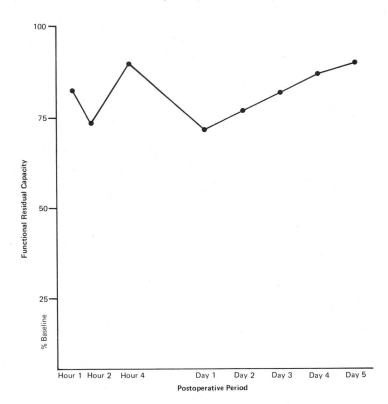

Figure 4–23. Composite curve of the mean values of the functional residual capacity (FRC) in the postoperative period. (From Drain, C.: Postanesthesia Lung Volumes in Surgical Patients AANA J, 49[3]:261–268, 1981, p. 264.)

seer after hour four, and baseline values are not restored until five days postoperatively. A possible explanation of the "peaks and valleys" of the FRC in the postoperative period may be that the first reduction in the FRC is associated with anesthesia and the latter reduction may be due to pain. General inhalational anesthesia and pain can dampen the physiologic sigh mechanism. Consequently, all patients who have undergone a surgical procedure, especially those who have their incision sites near the thorax or diaphragm, should be strongly encouraged to perform the SMI maneuver both in the PACU and on the surgical unit. The incentive spirometer can be used by the patient on the surgical unit; it is a device that is designed to encourage the patient by the use of positive feedback, to perform the SMI maneuver.

OXYGEN ADMINISTRATION IN THE POST ANESTHESIA CARE UNIT

The administration of oxygen to the patient in the post anesthesia care unit is an important facet in the emergence phase from anesthesia. Oxygen is given to the PACU patient primarily because he has a blunted or depressed response to carbon dioxide and low lung volumes. It is especially important that the patient who has received a general or spinal anesthetic be given supplemental oxygen during the recovery phase from anesthesia. The methods of oxygen administration are summarized in Chapter 18 (see Fig. 18–1).

PACU Nursing Care

A patent airway must be maintained throughout the administration of oxygen. The patient should be encouraged to cascade cough, perform the sustained maximal inspiration (SMI), and change positions according to the stir-up regimen discussed in this chapter and in Chapter 18. If a nasal catheter is utilized, the catheter should be removed every six hours to be cleaned and reinserted into the other nostril. Also, the nasal mucosa should be inspected periodically for dryness when a nasal catheter or prongs are used. Oxygen given in the dry gas form can cause drying and irritation of the mucosa, impair the ciliary action, and thicken secretions; therefore, oxygen should always be administered in the humidified form.

It is imperative for the PACU nurse to receive a report from the anesthesiologist or anesthetist or both as to the patient's preoperative pulmonary status. It is especially important to ascertain if the patient has a history of chronically retaining carbon dioxide, as occurs in chronic obstructive pulmonary disease. As described in this chapter, the patient with carbon dioxide retention who is receiving oxygen in the PACU should be monitored most carefully for any signs of hypoventilation, confusion, or becoming semicomatose. If any of these signs appear, the surgeon and anethesiologist or anesthetist should be notified immediately.

Oxygen Toxicity

When excessive concentrations of inspired oxygen (more than 60 percent) are administered to patients over prolonged periods of time, damage can be done to the eyes, lungs, and central nervous system.

The Eyes. Premature infants who receive high concentrations of oxygen for more than 24 hours are at risk for developing *retrolental fibroplasia*, caused by vasoconstriction of the blood vessels of the retina as a result of high oxygen concentrations in the blood. It presents in an acute form as a vascular retinopathy occurring at the developing edge of blood vessels in the premature infant's eye. This is followed by perivascular exudation, tissue hyperplasia, and scar tissue that exerts traction on the retina leading to retinal detachment and destruction of the infant's vision. Research indicates that the incidence of acute retrolental fibroplasia (RLF) is inversely proportional to birthweight. Because no quantitative data exist on the risk of RLF in tiny, sick, premature infants who are exposed to low to moderate concentrations (25 to 50 percent) of oxygen for a short duration, the PACU nurse should use her best informed judgment when caring for these infants. As with the adult, the infant who needs a high inspired oxygen concentration to provide adequate oxygenation should not be denied oxygen because of fear of complication.

The Lungs. Concentrations of oxygen over 60 percent will damage the lungs within three to four days. A 100 percent oxygen concentration administered for 24 to 48 hours also will cause pulmonary damage, the signs of which are manifested by Type II cell dysfunction in the lung. The Type II cells secrete surfactant, and the lack of surfactant in the alveoli will lead to alveolar collapse. The hyperoxic environment will also stop the ciliary action in the lungs. The early symptoms of this disorder include cough, nasal congestion, sore throat, reduced vital capacity (VC), tracheobronchitis, and substernal discomfort. The early signs of airway irritation may appear when a patient has received 80 to 100 percent oxygen continuously for eight hours or longer. The lung appears to tolerate oxygen concentrations lower than 40 percent indefinitely.

The Central Nervous System. When a PACU patient begins to show signs of oxygen toxicity, he may complain first of headache. If the oxygen toxicity continues, the patient will demonstrate some confusion. If a patient is receiving a high concentration of oxygen and has these signs and symptoms, the attending physician should be notified. Although convulsions usually are not seen in the post anesthesia care unit, they may occur when oxygen is given in conditions of above-normal atmospheric pressure, such as in hyperbaric oxygen chambers.

REFERENCES

1. Berger, A., Mitchell, R., and Severinghaus, J.: Regulation of respiration. N. Engl. J. Med., *297*:92;138;194, 1977.
2. Burrows, B., Knudson, R., Quan, S., and Kette, L.: Respiratory Disorders: A Pathophysiologic Approach. 2nd ed. Chicago, Year Book Medical Publishers, Inc., 1983.
3. Drain, C., and Vaughan, R.: Anesthetic considerations of morbid obesity. AANA J. 47:556–565, 1979.

4. Drain, C.: Postanesthesia lung volumes in surgical patients. AANA J, *49*:261–268, 1981.

5. Drain, C.: The anesthetic management of the patient: A broad view of the anesthetic consideration necessary regarding the respiratory system. AANA J, *50*:192–201, 1982.

6. Drain, C.: Managing postoperative pain . . . it's a matter of sighs. Nursing *14*(8):52–55, 1984.

7. Drain, C.: Comparison of two inspiratory maneuvers on increasing lung volumes in postoperative upper abdominal surgical patients. AANA J, *52*:379–388, 1984.

8. Flynn, J.: Oxygen and retrolental fibroplasia: Update and challenge. Anesthesiology, *60*(5):397–399, 1984.

9. Ganong, W.: Review of Medical Physiology. 12th ed. Los Altos, Lange Medical Publications, 1985.

10. Guyton, A.: Textbook of Medical Physiology. 7th ed. Philadelphia, W.B. Saunders Co., 1986.

11. Guenter, C., and Welch, M.: Pulmonary Medicine. Philadelphia, J. B. Lippincott Co., 1977.

12. Harper, R.: A Guide to Respiratory Care: Physiology and Clinical Applications. Philadelphia, J. B. Lippincott Co., 1981.

13. Hinshaw, H., and Murray, J.: Diseases of the Chest, 4th ed. Philadelphia, W. B. Saunders Co., 1980.

14. Keyes, J.: Blood-gases and blood-gas transport. Heart Lung, *3*(6):945–954, 1974.

15. Levitzky, M.: Pulmonary Physiology. 2nd ed. New York, McGraw-Hill, Inc. 1986.

16. Murray, J.: The Normal Lung. 2nd ed. Philadelphia, W. B. Saunders Co., 1986.

17. Shapiro, B.: Clinical Applications of Blood Gases. 3rd ed. Chicago, Year Book Medical Publishers, 1982.

18. Traver, G. (ed.): Respiratory Nursing: The Science and the Art. New York, John Wiley & Sons, 1982.

19. Wylie, W., and Churchill-Davidson, H.: A Practice of Anaesthesia. 4th ed. Philadelphia, W. B. Saunders Co., 1978.

5

Cardiovascular Anatomy and Physiology

Many drugs utilized for anesthesia depend on the cardiovascular system to produce their effects. Many of the same drugs also have effects upon the cardiovascular system. It is therefore imperative for the PACU nurse to understand the physiologic principles relating to the cardiovascular status of the patient who has received an anesthetic.

The basic anatomy of certain structures of the cardiovascular system will not be covered completely in this chapter, as basic nursing texts provide ample material on this subject.

Definitions

Adrenergic: a term describing nerve fibers that liberate norepinephrine.

Afterload: the impedance to left ventricular ejection. The afterload is expressed by total peripheral resistance (TPR).

Angina pectoris: chest pain caused by myocardial ischemia.

Arrhythmia: abnormal rhythm of the heart.

Arteriosclerosis: degenerative changes in the arterial walls resulting in thickening and loss of elasticity.

Bathmotropic: affecting the response of cardiac muscle (or any tissue) to stimuli.

Bigeminy: a premature beat along with a normal heart beat.

Bradycardia: a heart rate of 60 beats per minute or less.

Cardiac index: a "corrected" cardiac output used to compare that of patients with different body sizes. The cardiac index (CI) equals the cardiac output (CO) divided by the body surface area (BSA).

Cardiac output: the amount of blood pumped to the peripheral circulation per minute.

Cholinergic: a term describing nerve fibers that liberate acetylcholine.

Chronotropic: affecting the rate of the heart.

Cor pulmonale: pulmonary hypertension due to obstruction of the pulmonary circulation, causing right ventricular hypertrophy.

Cyanosis: bluish discoloration, seen especially on the skin and mucous membranes, due to a reduced amount of oxygen in the hemoglobin.

Diastole: period of relaxation of the heart, especially of the ventricles.

Dromotropic: affecting the conductivity of a nerve fiber, especially the cardiac nerve fibers.

Electrolyte: ionic substance found in the blood.

Embolism: a blood clot or other substance such as lipoid material in the bloodstream.

Fibrillation: ineffectual quiver of the atrium or ventricles.

Flutter: usually atrial, a condition in which the atria contract at a rate of 200 to 400 beats per minute.

Hypertension: persistently elevated blood pressure.

Hypervolemia: an abnormally large amount of blood in the circulatory system.

Infarction: a necrotic area due to an obstruction of a vessel.

Inotropic: affecting the force of contraction of muscle fibers, especially those of the heart.

Ischemia: local tissue anemia due to decreased blood flow.

Murmur: abnormal heart sound heard during systole, diastole, or both.

Myocardium: the muscular middle layer of the heart between the inner endocardium and the outer epicardium.

Normotensive: having a normal blood pressure.

Occlusion: obstruction of a blood vessel by a clot or foreign substance.

Pacemaker: the area in which cardiac rate commences, normally at the sinoatrial node.

Palpitation: abnormal rate, rhythm, or fluttering of the heart experienced by the patient.

Paroxysmal tachycardia: a period of fast heart beats that begins and ends abruptly.

Pericarditis: inflammation of the pericardium.

Peripheral resistance: resistance by the microcirculation.

Polycythemia: excessive amount of red blood cells, which is reflected in an abnormally high hematocrit.

Preload: the left ventricular end-diastolic volume (LVEDV).

Pulse deficit: the difference between the apical and radial pulses.

Syncope: fainting, giddiness, and momentary unconsciousness, usually due to cerebral anoxia.

Systole: period of contraction of the heart, especially the ventricles.

Thrombosis: formation of a clot (thrombus) inside a blood vessel or a chamber of the heart.

THE HEART

The Cardiac Cycle

The *heart* is a four-chambered mass of muscle that pulsates rhythmically, pumping blood into the circulatory system. The chambers of the heart are the atria and the ventricles. The atria, which are pathways for blood into the ventricles, are thin walled, have myocardial muscle, and are divided into the right and left atria by a partition down the middle. During each cardiac cycle, approximately 70 percent of the blood flows from the great veins through the atria and into the ventricles before the atria contract. The other 30 percent is pumped into the ventricles upon contraction of the atria. Upon contraction of the right atrium, the pressure in the heart will be 4 to 6 mm Hg. The contraction of the left atrium will produce a pressure of 7 to 8 mm Hg.

Three pressure elevations are produced by the atria, as depicted on the atrial pressure curve. They are termed the a, c, and v waves (Fig. 5–1). The *a wave* is a result of atrial contraction. The *c wave* is produced by both the bulging of atrial ventricular valves and the pulling of the atrial muscle when the ventricles contract. The *v wave* occurs near the end of ventricular contraction as the amount of blood in the atria slowly increases and the atrioventricular valves close.

The ventricles receive blood from the atria and then act as pumps to move blood through the circulatory system. During the first third of diastole, the atrioventricular valves open and blood rushes into the ventricles. This is referred to as the period of *rapid filling* of the ventricles. The middle third of diastole is referred to as *diastasis*, during which a small amount of blood moves into the ventricles. It is during the latter third of diastole that the atria contract and the other 30 percent of the ventricles fills. As the ventricles contract, the atrioventricular valves contract and then close, thereby preventing blood from flowing into the ventricles from the atria.

As the ventricles begin to contract during systole, the pressure inside the ventricles

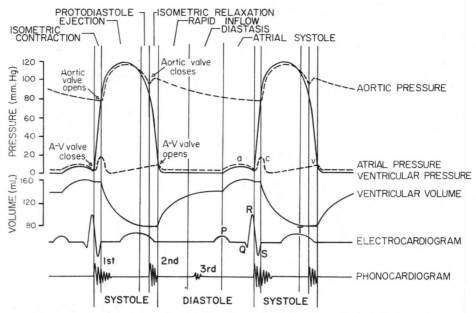

Figure 5–1. The events of the cardiac cycle, showing changes in left atrial pressure, left ventricular pressure, aortic pressure, ventricular volume, the electrocardiogram, and the phonocardiogram. (From Guyton, A. C.: Textbook of Medical Physiology. 5th ed. Philadelphia, W. B. Saunders Co., 1976, p. 164.)

increases, but no emptying of the ventricles occurs. During this time, referred to as the period of *isometric contraction*, the atrioventricular valves are closed. As the right ventricular pressure rises above 8 mm Hg and the left ventricular pressure exceeds 80 mm Hg, valves open to allow the blood to leave the ventricles. This period, termed the *period of ejection*, consumes the first three quarters of systole. The remaining fourth quarter is referred to as *protodiastole*, when almost no blood leaves the ventricles, yet the ventricular muscle remains contracted. The ventricles then relax, and the pressure in the large arteries pushes blood back toward the ventricles, which forces the aortic and pulmonary valves to close. This is the period of *isometric relaxation.*

At the end of diastole each ventricle usually contains approximately 120 ml of blood. This is the *end-diastolic volume*. During systole, each ventricle will eject 70 ml of blood, which is the *stroke volume*. The blood that remains in the ventricle at the end of systole is *end-systolic volume* and amounts to approximately 50 ml.

Cardiac Output

Cardiac output is the amount of blood ejected from the left or right ventricle in one minute. In the normal adult with a heart rate of 70, cardiac output is approximately 4900 ml. This estimate can be derived by taking the rate of 70 times the stroke volume of 70 ml. Because of "user friendly" sophisticated equipment, a patient's cardiac output can now be monitored in the PACU. The information derived from serial measurements of the cardiac output can be most helpful in the assessment of the general status of the cardiovascular system as well as in the determination of the appropriate amount and type of fluid therapy for the patient.

The cardiac output can be measured by a variety of techniques. Kaplan suggests that the thermodilution method, employing the Swan-Ganz catheter, is the clinical method of choice. To facilitate a higher degree of reproducibility, Kaplan suggests a technique of standardization in which the injectate temperature and volume, as well as the speed of injection, should be carefully controlled and duplicated. The most reproducible results have been obtained using injections of 10 ml of cold (1° to 2° C) 5 percent dextrose in water. It should be remembered that the thermal dilution technique measures right-sided cardiac outputs. Hence, patients with intracardiac shunts will usually have unreliable measurements of their cardiac output when the thermodilution technique is utilized.

Other methods of calculating the cardiac output are the Fick and Stewart techniques. The *Fick technique* involves calculations of the amount of blood required to carry oxygen taken up from the alveoli per unit time. This technique is said to be accurate within ±10 percent. In the *Stewart technique*, a known quantity of dye is injected and its concentration measured after the dye is dispersed per unit time.

Cardiac output can be influenced by *venous return*. As the *Frank-Starling law* of the heart states, "The heart pumps all the blood that it receives so that damming of the blood does not occur." If the heart receives an extra amount of blood from the veins (↑ preload), the cardiac muscle becomes stretched, and the stretched muscle will contract with an increased force to pump the extra blood out of the heart. If the heart receives less blood than normal (↓ preload), according to the Frank-Starling law of the heart, it will contract with less force. This concept is important to the PACU nurse. For example, if a patient is receiving mechanical ventilation and his lungs are being overinflated by too much positive end-expiratory pressure (PEEP), the venous return to the heart will be impeded by the increased pressure on the inferior vena cava and this will cause a decrease in the blood pressure. The blood pressure is derived from the following interacting factors: force of the heart, peripheral resistance, volume of blood, viscosity of blood, and the elasticity of the arteries. Thus, it can be seen that cardiac output plays a major role in the maintenance of a normal blood pressure.

Arterial Blood Pressure

The *arterial blood pressure* is composed of the systolic and diastolic arterial pressures.

The *systolic blood pressure* is the highest pressure that occurs within an artery during each contraction of the heart. The *diastolic blood pressure* is the lowest pressure that occurs within an artery during each contraction of the heart. The *mean arterial pressure* is the average pressure that pushes blood through the systemic circulatory system.

Some factors that affect the arterial blood pressure are the vasomotor center, renal system, vascular resistance, endocrine system, and chemical regulation. The *vasomotor center*, located in the pons and medulla, has the greatest control over the circulation. This center picks up impulses from all over the body and transmits them down the spinal cord and through vasoconstrictor fibers to most vessels of the body. These impulses may be excitatory or inhibitory. One type of pressoreceptor that sends impulses to the vasomotor center is the *baroreceptors*. They are located in the walls of the major thoracic and neck arteries, in particular the arch of the aorta. When these vessels are stretched by an increased blood pressure, they will send inhibitory impulses to the vasomotor center, which will result in a lowering of the blood pressure. The aortic and carotid bodies located in the bifurcation of the carotid arteries and along the aortic arch, when stimulated by a low PaO_2, can increase systemic pressure.

The renal regulation of arterial pressure occurs through the renin-angiotensin-aldosterone mechanism (discussed in Chapter 6).

The *vascular resistance* of the systemic vascular system can alter systemic pressure. As the total cross-sectional area of an artery decreases, the systemic vascular resistance increases. Therefore, as the blood flows out of the aorta, a decrease in the arterial pressure in each portion of the systemic circulation is directly proportional to the amount of vascular resistance. This is why the arterial pressure in the aorta is much higher than the pressure in the arterioles, which have a low cross-sectional area.

The nervous system, when stimulated by exercise or stress, will elevate the arterial pressure via sympathetic vasoconstrictor fibers throughout the body.

When the radial artery is to be cannulated for direct monitoring of blood pressure and the sampling of arterial blood gases, an *Allen test* should be performed in the PACU. This test is utilized to assess the risk of hand ischemia if occlusion of the cannulated vessel should occur. The Allen test is performed by having the patient make a tight fist, which will partially exsanguinate the hand. The nurse then occludes both the radial and the ulnar arteries with digital pressure. The patient is asked to open his hand and the compressed radial artery is then released. Blushing of the palm (post-ischemic hyperemia) should be observed. After about a minute the test should be repeated on the same hand with the nurse now releasing the ulnar artery while continuing to compress the radial artery. If the release of pressure over the ulnar artery does not lead to postischemic hyperemia, the contralateral artery should be similarly evaluated. The results of the Allen test should be reported as "refill time" for each artery.

The Valves of the Heart

The *semilunar valves* are the aortic and pulmonary valves. They consist of three symmetric valve cusps, which can open to the full diameter of the ring, yet provide a perfect seal when closed. During diastole, they prevent backflow from the aorta and pulmonary arteries into the ventricles.

The *atrioventricular valves* are the tricuspid and mitral valves. These valves prevent blood from flowing back into the atria from the ventricles during systole.

Attached to the valves are the *chordae tendineae*, which are attached to the papillary muscles, which in turn are attached to the endocardium of the ventricles. When the ventricles contract, so do the papillary muscles, pulling the valves toward the ventricles to prevent the bulging of the valves into the atria (Fig. 5–2).

The Heart Muscle

The heart muscle is composed of three major muscle types: atrial muscle, ventric-

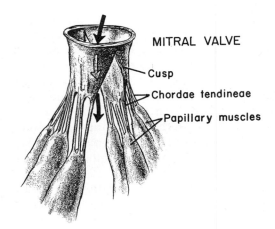

Figure 5–2. The mitral valve. (From Guyton, A. C.: Textbook of Medical Physiology. 5th ed. Philadelphia, W. B. Saunders Co., 1976, p. 166.)

ular muscle, and excitatory and conductive muscle fibers. The atrial and ventricular muscles act much like skeletal muscles. The excitatory and conductive muscles function primarily as an excitatory system for the heart and a transmission system for conduction of impulses throughout the heart.

The cardiac muscle fibers are arranged in a latticework; they divide and then rejoin. The constriction of the cardiac muscle fibers facilitates action potential transmission. The muscle is striated, and the myofibrils contain *myosin* and *actin filaments*. Cardiac muscle cells are separated by *intercalated discs*, which are actually the cardiac cell membranes and serve to separate the cardiac muscle cells from one another (Fig. 5–3). The intercalated discs do not hinder con-

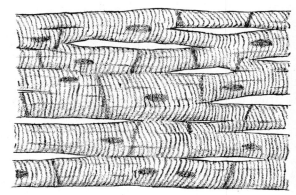

Figure 5–3. The "syncytial" nature of cardiac muscle. (From Guyton, A. C.: Textbook of Medical Physiology. 5th ed. Philadelphia, W. B. Saunders Co., 1976, p. 160.)

ductivity or ion transport between cardiac muscle cells to any great extent. When the cardiac muscle is stimulated, the action potential spreads to excite all the muscles. This is referred to as a *functional syncytium*. It can be divided into *atrial* and *ventricular syncytia*, which are separated by fibrous tissue. However, an impulse can be transmitted throughout the atrial syncytium and then via the *atrioventricular bundle* to the ventricular syncytium. The "all-or-nothing" principle is in effect: When one atrial muscle fiber is stimulated, all the atrial muscle fibers will react if the action potential is met. This applies to the entire ventricular syncytium as well.

The main properties of cardiac muscle are excitability (bathmotropism), contractility (inotropism), rhythmicity and rate (chronotropism), and conductivity (dromotropism.)

When cardiac muscle is excited, its action potential is reached and the muscle will contract. Certain chemical factors will alter the excitability and contractibility of cardiac muscle (Table 5–1).

Conduction of Impulses

Not only does the heart have a special system for generating the rhythmical impulses, but this system is able to conduct these impulses throughout the heart. This system for providing rhythmicity and conductivity consists of the sinoatrial node, the atrioventricular node, the atrioventricular bundle, and the Purkinje fibers (Fig. 5–4). The *sinoatrial (S-A) node* is situated at the posterior wall of the right atrium and just below the opening of the superior vena cava. The S-A node generates impulses by

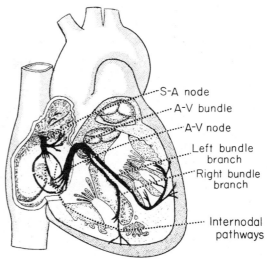

Figure 5–4. The S-A node and the Purkinje system of the heart. (From Guyton, A. C.: Textbook of Medical Physiology. 5th ed. Philadelphia, W. B. Saunders Co., 1976, p. 177.)

self-excitation, which is produced by the interaction of sodium and potassium ions. The S-A node provides a rhythmic excitation approximately 72 times per minute in the adult at rest. The action potential then spreads throughout the atria to the atrioventricular node.

The *atrioventricular (A-V) node* is located at the base of the wall between the atria. Its primary function is to delay the transmission of the impulses to the ventricles. This allows time for the atria to empty before the ventricles contract. The impulses then travel through the *A-V bundle*, sometimes referred to as the *bundle of His*. The A-V node is able to discharge impulses at a rate of 40 to 60 times per minute if not stimulated by an outside source.

The *Purkinje fibers* originate at the A-V node, form the A-V bundle, divide into the right and left bundle branches, and spread downward around the ventricles. The Purkinje fibers can transmit the action potential very rapidly, thus allowing immediate transmission of the cardiac impulse throughout the ventricles. The Purkinje fibers are able to discharge impulses at a rate between 15 and 40 times per minute if not stimulated by an outside source.

The parasympathetic nerve endings are distributed mostly at the S-A and A-V

TABLE 5–1. Chemical Factors That Affect Excitability and Contractility

Causing Increase
High pH
Alkalosis
High calcium concentration

Causing Decrease
High potassium concentration
High lactic acid concentration
Acidosis

nodes, over the atria, and, to a lesser extent, over the ventricles. If stimulated, they produce a decrease in the rate of rhythm of the S-A node and slow the excitability at the A-V node. The sympathetic nerves are distributed at the S-A and A-V nodes and all over the heart, especially the ventricles. Sympathetic stimulation will step up the S-A node rate of discharge, increase cardiac excitability, and increase the force of contraction.

The Coronary Circulation

The coronary arteries furnish the heart with its blood supply. The main coronary arteries are on the surface of the heart, but smaller arteries penetrate the heart muscle to provide it with nutrients. The inner surface of the heart derives its nutrition directly from the blood in its chambers.

The coronary arteries originate at two orifices just above the aortic valve. The right coronary descends by the right atrium and ventricle and usually terminates as the posterior descending coronary artery. The left coronary is usually about 1 cm in length and divides into the anterior descending and the circumflex arteries. The anterior descending artery usually terminates at the apex of the heart, anastomosing with the posterior descending artery. The anterior descending artery supplies part of the left ventricle, the apex of the heart, and most of the interventricular septum.

The left circumflex artery descends posteriorly and inferiorly down to and terminating in the left marginal artery or communicating with the posterior descending coronary artery. The venous drainage is by superficial and deep circuits. The superficial veins empty into either the coronary sinus or the anterior cardiac veins, both of which drain into the right atrium. The deep veins drain into the thebesian or sinusoidal channels.

The regulation of coronary blood flow is determined primarily by the oxygen tension of the cardiac tissues. The most powerful vasodilator of the coronary circulation is hypoxemia. Other factors that may affect coronary blood flow are carbon dioxide, lactate, pyruvate, and potassium, all of which are released from the cardiac muscle.

Stimulation of the parasympathetic nervous system will cause an indirect decrease in coronary blood flow. Direct stimulation is slight, owing to the sparse amount of parasympathetic nerve fibers to the coronary arteries. The sympathetic nervous system serves to increase coronary blood flow, both directly (as a result of the action of acetylcholine and norepinephrine) and indirectly (caused by a change in the activity level of the heart). The coronary arteries have both alpha and beta receptors in their walls (see Adrenergic and Cholinergic Receptors).

Because so much cardiac disease involves the coronary arteries, the anesthetic risk increases in patients with cardiac disease. A functional classification of cardiac patients is based on their ability to perform physical activities (Table 5–2).

Class III and Class IV patients represent a significant risk for surgery and anesthesia and should be completely monitored when they receive care in the PACU.

Myocardial Infarction

Acute myocardial infarctions are frequently encountered medical emergencies that can occur in the PACU. The objectives

TABLE 5–2. Functional Classification of Cardiac Patients

Class I:	No limitation. Ordinary physical activity does not cause undue fatigue, dyspnea, palpitation, or angina.
Class II:	Slight limitation of physical activity. Such patients will be comfortable at rest. Ordinary physical activity will result in fatigue, palpitation, dyspnea, or angina.
Class III:	Marked limitation of physical activity. Less than ordinary activity will lead to symptoms. Patients are comfortable at rest.
Class IV:	Inability to carry on any physical activity without discomfort. Symptoms of congestive failure or angina will be present even at rest. With any physical activity, increased discomfort is experienced.

From Perloff, J. K.: The clinical manifestations of cardiac failure in adults. Hosp. Pract., 5:43, 1970.

in the management of a patient with an acute myocardial infarction are to relieve pain, control complications, salvage ischemic myocardium, and return the patient to a productive life. The diagnosis of a myocardial infarction is made on clinical grounds, and therapy should be instituted immediately when it is suspected. (Cardiopulmonary resuscitation is discussed in Chapter 44.) An electrocardiogram performed in the PACU may reveal an injury pattern, but a normal electrocardiogram certainly does not exclude a diagnosis of a myocardial infarction.

Physical assessment of a patient with a suspected myocardial infarction may include the following subjective findings: (1) pain or pressure, which is usually substernal but may be manifested in the neck, shoulder, jaws, arms, or other areas; (2) nausea; (3) vomiting; (4) diaphoresis; (5) dyspnea; and (6) syncope. The onset of pain may occur with activity but may also occur at rest. The duration may be prolonged from 30 minutes to several hours. Objective findings may include hypotension, pallor, and anxiety. It must be remembered that the blood pressure, pulse, and heart sounds may be entirely normal in the patient who is suffering from an acute myocardial infarction. Upon auscultation of the chest, the abnormal cardiac findings may include atrial gallop, ventricular gallop, paradoxical second heart sound (S$_2$), friction rub, and abnormal precordial pulsations.

The electrocardiogram pattern may vary according to the location and extent of the infarction, but myocardial damage may occur without changes in the electrocardiogram. Some typical features of a transmural infarction are acute ST-segment elevation in leads reflecting the area of injury, abnormal Q waves, and T-wave inversion.

The laboratory data usually will reflect an elevated sedimentation rate and an elevated white blood count. The enzymes SGOT, LDH, and CPK may be elevated. Results of enzymatic studies in the patient with acute myocardial infarction do not indicate a specific cause, since other conditions and disease states may affect these enzymes. LDH and CPK isoenzyme studies may be necessary to differentiate the various disease abnormalities. Intramuscular injections may significantly elevate the level of CPK and therefore should be avoided.

Research has demonstrated that patients who have had a myocardial infarction (MI) within six months before surgery will have a recurrence rate of 54.5 percent for an MI that could occur during or after the surgical procedure. From six months to two years the rate of recurrence of infarction is between 20 and 25 percent, and between the second and third year the incidence of reinfarction is about 5 percent. Most studies indicate that after three years from the original myocardial infarction, the recurrence rate is about 1 percent, which equals the normal rate of MI for the general population. Hence, the chance of a patient's having an MI in the post anesthesia care unit can be considered significant. This is especially true for PACU patients who have had an MI within the last three years, or who have a documented MI risk factor such as angina, hypertension, or diabetes, or for those with some combination of the above.

PACU Nursing Care

The PACU nurse should be constantly alert for such things as anxiety, arrhythmias, shock, left ventricular failure, pulmonary embolism, and systemic embolism. Pain and apprehension may be relieved by morphine sulfate or meperidine hydrochloride (Demerol). Oxygen should be administered by nasal prongs, as a face mask may increase the patient's apprehension. Continuous cardiac monitoring should be instituted, and the patient should be kept in a quiet area. Drugs such as atropine, lidocaine, digitalis, quinidine, sodium nitroprusside, phentolamine, and nitroglycerin should be available. A machine for countershock should be immediately available. Fluid therapy and urine output should be monitored completely to prevent fluid overload. A Swan-Ganz catheter or central venous pressure monitor may be utilized to determine fluid replacement in patients with reduced intravascular volume and hypotension (see discussion of CVP and Swan-Ganz catheters below). There is no such thing as a benign infarction. All patients with a diagnosed myocardial infarction require constant, competent nursing care.

THE CIRCULATORY SYSTEM

The Red Blood Cell. The normal red blood cell is in the form of a biconcave disc, which can change its shape to move through the microcirculation. The major function of the red blood cell is the transport of oxygen to the tissue cells; it is also an important factor in carbon dioxide transport. The red blood cell is responsible for approximately 70 percent of the buffering power of whole blood in maintaining acid-base balance.

Red blood cells are produced by the bone marrow. The normal rate of production is sufficient to form about 1250 ml of new blood per month. This is also the normal rate of destruction. The average life span of a red blood cell is 120 days. The *hematocrit* is the percentage of red blood cells in the blood. The average is 47 ± 7 in men and 42 ± 5 in women. The normal amount of *hemoglobin* in the red blood cell is 16 grams of hemoglobin per dl of whole blood in men and 14 grams of hemoglobin per dl of whole blood in women.

The Blood Vessels. The circulatory system can be divided into the *systemic* and *pulmonary circulation*. The systemic or peripheral circulation is made up of arteries, arterioles, capillaries, venules, and veins.

The walls of the blood vessels, except the capillaries, are composed of three distinct coats: tunica adventitia, tunica media, and tunica intima. The outer layer, the tunica adventitia, consists of white fibrous connective tissue, which gives strength to and limits the distensibility of the vessel. The vasa vasorum, which supplies nourishment to the larger vessels, is in this layer. The middle layer, the tunica media, consists of mostly circularly arranged smooth muscle fibers and yellow elastic fibers. The innermost layer, the tunica intima, is a fine transparent lining that serves to reduce re-sistance to the flow of blood. The valves of the veins are formed by the foldings of this layer. The capillaries consist of a single layer of squamous epithelial cells, which is a continuation of the tunica intima.

The arteries are characterized by elasticity and extensibility. The veins have a poorly developed tunica media and, therefore, are much less muscular and elastic than arteries.

The Microcirculation. Microcirculation is the flow of blood in the finer vessels of the body. It involves the arterioles, capillaries, and venules. The arteries subdivide to the last segment of the arterial system, the arteriole. The *arteriole* consists of a single layer of smooth muscle in the shape of a tube to conduct blood to the capillaries. As the arterioles approach the capillaries, they lack the coating of smooth muscle and are termed *metarterioles*. At the point at which the capillaries originate from the metarterioles, a smooth muscle fiber, the *precapillary sphincter*, encircles the capillary. At the other end of the capillary is the *venule*, which is larger but has a much weaker muscular coat than the arteriole.

The capillaries are usually no more than 8 microns in diameter, which is barely large enough for corpuscles to pass through in single file. Blood moves through the capillaries in intermittent flow, caused by the contraction and relaxation of the smooth muscle of the metarterioles and precapillary sphincter. This motion is termed *vasomotion*. The metarterioles and precapillary sphincter open and close in response to oxygen concentration in the tissues—a form of local autoregulation.

The microcirculation serves three major functions: (1) transcapillary exchange of nutrients and fluids; (2) maintenance of blood pressure and volume flow; and (3) return of blood to the heart and regulation of active blood volume.

ADRENERGIC AND CHOLINERGIC RECEPTORS

The cardiovascular system and the concept of adrenergic and cholinergic receptors are closely related. It is very important for the PACU nurse to have an understanding of the pharmacodynamics of these receptors.

Functional Anatomy: The Mediators

Cholinergic is a term used to describe the nerve endings that liberate acetylcholine. The cholinergic neurotransmitter, acetylcholine, is present at all preganglionic parasympathetic fibers, all preganglionic sympathetic fibers, all postganglionic parasympathetic fibers, and all somatic motor neurons. Two exceptions to the general rule are postganglionic sympathetic fibers to the sweat glands and to the vasculature of skeletal muscle. These are considered sympathetic anatomically but cholinergic in terms of their neurotransmitter; that is, they release acetylcholine as their neurotransmitter.

The term *adrenergic* is used to describe nerves that release norepinephrine as their neurotransmitter. Epinephrine may be present in the adrenergic fibers in very small quantities, usually representing less than 5 percent of the total amount of both epinephrine and norepinephrine. The adrenergic fibers are the postganglionic sympathetic fibers, with the exception of the postganglionic sympathetic fibers to the sweat glands and to the efferent fibers to the skeletal muscle (Table 5–3).

The adrenal medulla should be considered separately, in that it is innervated by a preganglionic sympathetic fiber liberating the neurotransmitter acetylcholine; yet the postganglionic portion is the adrenal medulla, and behaves much like a postganglionic sympathetic fiber. The adrenal medulla is therefore stimulated by acetylcholine, which causes the release of both epinephrine and norepinephrine from its chromaffin cells. As opposed to the usual finding of a preponderance of norepinephrine at the postganglionic nerve fiber terminals, the distribution in the adrenal medulla is 80 percent epinephrine and 20 percent norepinephrine. Therefore, the neurotransmitter of the adrenal medulla is epinephrine.

Cholinergic Neurotransmitter: Biochemistry

The neurotransmitter acetylcholine is synthesized from choline and acetate through the enzymatic activity of choline acetylase to form acetylcholine (Table 5–4), and it is then stored in vesicles. When the acetylcholine is released from a preganglionic fiber it may then act on the membrane of the preganglionic fiber with a positive feedback mechanism, causing enhanced release of acetylcholine. The calcium ion facilitates this additional release of acetylcholine. This process is referred to as *excitation-secretion coupling* through calcium.

Adrenergic Neurotransmitter: Biochemistry

The adrenergic neurotransmitter, epinephrine, begins in the body as phenylalanine. This is hydroxylated to tyrosine, which is again hydroxylated to form dopa, an amino acid. This process is probably the weakest step in the biosynthetic chain and may be a possible site of action of an autonomic drug. A soluble enzyme, L-dopa decarboxylase, acts on dopa to form dopamine, which, in turn, is synthesized to norepinephrine. In the adrenal medulla, norepinephrine may be methylated in the cell to form the final product, epinephrine. This reaction is catalyzed by the enzyme phenylethanolamine - N - methyltransferase (Table 5–4).

TABLE 5–3. Cholinergic Nerves and Adrenergic Nerves

Mediator: Acetylcholine—Cholinergic Nerves
Effects:
All preganglionic parasympathetic fibers
All preganglionic sympathetic fibers
All postganglionic parasympathetic fibers
All somatic motor neurons
Postganglionic sympathetic fibers to sweat glands
Postganglionic sympathetic vasodilator fibers
  innervating skeletal muscle vasculature

Mediator: Nonepinephrine—Adrenergic Nerves
Effects:
All postganglionic sympathetic fibers

From Drain, C. B.: Current concepts on the pharmacodynamics of adrenergic and cholinergic receptors. J. Amer. Assoc. Nurse Anesthetists, 44:272–280, 1976.

TABLE 5–4. Synthesis of Neurotransmitters

Cholinergic

Choline + Acetate $\xrightarrow{\text{Choline acetylase}}$ Acetylcholine

Adrenergic

Phenylalanine $\longrightarrow$ Tyrosine $\xrightarrow{\text{tyrosine hydroxylase}}$ L-dopa

$\xrightarrow{\text{L-dopa decarboxylase}}$ Dopamine $\xrightarrow{\text{dopamine beta oxidase}}$

Norepinephrine $\xrightarrow{\text{Phenylethanolamine-N-methyltransferase}}$ Epinephrine

From Drain, C. B.: Current concepts on the pharmacodynamics of adrenergic and cholinergic receptors. J. Amer. Assoc. Nurse Anesthetists, 44:272–280, 1976.

The storage of norepinephrine in the adrenergic nerves appears to be in the intracellular granules. It is difficult to deplete the total content of norepinephrine through continued nerve stimulation, but through continuous chronic drug administration, a clinical hypotensive state may occur owing to the decreased sympathetic vasomotor tone.

The mechanism of release of norepinephrine from the adrenergic fibers and epinephrine from the adrenal medulla appears to be that of reverse pinocytosis. (Pinocytosis is a mechanism by which the membrane engulfs substances of the extracellular fluid.) Under the influence of the appropriate stimuli an opening is created through which the soluble contents of a portion of the storage granules are released.

The major means of inactivation of norepinephrine is through a mechanism known as uptake, in which the released neurotransmitter is recaptured into the neuronal system by the neuron that released it or neurons adjacent to it and in some cases by neurons associated with tissues some distance from the original site of release.

The norepinephrine not recaptured is metabolized eventually to vanillylmandelic acid. Epinephrine also goes through a number of steps in its biodegradation to vanillylmandelic acid. An increase in vanillylmandelic acid concentration in the urine is useful in the diagnosis of such conditions as pheochromocytoma and neuroblastoma (Fig. 5–5).

When a patient is receiving a drug that is a monoamine oxidase inhibitor such as isocarboxazid, phenelzine sulfate, or tranyl-cypromine, a buildup of epinephrine or norepinephrine can occur, leading to sympathetic hyperactivity. This is especially likely to occur when substances or drugs such as tyramine or indirect-acting vasopressors such as ephedrine are administered.

The Cholinergic Receptors

The pharmacologic and physiologic action of acetylcholine is apparently mediated by its combination with specific receptors, each of which serves as a drug recognition site. When a drug or neurotransmitter has an affinity for a specific receptor and this leads to a response, the neurotransmitter or drug is said to have *intrinsic* activity. A drug capable of eliciting a response is an *agonist*. Drugs that have affinity but no intrinsic activity at a specific receptor are called *antagonists*. However, if a drug occupies the receptor and the activity of the receptor is reduced, it is a *receptor-blocking agent*.

The actions of acetylcholine and drugs that mimic acetylcholine are mediated through two types of receptors: *nicotinic receptors* and *muscarinic receptors*.

When one stimulates the nicotinic receptors the following responses are observed:

1. Stimulation of autonomic ganglia—both parasympathetic and sympathetic.

2. Stimulation of the adrenal medulla, resulting in the release of both epinephrine and norepinephrine.

3. Stimulation of skeletal muscle at the motor end-plate.

The muscarinic responses elicited by muscarine as well as acetylcholine are:

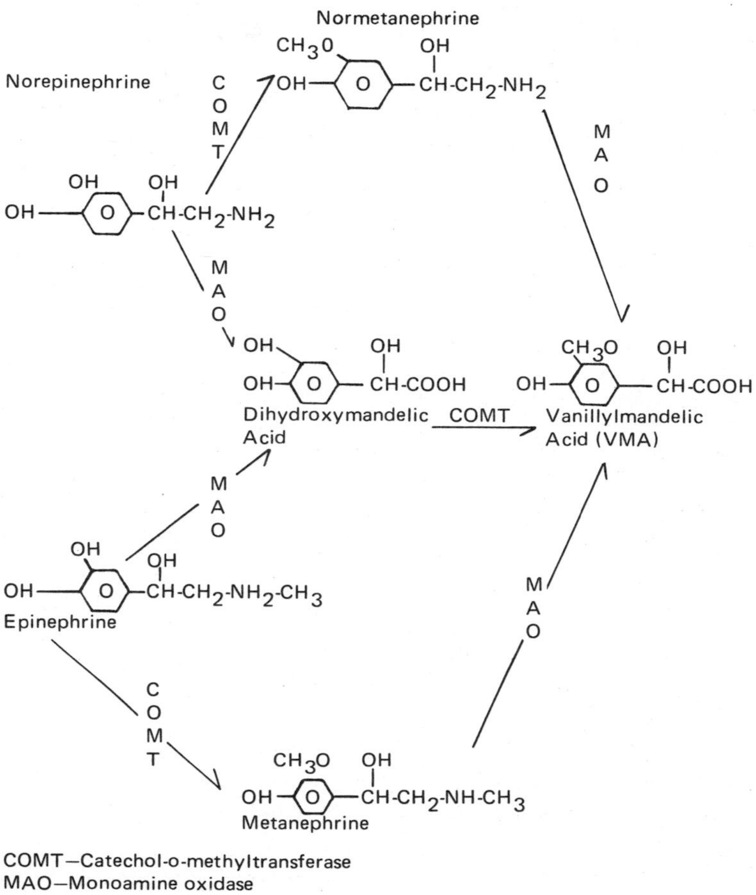

Figure 5–5. Metabolism of epinephrine and norepinephrine. (From Drain, C. B.: Current concepts on the pharmacodynamics of adrenergic and cholinergic receptors. J.A.A.N.A., 44[3]:272, 1976.)

COMT—Catechol-o-methyltransferase
MAO—Monoamine oxidase

1 Stimulation or inhibition of smooth muscle in various organs or tissues.

2 Stimulation of exocrine glands.

3 Slowing of cardiac conduction.

4 Decreased myocardial contractile force.

Nicotinic responses in terms of antagonism can be blocked by drugs such as ganglionic or neuromuscular blocking agents or both, whereas muscarinic responses are blocked by the class of drugs best typified by atropine.

Muscarine is a specific agonist at muscarinic receptors, while nicotine is a specific agonist at nicotinic receptors; however, acetylcholine is capable of stimulating both receptor types (Table 5–5).

There is a series of compounds specific in their ability to combine with acetylcholinesterase and inhibit its activity through competitive inhibition. The prototype compounds in this category would be neostigmine, physostigmine, pyridostigmine, and edrophonium.

Belladonna alkaloids such as atropine can and do have adverse effects that are peculiar to the PACU phase of the surgical experience. More specifically, belladonna alkaloids that cross the blood-brain barrier can cause disorientation, violent behavior, or somnolence. Physostigmine salicylate (Antilirium), an anticholinesterase that is capable of penetrating the blood-brain barrier, has been shown to be useful in the reversal of the adverse effects of belladonna alkaloids on the central nervous system. Physostigmine salicylate is also useful in reversing the disorientation or somnolence caused by such drugs as diazepam, phenothiazines, tricyclic antidepressants, antiparkinsonian drugs, promethazine, droperidol, and, in some cases, halothane. Pa-

TABLE 5–5. Cholinergic Receptors

Organ Stimulated by Cholinergic Agonist	Response	Type of Cholinergic Receptor Response
Heart		
S-A node	Negative chronotropic effect	Muscarinic
Atria	Decreased contractility and increased conduction velocity	Muscarinic
A-V node and conduction system	Decrease in conduction velocity—AV block	Muscarinic
Eye		
Sphincter muscle of the iris	Contraction (miosis)	Muscarinic
Lung		
Bronchial muscle	Contraction	Muscarinic
Bronchial glands	Stimulation	Muscarinic
Exocrine glands		
Salivary glands	Profuse, watery secretion	Muscarinic
Lacrimal glands	Secretion	Muscarinic
Nasopharyngeal glands	Secretion	Muscarinic
Adrenal medulla	Catecholamine secretion	Nicotinic
Autonomic ganglia	Ganglion stimulation	Nicotinic Muscarinic
Skeletal muscle		
Motor end-plate	Stimulation	Nicotinic (motor end-plate receptor)

From Drain, C. B.: Current concepts on the pharmacodynamics of adrenergic and cholinergic receptors. J. Amer. Assoc. Nurse Anesthetists, 44:272–280, 1976.

tients in the post anesthesia care unit who may benefit from treatment with physostigmine are those who have received a belladonna alkaloid or neuroleptic type of agent either preoperatively or intraoperatively, have demonstrated disorientation or restlessness or both for more than 30 minutes after anesthesia, and are difficult to arouse over an appropriate time period. Patients who demonstrate any one of these dysfunctions qualify for treatment and can be given 1 mg increments of physostigmine intravenously at 15 minute intervals, until they are conscious and oriented to time, place and person. Once treatment has begun, the PACU nurse should monitor the blood pressure and pulse immediately before and five minutes after the administration of physostigmine. Also, some patients may experience side effects from physostigmine, such as nausea, pallor, sweating and bradycardia. Because glycopyrrolate does not cross the blood-brain barrier, it is especially helpful in treating the side effects of physostigmine. Finally, patients who have been treated with physostigmine probably should remain in the post anesthesia care

unit for about an hour after the administration of the anticholinesterase.

In the skeletal muscle at the motor end-plate we can prevent the action of acetylcholine with neuromuscular blocking agents such as curare. Curare exerts its effects through competitive antagonism at the nicotinic receptor. Succinylcholine, on the other hand, causes a prolonged depolarization of the postsynaptic end-plate, which ultimately leads to skeletal muscle relaxation.

Adrenergic Receptors

The stimulation of the sympathetic nervous system can be both inhibitory and excitatory, which has caused considerable confusion. Originally there were theories postulated that this phenomenon dealt with the release of two different compounds. It was later discovered that the variation in the effects of stimulation was due not to the differences in chemical release but rather to a difference in the receptors' responses to the transmitter.

The adrenergic receptors, which respond to catecholamines, can be subdivided into three main types, the dopaminergic, alpha, and beta receptors. The *dopaminergic receptors* are primarily in the central nervous system and the mesenteric and renal blood vessels. The agonist for these receptors is dopamine. The *alpha receptors* can be further divided into alpha$_1$ (α_1) and alpha$_2$ (α_2) receptors. The postsynaptic alpha$_1$ receptors are excitatory in action, except in the intestine. The stimulation of the alpha$_1$ receptors causes smooth muscle contraction, which results in a vasoconstriction or pressor response. Hence, the alpha$_1$ receptor is activated by the release of norepinephrine, and this released norepinephrine also activates the presynaptic alpha$_2$ receptors to inhibit the further release of norepinephrine. Thus the α_1 receptor is activated by the release of norepinephrine, and the released norepinephrine in turn stimulates the α_2 receptor, producing inhibition of the release of norepinephrine, resulting in a negative feedback loop (Fig. 5–6).

It is believed that the drug clonidine (Catapres) stimulates the α_2 receptors, which lowers the sympathetic outflow of norepinephrine, which ultimately leads to a hypotensive effect. Besides lowering catecholamine levels, clonidine can reduce the plasma renin activity. This antihypertensive drug enjoys a significant degree of popularity, but it can have a negative impact upon the patient in the post anesthesia care unit. More specifically, the "clonidine withdrawal syndrome" has been reported when the drug has been abruptly stopped. The sequela of the syndrome resembles pheochromocytoma in that shortly after the withdrawal of the clonidine, the patient can experience hypertension, tachycardia, and increased blood levels of catecholamines. Treatment for this syndrome usually involves a reinstitution of the clonidine therapy and alpha-adrenergic blocking agents such as phentolamine.

Stimulation of the *beta receptor* causes vascular smooth muscle relaxation, which then leads to a decrease in blood pressure through a decrease in peripheral resistance. The beta receptor can be divided into two types: *beta$_1$* and *beta$_2$*. Beta$_1$-subtype receptors are found in all cardiac tissue except the coronary vasculature and are responsible for characteristic effects noted after stimulation of the heart by epinephrine: (1) increase in heart rate, (2) increase in contractile force, (3) increase in conduction velocity, and (4) shortening of the refractory period. Beta$_1$-subtype receptors mediate effects elicited by catecholamines.

The physiology of the beta receptor has many implications for the care of the PACU patient. Once the beta receptor has been activated by "first messengers," which are endogenous catecholamines or exogenous beta agonists such as isoproterenol, certain biochemical events occur (Fig. 5–7). The enzyme adenylate cyclase which is located on the plasma membrane is stimulated by beta-receptor activation. Then within the cell, adenosine triphosphate (ATP) is broken down to 3',5'-adenosine monophosphate (cyclic AMP). The cyclic AMP is then released into the cytoplasm of the cell and acts to modulate cellular activities. Hence, the cyclic AMP is considered to be the "second messenger." Cyclic AMP is inactivated to 5-AMP by the enzyme phosphodiesterase.

Clinically, isoproterenol or terbutaline may be administered to raise the cyclic AMP levels in the β_2 receptors in the bronchial

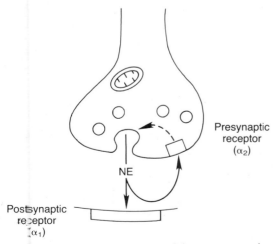

Figure 5–6. Pre- and postsynaptic alpha receptors at the ending of a noradrenergic neuron. (Adapted from Ganong, W. F.: Review of Medical Physiology. 12th ed. Palo Alto, Lange Medical Publications, 1985, p. 76.)

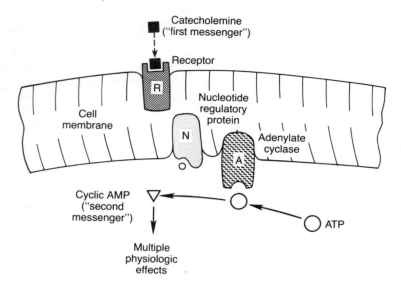

Figure 5–7. Catecholamine ("first messenger") binds to the beta receptor protein, which activates the enzyme adenylate cyclase via the nucleotide regulatory protein, which binds GMP. Via adenylate cyclase, ATP is broken down to cylic AMP. The cyclic AMP or "second messenger" then activates protein kinase, which ultimately produces a variety of physiologic effects. (Adapted from Catt, K., et al.: Regulation of peptide hormone receptors and gonadal steroidogenesis. Recent Prog. Horm. Res. 36:557, 1980.)

airways with the intended result of bronchodilatation. Another way to raise the cyclic AMP levels is to inhibit the action of phosphodiesterase. Caffeine and the methylxanthines such as aminophylline are inhibitors of the enzyme phosphodiesterase, and can be used alone or in combination (for synergistic effects) with the beta agonists to produce the desired bronchodilation in the patient. It should be remembered that other catecholamine effects are produced by the rise in cyclic AMP. Consequently, even though aminophylline is considered a bronchodilator, it does increase myocardial contractility and heart rate of the patient, thus mandating the PACU nurse to monitor both respiratory and cardiac function when methylxanthines are administered.

The coronary arteries contain α_1 and β_1 receptors and, therefore, also have the ability to vasoconstrict and vasodilate (Table 5–6). The endogenous catecholamines, norepinephrine and epinephrine, are capable of stimulating both the alpha and the beta receptors.

Site of Action of Autonomic Drugs

Methyldopa (Aldomet), which is the alpha-methylated analogue of L-dopa, is an antihypertensive drug. Methyldopa reduces

TABLE 5–6. Adrenergic Receptors

Response	Type of Adrenergic Receptor
Heart	
Positive inotropic effect	Beta$_1$
Positive chronotropic effect	Beta$_1$
Cardiac arrhythmias	Beta$_1$
Positive dromotropic effect	Beta$_1$
Vascular	
Arterial and arteriolar constriction	Alpha$_1$
Coronary dilatation	Beta$_2$
Arteriolar relaxation	Beta$_2$
GI Tract	
Intestinal relaxation	Alpha$_1$, Beta$_1$
Sphincter contraction (usually)	Alpha$_1$
Urinary Bladder	
Bladder relaxation (detrusor)	Beta$_2$
Bladder contraction (trigone and sphincter)	Alpha$_1$
Eye	
Contraction (mydriasis)	Alpha$_1$
Ciliary muscle of iris	Beta$_2$
Metabolic	
Liver glycogenolysis (hyperglycemia)	Alpha$_1$, Beta$_2$
Muscle glycogenolysis	Beta$_1$
Lipolysis	Beta$_1$
Oxygen consumption (increases)	Beta$_1$, Beta$_2$
Other Smooth Muscle	
Bronchial (relaxation)	Beta$_2$
Spleen (contraction)	Alpha$_1$
Ureter (contraction)	Alpha$_1$
Uterus (contraction)	Alpha$_1$
Uterus (relaxation)—non-pregnant condition	Beta$_2$

From Drain, C. B.: Current concepts on the pharmacodynamics of adrenergic and cholinergic receptors. J. Amer. Assoc. Nurse Anesthetists, 44:272–280, 1976.

the sympathetic nerve stimulation through the production of a selective agonist, α-methylnorepinephrine.

Guanethidine has the ability to prevent nerve stimulation, thus inhibiting norepinephrine release. Guanethidine interferes with the storage of norepinephrine and, if given chronically, will result in a decrease in the amount of norepinephrine stored in adrenergic nerves. Reserpine also shares this latter action with guanethidine. Thus, chronic use of guanethidine and reserpine will result in a relative depletion of the norepinephrine content from sympathetic nerves (Table 5–7).

· Recently, the *slow channel calcium blockers* have been found to have considerable value in the treatment of supraventricular tachycardias, angina pectoris, and myocardial infarction. The prototype slow channel calcium blockers are verapamil, nifedipine, and diltiazem. All three drugs depress calcium entry into conduction tissue and cardiac muscle, which results in a depression of conduction leading to a reduction of the circus movements. These calcium entry blockers produce hypotension by different mechanism: Nifedipine, like sodium nitroprusside, decreases the systemic vascular resistance with a compensatory tachycardia, and verapamil and diltiazem lower the cardiac output by exerting a negative dromotropic effect. The effects of the calcium channel blockers may be enhanced by inhalation anesthesia agents such as halothane. Consequently, in the post anesthesia care unit, patients who received an inhalational anesthetic and are being treated with a calcium channel blocker may experience some hypotension. Hence, the PACU nurse should vigorously monitor the cardiovascular parameters of these patients and report any confirmed hypotension to the attending physician.

Dopamine is a naturally occurring biochemical catecholamine precursor of norepinephrine. It exerts a positive inotropic effect and a minimal chronotropic effect on the heart. Therefore, the contractility of the heart is increased without changing the afterload (total peripheral resistance), which will lead to an increase in cardiac output. The increase is in the systolic and pulse pressure, with virtually no effect on the diastolic pressure. Dopamine is not associated with tachyarrhythmias and produces less of an increase in myocardial oxygen consumption than does isoproterenol. Blood flow to peripheral vascular beds may decrease while mesenteric flow increases. One of the major reasons for the increase in use of dopamine clinically is its dilatation of the renal vasculature. This action is secondary to the inotropic effect and decreased peripheral resistance. Therefore, the glomerular filtration rate is increased along with the renal blood flow and sodium excretion.

TABLE 5–7. Drugs That Interfere with Specific Steps in the Process of Chemical (Neurohumoral) Transmission

	Adrenergic Nerves	Cholinergic Nerves
Synthesis of the mediator	Methyldopa	Hemicholinium
Storage of the mediator	Reserpine	
Release of the mediator	Guanethidine	Botulinus toxin
Combination of the mediator with its receptor	Phenoxybenzamine (alpha receptor)	Atropine (muscarinic)
	Propranolol (beta receptors)	Nicotine (nicotinic)
Enzymatic destruction of the mediator	Pyrogallol (COMT inhibitor) Tranylcypromine (MAO inhibitor)	Physostigmine (cholinesterase-inhibitor)
Prevention of inactivation of the mediator (blocks the uptake)	Cocaine	—
Repolarization of the postsynaptic membrane (persistent depolarization)	—	Succinylcholine

From Drain, C. B.: Current concepts on the pharmacodynamics of adrenergic and cholinergic receptors. J. Amer. Assoc. Nurse Anesthetists, 44:272–280, 1976.

Hypotension Therapy

Hypotension in the immediate postoperative period is of great concern, and it deserves the prompt attention of the PACU nurse. When hypotension is detected in the postoperative patient, the nurse should first reaffirm the measurements. An improperly placed or improperly sized blood pressure cuff or malfunction of the stethoscope can yield incorrect measurements. If the hypotension is confirmed, hypovolemia should be considered as a possible cause. The clinical signs of hypotension due to hypovolemia include cold pale, clammy or diaphoretic skin; rapid, thready pulse; shallow, rapid respirations; disorientation, restlessness, or anxiety; and decreased central venous pressure and oliguria.

The nursing assessment of the hypotensive patient should include inspection of the dressings for excess bleeding and the evaluation of the clinical signs of hypovolemia. If the hypotension is 30 percent below preoperative baseline blood pressure readings, or one or more of the clinical signs of hypovolemia is present, the attending physician should be notified.

Usual therapy for hypotension in the PACU includes fluid infusion, reversal of residual anesthetic depressant effects, repositioning of the patient to facilitate venous return, and vasopressors or anticholinergics or both, such as glycopyrrolate (Robinul) or atropine, as indicated. It should be stated that the vasopressors exert their effect either directly or indirectly. The direct-acting vasopressor exerts its effect directly on the receptor. Conversely, the pharmacologic action of an indirect vasopressor facilitates the release of norepinephrine from its storage vesicles (primarily the terminal sympathetic nerve fibers) which stimulates the adrenergic receptor to achieve the desired effect. Therefore, a direct-acting vasopressor is probably necessary to achieve a response in patients who are depleted of catecholamines by such drugs as reserpine and guanethidine (Table 5–8).

Another area of consideration when selecting a vasopressor is the cardiotonic ac-

TABLE 5–8. Adrenergic Receptor Function

Stimulate	Inhibit
Beta₁	**Beta₂**
Heart—rate, contractility	Bronchial smooth
Respiratory center	muscle is relaxed
Glycogenolysis (muscle)	
Lipolysis	
Insulin release	Skeletal muscle
	vasomotion
	GI smooth muscle
	GU smooth muscle
Alpha₁	
Vascular smooth muscle (constriction):	
Skin	
Gut	
Kidney	
Liver	
Sphincters (constriction):	
GI	
GU	
Glycogenolysis (liver)	
(maybe beta)	

From Drain, C. B.: Current concepts on the pharmacodynamics of adrenergic and cholinergic receptors. J. Amer. Assoc. Nurse Anesthetists, 44:272–280, 1976.

tion desired. Metaraminol (Aramine), by its action of norepinephrine release, causes improved cardiac function as a result of its beta receptor activity. Conversely, phenylephrine (Neo-Synephrine) and methoxamine (Vasoxyl) possess little or no cardiac effect and exert a pressor action by pure alpha stimulation.

Hypertension Therapy

A hypertensive emergency may occur in the post anesthesia care unit. The patient may arrive in the PACU in a hypertensive state or may become hypertensive during the postoperative phase. If the diastolic blood pressure rises to about 120 to 140 mm Hg and the patient complains of headache and blurred vision and has papilledema along with disorientation, the physician should be notified immediately.

If the hypertension is due to acute anxiety with labile hypertension, the use of sedatives may dramatically reduce the blood pressure. If the patient has acute pulmonary edema caused by hypertensive heart disease, correction of the pulmonary edema usually brings the blood pressure down to acceptable limits.

If pharmacologic antihypertensive therapy is deemed necessary by the physician, the drugs listed in Table 5–9 will usually be instituted. Because these drugs are extremely potent and have their own complications, they will be discussed briefly.

Diazoxide (Hyperstat). This drug is avidly bound to and inactivated by serum proteins and thus must be given as a rapid (within 15 sec) intravenous (IV) bolus. Its action is immediate and is achieved through its direct vasodilating effects. Potential side effects are hypotension, hyperglycemia, sodium retention, and, occasionally, precipitation of congestive heart failure. It is usually advantageous to administer concurrently a loop-diuretic such as furosemide (40 to 80 mg IV), especially if the patient is edematous as a result of either cardiac or renal failure. Although the usual dose of diazoxide is 300 mg, in extremely large or small patients a dose of 5 mg per kg body weight may be given. A second dose may be given within 30 minutes if the first dose is not effective. With this second dose, the dose of concurrently administered diuretic is usually doubled. If the desired response is still not obtained, use of sodium nitroprusside should be considered. If diazoxide is effective, the drug is given at intervals of 4 to 24 hours, depending on the response. An oral medication should be started as soon as the blood pressure is lowered and stabilized. Blood glucose levels should be monitored and treated with tolbutamide if they become substantially increased. Nausea and vomiting may occur because of diazoxide's muscle-relaxing properties on the stomach. Withholding food for two hours before and after administration of diazoxide is advised.

Sodium Nitroprusside (Nipride). A compound of rather unusual chemical structure, this drug is immediately effective in all cases of severe hypertensive crises, including those resistant to diazoxide. Its action is thought to be due to the peripheral arteriolar dilatory effect of the drug. *Because of its ability to lower blood pressure rapidly, it requires careful intravenous administration with constant bedside arterial pressure monitoring.* The drug is extremely light-sensitive and must be administered through bottles and tubing that are wrapped and protected from the light. Only fresh solutions should be used, and those more than four hours old should be discarded because thiocyanates may be formed. Treatment is started with a solution of 500 ml of 5 percent dextrose in water and 50 mg of sodium nitroprusside using a microdrip regulator to ensure a precise flow rate. A dose of 1 to 3 μg per kg per min usually produces a prompt drop in blood pressure which will return to control levels within five minutes of stopping the drug. Because of its unique chemical structure, cyanide is released into the bloodstream when the drug is used. This is quickly converted to thiocyanate by the liver. Thiocyanate toxicity (fatigue, nausea, anorexia, muscle spasms, and disorientation) may result from prolonged use or high dosages; therefore, monitoring of serum thi-

TABLE 5–9. Drugs Used in Therapy of Hypertensive Crisis

Drug	Route	Initial Dose	Onset of Action	Duration of Action	Comment
Diazoxide (Hyperstat)	IV	300 mg or 5 mg/kg as a rapid bolus	Immediate	9 to 12 hours	
Sodium nitroprusside (Nipride)	IV	1 μg/kg	Immediate	< 5 minutes	Must titrate dose for desired effect
Phentolamine (Regitine)	IV	5–15 mg bolus 200–400 mg/liter infusion	Immediate	< 15 minutes	Must titrate dose for desired effect
Hydralazine (Apresoline)	IV or IM	10–20 mg or 100 mg/liter 10–50 mg	5–10 minutes 30 minutes	Approximately 12 hours	Given slowly when IV
Trimethaphan camsylate (Arfonad)	IV	0.5–2.0 mg/min	5–10 minutes	Effectiveness lost in 48 hours	

ocyanate levels is advised when the drug is used for more than 24 hours. Toxic symptoms appear with serum thiocyanate levels of 5 to 10 mg per dl and the compound can be rapidly removed by peritoneal dialysis. As with diazoxide, once blood pressure has been brought to control levels, concomitant use of oral medications such as guanethidine or methyldopa allows the gradual tapering and discontinuance of nitroprusside.

Phentolamine (Regitine). Phentolamine mesylate, an alpha-receptor blocker, is specifically indicated for managing hypertensive crises associated with increased circulating catecholamines. These may result from pheochromocytoma or the sudden release of tissue catecholamine stores caused by certain drugs or foods containing tyramine in patients receiving monoamine oxidase (MAO) inhibitors (pargyline derivatives, primarily Eutonyl). The antipressor effect of a single intravenous injection is short-lived, usually lasting less than 15 minutes. Therefore, it is desirable to administer phentolamine by intravenous infusion (200 to 400 gm per liter), titrating the dosage to achieve the desired pressure level, after the blood pressure has been controlled initially by a rapid IV dose of 5 to 15 mg. Since the drug blocks only alpha receptors, beta-mediated effects of the circulating catecholamine upon the heart must be controlled with the specific beta-blocker, propranolol hydrochloride.

With rare exception, these three drugs can be considered the mainstays of modern therapy in acute hypertensive crises. The others listed and discussed here should be considered second-line drugs. Their primary disadvantages include slower onset of action, rapid development of tachyphylaxis, and marked central nervous system depressant effects. In most instances, their use should be to supplement and initiate long-term control once the acute crisis is resolved by the primary drugs.

Hydralazine (Apresoline). Hydralazine is not effective in hypertensive encephalopathy complicating acute or chronic glomerulonephropathies; it is used in encephalopathy that has chronic essential hypertension

as an underlying cause. Reduction in blood pressure is accomplished through vasodilation, which reduces resistance of vessels. This results in a marked increase in cardiac output and heart rate that can aggravate underlying angina and cardiac failure. The determining factor in this situation is the net change in myocardial oxygen consumption achieved by lowering the elevated afterload. On the other hand, a decrease of blood pressure produced by hydralazine is not accompanied by a commensurate decrease in renal blood flow, so that it is especially suited for managing hypertensive emergencies associated with renal insufficiency. The initial parenteral dose of 20 to 40 mg may be repeated every 30 to 60 minutes until diastolic pressure is obtained or 100 mg has been given. Alternatively, one may increase the drug dose in 5 mg increments up to 20 mg. Maintenance dose depends on patient response but is generally 5 to 20 mg IV every four to six hours.

Trimethaphan Camsylate (Arfonad). This ganglionic vasodepressor blocks both sympathetic and parasympathetic systems at the autonomic ganglia. The effect is primarily orthostatic, so that large doses must be employed to reduce blood pressure in supine patients. The head of the bed should be elevated (reverse Trendelenburg), if possible, to augment the antipressor action. Complications of such ganglionic blockade include atony of the bowel and bladder and paralytic ileus, especially when used for more than 24 hours. Because of the commensurate fall in glomerular filtration rate when blood pressure is lowered by the use of this agent, it is not recommended for use in cases in which renal insufficiency complicates the hypertensive crisis. Its major disadvantage, however, is that it rapidly loses effectiveness after 24 to 72 hours and another agent must be substituted. Use of the drug requires extremely close monitoring by the PACU nurse.

Nitroglycerin. This potent vasodilator produces relaxation of both arterial and venous smooth muscle. The pharmacologic effects of nitroglycerin are mainly on the venous side of the circulation. It produces an increase in venous capacitance which leads to a reduction in venous return and a fall in right atrial and pulmonary capillary wedge pressures. Therefore, the main effect of nitroglycerin is to reduce the preload. Also, the myocardial oxygen demand is decreased owing to the fall in myocardial wall tension.

Intravenous nitroglycerin may be indicated in the treatment of myocardial ischemia, to control hypertension, to relieve angina pectoris, and to produce vasodilation for patients in severe congestive heart failure.

When intravenous nitroglycerin is administered in the PACU, an automated infusion pump should be utilized. The usual dosage is between 25 to 300 μg per minute. The patient should be continuously monitored for hypotension. Should hypotension occur, an alpha agonist such as methoxamine may be used to ensure that the patient's coronary perfusion pressure is maintained. It should also be stated that nitroglycerin does migrate into plastic. Hence, the PACU nurse should periodically change the plastic tubing on the automated infusion pump along with ensuring that only glass bottles are used for dilution.

REFERENCES

1. Alspach, J., and Williams, S.: AACN: Core Curriculum for Critical Care Nursing. 3rd ed. Philadelphia, W. B. Saunders Co., 1985.
2. Brown, B. (ed.): Contemporary Anesthesia Practice: Anesthesia and the Patient with Heart Disease. Philadelphia, F. A. Davis Co., 1980.
3. Cullen, D. J.: Recovery room management of the surgical patient. Cur. Rev. Recovery Room Nurses, 3(19):146–151, 1981.
4. Drain, C.: Current concepts on the pharmacodynamics of adrenergic and cholinergic receptors. J. Amer. Assoc. Nurse Anesthetists, 44:272–280, 1976.
5. Ganong, W.: Review of Medical Physiology. 12th ed. Los Altos, Lange Medical Publications, 1985.
6. Goodman, L. S., and Gilman, A.: The Pharmacological Basis of Therapeutics. 6th ed. New York, Macmillan Publishing Company, 1980.
7. Gordon, R., Ravin, M., and Daicoff, G.: Cardiovascular Physiology for Anesthesiologist. Springfield, Charles C Thomas, Publisher, 1979.
8. Gray, C., Nunn, J., and Letting, J.: General Anaesthesia. 4th ed. London, Butterworth & Co., Ltd., 1982.
9. Guyton, A. C.: Textbook of Medical Physiology. 7th ed. Philadelphia, W. B. Saunders Co., 1986.
10. Kaplan, J.: Cardiac Anesthesia: Cardiovascular Pharmacology, Vol. 2. New York, Grune & Stratton, Inc., 1983.
11. Messick, J.: Allen's test—neither positive nor negative. Anesthesiology, 54:523, 1981.
12. Miller, R.: Anesthesia. 2nd ed. New York, Churchill Livingstone Inc., 1986.
13. Orkin, L., and Cooperman, L.: Complications in Anesthesiology. Philadelphia, J. B. Lippincott Co., 1983.
14. Philbin, D.: Anesthetic management of the patient with cardiovascular disease. Int. Anesthesiol. Clin. 17(1):1–196, 1979.
15. Reves, J.: The relative hemodynamic effects of Ca++ entry blockers. Anesthesiology, 61:3–5, 1984.
16. Wood, M., and Wood, A. (eds.): Drugs and Anesthesia: Pharmacology for Anesthesiologists. Baltimore, Williams & Wilkins, 1982.

6

Renal Anatomy and Physiology

Most of the drugs used in anesthesia are excreted unchanged or as a metabolic by-product by the kidneys. Homeostasis is maintained by proper kidney function, since the kidneys regulate the balance of acid-base, electrolyte, and fluid volumes and remove waste materials and toxic substances from the body.

Kidney function is sometimes difficult to assess in the post anesthesia care unit (PACU), especially in the uncatheterized patient. In patients who do have urinary catheters in place after surgery, assessment of kidney function should be part of the PACU nursing care. It is important to understand renal anatomy and physiology so that total PACU nursing care can be rendered to the patient.

Definitions

Acetonuria: appearance of acetone in the urine. It is present when excessive fats are consumed or when an inadequate amount of carbohydrates is metabolized.

Albuminuria: presence of protein in the urine, also referred to as proteinuria. Albumin is the most common protein found in the urine. This condition is usually indicative of malfunction in glomerular filtration.

Azotemia: presence of nitrogenous products in the blood, usually due to decreased kidney function.

Cystitis: inflammation of the bladder.

Dysuria: painful or difficult urination.

Enuresis: involuntary discharge of urine.

Glycosuria: presence of glucose in the urine.

Hematuria: presence of blood in the urine.

Incontinence: inability to retain urine in the bladder.

Nephritis: inflammation of the kidney; called Bright's disease.

Nephrosis: degeneration of the kidney without the occurrence of inflammation.

Oliguria: decrease in the normal amount of urine formation.

Pyelitis: inflammation of the renal pelvis and calyces.

Retention: failure to expel urine from the bladder.

Stricture: abnormal narrowing of the ureter or urethra.

Uremia: toxic condition usually due to renal insufficiency and retention of nitrogenous substances in the blood.

ANATOMY OF THE KIDNEYS

The kidneys are two bean-shaped organs in the retroperitoneal spaces near the upper lumbar area. The right kidney is at a slightly lower level than the left. Each kidney weighs approximately 150 grams. The notched portion of the kidney is called the *hilum*, and it is here that the ureter, the renal vein, and the renal artery enter the kidney (Fig. 6–1).

The ureter opens into a large cavity called the *pelvis*. From the pelvis, two to five *major calyces* project deeper into the kidney. The major calyces branch out to form six to ten *minor calyces*. The ends of the minor calyces are capped by the *renal papillae*.

The *medulla* is the inner portion of the kidney. It is made up of several *pyramids*, which correspond to the number of minor calyces. The base of the pyramid projects toward the outer portion of the kidney, which is termed the *cortex*. The apex of the pyramid forms the papillae, which cap each minor calyx.

Blood is supplied to the kidney by the *renal artery*. The rate of blood flow through both kidneys of a 70 kg man is about 1200 ml per minute, or about 21 percent of the cardiac output. As the renal artery enters the kidney at the hilum, it divides into the interlobar arteries in the medulla; then, as

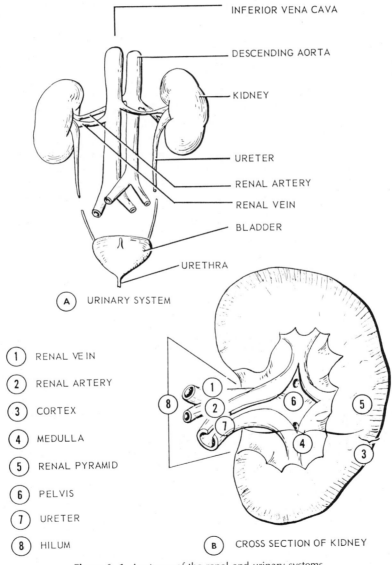

(A) URINARY SYSTEM

1. RENAL VEIN
2. RENAL ARTERY
3. CORTEX
4. MEDULLA
5. RENAL PYRAMID
6. PELVIS
7. URETER
8. HILUM

(B) CROSS SECTION OF KIDNEY

Figure 6–1. Anatomy of the renal and urinary systems.

they enter the cortex, they divide into the *arciform (arcuate) arteries.* The afferent arteries project from the interlobar arteries and go to the nephron, where they divide into capillaries. The capillaries form the efferent arterioles, which then divide to form the *peritubular capillaries,* which help supply the nephron, a portion of the tubular capillaries, and the vasa recta, which descend around the loop of Henle, in the case of juxtamedullary nephrons. These nephrons, which are close to the renal medulla, have a long, extended loop of Henle that dips deep into the medulla. They then return to the venules as do the tubular capillaries (Figs. 6–2 and 6–3).

The *nephron* is the functional unit of the kidney. The two kidneys contain approximately 2.4 million nephrons. Each nephron can be divided into three major portions: the renal corpuscle, the renal tubule, and the collecting ducts. The blood enters the afferent arteriole and goes into the glomerulus in the cortex. It consists of a network of 50 parallel capillaries encased in Bowman's capsule. This structural component is the renal capsule.

The renal tubules begin in Bowman's cap-sule. A pressure gradient forces fluid to leave the glomerulus and enter Bowman's capsule. The fluid then flows into the proximal tubule, which is still in the cortex of the kidney, and then into the loop of Henle. The loop of Henle is at first thick-walled but becomes thin-walled at the distal segment in the medulla of the kidney. The fluid then flows into the distal tubule, located in the cortex of the kidney, and passes into the collecting ducts, which go from the cortex to the medulla where they form papillary ducts (ducts of Bellini) and into the renal pelvis, by way of the renal calyces. It is at this point that the fluid in the renal pelvis is termed urine.

RENAL PHYSIOLOGY

The constituents of urine are formed by filtration, reabsorption, and secretion. *Filtration* occurs as the blood passes through the glomerulus. The force of filtration is a pressure gradient pushing fluid through the glomerular membrane. Approximately 180 liters of water every 24 hours are filtered out of plasma with other substances (Table 6–1). Blood cells and colloidal substances

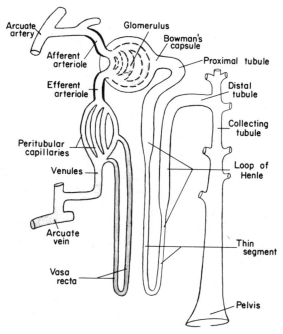

Figure 6–2. The functional nephron. (From Guyton, A. C.: Textbook of Medical Physiology. 5th ed. Philadelphia, W. B. Saunders Co., 1976, p. 440.)

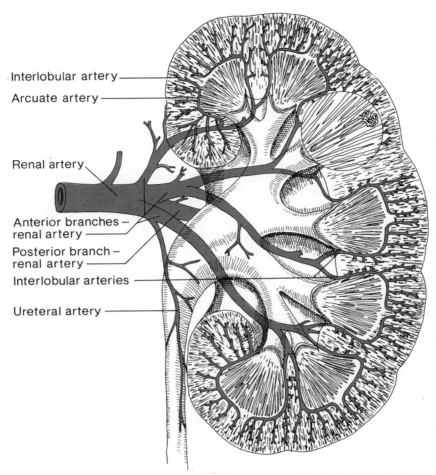

Interlobular artery

Arcuate artery

Renal artery

Anterior branches – renal artery

Posterior branch – renal artery

Interlobular arteries

Ureteral artery

Figure 6–3. Arterial supply to the kidney. Soon after entering the hilum of the kidney, the renal artery divides into several anterior and posterior branches. The branches then divide into interlobar arteries, which course between the medullary pyramids. The interlobar arteries then give off the arcuate arteries, which course between the cortex and medulla. From this arcuate complex arise the interobar arteries, which give off the afferent arterioles to the glomeruli. (From Wilson, R. F.: Principles of Critical Care. The Upjohn Company, 1976.)

TABLE 6–1. The Measure of Reabsorption by the Kidney

Substance	Filtered mEq/24 hr/170 L	Reabsorbed mEq/24 hr/169 L	Excreted mEq/24 hr/45 L
Sodium	24500	24350	150
Chloride	17800	17700	150
Bicarbonate	4900	4900	1
Potassium	700	600	24
Glucose	780	780	0
Urea	870	460	410
Creatinine	12	0	12
Uric acid	50	45	5

are usually retained in the blood, as they are too large to pass through the epithelium. The presence of red blood cells or protein in the urine is usually indicative of some pathologic process occurring in the kidney.

Reabsorption occurs in the proximal and distal tubules. Approximately 99 percent of the water is reabsorbed. Many substances in the water are reabsorbed by active or passive transport. Active transport requires energy for movement of the substance across the membrane. Passive transport can be regarded as simple diffusion that is devoid of energy.

Substances such as glucose, amino acids, sodium, potassium, calcium, and magnesium, which are important constituents of body fluids, are almost entirely reabsorbed. Certain substances are reabsorbed in limited quantities and consequently appear in the urine in considerable amounts. Some of these substances are urea, creatinine, and the phosphates.

The last mechanism in the formation of urine is *secretion*. Various substances, including hydrogen, potassium, and urate ions, are secreted directly into the tubular fluid through the epithelial cells lining the renal tubules.

REGULATION OF KIDNEY FUNCTION

The formation of urine and the retention of substances needed for proper body function are aided by three physiologic mechanisms: the counter-current mechanism, autoregulation, and hormone control.

Counter-current Mechanism. The counter-current mechanism is utilized by the kidneys to concentrate urine. This mechanism is aided by the anatomic arrangement of the loops of Henle of the juxtamedullary nephrons, which go deep into the medulla, and the peritubular capillaries, called the vasa recta. The osmolality of the interstitial fluid increases as one goes more deeply into the medulla; this greater osmolality results in active transport of solutes into the interstitial fluid. This counter-current mecha-

nism is useful when the body needs to excrete a large amount of waste products and yet reabsorb the normal amount of solutes. This is also true when the water in the body needs to be conserved, as in conditions of inadequate water supply. Therefore, water is conserved while waste products are eliminated.

Autoregulation. Autoregulation helps to keep the glomerular filtration at a near-normal rate despite fluctuations in arterial pressure. In fact, over the blood pressure range of 80 to 180 torr, there is little change in either renal plasma flow or glomerular filtration rate. Consequently, as the arterial pressure rises, the sympathetic innervation to the afferent arterioles causes constriction, keeping the glomerular filtration rate constant. The reverse is also true. When the arterial pressure is low, dilation of the afferent arterioles serves to keep the glomerular filtration rate constant.

Hormone Control. The antidiuretic hormone (ADH) is secreted by the posterior pituitary gland. The secretion of this hormone is influenced by plasma osmolality. If hypertonicity of the blood occurs, ADH is secreted and water is retained by the kidneys. If the blood is hypotonic, less ADH is formed and the kidneys release water. This hormone acts on the distal tubule and collecting tubules by altering their permeability to water.

The *juxtaglomerular apparatus* is located just before the glomerulus. If the sodium concentration is low, if the pressure in the afferent arteriole is low, or if a reduced glomerular filtration rate or increased sympathetic stimulation exists, an enzyme, renin, will be released from the juxtaglomerular cells. The renin probably plays an important role in conserving sodium in hypotensive states and controlling fluid volume excretion. The renin, when released in the blood, will catalyze the splitting of angiotensin I from a renin substrate. As the angiotensin I passes through the lungs it is converted to angiotensin II (Fig. 6–4). The *angiotensin II* is a highly effective pressor agent and a major stimulus to the secretion of aldosterone. *Aldosterone*, a mineralocor-

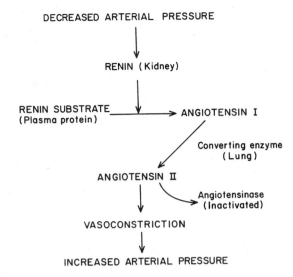

Figure 6–4. The renin-angiotensin-vasoconstrictor mechanism for arterial pressure control. (From Guyton, A. C.: Textbook of Medical Physiology. 5th ed. Philadelphia, W. B. Saunders Co., 1976, p. 231.)

ticoid, appears to act on the distal tubule and the thick segment of the ascending loop of Henle. When secreted, it controls the reabsorption of some of the sodium and water. Because the renin-angiotensin system causes this reabsorption of water and sodium, it plays a role in the control of arterial blood pressure.

RENAL ROLE IN REGULATION OF BODY HOMEOSTASIS

The kidneys play a role in regulation of body fluids. For the most part, they determine the adjustment of blood volume, extracellular fluid volume, and osmolality of the extracellular fluids, electrolytes and ions; they remove waste products and toxic substances; they maintain the acid-base balance.

The kidneys regulate blood volume in the following manner. When the circulating blood volume is excessive, the cardiac output and arterial pressure increase, causing stimulation of volume receptors located in the left and right atria and the baroreceptors located in the carotid, aortic, and pulmonary regions. The net effect is an increase in urine formation, returning blood volume to a normal range. Aldosterone and the antidiuretic hormone also have a role in

improving the economy of blood volume and electrolytes.

If the patient is hypovolemic, the kidney will conserve fluid and thus return the blood volume to normal limits.

The normal intake of water into the body in 24 hours is 2500 ml. Of this, 1200 ml is ingested liquids and 1000 ml is water in solid food. The remaining 300 ml is water derived from oxidation of food in the tissue cells. Table 6–2 shows the avenues by which water is lost in a 24-hour period.

The extracellular fluid volume is controlled by the kidneys as they control the blood volume. The relative ratio of the extracellular fluid volume to blood volume depends upon the physical properties of the circulation and of the interstitial spaces, including their compliances and their dynamics.

The kidney maintains the osmolality of the extracellular fluid mainly by regulating

TABLE 6–2. Average Water Loss per 24 Hours at Average Temperature and Humidity

Route	Amount
Through the skin	500 ml
Through the lungs	350 ml
Through the kidneys	1500 ml
Through the feces	150 ml

the extracellular sodium concentration. Extracellular sodium controls 90 to 95 percent of the effective osmotic pressure of extracellular fluid.

The kidneys also control the extracellular concentration of other electrolytes such as potassium, calcium, magnesium, and phosphate ions.

COMPONENTS OF URINE

The end product of excretion by the kidneys is urine, which is 95 percent water and 5 percent solids. The solids, which account for approximately 60 grams per liter of urine, are listed in Table 6–3. *Urea* is derived mostly from the catabolism of amino acids. *Creatinine* is thought to be derived from creatine, a nitrogenous substance found in muscle tissue. Because it is not resorbed by the tubular mechanism of the kidney, creatinine is a good indicator of kidney function. Creatinine and sulfates are considered nonthreshold substances because they are excreted in their entirety. *Uric acid* is an end product of purine metabolism, formed from purines ingested as food and from those formed in the body.

High-threshold substances are almost entirely reabsorbed in the kidney. They are an important portion of the blood and are excreted only if they are in an excess concentration. Some of the high-threshold substances are glucose, potassium, calcium, and magnesium. Low-threshold substances, such as urea, uric acid, and phosphates, are only minimally reabsorbed by the kidney.

In considering the substances found in urine, it is useful to know the characteristics of normal urine. Normal urine should be amber in color, owing to the pigment urochrome, and it should also be clear and transparent. It usually is acidic, with a pH of about 6, owing to the presence of sodium acid phosphate. The specific gravity is between 1.003 and 1.025. The volume of urine excreted every 24 hours is about 1500 ml.

ACID-BASE BALANCE

The kidneys play a major role in acid-base balance. Although they are the most powerful acid-base regulators, they require several hours to one day to return the hydrogen ion concentration to a normal range. The buffer systems (bicarbonate, phosphate, and protein buffer systems) can react within a fraction of a second to alterations of hydrogen ion concentration. The respiratory system usually takes one to three minutes to react.

The pH is a negative logarithmic expression of the hydrogen ion concentration in the body fluids (see Chapter 4, p. 48). Bicarbonate and carbon dioxide are also factors. The bicarbonate is mainly under renal control and the carbon dioxide is under respiratory control, and because there is approximately 20 times more bicarbonate than carbon dioxide in the plasma, a 20-to-1 ratio exists. Thus, it can be said that any change in the 20-to-1 ratio will affect the pH. Any change that negates the functioning of the kidneys or the rest of the body may affect the bicarbonate portion of the ratio and is a metabolic problem. Conversely, any change in the function of the lungs, which usually affects the carbon dioxide portion of the ratio, is a respiratory problem.

If, for example, a large amount of a bicarbonate solution were rapidly infused into a patient and his ventilation did not change (PCO_2 stays constant), the result would be a higher value for the bicarbonate and no change in the PCO_2. The net result would

TABLE 6–3. Principal Constituents of Urine

Organic Constituents	gm/L
Urea	20.0–300
Uric acid	0.6–0.75
Creatinine	1.5
Others	2.6
Inorganic Constituents	
Sodium chloride	9.0
Potassium chloride	2.5
Sulfuric acid	1.8
Phosphoric acid	1.8
Ammonia	0.5–15
Calcium	0.2
Magnesium	0.2

be a higher pH, which would constitute alkalosis, in this case termed *metabolic alkalosis*. On the other hand, if an acid were infused, the ratio would become smaller and the pH would fall, indicating acidosis, which would be termed *metabolic acidosis*.

Respiratory acidosis occurs when the P_{CO_2} is increased, as in acute hypoventilation, for example. The pH will be lowered because the ratio will become smaller. Conversely, if the patient hyperventilates, the P_{CO_2} will drop and the ratio will rise, thus increasing the pH and producing *respiratory alkalosis*.

The kidneys regulate pH by increasing or decreasing the bicarbonate ion concentration in the body fluid. This is done by a complex series of reactions, which begin with hydrogen ions being secreted into the tubular fluid. Carbon dioxide, an end product of tubular cell metabolism, combines with water to form carbonic acid (H_2CO_3). The carbonic acid dissociates to form hydrogen (H^+) and bicarbonate (HCO_3^-). The hydrogen ion is taken by active transport to the renal tubule and usually exchanges in the tubule with sodium. By active transport the sodium moves to the extracellular fluid, where it combines with the bicarbonate that was reabsorbed into the extracellular fluid to form sodium bicarbonate ($NaHCO_3$). In the tubules, the hydrogen ion that was actively transported to the tubule combines with the filtrate bicarbonate to form carbonic acid. The carbonic acid dissociates to form carbon dioxide and water. The carbon dioxide is reabsorbed into the extracellular fluid and eventually excreted by the lungs, while the water is excreted as part of the urine.

The kidneys correct alkalosis by decreasing the bicarbonate in the extracellular fluid. This occurs because fewer hydrogen ions enter the tubules, owing to a low carbon dioxide concentration, and there is a high bicarbonate concentration in the tubules. The bicarbonate cannot be reabsorbed without first combining with the hydrogen; therefore, the excess bicarbonate ions will be lost to the urine as will other positive ions such as sodium and hydrogen. Cellular potassium may exchange with the sodium instead of the cellular hydrogen to conserve the hydrogen, which may help to return the pH to normal limits.

Renal correction of acidosis is done by increasing the amount of bicarbonate in the extracellular fluid. There is an excess of hydrogen ions as compared with the bicarbonate filtration into the tubules. The excess hydrogen ions are secreted into the tubules, where they combine with phosphate buffer systems or the ammonia buffer system. The sodium ions in the tubules move by active transport to the extracellular fluid and combine with the bicarbonate ion to form sodium bicarbonate, which helps correct the acidosis. The urine will be acidic because the kidney is excreting the excess hydrogen ions.

DIURETIC THERAPY IN THE POST ANESTHESIA CARE UNIT

In the PACU, diuretics are commonly used to reduce brain size and intracranial pressure, to treat hypervolemia, to prevent oliguria, or to help in diagnosing the cause of the oliguria. The major side effects of diuretic therapy are related to the contraction of the extracellular fluid volume and the alterations in potassium concentrations. Because the use of diuretics is so important in the PACU, a brief review of the major types of diuretics will be presented.

Osmotic Diuretics. Osmotic diuretics are used to evaluate the etiology of oliguria, to reduce intracranial pressure and brain size, and to protect the kidneys against the development of acute renal failure. Mannitol, a six-carbon sugar, is the prototype of the osmotic diuretics. This high molecular weight drug, when given intravenously, will increase the plasma osmolality, with a resulting expansion of the intravascular volume by means of drawing fluid from the intracellular space into the extracellular space. In the kidneys, mannitol's osmotic effect on the tubules leads to a diuretic effect. The major concern with mannitol therapy is an increased extracellular fluid volume. This can be of grave consequence in patients with impending pulmonary edema. Hence, the PACU nurse should frequently assess the pulmonary parameters in patients receiving mannitol in whom pulmonary edema is a possibility. An early sign of pulmonary edema is wheezing. Wheezing is usually indicative of interstitial edema. If wheezing is detected in a non-asthmatic patient, the attending physician should be notified immediately. As the edema formation progresses, wet basilar rales or crackles may be heard during auscultation of the chest. The crackles will become coarser as the pulmonary edema worsens.

Thiazide Diuretics. Thiazide diuretics are mainly used in the treatment of hypertension, edema, and diabetes insipidus. These diuretics are secreted in the proximal convoluted tubule and have their major effect in the loop of Henle, where chloride reabsorption is inhibited. This results in diluting defects and increased distal delivery of salt and water. Patients on long-term thiazide diuretic therapy can experience increased urinary losses of water, sodium, chloride, and potassium, and some loss of bicarbonate. Hence, these patients are particularly susceptible to hypochloremic, hypokalemic metabolic alkalosis. Some of the common thiazide diuretics are chlorothiazide and hydrochlorothiazide.

The most common untoward effect of thiazide diuretics is hypokalemia. Hypokalemia, which is a reduced serum potassium, can cause paralytic ileus, severe weakness or flaccid paralysis, hypotension, atrial and ventricular dysrhythmias, and potentiation of digitalis toxicity. If it is determined that treatment for hypokalemia be instituted, intravenous potassium replacement may be given in the PACU. *If the infusion rates of the potassium replacement exceed 40 mEq/hr or if the concentration of potassium in the individual intravenous container is greater than 40 mEq/L, continuous electrocardiographic monitoring should be instituted to detect any dysrhythmias.* Also, if the potassium chloride is added to solutions in flexible plastic bags in the PACU, the nurse should ensure that it is properly mixed in the infusion solution.

This will prevent the patient's receiving an inadvertent bolus of potassium chloride. Other untoward side effects of thiazide diuretics are dermatitis, bone marrow depression, and reduced liver function.

Potassium-Sparing Diuretics. This class of diuretics acts on the distal convoluted tubule. The product of their actions is an increased urinary output without potassium loss. The most popular potassium-sparing diuretics include triamterene, amiloride, and spironolactone. The major side effect of this class of diuretics is hyperkalemia, which can occur because of excess usage along with the overuse of potassium supplementation. The symptoms of hyperkalemia include muscular weakness, conduction defects, ventricular dysrhythmias, and ileus. To reduce the effects of hyperkalemia, calcium gluconate or calcium chloride may be administered. Also, to reduce the high potassium levels, sodium bicarbonate, glucose, or insulin and glucose may be given.

Loop Diuretics. The loop diuretics, of which ethacrynic acid and furosemide are the prototype drugs, are utilized primarily in the treatment of pulmonary edema and general edema and in the diagnosis of acute renal failure. The loop diuretics are secreted into the tubule and have their major action on the medullary concentrating segment where chloride transport is inhibited. Consequently, the concentrating and diluting mechanisms of the kidneys are interfered with, which results in the production of isotonic urine. Also with these drugs, because of the increased delivery of salt, potassium secretion is increased. Hence, the major problems with these drugs are in the realm of deafness (caused by ethacrynic acid), hepatic dysfunction, hypokalemia, alkalosis, extracellular fluid volume contraction, and electrolyte imbalance. Owing to their high potency and their ability to take effect rapidly, loop diuretics are usually the diuretic of choice, when indicated, for the patient in the post anesthesia care unit. The two major concerns when one of these drugs is administered are hypokalemia and hypovolemia. The effects and treatment of hypokalemia were discussed in the section that dealt with thiazide diuretics. The objective findings that indicate hypovolemia (contraction of the extracellular fluid volume) are hypotension, tachycardia, and low right and left ventricular filling pressures. Treatment can include repositioning the patient with the legs elevated or the administration of intravenous salt-containing solutions, or both.

EFFECTS OF ANESTHESIA ON RENAL FUNCTION

In patients with normal renal function who receive general inhalational anesthesia, some depression of renal function will occur. This is because all of the general anesthetics depress such functions as glomerular filtration rate (GFR), renal blood flow, and urinary flow. The depression in renal function is due to direct and indirect effects of the general anesthetic agents. In regard to the vascular effects, during general anesthesia, the renal blood flow may be depressed owing to renal vasoconstriction or systemic hypotension, or both. Of interest is that droperidol, the tranquilizer component of Innovar, has the smallest effect on the changes on renal function. It should be stated that, in most cases, the renal depression due to the anesthetic agents is completely reversible at the end of the operative procedure.

It appears that patients who are anesthetized in lighter planes of anesthesia may experience some manifestations of the stress response. One of the hormones that is released in response to a stressor is antidiuretic hormone (ADH). This hormone is the most important regulator of urine volume. When ADH is released, it promotes an increase in tubular reabsorption of water, which results in a fall in urine volume and an increase in urine concentration. Other biochemical products of the stress response, namely epinephrine, norepinephrine, and the renin-angiotensin system, also affect the renal system. More specifically, when these amines are liberated, renal blood flow is decreased. Because some patients can undergo a stress response under anes-

thesia, it is important for the PACU nurse to monitor renal function during the emergence phase of the anesthesia. It is not uncommon for patients who have undergone major abdominal or thoracic surgery to experience some diuresis during the immediate postoperative period. Hence, urine volume and concentration should be monitored in all patients who (1) have undergone a major surgical procedure, (2) have received general anesthesia for more than two hours, (3) have compromised cardiovascular or renal system, or both, and (4) have had a significant blood volume replacement during the preoperative or intraoperative phase of the anesthetic experience.

EFFECTS OF DRUGS IN PATIENTS WITH COMPROMISED RENAL FUNCTION

Patients with severe renal disease will usually have anemia, body fluid relocation, abnormal cell membrane activity, and alterations in blood albumin and electrolytes. It also should be noted that these patients are usually debilitated and, if in the uremic state, central nervous system (CNS) depression is usually present. Drugs that are not metabolized in the body and are therefore excreted unchanged by the kidneys should be avoided in patients with severe renal disease. Hence, the long-acting barbiturates barbital and phenobarbital and the skeletal muscle relaxants decamethonium and gallamine, along with digoxin and lanatoside C, should be avoided in these patients. Because about half of the administered dose of the belladonna alkaloids atropine and hyoscyamine is excreted unchanged, the dosage should be modified depending on the degree of severity of the renal impairment. When CNS depression is present in the patient with renal impairment, the actions of narcotics are intensified and prolonged. Along with this, diazepam, which has a 24 hour half-life, is probably not a good choice because of its additive effect upon the CNS depression. In patients with mild to moderate renal dysfunction, all inhalational anesthetics except methoxyflurane and possibly enflurane can be utilized in the usual clinical dose range. Because thiopental depends on redistribution for the termination of its action, it may be used in patients with renal impairment. However, the sleeping time is increased in proportion to the degree of uremia. Along with this, the skeletal muscle relaxants succinylcholine, curare and pancuronium are also acceptable for use in the patient with compromised kidney function. Neuroleptanalgesia, which derives from the combination of a narcotic and a tranquilizer, when achieved with nitrous oxide and oxygen, is an acceptable technique for the uremic patient. It should be pointed out that if a patient has received Innovar, which is the prototype neuroleptanalgesic drug, the PACU nurse should monitor the patient for prolonged depressant effects of the drug. More specifically, the tranquilizer component of Innovar, droperidol, has a very long half-life; therefore, its prolonged effects, coupled with CNS depression from the uremia, may cause the patient to be slow to arouse in the immediate postoperative emergence phase. Consequently, airway patency and the cardiovascular parameters should be monitored closely for an extended period of time when droperidol has been administered to the patient in either the preoperative or the intraoperative phase of the anesthetic experience.

RENAL SHUTDOWN OR FAILURE

Acute renal failure can occur in the post anesthesia care unit owing to a variety of reasons such as hemorrhage and circulatory failure from trauma or extensive surgery, acute glomerulonephritis, vascular occlusions, or toxicity from drugs.

The most common cause of acute renal failure is acute tubular necrosis (ATN). Oliguria produces the clinical setting in which renal cell necrosis may develop. Persistent oliguria, below 25 ml of urine per hour for more than two hours, constitutes a true medical emergency, and the surgeon should be notified immediately. The urine volume may be abnormally high in conditions in which the glomerular filtration rate is reduced to the point of renal failure, and the increased urine volume represents a supplemental failure of tubular function. In patients with mild to moderate renal dysfunction, enflurane may potentially cause nephrotoxicity. This is because enflurane is metabolized to inorganic fluoride. However, clinical studies have not been able to demonstrate this possibility. Nephrotoxicity is characterized by polyuria and azotemia. Therefore, the accurate and continuous measurement of urine volume is essential in the postoperative nursing care of the patient with suspected renal failure.

Creatinine clearance is a laboratory test that provides an excellent index to measure the quantity of glomerular filtrate. Creatinine is a component of urine not resorbed by tubular mechanisms. Hence, every milliliter of glomerular filtrate should contain precisely the same quantity of creatinine as 1 ml of plasma.

Measurement of *urinary sodium* will yield information on sodium absorption. The *urine plasma osmolar ratio* provides an index of water resorption in the collecting tubules and is an excellent measurement of tubular function. The quality rather than the quantity of the urine provides useful information as to the renal state of the patient (Fig. 6–5).

PACU NURSING CARE

PACU nursing care centers on recognition and care of the patient in impending renal failure. Urinary output should be monitored by an indwelling urethral catheter. It will provide moment-to-moment information concerning urine output and its constituents that can be measured. Modern collecting devices provide a closed system between the catheter and a graduated measuring flask that can be emptied from the bottom without disconnecting the catheter. In this way, the danger of gross contamination is minimized while the necessary monitoring facility is still provided.

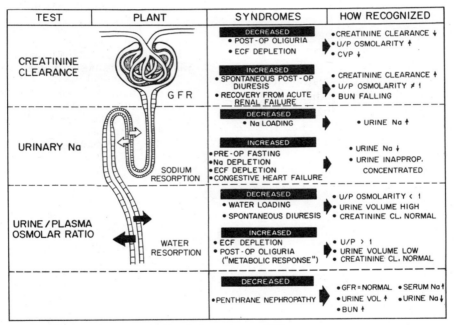

TEST	PLANT	SYNDROMES	HOW RECOGNIZED
CREATININE CLEARANCE	G F R	**DECREASED** • POST-OP OLIGURIA • ECF DEPLETION	• CREATININE CLEARANCE ↓ • U/P OSMOLARITY ↑ • CVP ↓
		INCREASED • SPONTANEOUS POST-OP DIURESIS • RECOVERY FROM ACUTE RENAL FAILURE	• CREATININE CLEARANCE ↑ • U/P OSMOLARITY ≠ ↑ • BUN FALLING
URINARY Na	SODIUM RESORPTION	**DECREASED** • Na LOADING	• URINE Na ↑
		INCREASED • PRE-OP FASTING • Na DEPLETION • ECF DEPLETION • CONGESTIVE HEART FAILURE	• URINE Na ↓ • URINE INAPPROP. CONCENTRATED
URINE / PLASMA OSMOLAR RATIO	WATER RESORPTION	**DECREASED** • WATER LOADING • SPONTANEOUS DIURESIS	• U/P OSMOLARITY < ↑ • URINE VOLUME HIGH • CREATININE CL. NORMAL
		INCREASED • ECF DEPLETION • POST-OP OLIGURIA ("METABOLIC RESPONSE")	• U/P > ↑ • URINE VOLUME LOW • CREATININE CL. NORMAL
		DECREASED • PENTHRANE NEPHROPATHY	• GFR = NORMAL • SERUM Na ↑ • URINE VOL ↑ • URINE Na ↓ • BUN ↑

Figure 6–5. Alterations in renal function that result from a normal kidney acting to correct or preserve an abnormal internal environment. The quantity and quality of urine are appropriate for preserving the entire organism but may, if uncorrected, result in renal damage. (From Kinney, J. M., et al.: Manual of Preoperative and Postoperative Care. 2nd ed. Philadelphia, W. B. Saunders Co., 1971, p. 244.)

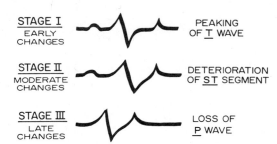

STAGE I EARLY CHANGES		PEAKING OF <u>T</u> WAVE
STAGE II MODERATE CHANGES		DETERIORATION OF <u>ST</u> SEGMENT
STAGE III LATE CHANGES		LOSS OF <u>P</u> WAVE

Figure 6–6. Stages of electrocardiographic evidence of hyperkalemia. (From Kinney, J. M., et al.: Manual of Preoperative and Postoperative Care. 2nd ed. Philadelphia, W. B. Saunders Co., 1971, p. 256.)

Continuous electrocardiographic monitoring should be done because the patient in acute renal failure will probably have hyperkalemia, which can lead to cardiac arrest. The ECG changes indicative of hyperkalemia are initially high peaked T waves and depressed S-T segments. Subsequent disappearance of T waves, heart block, and diastolic cardiac arrest occur with increasing levels of potassium (Fig. 6–6).

Osmotic diuretics, such as mannitol, or one of the loop diuretics, such as ethacrynic acid or furosemide, may be used in the treatment of tubular necrosis. A central venous pressure monitor may be inserted to measure blood volume. If renal failure continues, dialytic therapy will probably be necessary.

REFERENCES

1. Guyton, A.: Textbook of Medical Physiology. 7th ed. Philadelphia, W. B. Saunders Co., 1986.
2. Katz, J., Benumof, J., and Kadis, L.: Anesthesia and Uncommon Diseases. 2nd ed. Philadelphia, W. B. Saunders Co., 1981.
3. Miller, R.: Anesthesia. 2nd ed. New York, Churchill Livingstone, Inc., 1986.
4. Schramm, S. M. A.: Anatomy and Physiology of the Kidney. J. AANA, 43(1):39, 1975.
5. Walsh, P. C., Perlmutter, A. D., Gittes, R. F., et al.: Campbell's Urology. 5th ed. Philadelphia, W. B. Saunders Co., 1986.

7

Gastrointestinal Anatomy and Physiology

Because so many surgical procedures involve the gastrointestinal tract, it is important for the PACU nurse to understand some functions of the organs of this system. This chapter will discuss the overall function of each organ and the possible postoperative complications that may involve the gastrointestinal tract.

THE ESOPHAGUS

The esophagus is a muscular tube extending from the pharynx to the stomach (Fig. 7–1). It is located behind the trachea and in front of the thoracic aorta and traverses the diaphragm to enter the esophagogastric junction, sometimes referred to as the cardia. Approximately 5 cm above the junction with the stomach is the gastroesophageal sphincter, which functions to prevent the reflex of stomach contents into the esophagus. Ordinarily, it remains constricted except in the act of swallowing. Another factor preventing reflux of gastric contents into the esophagus is physiologic compression by intra-abdominal pressure on the esophagus just below the diaphragm. Guyton refers to this mechanism as a flutter valve closure. The main function of the esophagus is to conduct ingested material to the stomach. The innervation of the esophagus appears to originate from the vagus.

Disorders of the Esophagus

Esophageal achalasia, a disease of unknown origin, is characterized by an absence of peristalsis in the esophagus and by constriction of the cardia sphincter. The patient with this disorder will usually have hypermotility of the esophagus and diffuse spasms of the esophagus.

A problem every PACU nurse should watch for is *regurgitation under anesthesia*. When a patient is anesthetized with a general anesthetic, the swallowing mechanism is abolished. Foodstuffs or fluids can be passively or actively vomited. The vomitus may then be aspirated into the trachea and lungs. In some instances, this type of aspiration is called *Mendelson's syndrome,* and inspiring vomitus can lead to *aspiration pneumonia.* It can occur during the induction of anesthesia, during the operation, or in the immediate PACU phase as the patient emerges from anesthesia.

If a patient begins vomiting, he or she should be placed in a head-down position and given oxygen immediately. Fluid should be suctioned rapidly while administration of oxygen continues. If the patient's airway is obstructed by large particles, finger or forceps should be used to clear the debris and then oxygen should be administered. The physician or anesthetist should be notified immediately.

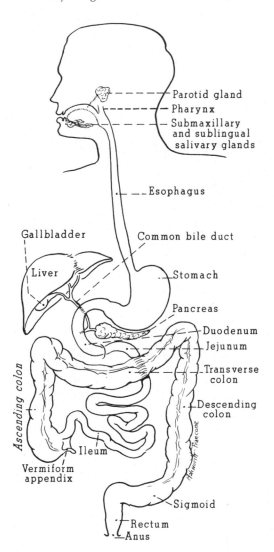

Figure 7–1. The digestive system and its associated structures. (From Jacob, S. W., Francone, C. A., and Lossow, W. J.: Structure and Function in Man. 4th ed. Philadelphia, W. B. Saunders Co., 1978, p. 453.)

Further treatment may include intubation and instillation of a weak solution of bicarbonate or saline through the endotracheal tube to aid in the neutralization of acidic gastric fluid in the respiratory tract. Steroids and antibiotics may also be administered.

A patient recovering from a general anesthetic should be assessed for possible *passive regurgitation,* especially if the patient was not intubated during surgery. Clinical signs include dyspnea, cyanosis of varying degrees, and tachycardia. Upon auscultation of the lungs abnormal sounds will usually be heard. If the assessment indi-

cates the possibility of this syndrome, oxygen should be administered and the physician notified at once.

Patients who had a "full stomach" at induction of anesthesia, or have had bowel surgery or emergency surgery, or have a suspected hiatal hernia have a higher incidence of this syndrome. The best treatment is prevention. These patients should have a complete return of consciousness before the endotracheal tube is removed. If the endotracheal tube is to be removed in the PACU, the patient should be placed in a lateral position with the head down. Oxygen should be administered and suction should be available for immediate use before the extubation is performed.

Hiatal hernia can occur where the esophagus traverses the diaphragm. Ultimately, a lower esophageal stricture may occur that can cause such symptoms as heartburn, pain, and vomiting. Patients who have a diagnosed hiatal hernia require constant observation for active and passive vomiting during the emergence phase of anesthesia. This is especially important if the surgery was performed on an emergency basis when the patient had a full stomach.

THE STOMACH

The stomach can be anatomically divided into three portions: the fundus, the body, and the pyloric portion (Fig. 7–2). The *fundus* is the dome of the stomach, where peptic juice is secreted. The *body* is the middle portion of the stomach and is lined with gastric glands that secrete hydrochloric acid. The pH of the solution as secreted is approximately 0.8, which is extremely acidic. If vomiting occurs and some gastric juice is aspirated into the lungs, the acidic gastric juice can devastate the tissue of the respiratory tract. The third portion of the stomach is the *pyloric portion,* sometimes called the *pyloric antrum.* Here, a thick, viscous mucus and the hormone gastrin are secreted. At the end of the antrum is the pylorus, an opening surrounded by a strong band of sphincter muscle, which controls the amount of gastric contents entering the duodenum.

The *vagus nerve* (parasympathetic nervous system) provides the nerve supply to the stomach. When the vagus is stimulated, it causes increased motility of the stomach and the secretion of acid, pepsin, and gastrin. Thus, a vagotomy is sometimes performed during gastric surgery to decrease gastric motility and acid production.

THE INTESTINES

The *duodenum,* which is a part of the small intestine, arises at the pylorus of the stomach and ends at the duodenojejunal junction. The duodenum is divided into four segments: superior, descending, transverse, and ascending. The common bile duct and the main pancreatic duct empty into the descending duodenum. The main function of the stomach and the first portion of the duodenum is to alter the form of food and to supply enzymes for digestion.

The *jejunum* begins at the descending duodenum at the duodenojejunal angle. It

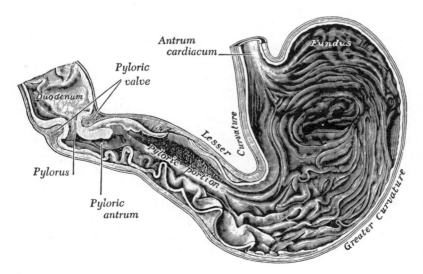

Figure 7–2. Interior of the stomach. (From Clemente, C. [ed.]: Gray's Anatomy of the Human Body. 30th ed. Philadelphia, Lea & Febiger, 1985, p. 1225.)

composes the first two fifths of the small intestine, and the ileum occupies the distal three fifths of the small intestine. The mesentery, which contains blood vessels, nerves, lymphatics, lymph nodes, and fat, stabilizes the small bowel and prevents it from twisting and constricting its blood supply.

The digestive glands secrete large quantities of water to aid in the digestive process. It has been estimated that between 5 and 10 liters of water enter the small intestine and only about 500 ml leave the ileum and enter the colon. Among the important materials absorbed from the small intestine are sodium, bicarbonate, chloride, calcium, iron, carbohydrates, fats, and amino acids.

Sodium is absorbed by the small intestine at a rate of 25 to 35 grams per day. This accounts for approximately one seventh of all the sodium in the body. When a patient is experiencing extreme diarrhea, sodium can be depleted to a lethal level within a few hours.

THE COLON AND RECTUM

At the end of the small intestine is the *ileocecal valve,* which functions to prevent backflow of fecal material from the colon into the small intestine.

The colon is divided anatomically into the cecum, ascending colon, transverse colon, and descending and sigmoid colon. The function of the colon is the absorption of water and electrolytes, which occurs principally in the proximal half of the colon, and the storage of fecal material, which occurs in the distal colon. The contents of the cecum are mainly liquid, as compared with the solid material contained in the sigmoid colon. Therefore, if a patient has had a colostomy, it is important to know from which portion of the colon the stoma originates, so as to determine if the excreted fecal material has the normal amount of water content.

Of surgical importance is the *appendix,* which arises from the cecum at its inferior tip. It represents a special type of intestinal obstruction when it becomes inflamed ow-

ing to hyperplasia of submucosal lymphoid follicles, fecoliths, foreign bodies, or tumors.

The rectum functions entirely as an excretory canal and has no digestive function. It begins anatomically at the distal end of the sigmoid colon and ends at the anus. It is tubular and has two layers. The innermost layer is the tract, and the outermost layer is skeletal muscle of the pelvic floor. The muscle is innervated by the parasympathetic nervous system.

THE ANUS

The anus is the termination of the alimentary canal. It is encircled by striated muscle and innervated by somatic sympathetic and parasympathetic fibers. Owing to the parasympathetic innervation of the rectum and anus, parasympathetic stimulation may occur during a rectal examination or surgical procedure. This parasympathetic reflex can also occur when a patient is recovering from a general anesthetic. If a physician deems it necessary to perform a rectal examination, the PACU nurse should be prepared to monitor the patient for bradycardia and laryngospasm, as they may result from stimulation of the anus and rectum.

THE LIVER

The importance of the liver is generally underestimated. In Chinese medicine, the liver is considered the most important organ of the body. It is one of the basic homeostatic organs, as it maintains the consistency of the blood on a minute-to-minute basis.

The liver is located in the right upper quadrant of the abdomen. It has a dual blood supply, consisting of the hepatic artery and the portal vein. Both carry oxygen and foodstuffs to the liver for assimilation. The *sinusoids,* which surround the liver cells, empty into a venous system that eventually forms the hepatic vein and empties into the inferior vena cava. About 1400 ml of blood per minute flow through the liver.

The liver is the body's most important storage organ. It is able to absorb glucose in the form of glycogen and it maintains a normal glucose concentration in the body. The liver also stores amino acids, iron, and vitamins. The liver can store up to 400 ml of blood in the sinusoids. If a person loses an appreciable amount of blood, the liver can release stored blood into the circulation to replace that which was lost.

Certainly the liver performs many vital physiologic functions that have a significant impact on the pharmacologic actions of many of the drugs used in the perioperative period. Consequently, knowledge of bilirubin metabolism, protein synthesis, and drug biotransformation is of critical importance to the PACU nurse.

Bilirubin Metabolism. Bilirubin is made from one of the by-products of red blood cell hemolysis—hemoglobin. The reticuloendothelial system converts the hemoglobin to unconjugated bilirubin. The bilirubin is transported to the liver via serum albumin. In the liver the bilirubin is then removed from the albumin and is conjugated with glucuronic acid. Conjugated bilirubin is highly water soluble and easily excreted in the urine. The other type of bilirubin, which is unconjugated, is lipid soluble and not excreted in the urine. Conditions such as sickle cell disease, thalassemia minor, drug-induced hemolysis, and breakdown of red blood cells following massive transfusions can cause an increase in unconjugated bilirubin. This will eventually lead to an increase in bilirubin production. *Jaundice,* a yellowish tint to the body tissues, can be caused by a high concentration of bilirubin in the extracellular fluids. Consequently, diseases that are considered prehepatic will cause an increase in unconjugated bilirubin and eventually lead to what is known as *hemolytic jaundice. Obstructive jaundice* occurs when the outflow of bile is blocked by an obstruction such as gallstones, stricture, or compression from external masses. In this case, the conjugated bilirubin will increase in the serum. The third type of jaundice, *toxic jaundice,* usually follows damage to the liver cells. Use of chloroform can cause this type of jaundice, as can use of carbon tetrachloride.

Protein Synthesis. The liver is responsible for the synthesis of most of the proteins found in the plasma. Albumin is the most notable of the plasma proteins synthesized by the liver. Albumin synthesis is regulated by the state of nutrition and, therefore, a nutritional deficit will result in reduced albumin production. Because many drugs used in anesthesia are protein bound, a reduction in albumin can have a significant impact on the pharmacologic action of the drugs. Because the protein-binding sites are reduced, the unbound fraction of the drug will be increased, which will ultimately lead to an increased sensitivity to the drug or a prolonged action. This is particularly true for the highly protein-bound barbiturates. Hence, in the PACU, hyponatremic patients who have received thiopental intraoperatively should be closely monitored for respiratory and cardiovascular depression due to the prolonged action of the ultra–short-acting barbiturate. The liver also synthesizes the enzyme pseudocholinesterase (plasma cholinesterase). This protein is the principal enzyme in the metabolism of succinylcholine and the ester-type local anesthetics. Succinylcholine, which is the principal depolarizing skeletal muscle relaxant in use, demonstrates an inverse correlation between duration of action and pseudocholinesterase levels. Therefore, any patient with suspected liver dysfunction who has received succinylcholine intraoperatively should be closely monitored for respiratory depression in the immediate postoperative period. Finally, the liver produces a large proportion of the protein substances used in coagulation.

Drug Biotransformation. The enzymes required for oxidation and conjugation in the liver are referred to as the microsomal enzymes. Exposure to certain drugs, including barbiturates and some anesthetics, can lead to an increase in the microsomal enzymes. This process is commonly called *enzyme induction.* When enzyme induction occurs, the result will be an increase in the rate of drug biotransformation. Patients with severe liver disease may have reduced microsomal activity in the liver. Hence, drugs such as thiopental, diazepam, and meperidine will have a prolonged action owing to a decreased rate of drug biotransformation by the microsomal enzymes. Consequently, patients with severe hepatic disease should be closely monitored for respiratory and cardiovascular depression in the post anesthesia care unit phase of their anesthetic experience.

Acute Hepatic Failure

This rare syndrome may be seen if the patient has undergone a period of severe hypotension (≤40 mm Hg systolic) during anesthesia. Because of the hypotension, the liver cells die and the patient will appear lethargic and drowsy postoperatively. Persistent oliguria, which leads to anuria within 24 to 48 hours, is the cardinal symptom of this syndrome. The signs of liver damage will ensue and include headache, anorexia, malaise, vomiting, and pyrexia. The syndrome progresses to persistent vomiting and by the end of the first week jaundice may be present. The final stages of this disease are marked by delirium, coma, and death.

Treatment of this syndrome is entirely symptomatic and includes maintenance of fluid and electrolyte balance, treatment of the anemia, and a high carbohydrate diet.

GALLBLADDER

The gallbladder is a thin-walled, pear-shaped organ attached to the inferior surface of the liver (Fig. 7–3). It is 7 to 10 cm long and 3 to 5 cm wide. It has a capacity of 30 to 60 ml of fluid. Anatomically, it is divided into the *fundus,* the distal tip; the *corpus,* the middle body portion; the *infundibulum,* a pouchlike structure; and the *neck,* which leads to the cystic duct. The cystic duct joins the common hepatic duct to form the common bile duct. The common bile duct and the main pancreatic duct of Wirsung usually join at the choledochoduodenal junction, which is a passageway through the duodenal wall. The muscle of the choledochoduodenal junction is the *sphincter of Oddi,* which regulates the flow

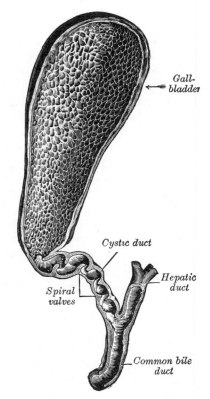

Figure 7–3. The gallbladder and bile ducts laid open (Spalteholz). (From Clemente, C. [ed.]: Gray's Anatomy of the Human Body. 30th ed. Philadelphia, Lea & Febiger, 1985, p. 1254.)

of bile into the duodenum. Many common narcotic analgesics can produce spasm of the sphincter of Oddi and the duodenum and can increase the pressure in the biliary tree.

THE PANCREAS

The pancreas is situated in the upper abdomen behind the stomach. It is a slender organ, which consists of a head, body, and tail (Fig. 7–4). Its main duct, through which pass the pancreatic enzymes, runs the entire length of the gland and opens into the duodenum along with the common bile duct. Scattered throughout the pancreas are small clusters of cells called the *islets of Langerhans.* They are responsible for the production and secretion of hormones that they empty directly into the bloodstream; therefore, the islets of Langerhans are con-

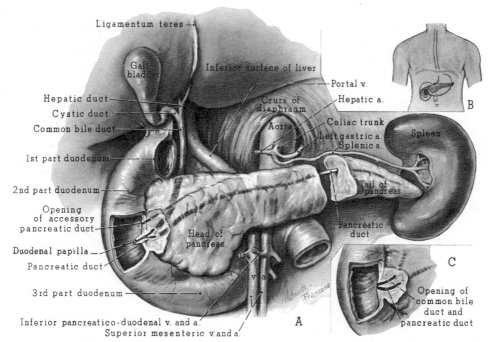

Figure 7–4. *A*, Relationship of the pancreas to the duodenum, showing the pancreatic and bile ducts joining at the duodenal papilla. A section has been removed from the pancreas to expose the pancreatic duct. *B*, Anatomic position of the pancreas. *C*, Common variation. (From Jacob, S. W., Francone, C. A., and Lossow, W. J.: Structure and Function in Man. 4th ed. Philadelphia, W. B. Saunders Co., 1978, p. 466.)

sidered an endocrine gland. Three types of cells are found in the islets of Langerhans: alpha, beta, and delta. The alpha cells are associated with the production of the hormone *glucagon* and the beta cells with *insulin.* The physiologic significance of the delta cells has not been determined.

Insulin is secreted in response to an increase in concentration of glucose. The secretion of insulin is inhibited when a low concentration of glucose exists. Glucagon is frequently called *hyperglycemic factor* because it causes hyperglycemia by stimulating the breakdown of liver glycogen with consequent release of glucose into the circulation. It also stimulates gluconeogenesis, which is the formation of glucose from noncarbohydrate sources.

The pancreas excretes juice for digesting all three major types of food: carbohydrates, fats, and proteins. The pancreatic juice also contains large amounts of bicarbonate ions, which help neutralize the acidic chyme as it passes into the duodenum from the stomach.

Pancreatitis

Acute pancreatitis is a serious complication of surgery on the biliary tract. It can occur as a result of common duct exploration during gallbladder surgery. Acute postoperative pancreatitis should be suspected if there is excessive pain, vomiting, fever, tachycardia, persistent ileus, or jaundice. The PACU nurse should be aware of these symptoms and, if detected, they should be reported to the surgeon. Treatment of this disorder may include nasogastric suction, anticholinergic drugs, antibiotics, and replacement of fluids and electrolytes.

THE SPLEEN

Because of its anatomic location, not its physiologic functions, the spleen will be discussed here (see also Chapter 27).

The spleen is an oval organ located in the upper left quadrant of the abdominal cavity. Its physiologic functions include filtering blood and foreign material, hematopoiesis, and, in some instances, the production of lymphocytes and antibodies.

The spleen is a highly vascular organ, and approximately 350 liters of blood normally flow through it daily. The spleen acts as a reservoir of blood. It can store so many red cells that splenic contraction can cause the hematocrit of the systemic blood to increase as much as 3 to 4 percent.

Normal health is possible after splenectomy, as other tissues can assume the functions the spleen normally performs. Splenectomy is usually performed for the cure or alleviation of hematologic disease or for traumatic rupture of the spleen. Because the spleen is friable and vascular, blood loss from a splenectomy can be high. It is im-

portant, therefore, for the PACU nurse to assess the blood loss during the recovery phase as well as the cardiovascular status of the patient.

REFERENCES

1. Guyton, A.: Textbook of Medical Physiology. 7th ed. Philadelphia, W. B. Saunders Co., 1986.
2. Katz, J., Benumof, J., and Kadis, L.: Anesthesia and Uncommon Diseases: Pathophysiologic and Clinical Correlations. 2nd ed. Philadelphia, W. B. Saunders Co., 1981.
3. Miller, R. (ed.): Anesthesia. 2nd ed. New York, Churchill Livingstone, Inc., 1986.
4. Sabiston, D. (ed.): Textbook of Surgery. 13th ed. Philadelphia, W. B. Saunders Co., 1986.

8

Integumentary Anatomy and Physiology

The recovery room nurse should have a basic understanding of the integumentary system. This body system performs many functions that will influence the nursing care rendered to the post anesthesia care unit (PACU) patient. Aseptic technique, intravenous cannulation, and care of the burn patient are discussed in this chapter because of their involvement with the integumentary system.

INTEGUMENTARY ANATOMY

The skin, or integument, provides a boundary between the internal and external environments of the body. The surface area covered by the skin is about 1.8 square meters in the average male and 1.6 square meters in the average female. The skin accounts for 15 percent of the total body weight. It is divided into two major layers, the *epidermis* and the *dermis* or *corium*. The epidermis consists of stratified squamous epithelium and has no blood vessels. The cells of the innermost or basal layer (stratum basale or stratum germinativum) of the epidermis are constantly dividing and producing cells of the outer layers. It is from this layer that basal cell cancer develops. The prickly layer, or *stratum spinosum*, located immediately above the basal layer, consists

of cells that are connected by intercellular bridges. It is from this layer that squamous cell cancer arises (Fig. 8–1).

The granular layer, or *stratum granulosum*, contains three or four layers of cells. Squamous epithelial cells are converted here into hard material by a process called *cornification*.

The next layer, the *stratum lucidum*, develops only on the palms of the hands and the soles of the feet. Above this layer is the outermost epidermal layer, which is called the horny layer or *stratum corneum*. It is composed of dead cells, keratin, surface lipids, and dirt. Dead cells are shed at a fairly constant rate, a process referred to as *desquamation*.

The epidermis has keratinizing appendages, which comprise the hair and the nails; and glandular appendages, which include sweat, scent, and sebaceous glands.

The dermis, or corium, lies below the epidermis and consists of collagen, elastic, and reticular fibers. It also contains blood vessels, nerves, lymphatics, and smooth muscle.

INTEGUMENTARY FUNCTIONS

The skin has many important functions, the most important of which is to act as a

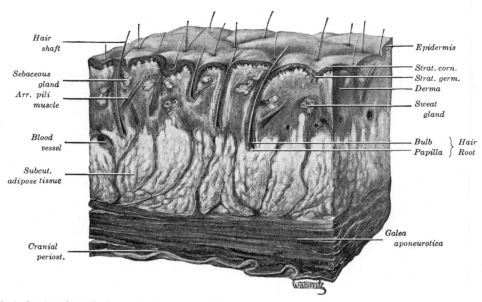

Figure 8–1. Section through the scalp of an adult cadaver (×5). (From Clemente, C. [ed.]): Gray's Anatomy of the Human Body. 30th ed. Philadelphia, Lea & Febiger, 1985, p. 1106.)

barrier between internal and external environments. In addition, it plays an important part in body temperature regulation, fluid regulation, excretion, secretion, vitamin D production, sensation, appearance, and many other functions that have yet to be identified.

Protection

The skin functions to protect the body from injurious stimuli, which can be physical, chemical, electrical, thermal, or biologic. Of particular importance to the PACU nurse is the presence of bacteria on the skin that may cause sepsis when the barrier is broken. Some of the normal flora of the skin are gram-positive cocci and rods. A number of diphtheroids are widely distributed on the skin, especially in moist areas. The normal pH of the skin is 4 to 6, which derives from lactic acid and amino acid residues of keratinization.

When intact, the skin stops pathogenic organisms from entering the body and at the same time prevents the loss of *water*, *electrolytes*, and *proteins* to the external environment. Once the skin is broken, for example, by surgical incision or venipunc-

ture, the barrier between the internal and external environments is broken. This is why aseptic technique is important whenever opening of the skin is anticipated or has occurred.

Thermoregulation

The skin functions to regulate body temperature by conserving heat in a cold environment. By sweating it can lower the body temperature in hot environments. The sweat glands are innervated by the sympathetic and parasympathetic nervous systems. Sweat has a pH of 3.8 to 6.5 and contains sodium, chloride, potassium, calcium, and lactic acid as well as urea. Therefore, sweating is an act of excretion as well as secretion.

IMPORTANCE OF ASEPTIC TECHNIQUE

Since all skin has pathogenic organisms on it, skin can never be sterile. Precautions should be taken to reduce the number of pathogenic organisms that may be introduced into a wound. Handwashing technique is most important. This should be accomplished before care is given to the patient. A good mechanical scrub with a skin antiseptic, such as a soap containing iodine, should be done.

The surgical wound site should be kept clean and the dressings should remain sterile. If there is any question about sterility because of excess bleeding, fluid, or physical contamination, the dressing should be changed. Special precautions to reduce the introduction of pathogenic organisms should be taken with patients who are prone to infection. This includes patients who are obese, anemic, or debilitated; those with vascular insufficiency, chronic obstructive pulmonary disease (COPD), and diabetes mellitus; and those with an immune deficiency, including patients who are on chemotherapy. Aseptic technique in wound care of these patients should include the wearing of a surgical mask and the use of sterile gloves and drapes.

Sterile Technique for Intravenous Therapy

Establishing an intravenous infusion should be accomplished with sterile technique. The site chosen for cannula (needle) placement should be prepared in a suitable fashion. An excellent method utilizes 1 percent iodine in 70 percent isopropyl alcohol. After at least 30 seconds' drying time, the iodine solution should be washed off with 70 percent isopropyl alcohol. Both agents should be applied with friction, working from the center of the field to the periphery. An iodophor skin preparation may be substituted in patients with sensitive skin but should not be washed off with alcohol, as its antibacterial action may depend in part on the sustained release of free iodine. In the rare case in which iodine preparations cannot be tolerated at all, vigorous, prolonged (more than 1 minute) washing with 70 percent isopropyl alcohol is acceptable.

After the intravenous administration route is established, the cannula (needle) should be securely anchored to prevent irritating to-and-fro motion and to avoid potential transport of cutaneous bacteria into the puncture wound. Although evidence is not conclusive, additional protection from infectious complications may follow topical antimicrobial applications to the infusion site. Since studies have demonstrated that antibiotic ointments may actually favor the selective growth of fungi, the use of topical antiseptic iodophor ointment should be considered. The intravenous site should be covered with a sterile dressing.

Overview of Burn Injuries

The care of the postoperative burn patient can be most challenging to the PACU nurse. These patients usually present a very complex array of pathophysiologic difficulties, from deranged fluid and electrolyte balance, respiratory complications, and disrupted temperature regulation to psychologic disturbances. A burn, no matter how small, represents a total body assault. Infection is the most common and the most dreaded complication following a burn injury; therefore, aseptic skin care is of primary importance. The PACU nursing care of the patient with a burn injury is very complex; Chapter 33 will present specific pathophysiologic processes, assessment, and nursing interventions for the burn patient.

There are four main types of burn injuries: cold, chemical, electrical and thermal. A *cold* injury is trauma caused by exposure to cold. Such conditions as frostbite, chilblain, immersion foot, and trench foot are the result. *Frostbite* results from the crystallization of tissue fluids in the skin or subcutaneous tissue. *Chilblain* results from exposure to cold temperatures above freezing associated with high humidity. *Immersion foot* occurs when the skin of the foot is exposed to water which is below 50°F for a long period of time.

Chemical burns are produced by caustic agents, either acid or base. They are devastating because without appropriate emergency treatment these agents continue to cause destruction of fascia, fat, muscle, and bone.

Electrical burns, which result from direct contact with electrical voltage, are quite deceiving in appearance. Although the only visible wounds may be those of entrance and exit, massive damage is often sustained as the high energy sources follow conductive muscle and nerves, causing damage that may require amputation of extremities. Thermal injury often occurs from the heat of arcing, and clothing igniting.

The most common type of burn injury is the *thermal burn*. It is caused by excessive heat and can cause metabolic derangement as well as problems in maintaining thermal control. Unless otherwise indicated, this discussion will cover thermal burns. Various terms are currently in use to classify burns. The most common trend today is the use of the terms "partial-thickness," "deep dermal," and "full-thickness" in describing burns. The terms, "first degree," "second degree," "third degree," and sometimes "fourth degree" burns are based on the characteristics and the surface appearance of the burn wound.

A *partial-thickness burn* is a wound that has the ability to heal without grafting. Because only part of the skin has been damaged or destroyed, enough epithelial cells remain in the skin to provide new epidermis, which includes hair follicles and sweat glands. The partial-thickness burn can also be referred to as a first or second degree burn. Partial-thickness burns can be divided into three categories: (1) *superficial*

burns, in which there is partial skin loss but no dermal death and, therefore, no slough forms; (2) *intermediate partial-thickness burn,* characterized typically by healing from the level of the hair follicles; and (3) *deep partial-thickness burn,* which heals typically from the level of the sweat ducts. A *deep dermal burn* is a partial-thickness burn that can heal without grafting. However, if it is complicated by infection or mechanical trauma, it is likely to be converted into a full-thickness burn.

Full-thickness burns cause all the skin to be destroyed. No viable epithelial elements are present, and there may be destruction of the subcutaneous tissue, muscles, and bones. The wound must be grafted, as the skin will not regenerate. The full-thickness burn is equivalent to the *third degree burn.* When the destruction of the full-thickness burn extends to the structures underneath the skin to include the bone, it can be called a *fourth degree burn.*

REFERENCES

1. Boswick, J., Thompson, J., and Kershner, C.: Critical care of the burned patient. Anesthesiology, 47:164–170, 1977.
2. Guyton, A.: Textbook of Medical Physiology. 7th ed. Philadelphia, W. B. Saunders Co., 1986.
3. Moncrief, J.: Burns. N. Engl. J. Med., 288:444–454, 1973.
4. Sabiston, D. (ed.): Textbook of Surgery. 13th ed. Philadelphia, W. B. Saunders Co., 1986.

9

Central Nervous System Anatomy and Physiology

Marie H. Dutton, R.N., M.S.N.

The central nervous system (CNS) is composed of the brain and spinal cord and is exceedingly complex, both anatomically and physiologically, and no structure in the CNS functions in an isolated manner. Neural activity at any level of the CNS always modifies or is modified by influences from other parts of the system. This accounts for the unique nature and extreme complexity of the CNS, much of which remains to be clearly understood.

The central nervous system is affected not only by surgery carried out on it directly but also by regional and general anesthetics. Hence, most patients in the post anesthesia care unit (PACU) are experiencing some alteration in CNS function. Consequently, it is important for the PACU nurse to have an understanding of some of the basic anatomic and physiologic principles that are operative in the central nervous system.

Definitions

Afferent: carrying sensory impulses toward the brain.

Autoregulation: an alteration of the diameter of the resistance vessels to maintain a constant perfusion pressure during changes in blood flow.

Cistern: a reservoir or cavity.

Commissure: white or gray matter that crosses over in the midline and connects one side of the brain or spinal cord with the other.

Decussate: commonly refers to crossing of parts.

Dorsal: posterior.

Efferent: carrying motor impulses away from the brain.

Estrus: the cycle of changes in the female genital tract produced as a result of ovarian hormonal activity.

Inferior: beneath. Also used to indicate the lower portion of an anatomic part.

Lower motor neurons: The neurons of the spine and cranium that directly innervate the muscles (e.g., those found in the anterior horns or anterior roots of the gray matter of the spinal cord).

Metabolic regulation: a change in blood flow in response to the metabolic requirements of tissues.

Neuroglia: the supporting structure of nervous tissue, consisting of a fine web of tissue made up of modified ectodermic elements. It encloses branched cells known as neuroglia cells, or glia cells, but lacks nerve fibers itself. It performs less specialized functions of the nerve network.

Plexus: a network of nerves.

Postural reflexes: reflexes that are basically proprioceptive, being concerned with the position of the head in relation to the trunk and with adjustments of the extremities and eyes to the position of the head.

Proprioception: the awareness of posture, movement, and changes in equilibrium.

Ramus (rami): primary division of a nerve.

Righting reflexes: reflexes that maintain the head in an upright position in relation to the environment, through the utilization of the eyes, inner ears, and muscles of the neck and trunk.

Upper motor neurons: The neurons in the brain and spinal cord that activate the motor system (e.g., the descending fibers of the pyramidal and extrapyramidal tracts).

Ventral: anterior.

THE BRAIN

The human brain serves both structurally and functionally as the primary center for control and regulation of all nervous system functions. As such, it is the highest level of control and integration of sensory and motor information in the entire body.

The *brain (encephalon)* is divided into three large areas based on its embryologic development. The *forebrain (proencephalon)* contains the *cerebrum* with its hemispheres and the *diencephalon*. The *midbrain (mesencephalon)* contains the *cerebral peduncles*, the *corpora quadrigemina*, and the *cerebral aqueduct*. The *hindbrain (rhombencephalon)* consists of the *medulla oblongata*, the *pons*, the *cerebellum*, and the *fourth ventricle*.

The Cerebrum

The cerebrum is the largest part of the brain. It fills the entire upper portion of the cranial cavity and consists of billions of neurons that synapse to form a complex network of neural pathways.

The cerebrum consists of two hemispheres interconnected only by a large band of white fiber tracts known as the *corpus callosum*. Each hemisphere is further subdivided into four lobes corresponding in name to the overlying bones of the cranium. These are the *frontal, parietal, temporal,* and *occipital lobes*. Both hemispheres consist of an *external cortex* of gray matter, the underlying *white matter tracts,* and the *basal ganglia (cerebral nuclei)*. Each hemisphere also contains a *lateral ventricle*, which is an elongated cavity concerned with the formation and circulation of cerebrospinal fluid.

The Cerebral Cortex

The cerebral cortex has an elaborate mantle of *gray matter* and is the most highly integrated area in the nervous system. It is arranged in a series of folds dipping down into the underlying regions. These folds greatly expand the surface area of the gray matter within the limited confines of the skull. Each fold is known as a *convolution* or *gyrus*. Deeper grooves exist between these convolutions. A shallow one is known as a *sulcus*, while a deeper one is known as a *fissure*.

The cerebral hemispheres are separated from each other by the *longitudinal fissure* anteroposteriorly. The *transverse fissure* separates the cerebrum from the cerebellum beneath it.

Each hemisphere has three sulci between the lobes. The *central sulcus* (also known as the fissure of Rolando) separates the frontal and parietal lobes. The *lateral sulcus* (fissure of Sylvius) lies between the frontal and parietal lobes above and the temporal lobe below. The small *parieto-occipital sulcus* is located between its corresponding lobes (Figs. 9–1 and 9–2).

The *white matter* of the cerebrum is situated below the cortex and is composed of three main groups of myelinated nerve fibers arranged in related bundles or tracts. The *commissural neurons* transmit impulses between the hemispheres. The largest of

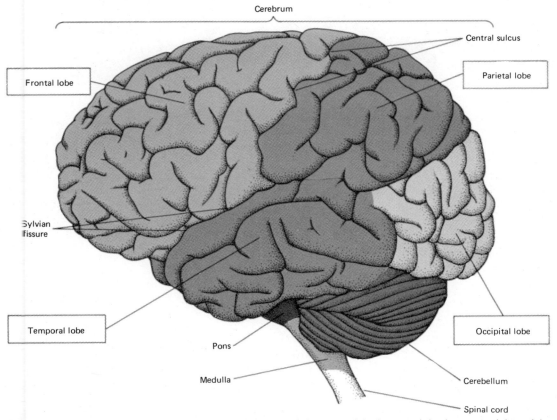

Figure 9–1. Left lateral view of the brain, showing the principal divisions of the brain and the four major lobes of the cerebrum.

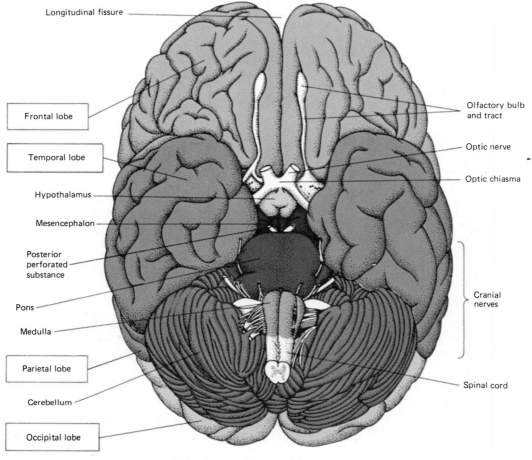

Longitudinal fissure

Frontal lobe

Temporal lobe

Hypothalamus

Mesencephalon

Posterior perforated substance

Pons

Medulla

Parietal lobe

Cerebellum

Occipital lobe

Olfactory bulb and tract

Optic nerve

Optic chiasma

Cranial nerves

Spinal cord

Figure 9–2. Basal view of the brain.

these is the corpus callosum. The *projection fibers* ascend and descend to transmit impulses from one level of the CNS to another. A notable example is the internal capsule that surrounds most of the basal ganglia and connects the thalamus and the cerebral cortex. The *association fibers* disseminate impulses from one part of the cortex to another within the same hemisphere.

The Basal Ganglia (Cerebral Nuclei)

A cerebral nucleus is a group of neuron cell bodies lying within the CNS. Four of these deep-lying masses of gray matter are located within the white matter of each hemisphere and are collectively known as the *basal ganglia* (Fig. 9–3). These are the *caudate nucleus*, the *lentiform nucleus*, the *amygdaloid body*, and the *claustrum*. Together, they exert a steadying influence on muscle activity. Along with that portion of the internal capsule that lies between them, the caudate and lentiform nuclei compose the *corpus striatum*, the most significant functional unit of the basal ganglia. The basal ganglia are an important part of the extrapyramidal motor pathway connecting nuclei with each other, with the cortex, and with the spinal cord. The ganglia also connect with areas in the hindbrain (the red nucleus and the substantia nigra) to assist in carrying out their role in smoothing and coordinating muscle movements. Disturbances in these ganglia result in tremor, rigidity, and loss of expressive and walking movements, as seen in *Parkinson's syndrome*.

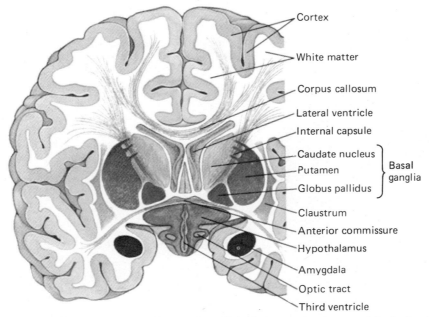

Figure 9–3. A coronal section of the cerebrum in front of the thalamus, showing especially the basal ganglia.

Functional Aspects of the Cerebrum

Nearly every portion of the cerebral cortex is connected with subcortical centers, and there are no areas in the cortex that are exclusively motor (expressive) or exclusively sensory (receptive) in nature. However, there are some regions that are primarily concerned with the expressive phase of cortical functioning and others that are primarily receptive in nature. The activities of these areas are integrated by association fibers that compose the remainder of the cerebral cortex. Association fibers play important roles in complex intellectual and emotional processes.

Motor Areas

There is no single area of motor control within the brain, because the integration and control of muscle activity is dependent upon the harmonious activities of several areas, including the cerebral cortex, the basal ganglia, and the cerebellum.

The Primary Motor Area

The primary motor area of the cerebral cortex is located in the precentral gyrus of the frontal lobe, just anterior to the central sulcus, and is concerned mainly with the voluntary initiation of finely controlled movements, such as those of the hands, fingers, lips, tongue, and vocal cords. Skeletal muscles responsible for these discrete movements are largely represented by neurons in the motor cortex. Muscles of the arms, legs, and trunk are served by a comparatively small group of neurons, so that this part of the motor cortex controls larger groups of muscles and produces grosser movements (Fig. 9–4).

The axons of the pyramidal cell bodies in the primary motor area descend through the internal capsule, midbrain, and pons to the medulla, where the majority of them decussate, or cross, to the opposite side and continue down into the spinal cord, where they are known as the *crossed pyramidal* or *lateral corticospinal tracts*. Fibers that have not crossed are known as the *uncrossed pyramidal* or *ventral corticospinal tracts*. Most of these eventually do decussate at lower levels within the cord. Pyramidal cell axons also connect within the brain with the basal ganglia, the brainstem, and the cerebellum. All of the complex connections of the py-

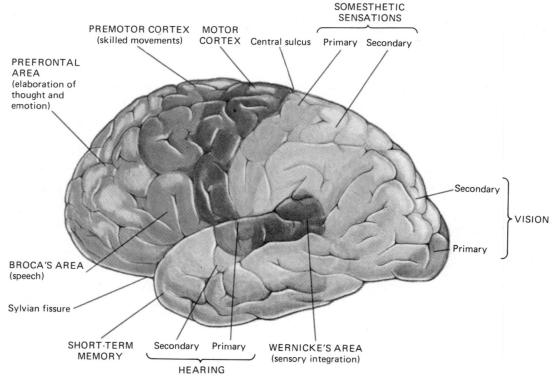

Figure 9–4. The functional areas of the cerebral cortex.

ramidal cells play important roles in the overall coordination and control of skeletal muscle activity.

The Premotor Area

The premotor area of each hemisphere is located in the cortex immediately anterior to the precentral gyrus in the frontal lobe. On the whole, it is concerned with movement of the opposite side of the body, especially with control and coordination of skilled movements of a complex nature. In addition to its subcortical connections with the primary motor area, its neurons also have direct connections with the basal ganglia and related nuclei in the brainstem, for example, the reticular formation. Many of the axons from these subcortical centers cross to the opposite side before descending as *extrapyramidal tracts* in the spinal cord. Collectively, the connections from the premotor area to these related nuclei make up the extrapyramidal system, which coordinates gross skeletal muscle activities that

are largely automatic in nature. Examples are postural adjustments, chewing, swallowing, gesticulating, and associated movements that accompany voluntary activities. Certain portions of the extrapyramidal tract also have an inhibitory effect on spontaneous movements initiated by the cerebral cortex. They serve to prevent tremors and rigidity. Complete structural and functional separation of the pyramidal and extrapyramidal systems is impossible, as they are so closely connected in the harmonious work of executing complex coordinated movements (Fig. 9–3).

Of interest to the PACU nurse is that drugs used to produce neuroleptanesthesia can cause extrapyramidal reactions. More specifically, the neuroleptics such as the phenothiazines, of which chlorpromazine (Thorazine) is the prototype drug, and the butyrophenones, as typified by droperidol (Inapsine) and haloperidol (Haldol), are known to produce extrapyramidal reactions. There are four varieties of extrapyramidal reactions. They are drug-induced parkinsonism, akathisia, acute dystonic reactions, and tardive dyskinesia.

Drug-induced parkinsonism, which can occur from one to five days after the administration of the neuroleptic drug, is typified by a generalized slowing of automatic and spontaneous movements (bradykinesia), with a mask-like facial expression and a reduction in arm movements. The most noticeable signs of the drug-induced parkinsonism syndrome are rigidity and oscillatory tremor at rest. Treatment is with antiparkinsonian agents such as levodopa (Larodopa), trihexyphenidyl (Artane), and benztropine (Cogentin). *Akathisia,* which can occur 5 to 60 days after the administration of a neuroleptic drug, is a term that refers to a subjective feeling of restlessness accompanied by a need on the part of the patient to move about and to pace back and forth. Treatment requires a reduction in the dose of the offending drug. *Acute dystonic reactions* can occur after the administration of some psychotropic drugs and are characterized by torsion spasms such as facial grimacing and torticollis. These reactions are occasionally seen when a phenothiazine is first administered and are associated with oculogyric crises. Acute dystonic reactions can be mistaken for hysterical reactions or seizures and can usually be reversed by anticholinergic antiparkinsonian drugs such as benztropine (Cogentin) or trihexyphenidyl (Artane). *Tardive dyskinesia* is a late-appearing neurologic syndrome and is characterized by stereotypical involuntary rapid and rhythmically repetitive movements, such as continual chewing movements, and darting movements of the tongue. Treatment is not always satisfactory, as antiparkinsonian drugs sometimes exacerbate tardive dyskinesia. Tardive dyskinesia often persists despite discontinuation of the offending drug.

Two important structural aspects of the premotor area are worth noting for those caring for neurosurgical patients. The first is that fibers from both the primary motor and the premotor areas are funnelled through the narrow *internal capsule* as they descend to lower areas of the CNS. This is significant because the internal capsule is a frequent site of cerebrovascular accidents (CVAs). The second is that lesions within one side of the internal capsule will result in paralysis of the skeletal muscles on the opposite side of the body, owing to the crossing of fibers within the medulla.

The Motor Speech Area

The motor speech area is only one point in the complicated network required to form spoken and written words. It lies at the base of the motor area and slightly anterior to it in the inferior frontal gyrus and is also known as Broca's area. In right-handed individuals (the majority) the language and speech areas are usually located in the left hemisphere. In those who are left-handed, these areas may lie within the right or the left hemisphere.

The Prefrontal Area

The prefrontal area of the frontal lobe lies anterior to the premotor area. It has extensive connections with other cortical areas and is believed to play an important role in complex intellectual activities such as mathematical and philosophic reasoning, abstract and creative thinking, learning, judgment and volition, and social, moral, and ethical values. The prefrontal area also influences certain autonomic functions of the body through the conduction of impulses directly or indirectly through the thalamus to the hypothalamus, which makes possible certain physiologic responses to feelings such as anger, fear, and lust.

Sensory Areas

Sensory information from one side of the body is received by the *general sensory (or somasthetic) area* of the opposite hemisphere. It is located in the parietal lobe in the area of the postcentral gyrus. Crude sensations of pain, temperature, and touch can be experienced at the level of the thalamus, but true discrimination of these sensations is a function of the parietal cortex. The activities of the general sensory area allow for proprioception; for the recognition of the size, shape, and texture of objects; and for the comparison of stimuli as to intensity and location.

The *auditory area* lies in the cortex of the superior temporal lobe. Each hemisphere receives impulses from both ears. The *visual area* is located in the posterior occipital lobe, where extremely complex transformations in the signals conveyed by the optic nerve occur. The right occipital cortex receives impulses from the right half of each eye, and the left occipital cortex receives impulses from the left half of each eye. It is believed that the *olfactory area* (sense of smell) is located in the medial temporal lobe and that the *gustatory area* (sense of taste) is located nearby at the base of the postcentral gyrus.

The Association Areas

Large areas of the cortex remain for which no discrete function is known. They are referred to as association areas. They play a major role in the integration of the sensory and motor phases of cortical function by providing complex connections between them.

The Limbic System

The principal structural and functional units of the limbic system are the two rings of limbic cortex and a number of related subcortical nuclei, the anterior thalamic nuclei, and portions of the basal nuclei (Fig. 9–5). The terms limbic system, limbic lobe, and rhinencephalon are often used interchangeably. Generally speaking, the limbic system is concerned with a wide variety of autonomic somatosensory and somatomotor responses, especially those involved with emotional states and other behavioral responses.

The limbic system, acting in close concert with the hypothalamus, can evoke a wide variety of autonomic responses, including changes in heart rate, blood pressure, and respiratory rate. It plays an intimate role in the genesis of emotional states, particularly anxiety, fear, and aggression. Stimulation of the limbic system also evokes complex motor responses directly related to feeding behavior. It has been demonstrated that the limbic system has major relationships with the reticular formation of the brainstem and is presumed to have a role in the alerting or arousal process. It is also implicated in the hypothalamic regulation of pituitary ac-

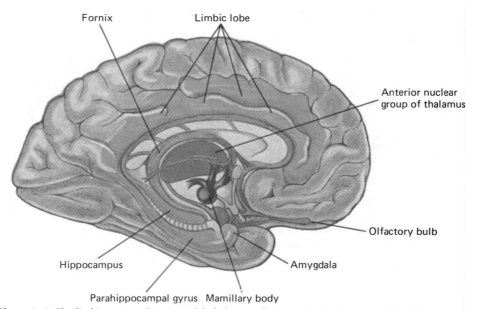

Figure 9–5. The limbic system. Structures labeled generally considered to be part of the limbic system.

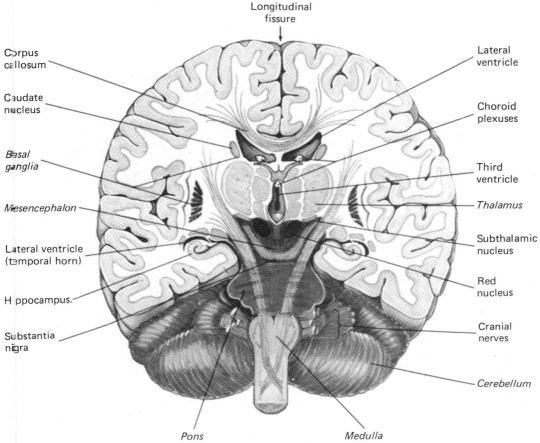

Figure 9–6. A coronal view of the cerebrum looking from anteriorly backward. This section was made immediately anterior to the lower brain stem and through the middle of the thalamus.

tivity. It may be associated somehow with the memory process for recent events as well. In addition, it is intimately concerned with such complex phenomena as the control of various biologic rhythms, sexual behavior, and motivation.

The Diencephalon

The second major division of the forebrain is the diencephalon (Fig. 9–6). It consists of the thalamus, the epithalamus, the subthalamus, and the hypothalamus. The diencephalon also contains the third ventricle and is almost completely covered by the cerebral hemispheres. This portion of the brain has a primary role in sleep, emotion, thermoregulation, autonomic activity, and endocrine control of ongoing behavioral patterns.

The *thalamus* consists of right and left egg-shaped masses that make up the greatest bulk of the diencephalon and form the lateral wall of the third ventricle. Each thalamus serves as a relay center for all incoming sensory stimuli except taste and smell. These impulses are then grouped and transmitted to the appropriate area of the cerebral cortex. Because of its interconnections with the hypothalamus, the limbic system, and the frontal, temporal, and parietal lobes, this structure is also integrally involved with emotional activities, instinctive responses, and attentive processes.

The *epithalamus* contains the pineal body (or gland), which is known to secrete melatonin. Melatonin inhibits gonadal development and regulates estrus. Its most important function is to slow maturation. It is believed that melatonin has its greatest effect on brain tissue rather than on the gonads themselves.

Situated below the thalamus and above the midbrain, the *subthalamus* serves as a correlation center for the optic and vestibular impulses. Stimulation of centers in or around the subthalamic nuclei produce the excitation of appropriate patterns of action in the brainstem and spinal cord, which results in rhythmic motions of forward progression necessary in the act of walking. Damage to the subthalamic nuclei on one side is known to cause violent involuntary movements of the limbs of the opposite side of the body, brought about by contractions of their proximal muscles.

The *hypothalamus* is a group of bilateral nuclei that form the floor and part of the lateral walls of the *third ventricle*. Extremely complex in function, it has extensive connections with the autonomic nervous system as well as with other parts of the CNS. It also influences the endocrine system by virtue of direct and indirect connections with the pituitary gland and the release of its own hormones. In association with these other structures, it participates in the regulation of appetite, water balance, carbohydrate and fat metabolism, growth, sexual maturity, body temperature, pulse rate, blood pressure, sleep, and aspects of emotional behavior. Because of the connection of the hypothalamus with the thalamus and cerebral cortex, it is possible for emotions to influence visceral responses on certain occasions.

The Midbrain

The midbrain, or mesencephalon, is a short, narrow segment of nervous tissue connecting the forebrain with the hindbrain (Fig. 9–7). The midbrain is vital as a conduction pathway and as a reflex control center. Passing through the center of the midbrain is the *cerebral aqueduct,* a narrow canal that serves to connect the third ventricle of the diencephalon with the fourth ventricle of the hindbrain for the circulation of cerebrospinal fluid (CSF).

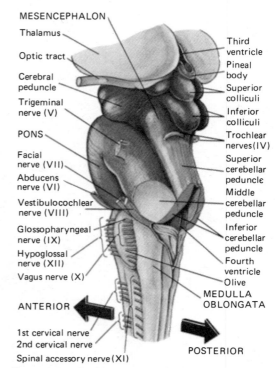

Figure 9–7. The brainstem, including portions of the diencephalon, the midbrain, and the hindbrain.

The *cerebral peduncles* are located in the anterior portion of the midbrain and consist of multiple projectional fibers that connect the cerebral cortex with other structures in the brainstem. Their dorsal aspect (the *tegmentum*) contains the motor nuclei of the oculomotor, trigeminal, and trochlear nerves. The ventral aspect contains the *red nucleus,* a part of the reticular formation, and the origin of a portion of the extrapyramidal system.

The *corpora quadrigemina* is a group of cells divided in the midline and transversely to form four distinct areas or *colliculi*. The inferior colliculi are vital components of the auditory pathway and are responsible for complex acoustic reflexes. The superior colliculi are optic reflex centers.

The centers for postural and righting reflexes are found in the midbrain. The dorsal, or posterior, portion of the midbrain is concerned with visual and auditory reflexes, such as movement of the eyes in accordance with changes in head position, the pupillary light reflex, and turning the head in the direction of a noise. Key structures of the reticular formation also originate in this area. Also, cranial nerves III (oculomotor) and IV (trochlear) originate in the ventral aspect of the midbrain.

The Hindbrain

The hindbrain, or rhombencephalon, consists of the pons, the medulla oblongata, the cerebellum, and the fourth ventricle (Fig. 9–8).

The Pons

Lying in front of the fourth ventricle and separating it from the cerebellum, the pons is literally the bridge between the midbrain and the medulla oblongata. It receives many ascending and descending fibers en route to other points in the CNS. It also contains the motor and sensory nuclei of cranial nerves V (trigeminal), VI (abducens), VII (facial), and VIII (acoustic). The pontine nuclei of the pons are composed of gray matter. White fiber tracts connect the medulla below with the cerebrum above. These

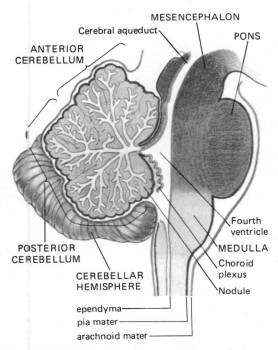

Figure 9–8. Relationship of the cerebellum to the brainstem.

are the so-called *corticospinal tracts*. White fiber (*corticobulbar*) tracts also connect the cerebellum with the pons. The roof of the pons contains a portion of the reticular formation, and the lower pons assists in the regulation of respiration.

The Medulla Oblongata

The medulla oblongata is an expanded continuation of the spinal cord and is located between the foramen magnum and the pons. It is anatomically complex and not usually amenable to surgery. Many of the white fiber tracts between the brain and spinal cord decussate as they pass through the medulla. Centers for many complex reflexes are located in the medulla oblongata and include those for swallowing, vomiting, coughing, and sneezing. The originating nuclei of cranial nerves IX (glossopharyngeal), X (vagus), XI (accessory), and XII (hypoglossal) are found in the medulla oblongata (Table 9–1 and Fig. 9–7). Because of this, the medulla plays an essential role in the regulation of cardiac, respiratory, and vasomotor reflexes. Injuries to the medulla, such as those accompanying basilar skull fracture, frequently prove fatal.

The Cerebellum

Having two hemispheres and a constricted central portion, the cerebellum overlaps the pons and the medulla oblongata dorsally and is located just below the occipital lobes of the cerebrum. It is separated from the cerebrum by the tentorium above it and has a two-layered cortex composed of gray matter. Beneath the gray matter are white fiber tracts that extend like branches of a tree to all parts of the cortex. Deep within the white matter are masses of gray matter called the cerebellar nuclei. These connect the cerebellar hemispheres with each other and with areas in the cerebrum, the hindbrain, and the spinal cord.

The cerebellum has no sensory function and does not initiate movement as the cerebrum does. Functionally, it does coordinate muscle tone and voluntary movements through important connections via the spinal cord with the proprioceptor endings

TABLE 9–1. Cranial Nerves and Their Function

Number	Name	Type	Function
I	Olfactory	Sensory	Smell
II	Optic	Sensory	Vision
III	Oculomotor	Mixed—mainly motor	Motion of eye up, in, and down Raising of eyelid Constriction of pupil Accommodation of pupil to distance Proprioceptive impulses
IV	Trochlear	Mixed—mainly motor	Motion of eye down and out Proprioceptive impulses
V	Trigeminal: Ophthalmic branch Maxillary branch Mandibular branch	Mixed	Motor: muscles of mastication Sensory: face, nose, mouth Proprioceptive impulses from teeth sockets and jaw muscles
VI	Abducens	Mixed—mainly motor	Outward motion of eye Proprioception from eye muscles
VII	Facial	Mixed—mostly motor; some sensory and autonomic	Motor: movement of facial muscles, ear, nose, and neck Sensory: taste, anterior two thirds of tongue Autonomic: secretion of saliva, tears
VIII	Acoustic: Cochlear branch Vestibular branch	Sensory	Cochlear: hearing Vestibular: maintenance of equilibrium and posturing of head
IX	Glossopharyngeal	Mixed—motor, sensory, and autonomic	Motor: muscles of swallowing Sensory: taste, posterior third of tongue; sensation from pharynx Autonomic: impulses to parotid glands; decrease blood pressure and pulse
X	Vagus	Mixed—motor, sensory, and autonomic	Motor, sensory, and autonomic information to/from larynx, pharynx, trachea, esophagus, heart, and abdominal viscera
XI	Spinal accessory	Mixed—mostly motor	Cranial portion: motor and sensory information to/from voluntary muscles of pharynx, larynx, and palate (swallowing) Spinal portion: motor information to sternocleidomastoid and trapezius muscles May form components of cardiac branches of vagus
XII	Hypoglossal	Mixed—mostly motor	Motor and sensory information to/from tongue muscles Position sense

in skeletal muscles, tendons, and joints. In addition, the cerebellum is involved in reflexes necessary for the maintenance of equilibrium and posture, through its connections with the vestibular apparatus of the inner ear. The cerebellum also receives optic and acoustic information, but the anatomic pathways involved have not yet been discerned.

Damage to the cerebellum does not result in paralysis or sensory loss. The outcome of damage depends on which portion of the structure is involved. Damage to one part may result in loss of balance, nystagmus, and/or a reeling gait (cerebellar ataxia). Damage to another area can cause disturbances in the postural reflexes. Posterior lobe disturbances result in such changes in voluntary movements as discrepancies in force, direction, and range of movements, lack of precision in movements, and, possibly, intention tremors.

The Fourth Ventricle

The fourth ventricle is a diamond-shaped space between the cerebellum posteriorly and the pons and medulla oblongata anteriorly and contains cerebrospinal fluid.

The Brainstem

There is some disagreement among authors as to what structures collectively constitute the brainstem. All agree that it includes the *midbrain,* the *pons,* and the *medulla oblongata.* Some believe that the *diencephalon* rightly belongs in the group also. Whichever grouping is used, all functions of each structure within it can be considered to be basic activities of the brainstem. Noteworthy is the fact that all of the cranial nerves are attached to the brainstem (if the diencephalon is included), with the exception of the olfactory nerve and the spinal portion of the accessory nerve.

The Reticular Formation

The reticular formation lies within the brainstem (including the diencephalon). An important function of the reticular formation is its action as an intermediary between the upper and lower motor neurons of the extrapyramidal system. In this way it facilitates or augments reflex activity as well as voluntary movements. Its motor neurons can be excitatory or inhibitory in action. For example, by inhibiting extensor muscles it facilitates the action of flexor muscles.

Every pathway that carries information to the brain also contributes afferent fibers to the reticular formation, so that it is kept well informed of conditions both of the outside world and of the internal organs. Efferent impulses leaving the reticular formation travel to the cerebral cortex and to the spinal cord. By virtue of its location in and connections with the brainstem and diencephalon, it participates integrally in their activities.

Another important function of the reticular formation is the activation and regulation of those brain activities related to attention-arousal and consciousness. For this reason it is frequently referred to as the reticular activating system (RAS).

Damage to the reticular formation results in greatly decreased levels of consciousness. When the cerebral cortex is isolated from the RAS by disease or injury of the upper portion of the midbrain, decerebrate rigidity occurs. This abnormal posturing results from the dominant effect of the extensor muscles and a lack of inhibition from opposing motor neurons and flexor muscles. This rigidity is accompanied by a profoundly reduced level of consciousness.

Protection of the Brain

The brain is protected by the cranial bones, the meninges, and the cerebrospinal fluid (CSF) (Figs. 9–9 and 9–10).

The Cranial Bones

There are eight cranial bones that encase the brain, supporting it and protecting it from most ordinary bumps and jarring. In the adult, immovable fibrous joints, or sutures, fuse these bones together to form the rigid walls of the box known as the cranium. The base of the cranium is both thicker and stronger than its roof or walls.

The bones of the cranium are the frontal, right and left parietal, occipital, sphenoid, ethmoid, and right and left temporal bones. The frontal bone forms the anterior roof of the skull and the forehead. Within the frontal bone are the frontal sinuses, which communicate with the nasal cavities. The parietal bones form much of the top and sides of the cranium. The occipital bone forms the back and a large portion of the base of the skull. The two temporal bones are complicated and form part of the sides and a part of the base of the skull. Their inner surfaces are not as smooth and regular as the bones previously mentioned. Parts of the temporal bones articulate with the condyles of the lower jaw, and air cells in the mastoid portions of the temporal bones communicate with the middle ear. The sphenoid bone occupies a central portion of the floor of the skull. It alone articulates with each of the other cranial bones. Its middle portion contains the sphenoid sinuses that open into the nasal cavity. The upper portion of the sphenoid has a marked

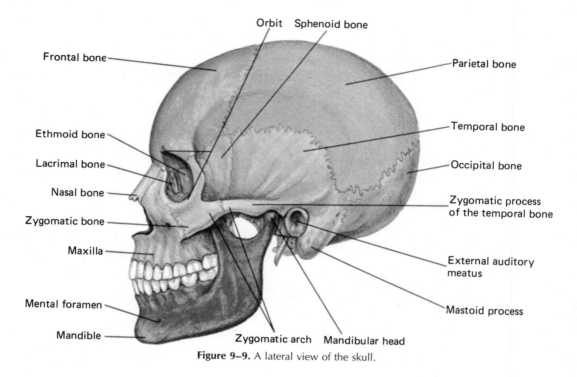

Figure 9–9. A lateral view of the skull.

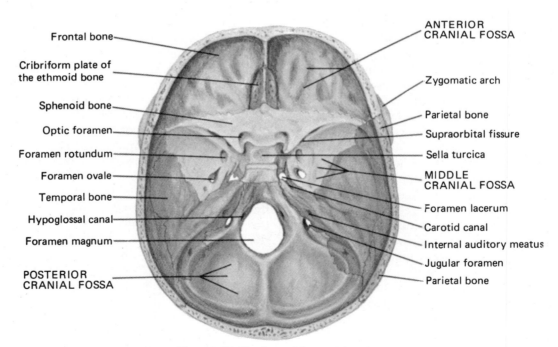

Figure 9–10. The floor of the cranial cavity.

saddle-like depression, the sella turcica, which holds the pituitary gland. The ethmoid bone is light and has a spongy structure. It is located between the orbital cavities. It is a cribriform plate that forms the roof of the nasal cavity and part of the base of the cranium. The ethmoid sinuses open into the nasal cavities.

Several features of the cranial bones are particularly noteworthy for the PACU nurse. Among these are the fact that the air cells in the mastoid portion of the temporal bone can become infected secondary to otitis media or following surgery on the middle or inner ear. This mastoiditis can cause severe complications if it extends through the thin plate of bone that separates it from the cranial meninges. Another point of interest is that surgical access to the pituitary gland is commonly accomplished through the sphenoid bone via the nostrils; one example is trans-sphenoidal hypophysectomy. Lastly, nasal suctioning is absolutely contraindicated in the cranial surgery patient because of the danger of perforating the cribriform plate of the ethmoid bone, which would result in leakage of CSF and would permit direct access to the brain by infectious organisms.

There is one main opening at the base of the skull called the *foramen magnum.* It marks the point at which the brainstem changes structure and becomes identified inferiorly as the spinal cord. Many smaller openings in the skull allow the cranial nerves and some blood vessels to pass through it to and from the face, jaw, and neck. The atlas of the vertebral column (the first cervical vertebra) supports the skull and forms a moveable joint with the occipital bone.

The Meninges

The meninges (Fig. 9–11) are three fibrous membranes between the skull and the brain and between the vertebral column and the spinal cord. The outer membrane is the dura mater, the inner one is the pia mater, and between them lies the arachnoid.

The Dura Mater. The dura mater is a shiny, tough, inelastic membrane that envelops and supports the brain and spinal cord and, by various folds, separates parts of the brain into adjoining compartments. The portion within the skull differs from the dura of the spinal cord in three ways. First, the cranial dura is firmly attached to the skull. The spinal dura has no attachment to the vertebrae. Second, the cranial dura consists of two layers: It not only covers the brain (meningeal dura) but also lines the interior of the skull bones (perios-

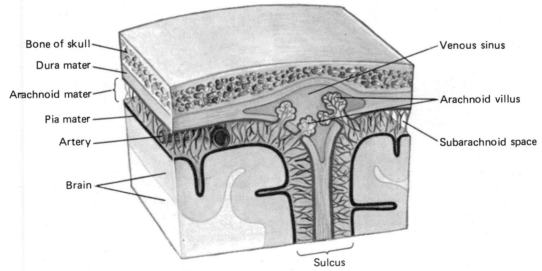

Bone of skull
Dura mater
Arachnoid mater
Pia mater
Artery
Brain
Venous sinus
Arachnoid villus
Subarachnoid space
Sulcus

Figure 9–11. An expanded view of the meninges covering a section of the brain. Note also the venous sinus with arachnoid villi protruding into it.

teal dura). Third, the two layers of the cranial dura are in contact with each other in some places but separate in others where the inner layer dips inward to form the protective partitions between parts of the brain. Also, the spaces or channels formed by these separations of dural layers are filled with venous blood leaving the brain and are called cranial venous sinuses, an elaborate network unique to the brain (Fig. 9–12).

There are three major partitioning folds of the meningeal dura. The falx cerebri separates the right and left hemispheres of the cerebrum. The tentorium cerebelli supports and separates the occipital lobes of the cerebrum from the cerebellum. The falx cerebelli separates the two cerebellar hemispheres. The tentorium separates the posterior cranial chamber from the remainder of the cranial cavity and serves as a line of demarcation for describing the site of a surgical procedure or a lesion as either supratentorial or infratentorial.

Encased between the two dural layers are two major groups of venous channels draining blood from the brain. None of these vascular channels possesses valves, and their walls are extremely thin owing to the absence of muscular tissue. The superior-posterior group consists of one paired and four unpaired sinuses. The anterior-inferior group consist of four paired sinuses and one plexus. The sinuses function to drain venous blood into the internal jugular veins, which are the principal vessels responsible for the return of the blood from the brain to the heart (Fig. 9–13).

The Arachnoid. The arachnoid is a fine membrane between the dura mater and the pia mater. Between the arachnoid and the dura is the subdural space, a noncommunicating space filled with CSF. The cerebral blood vessels traversing this space have

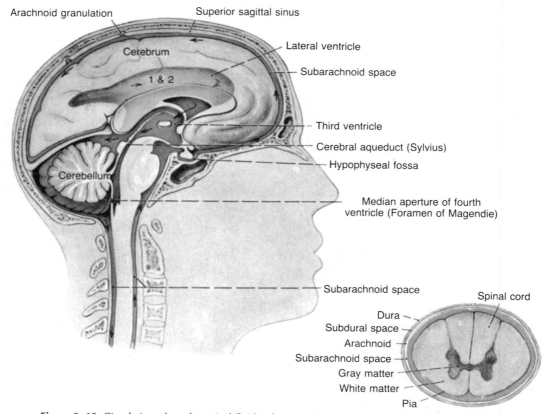

Figure 9–12. Circulation of cerebrospinal fluid in brain and spinal cord. Note superior sagittal sinus.

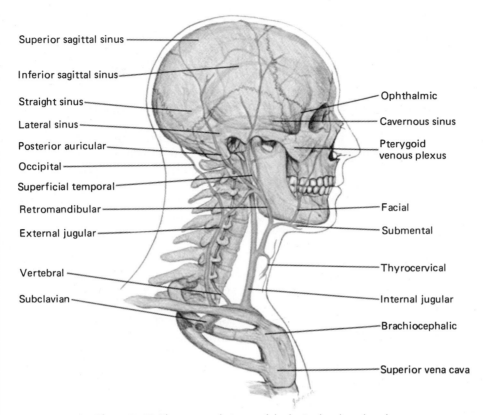

Superior sagittal sinus

Inferior sagittal sinus

Straight sinus

Lateral sinus

Posterior auricular

Occipital

Superficial temporal

Retromandibular

External jugular

Vertebral

Subclavian

Ophthalmic

Cavernous sinus

Pterygoid venous plexus

Facial

Submental

Thyrocervical

Internal jugular

Brachiocephalic

Superior vena cava

Figure 9–13. The venous drainage of the brain, head, and neck.

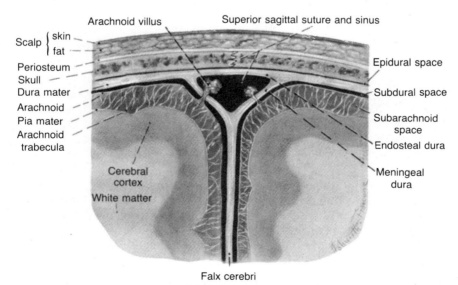

Arachnoid villus

Superior sagittal suture and sinus

Scalp { skin
        { fat

Periosteum

Skull

Dura mater

Arachnoid

Pia mater

Arachnoid trabecula

Cerebral cortex

White matter

Epidural space

Subdural space

Subarachnoid space

Endosteal dura

Meningeal dura

Falx cerebri

Figure 9–14. Coronal section of skull, brain, meninges, and superior sagittal sinus.

little supporting structure, making them particularly vulnerable to insult at this point.

The arachnoid forms a type of roof over the pia mater, to which it is joined by a network of trabeculae in the subarachnoid space. It does not follow the depressions of the surface architecture. The arachnoid sends small tuft-like extensions through the meningeal layer of the dura into the cranial venous sinuses. These are called the *arachnoid granulations* or *arachnoid villi*. The arachnoid villi serve as a pathway for the return of CSF to the venous blood system. Subarachnoid CSF is most abundant in the grooves between the gyri, particularly at the base of the brain, where the more freely communicating compartments form six subarachnoid cisternae, or reservoirs.

The Pia Mater. The inner layer of the meninges, the pia mater, is a very fine membrane rich in blood (choroid) plexuses and mesothelial cells. It is closely associated with the arachnoid and covers the brain intimately, following the invaginations and convolutions of the brain surface. The veins of the brain lie between thread-like trabeculae in the subarachnoid space. Branches of the cortical arteries in the subarachnoid space are carried with the pia mater and enter the brain substance itself (Fig. 9–14).

The Cerebrospinal Fluid System

The cerebrospinal fluid is a clear, colorless, watery fluid with a specific gravity of 1.007. A principal function of this fluid is to act as a cushion for the brain. Since both brain tissue and CSF have essentially the same specific gravity, the brain literally floats within the skull. CSF also serves as a medium for the exchange of nutrients and waste products between the bloodstream and the cells of the CNS.

Cerebrospinal fluid is found within the ventricles of the brain, in the cisterns surrounding it, and in the subarachnoid spaces of both the brain and the spinal cord. Largest of the cisterns is the *cisterna magna,* located beneath and behind the cerebellum (Figs. 9–15 and 9–16).

Although some CSF is formed by filtration through capillary walls throughout the brain's vascular bed, its primary site of formation is in the choroid plexuses within the ventricles. This is achieved by a system of secretion and diffusion. The choroid plexuses are highly vascular tufted structures composed of many small granular pouches that project into the ventricles of the brain. CSF is formed continuously and reabsorbed at a rate of approximately 750 ml per day. The net pressure of the CSF is regulated, in part, by a balance between formation and reabsorption.

The four ventricles of the brain communicate directly with each other. The first and second (lateral) ventricles are elongated cavities that lie within the cerebral hemispheres. The third ventricle is a slit-like cavity beneath and between the two lateral ventricles. The fourth ventricle is a diamond-shaped space between the cerebellum posteriorly and the pons and medulla oblongata anteriorly.

The circulation of cerebrospinal fluid is as follows: Each lateral ventricle contains a large choroid plexus that forms CSF. From the lateral ventricles, the fluid passes through an interventricular foramen (foramen of Monro) into the third ventricle. Together with the additional fluid formed there, the CSF travels posteriorly through the cerebral aqueduct (aqueduct of Sylvius) into the fourth ventricle, where more fluid is produced. The combined CSF volumes then pass through three openings leading from the fourth ventricle to the cranial subarachnoid space of the cisterna magna. These openings are the two lateral foramina of Luschka and the medial foramen of Magendie. From the cisterna magna, CSF flows freely within the entire subarachnoid space of the brain and spinal cord.

The main route of reabsorption of excess CSF is through the arachnoid villi that project from the subarachnoid spaces into the venous sinuses of the brain, particularly those of the superior sagittal sinus. The arachnoid villi provide highly permeable regions that allow free passage of CSF, including protein molecules and some small

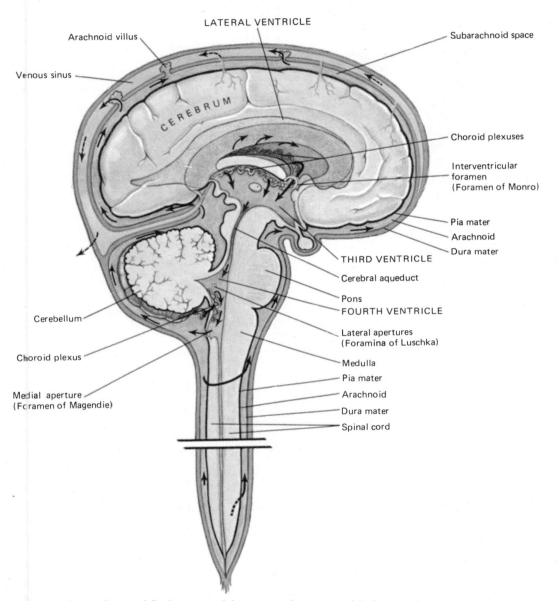

Figure 9–15. The cerebrospinal fluid system and the meningeal coverings of the brain and cord. Note the directions of flow of cerebrospinal fluid indicated by the arrows.

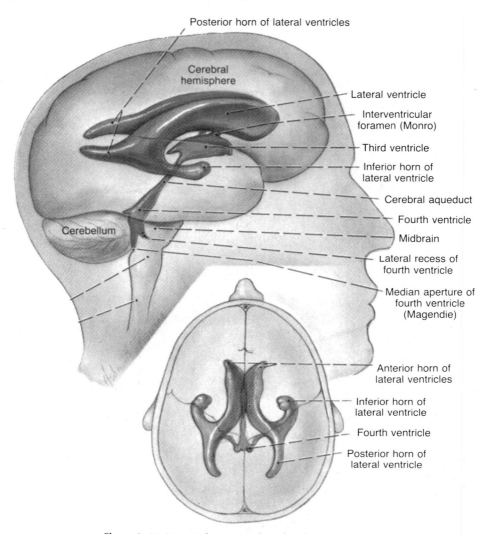

Figure 9–16. Ventricular system, lateral and superior views.

particulate matter contained within it. It is believed that the process of osmosis is mainly responsible for the reabsorption of the fluid.

Blood-Brain and Blood-CSF Barriers of the CNS

Throughout the body, the constancy of the composition of the extracellular fluid is maintained by multiple homeostatic mechanisms. Because of the exquisite sensitivity of the neurons of the central nervous system, additional mechanisms are necessary to prevent the far-reaching consequences that even minor fluctuations in their chemical environment would cause. In health,

the unique blood-brain and blood-CSF barriers present in most regions of the CNS have evolved to accomplish this task. The development of the blood-brain barrier occurs gradually during the first several years of childhood.

The site of the blood-brain barrier is *not* at the surface of the neurons themselves. Rather, it is located between the plasma within the capillaries and the extracellular space of the brain. It is generally believed that the exchange of many physiologically important substances within the capillaries of the CNS is slowed or practically prohibited by several anatomic factors, rather than by any one alone. It is also likely that these structures form a sequence of morphologic barriers acting in concert to prevent the rapid transport of substances from the blood to the nervous tissue. These include the tight intercellular junctions between the epithelial cells of the capillaries that appear to effectively reduce permeability. There is also a substantial basement membrane surrounding the capillaries and an external membrane provided by the end-feet of the astrocytes between the neurons and the capillaries. These appear to have a major role in retarding or preventing the passage of foreign substances into the brain tissue.

Despite the uncertainty as to the ultimate site of the blood-brain barrier, it has been firmly established that the rapidity with which substances penetrate brain tissue is inversely related to their molecular size and directly related to their lipid solubility. Only water, carbon dioxide, and oxygen cross the blood-brain barrier rapidly and readily, whereas glucose crosses more slowly and by a facilitated transport mechanism. Water-soluble compounds, electrolytes, and protein molecules generally cross very slowly. Most general anesthetics effectively cross the blood-brain barrier because of their high lipid solubility.

Of critical clinical importance is the fact that the effectiveness of the blocking mechanism of the blood-brain barrier can break down in areas of the brain that are infected, traumatized, irradiated, or contain tumors. It is also important to note that, as effective as the blood-brain barrier is, no substance is completely excluded from reaching the central neurons. Instead, it is the *rate* of transport of substances through the barrier that is of major significance in maintaining the constancy of the internal environment of the brain.

There are a limited number of structures in the brain that have unique capillaries and that are not restricted by the blood-brain barrier. These organs appear to function as chemoreceptors and, as such, must be in intimate contact with the chemical substances within the blood. The posterior pituitary is one of these structures. The blood-CSF barrier is located at the choroid plexus.

As in the case of the blood-brain barrier, the rate of transport of substances across the blood-CSF barrier is controlled by molecular size and lipid solubility.

The routes whereby substances leave the CSF are different from those by which they enter. They may leave rapidly via the arachnoid villi regardless of their molecular size or lipid solubility. Alternatively, the bulk circulation of the CSF throughout the brain enhances the direct removal of certain lipid-soluble substances across the blood-brain barrier.

The Arterial Blood Supply to the Brain

The entire arterial blood supply to the brain, with the exception of a small amount that flows in the anterior spinal artery to the medulla, is carried through the neck by four vessels—the two *vertebral arteries,* and the two *carotid arteries* (Figs. 9–17 and 9–18).

The two vertebral arteries supply the posterior portion of the brain. They ascend in the neck through the transverse foramina on each side of the cervical vertebrae, enter the skull through the foramen magnum, and anastomose near the pons to form the *basilar artery* of the hindbrain. A relatively small volume of the total blood flow to the brain is carried by the vertebral or basilar arteries. The *circle of Willis* in turn is formed by the union of the basilar artery and the two internal carotids. Before they join the circle of Willis, these arteries send essential branches to the brainstem, cerebellum, and falx cerebelli.

The circle of Willis is a ring of blood vessels that surrounds the optic chiasm and the pituitary stalk. Three pairs of large arterial vessels that supply the cerebral cortex originate from the circle of Willis. They are the anterior, the middle, and the posterior cerebral arteries. Each supplies specific areas of the brain.

The anterior cerebral arteries supply about half of the frontal and parietal lobes, including much of the corpus callosum. The middle cerebral arteries perfuse most of the

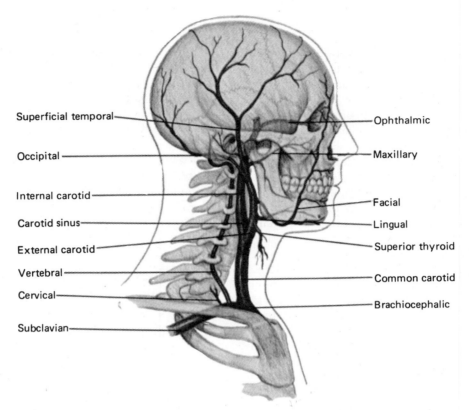

Figure 9–17. The arterial supply of the neck and head.

Superficial temporal
Occipital
Internal carotid
Carotid sinus
External carotid
Vertebral
Cervical
Subclavian

Ophthalmic
Maxillary
Facial
Lingual
Superior thyroid
Common carotid
Brachiocephalic

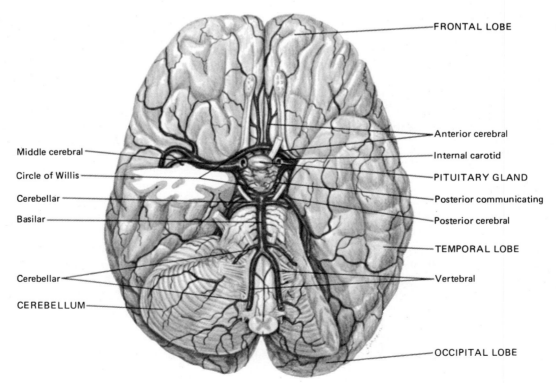

Figure 9–18. The arteries of the brain.

Middle cerebral
Circle of Willis
Cerebellar
Basilar
Cerebellar
CEREBELLUM

FRONTAL LOBE
Anterior cerebral
Internal carotid
PITUITARY GLAND
Posterior communicating
Posterior cerebral
TEMPORAL LOBE
Vertebral
OCCIPITAL LOBE

lateral surfaces of the hemispheres and send off branches to the corpus striatum and the internal capsule. The posterior cerebral arteries supply the occipital lobes and the remaining portions of the temporal lobes that are not supplied by the middle cerebral arteries.

Intracranial Pressure Dynamics

Intracranial pressure (ICP) is that pressure exerted against the skull by its contents: cerebrospinal fluid, blood, and brain. The volumes of these may fluctuate slightly, but, despite variations, the total volume and intracranial pressure remain nearly constant. Compensatory mechanisms account for this stability of the overall intracranial pressure.

In health, the cerebrospinal fluid pressure system is a dynamic one, allowing the pressure to vary only slightly by means of a compensatory mechanism that shunts CSF into the spinal subarachnoid space. The spinal dura covers the cord loosely and does not adhere to the vertebrae, which allows it to expand, whereas the cranial dura cannot. When CSF pressure becomes too great within the cranium, owing to an increase in volume of any of its contents, CSF is shunted out of the cranium, decreasing cranial volume and CSF pressure. In addition, CSF may be absorbed at an increased rate, which further aids in maintaining normal pressure.

Autoregulation of cerebral blood volume is another compensatory mechanism responsible for maintaining cerebral perfusion pressure (CPP) at a constant level. It is an alteration of the diameter of the resistance vessels aimed at maintaining a constant perfusion pressure during changes in blood flow. When autoregulation is intact, vaso-

dilation occurs in response to moderate degrees of hypercapnia, hypoxia, hyperthermia, and raised ICP. The normal ICP ranges from 4 to 15 mm Hg. Normal CPP is 80 to 90 mm Hg.

Under normal conditions, CPP and resultant blood flow are determined by the difference between the inflow pressures and the outflow pressures. Inflow pressures are represented by the mean systemic arterial pressure (MSAP), and under normal conditions the mean outflow pressure is equivalent to the mean venous pressure. In situations in which ICP is greater than venous pressure,

$$CPP = MSAP - ICP$$

It is readily apparent that any increase in ICP or reduction in MSAP will reduce cerebral perfusion pressure and the resulting cerebral blood flow.

Autoregulation is capable of maintaining a constant CPP only until the finite limit of CSF compensation is reached (Fig. 9–19). The spinal subarachnoid space is capable of holding only a limited amount of fluid and, despite its inability to hold any additional displaced fluid, autoregulation continues. In this event, autoregulation ceases to be beneficial or effective in preventing further increases in intracranial pressure.

THE SPINAL CORD

Protection of the Spinal Cord

The Bones of the Spine

The spine is composed of a series of irregular bony vertebrae "stacked" one atop the other to form a strong but flexible column. They are joined by a series of ligaments and intervening cartilages and have

Figure 9–19. CSF shunting and autoregulation as effective compensatory mechanisms. ICP = intracranial pressure; CPP = cerebral perfusion pressure; CSF = cerebrospinal fluid.

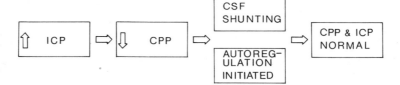

two primary functions. Together these structures support the head and trunk. The spine also protects the spinal cord and its 31 pairs of spinal nerve roots by encasing them in a long canal formed by openings in the center of each vertebra. This vertebral canal extends the entire length of the spine and conforms to the various spinal curvatures as well as to the variations in size of the spinal cord itself.

There are 7 cervical, 12 thoracic, and 5 lumbar vertebrae. In the adult, the sacrum consists of 5 vertebrae fused to form one bone. Similarly, the coccyx results from the fusion of four or five rudimentary vertebrae.

Despite variations in their structure, all but two vertebrae share certain anatomic and functional aspects. With the exception of the first and second cervical vertebrae, all have a solid drum-shaped *body* anteriorly that serves as the weight-bearing segment. The posterior segment of the vertebra is called the *arch*, and each one consists of two pedicles, two laminae, and seven processes (four articular, two transverse, and one spinous). Projecting from the upper part of the body of each vertebra are a pair of short, thick *pedicles*. The concavities above and below the pedicles are the four *intervertebral notches*. When the vertebrae are articulated, the notches of each adjacent pair of bones form the oval *intervertebral foramina*, which communicate with the vertebral canal and transmit the spinal nerves and blood vessels.

Arising from the pedicles are two broad plates of bone, the *laminae*, which meet and fuse at the midline posteriorly to form an arch. Projecting backward and downward from this junction is the *spinous process*, a knobby projection easily palpated under the skin of the back. Lateral to the laminae, near their junction with the pedicles, are paired *articular processes*, which facilitate movement of the vertebral column. The two superior processes of each vertebra articulate with the inferior processes of the vertebra immediately above it. The small surfaces where they articulate are called *facets*. The *transverse processes* are located somewhat anterior to the junction of the pedicles

and the laminae. They are between the superior and inferior articular processes. These and the spinous processes provide sites for the attachment of muscles and ligaments. The hollow opening formed by the body of the vertebra and the arch is termed the *vertebral foramen*, a protected space through which the spinal cord passes.

Between each of the vertebrae and atop the sacrum is an *intervertebral disc* composed of compressible, tough, fibrous cartilage concentrically arranged around a soft, pulpy substance called the *nucleus pulposus*. Each disc acts as a cushion-like shock absorber between vertebrae. When the intervertebral disk is ruptured, the soft nucleus pulposus may protrude into the vertebral canal, where it can exert pressure on a spinal nerve root, causing disturbances in motor and sensory function. This herniated nucleus pulposus (HNP) may require surgical excision through a laminectomy, if the herniation is severe enough.

Many important variations exist among the regional vertebrae. For example, the first cervical vertebra, or *atlas*, is ring-shaped and supports the cranium. It has no body or spinous process and allows for nodding motion of the head. The second cervical vertebra, or *axis*, is most striking because of the *odontoid process*, or *dens*, that arises perpendicularly to articulate with the atlas and allows rotation of the head. The cervical spine as a whole is extremely mobile and is therefore particularly susceptible to acceleration-deceleration and torsion injuries that hyperflex or hyperextend the neck. Also, the spinal cord is relatively large in this area and therefore sustains damage fairly easily after injury to the cervical spine (Fig. 9–20).

The 12 thoracic vertebrae increase in size as they approach the lumbar area. They are distinctive in that they have facets on their transverse processes and bodies for articulation with the ribs. The thoracic spine is fixed by the ribs but the lumbar spine is not. This creates a vulnerability that is responsible for an increased incidence of fracture-dislocations at the twelfth thoracic and the first and second lumbar vertebrae.

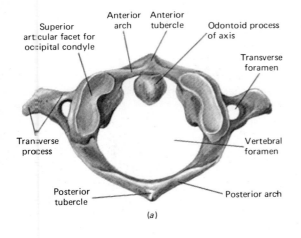

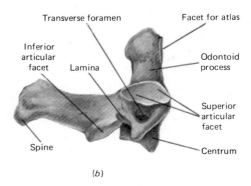

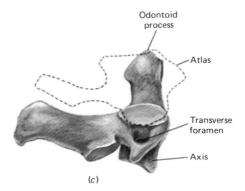

Figure 9–20. (a) Superior view of the atlas. (b) Lateral view of the axis. (c) How the atlas and axis articulate.

These injuries are typically found in motor vehicle accident victims who had been wearing lap seatbelts without shoulder restraints.

The five lumbar vertebrae are large and massive because of their prominent role in weight bearing. They have no transverse foramina. The sacrum, with its five fused vertebrae, is large, triangular, and wedge-shaped. It forms the posterior wall of the pelvis and articulates with the fifth lumbar vertebra, the coccyx, and the iliac portions of the hips. The triangular coccyx is formed by four small segments of bone, the most rudimentary part of the vertebral column.

The Spinal Meninges

In addition to the bony vertebral column, the spinal cord is covered and protected by the continuous downward projection of the three meninges that perform the same protective function for the brain. The dura mater is the outermost membrane, a strong but loose and expandable sheath of dense fibrous connective tissue that ends in a blind sac at the end of the second or third segment of the sacrum, and protects the cord and the spinal nerve roots as they leave the cord. The dura does not extend beyond the intervertebral foramina. In contrast to the cranial dura, the spinal dura is not attached to the surrounding bone, consists of only one layer, and does not send partitions into the fissures of the cord.

The *epidural space* is located between the outer surface of the dura and the bones of the vertebral canal. It contains a quantity of loose areolar connective tissue and a plexus of veins. The *subdural space* is a potential space that lies below the inner surface of the dura and the arachnoid membrane. It contains only a limited amount of cerebrospinal fluid.

The middle meningeal layer is the arachnoid membrane. Thin, delicate, and nonvascular, it is continuous with the cranial arachnoid and follows the spinal dura to the end of the dural sac. For the most part, the dura and arachnoid are unconnected, though they are in contact with each other.

The arachnoid is attached to the pia mater by delicate filaments of connective tissue. The considerable space between these two meningeal layers is called the *subarachnoid space*. It is continuous with that of the cranium and is largest at the lower end of the spinal canal, where it encloses the masses of nerves that form the cauda equina. The spinal subarachnoid space contains an abundant amount of CSF and is capable of expansion to the point of completely filling the entire space included in the dura mater. It plays a vital role in the regulation of intracranial pressure by allowing for the shunting of CSF away from the cranium. When spinal anesthesia is used, the local anesthetic agent is deposited into the subarachnoid space. Because the CSF in the subarachnoid space bathes the spinal nerves before they exit, the local anesthetic effectively blocks spinal nerve conduction.

The third and innermost meningeal layer of the spine is the delicate pia mater. Though it is continuous with the cranial pia mater, it is less vascular, thicker, and denser in structure than the pia mater of the brain. The pia mater intimately invests the entire surface of the cord and, at the point where the cord terminates, it contracts and continues down as a long slender filament (central ligament) through the center of the bundle of nerves of the cauda equina and anchors the cord at the base of the coccyx.

Lumbar Puncture. The examination of cerebrospinal fluid and determination of CSF pressure are frequently of great value in the diagnosis of neurologic and neurosurgical conditions. The collection of CSF is ordinarily accomplished through the insertion of a long spinal needle between the third and fourth or fourth and fifth lumbar vertebrae, through the dura and arachnoid into the subarachnoid space. Since the spinal cord in adults ends at the level of the disc between the first and second lumbar vertebrae, there is minimal danger of injuring the cord through this procedure. In children, the spinal cord may extend below the third lumbar vertebra so that the subarachnoid space is usually safely entered in the areas between L4 and L5. In both adults and children, flexion of the spine raises the cord superiorly somewhat farther, minimizing the risk of damage to the cord. Because the most superior points of the iliac crests are at the level of the upper border of the spine of the fourth lumbar vertebra, they are used as anatomic reference points in selecting the site for lumbar puncture.

Structure and Function of the Spinal Cord and the Spinal Nerve Roots

It is in the spinal cord that the lowest level of the functional integration of information in the CNS takes place. Here information is received in the form of afferent (sensory) nerve impulses from the periphery of the body. This information may be acted on locally within the cord but more often is relayed to higher brain centers for additional processing and modification, resulting in sophisticated and elaborate motor (efferent) responses. A discussion of the spinal cord involves primarily the consideration of its function as a relay system for both afferent and efferent impulses.

The spinal cord is the elongated, slightly ovoid mass of central nervous tissue that occupies the upper two thirds of the vertebral canal. In the adult, it is approximately 45 cm (17 inches) long, although this varies somewhat from individual to individual depending upon the length of the trunk. The cord is actually an inferior extension of the medulla oblongata and begins at the level of the foramen magnum of the occipital bone. From there it continues downward to the upper level of the body of the second lumbar vertebra, where it narrows to a sharp tip called the *conus medullaris*. From the end of the conus an extension of the pia mater known as the *filum terminale* continues to the first segment of the coccyx, where it attaches (Fig. 9–21).

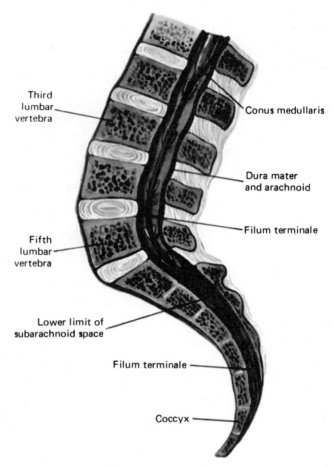

Third
lumbar
vertebra

Conus medullaris

Dura mater
and arachnoid

Filum terminale

Fifth
lumbar
vertebra

Lower limit of
subarachnoid space

Filum terminale

Coccyx

Figure 9–21. Median sagittal section of the lumbosacral portion of the vertebral column showing the conus medullaris and filum terminale. The subarachnoid space has been exposed inferiorly to the level of the first sacral vertebra to show the filum terminale.

The small central canal of the spinal cord contains CSF. This cavity extends the entire length of the cord and communicates above directly with the fourth ventricle of the medulla oblongata.

The spinal cord (Fig. 9–22) is composed of 31 horizontal segments of varying lengths. There are 8 cervical, 12 thoracic, 5 lumbar, 5 sacral, and 1 coccygeal segment, each with a corresponding pair of spinal nerves attached.

During the growth of the fetus and young child, the spinal cord does not continue to lengthen as the vertebral column lengthens. Consequently, the cord segments, from which spinal nerves originate, are displaced upward from their corresponding vertebrae. This discrepancy becomes greater with each downward segment. For example, the cervical and thoracic nerve roots

take an almost horizontal course as they leave the spinal cord and emerge through the intervertebral foramina. The lumbar and sacral nerve roots, however, are extremely long and take an oblique, downward course before finally emerging from their appropriate lumbar or sacral intervertebral foramina. The large bundle of nerves lying within the inferior vertebral canal is called the *cauda equina* for its resemblence to a horse's tail (Fig. 9–22). Several longitudinal grooves divide the spinal cord into regions. The deepest of these is the anterior median fissure. Opposite this, on the posterior surface of the cord, is the posterior median fissure. These divide the cord into symmetric right and left halves that are joined in the central midportion (Fig. 9–23).

Like the brain, the spinal cord is composed of areas of gray matter and areas of

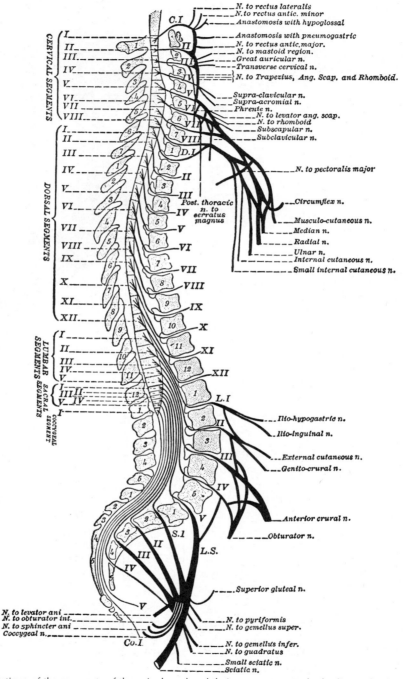

Figure 9–22. Relations of the segments of the spinal cord and their nerve roots to the bodies and spinous processes of the vertebrae. (From Anson, B. J., and McVay, C. B.: Surgical Anatomy. 5th ed. Philadelphia, W. B. Saunders Co., 1971, p. 934.)

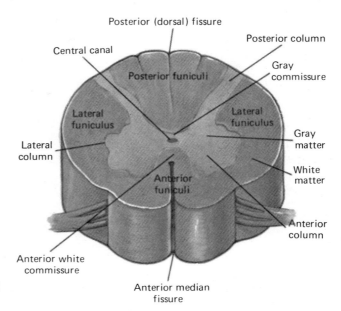

Figure 9–23. Cross section through the spinal cord.

white matter. Unlike their locations in the brain, the gray matter of the cord is situated deep in its center, while the white matter is on the surface. The gray matter of the cord is composed of large masses of nerve cell bodies, along with dendrites of association and efferent neurons, and unmyelinated axons, all embedded in a framework of neuroglia cells. It is also rich in blood vessels. The gray matter has two main functions: First, synapses within the gray matter relay signals between the periphery and the brain, sometimes via the white matter of the cord. Secondly, nuclei in the gray matter also function as centers for all spinal reflexes, and even integrate some motor activities within the cord itself (such as the "knee jerk" stretch reflex).

The white matter of the cord completely invests the gray matter. It consists primarily of long myelinated axons in a network of neuroglia and blood vessels. Its fibers are arranged into bundles called tracts, columns, or pathways that pass up and down, linking various segments of the cord and connecting the spinal cord with the brain, thus integrating and coordinating sensory and motor functions to or from any level of the CNS.

When viewed in cross section, the gray matter of the cord looks like the letter H,

two crescent-shaped halves joined together by the gray commissure surrounded by white matter. For descriptive purposes, the four segments of the H are referred to as right and left anterior (ventral) and posterior (dorsal) horns. The *anterior motor (efferent) neurons* lie within the anterior (ventral) gray horns and send fibers through the spinal nerves to the skeletal muscle. The nerve cell bodies making up the posterior (dorsal) gray horns receive sensory (afferent) signals from the periphery via the spinal nerve roots. The lateral gray horns project from the intermediate portion of the H. The nerve cells in these horns (called preganglionic autonomic neurons) give rise to fibers that lead to the autonomic nervous system.

The white matter of each half of the cord is divided into three columns (or funiculi). They are the ventral, the lateral, and the dorsal columns. Each column is subdivided into tracts, which are large bundles of nerve fibers that are arranged in functional groups. The ascending or sensory projection tracts transmit impulses to the brain, and the descending or motor projection tracts transmit impulses away from the brain to various levels of the spinal cord. Some short tracts travel up or down the cord for only a few segments of the cord.

These propriospinal (association or inter-segmental) tracts connect and integrate separate cord segments of gray matter with one another and, consequently, have important roles in the completion of various spinal reflexes.

There are 31 pairs of symmetrically arranged spinal nerves. Each nerve contains several types of fibers and arises from the spinal cord by two roots: a posterior (dorsal) and an anterior (ventral) root (Fig. 9–24). The axons that make up the fibers in the anterior roots originate from the cell bodies and dendrites in the anterior and lateral gray horns. The *anterior (ventral) root* is the *motor root*, conveying impulses from the CNS to the skeletal muscles. The *posterior (dorsal) root* is known as the *sensory root*. Sensory fibers originate in the *posterior root ganglia* of the spinal nerves. Each ganglion is an oval enlargement of the root lying just medial to the intervertebral foramen and contains the accumulated cell bodies of the axons making up the sensory fibers. One

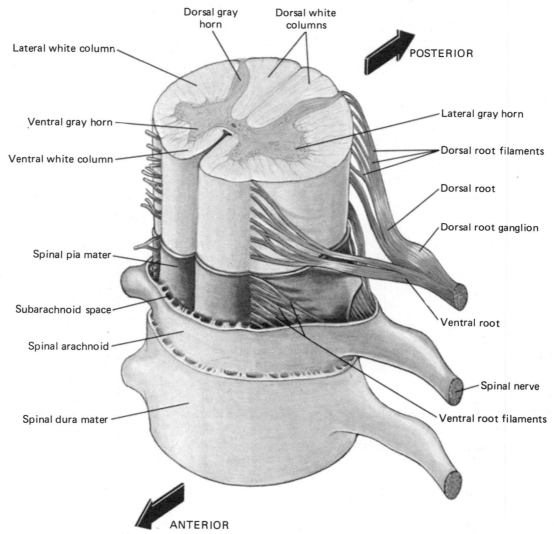

Figure 9–24. Structure of the spinal cord, and its connections with the spinal nerves by way of the dorsal and ventral spinal roots. Note also the coverings of the spinal cord, the meninges.

branch of the ganglion extends into the posterior gray horn of the cord. The other branch is distributed to both visceral and somatic organs and mediates afferent impulses to the CNS. The cutaneous (skin) area innervated by a single posterior root is called a dermatome. Knowledge of dermatome levels is useful clinically in determining the level of anesthesia after spinal or regional anesthesia (see Chapter 15).

The lateral gray horns of the spinal cord give rise to fibers that lead into the autonomic nervous system (ANS) controlling many of the internal (visceral) organs. Sympathetic fibers from the thoracic and lumbar cord segments are distributed throughout the body to the viscera, blood vessels, glands, and smooth muscle. Parasympathetic fibers, present in the middle three sacral nerves, innervate the pelvic and abdominal viscera. Hence, the ventral (anterior) root of the spinal nerve is often referred to as the motor root, though it is also responsible for the preganglionic output of the autonomic nervous system.

The anterior and posterior roots extend to the intervertebral foramen corresponding to their spinal cord segment of origin. As they reach the foramen the two roots unite to form a single mixed spinal nerve containing both motor and sensory fibers. As the nerve emerges from the foramen it gives off a small meningeal branch that turns back through the same foramen to innervate the spinal cord membranes, blood vessels, intervertebral ligaments, and spinal joint surfaces. The spinal nerve then branches into two divisions that are called *rami*. Each ramus contains fibers from both roots. The posterior rami supply the skin and the longitudinal muscles of the back. The larger anterior rami supply the anterior and lateral portions of the trunk and all of the structures of the extremities. However, the anterior rami (except those of the 11 thoracic nerves) do not go directly to their destinations. Instead, they are first rearranged without intervening synapses to form intricate networks of nerve fibers called *plexuses*.

There are five major plexuses: cervical, brachial, lumbar, sacral, and pudendal. Peripheral nerves emerge from each plexus and are named according to the region that they supply.

The cervical plexus is composed of the first four cervical spinal nerves. The phrenic nerve is the most important branch of the cervical plexus, as it supplies motor impulses to the diaphragm. Any injury to the spinal cord above the origin of the phrenic nerve (fourth cervical vertebra) will result in paralysis of the diaphragm and death. Selective anesthesia of the brachial or pudendal plexuses is frequently utilized in regional anesthesia. By depositing the local anesthetic at or near the brachial plexus, the musculocutaneous, median, ulnar, and radial nerves can be anesthetized, allowing painless surgery from the elbow to the fingers. The pudendal nerve, which supplies motor and sensory fibers to the perineum, can be anesthetized by a pudendal plexus block. This type of nerve block is effective in relieving some of the pain of childbirth. Among the nerves given off by the lumbar plexus are the ilioinguinal, genitofemoral, obturator, and femoral nerves. Among those given off by the sacral plexus are the superior and the inferior gluteal nerves.

Anterior rami from the thoracic area do not form a plexus but lead instead to the skin of the thorax and to the intercostal muscles directly. The thoracic and upper lumbar spinal nerves also give rise to white rami (visceral efferent branches), or preganglionic autonomic nerve fibers. Parts of this ramus join the spinal nerves to the sympathetic trunk. The gray ramus is present in all spinal nerves.

The term *final common pathway* is seen frequently in the literature. It refers to the motor neurons in the anterior gray horns. All excitatory or inhibitory impulses controlling movement, from the cerebral cortex to the proprioceptors, influence the motor neurons of the anterior horn either directly or indirectly. Thus, all neural impulses arising in receptors, as well as in the brain and spinal cord, must ultimately converge in this area before movement of skeletal muscle can be integrated. Hence, the term final common pathway.

Vascular Network of the Spinal Cord

The spinal cord derives its rich arterial blood supply from the vertebral arteries and from a series of spinal arteries that enter the cord at successive levels. Segmentally, the spinal arteries that enter the intervertebral foramina are given off by the intercostal vessels and by the lateral sacral, iliolumbar, inferior thyroid, and vertebral arteries.

The venous supply inside and outside the entire length of the vertebral canal is derived from a series of venous plexuses that anastamose with each other and end in intervertebral veins. The intervertebral veins leave the cord through the intervertebral foramina with the spinal nerves.

REFERENCES

1. Chaffee, E., and Lytle, I.: Basic Physiology and Anatomy. 4th ed. Philadelphia, J. B. Lippincott Co., 1980.
2. Chusid, J.: Correlative Neuroanatomy and Functional Neurology. 19th ed. Los Altos, Calif. Lange Medical Publications, 1985.
3. Conway-Rutkowski, B.: Carini and Owens Neurological and Neurosurgical Nursing. 8th ed. St. Louis, C. V. Mosby Co., 1982.
4. Ganong, W.: Review of Medical Physiology. 12th ed. Los Altos, Calif. Lange Medical Publications, 1985.
5. Guyton, A. C.: Anatomy and Physiology. Philadelphia, W. B. Saunders Co., 1985.
6. Hanlon, K.: Description and use of intracranial pressure monitoring. Heart Lung, 5:277, 1976.
7. Jacob, S., Francone, C., and Lossow, W.: Structure and Function in Man. 5th ed. Philadelphia, W. B. Saunders Co., 1982.
8. Jensen, D.: The Principles of Physiology. New York, Appleton-Century-Crofts, 1976.
9. Nauta, W., and Feirtag, M.: The organization of the brain. Sci. Am., 241(3):88–111, 1979.
10. Netter, F.: The CIBA Collection of Medical Illustrations, Volume One, The Nervous System. Summit, N.J., CIBA Pharmaceutical Co., 1972.
11. Pick, T., and Howden, R. (eds.): Gray's Anatomy. New York, Bounty Books, 1977.
12. Solomon, E., and Davis, P.: Human Anatomy and Physiology. Philadelphia, W. B. Saunders Co., 1983.

10

Endocrine Physiology

The essence of physiology is regulation and control. The physiologic functions of the body are regulated by the two major control systems—the nervous and the endocrine systems. Along with this, many interrelationships exist between the endocrine and the nervous systems. Dysfunction of the endocrine system is associated with over- or underproduction of a single hormone or multiple hormones. This dysfunction may be the primary reason for surgery, or it may coexist in patients requiring surgery on other organ systems. To assure the provision of appropriate nursing interventions for the patient with endocrine dysfunction, the post anesthesia care unit (PACU) nurse must understand the physiology and pathophysiology of the endocrine system.

Definitions

Endocrine gland: a group of hormone-producing cells.

Gluconeogenesis: the conversion of amino acids into glucose.

Glycogenesis: the deposition of glycogen in the liver.

Hormone: a biochemical substance that is secreted by a specific endocrine gland and is transported in the blood to distant points in the body, where it regulates rates of specific processes.

Lipolysis: the mobilization of depot fat.

Stress: a chemical or physical disturbance in the cells or tissues produced by a change, occurring either in the external environment or within the body, that requires a response to counteract the disturbance.

Tropic hormones: a hormone that regulates the blood level of a hormone secreted from another endocrine gland.

Target organs: the glands whose activities are regulated by tropic hormones.

Releasing factor (RF): a proposed hormone that is secreted from the hypothalamus.

Releasing hormone (RH): a proven hormone that is secreted from the hypothalamus.

THE MEDIATORS OF THE ENDOCRINE SYSTEM—THE HORMONES

A hormone is a biochemical substance that is synthesized in an endocrine gland and secreted into the body fluids to regulate or control physiologic processes of other cells of the body. Biochemically, hormones are either proteins (or derivatives of proteins or amino acids) or steroids. Protein hormones, such as the releasing hormones, catecholamines, and parathormone, fit the *fixed receptor model* of hormone action. In this model, the stimulating hormone, called the *first messenger*, combines with a specific receptor for that hormone on the surface of the target cell. This hormone-receptor combination activates the enzyme adenylate cyclase in the membrane, and that portion of the adenylate cyclase which is exposed to the cytoplasm will cause the immediate conversion of cytoplasmic ATP into cyclic AMP. The cyclic AMP then acts as a *second messenger* and initiates any number of cellular functions. In the *mobile receptor model*, a steroid hormone, because of its lipid solubility, will pass through the cell membrane into the cytoplasm, where it binds with a specific receptor protein. The combined receptor protein–hormone either diffuses or is transported through the nuclear membrane, transferring the steroid hormone to a smaller protein. In the nucleus, the hormone activates specific genes to form the *messenger RNA*. The messenger RNA then passes out of the nucleus into the cytoplasm, where it promotes the translation process in the ribosomes to form new proteins. Hormones that fit the fixed receptor model produce an almost instantaneous response on the part of the target organ. In contrast, because of their action on the genes to cause protein synthesis, when the steroid hormones are secreted there is a characteristic delay in the initiation of hormone response that varies from minutes to days.

THE PHYSIOLOGY OF THE ENDOCRINE GLANDS

Pituitary Gland

The pituitary gland rests in the sella turcica of the sphenoid bone at the base of the brain. This gland is divided into the anterior and posterior lobes. Because of its glandular nature, the anterior lobe is called the *adenohypophysis*; the posterior lobe, which is an outgrowth of a part of the nervous system—the hypothalamus—is called the *neurohypophysis*. The pituitary gland receives its arterial blood supply from two paired systems of vessels: (1) the right and left superior hypophyseal arteries from above, and (2) the right and left inferior hypophyseal arteries from below. However, the anterior lobe receives no arterial blood supply. Instead, its entire blood supply is derived from the hypophyseal portal veins. This rich capillary system facilitates the rapid discharge of releasing hormones that have target cells in the anterior hypophysis.

Although the pituitary gland is called the master gland, it is actually regulated by other endocrine glands and by the nervous system. The secretion of the hormones of the anterior hypophysis is primarily influenced and controlled by the higher centers in the hypothalamus. Releasing hormones are elaborated by the hypothalamic nuclei via the infundibular tract to the portal venous system of the pituitary gland to their respective target cells of the adenohypophysis. Consequently, the hypothalamus brings about fine regulation of the action of the anterior pituitary, and still higher nervous centers apparently modulate further the production of the releasing factors. Hence, the many influences coming into the brain and central nervous system (CNS) impinge on the anterior pituitary either to enhance or to dampen its activity. The hormonal control of the pituitary involves certain feedback systems. For example, corticotropin-releasing hormone will stimulate the production and release of adrenocorticotropic hormone (ACTH). The increased concentration of ACTH causes the hypothalamus to decrease its production of corticotropin-releasing hormone, which in turn reduces ACTH production, ultimately reducing the blood level of adrenocorticotropic hormone. Therefore, when exogenous corticoids are administered over time, ACTH secretion will be reduced and the adrenal cortex will atrophy. On the other hand, the removal of endogenous corticoids by a bilateral adrenalectomy can result in a tumor of the pituitary gland owing to the absence of the feedback depression of the corticotropin-releasing hormone.

The posterior lobe of the pituitary gland is made up of an abundant nerve supply. The nerve cell bodies in the posterior lobe produce two neurosecretions (antidiuretic hormone and oxytocin) which are stored as granules at the site of the nerve cell bodies. When the hypothalamus detects a need for either neurohypophyseal hormone, nerve impulses are sent to the posterior lobe and the hormone is released by granules into the neighboring capillaries. Consequently, the hormonal function of the posterior lobe is under direct nervous system regulation.

Hormones of the Adenohypophysis

Growth Hormone (GH) or Somatotropin. This hormone is unique in that it has no target gland to stimulate, but acts on all tissues of the body. Its primary functions are to maintain blood glucose levels and to regulate the growth of the skeleton. Growth hormone conserves blood glucose by increasing fat metabolism. It steps up the active transport of amino acids into cells, increases the rate of protein synthesis, and promotes cell division. In addition, growth hormone enhances the formation of somatomedin, which acts directly on cartilage and bone to promote their growth. The active secretion of growth hormone is regulated in the hypothalamus via growth hormone–releasing hormone (GRH). Stimuli such as hypoglycemia, exercise, and trauma will cause the hypothalamus to secrete GRH, which is transported to the anterior lobe of the pituitary gland, causing growth hormone to be released into the blood. The secretion of GH can be inhibited by somatostatin, which is also referred to as *growth hormone–inhibiting hormone (GIH)* and is secreted from the hypothalamus and the delta cells of the pancreas.

Hypofunction of the growth hormone before puberty leads to *dwarfism* or a failure to grow. After puberty, growth hormone hypofunction may result in the condition known as *Simmonds' disease.* This disease is characterized by premature senility, weakness, emaciation, mental lethargy, and wrinkled, dry skin. *Giantism* is the result of growth hormone hyperfunction before puberty. After puberty, when the epiphyses of the long bones have closed, growth hormone hyperfunction leads to *acromegaly.* In this disease, the face, the hands, and the feet become enlarged. Patients with acromegaly are prone to airway obstruction owing to their protruding lower jaw and enlarged tongue. Hence, in the post anesthesia care unit, constant vigilance as to the respiratory status of these patients is essential.

Thyroid-Stimulating Hormone (TSH) or Thyrotropin. The follicular cells of the thyroid are the target for thyroid-stimulating hormone (TSH). This hormone promotes the growth and secretory activity of the thyroid gland. Production of TSH is regulated in a reciprocal fashion by the blood levels of thyroid hormone and the formation of a *thyrotropin-releasing hormone (TRH)* in the hypothalamus.

Adrenocorticotropin (ACTH). This hormone promotes the growth and secretory activity of the adrenal cortex, which produces the glucocorticoids, mineralocorticoids, and androgenic steroids. This hormone is released in response to such stimuli as pain, hypoglycemia, hypoxia, bacterial toxins, hyperthermia, hypothermia, and physiologic stress. More specifically, the hypothalamus monitors for these various stressors, and upon excitation *corticotropin-releasing hormone (CRH)* is secreted which stimulates ACTH secretion from the adenohypophysis. The blood levels of certain adrenocortical hormones regulate the secretion of ACTH by a hypothalamic feedback mechanism.

Gonadotropic Hormones. These hormones regulate the growth, development, and function of the ovaries and testes. The gonadotropic hormones are the *follicle-stimulating hormone (FSH)* and *luteinizing hormone (LH).* Secretion of the gonadotropic hormones is stimulated by *gonadotropin-releasing hormone (GnRH)*, which is secreted by the hypothalamus.

Prolactin (PRL) or Lactogenic Hormone. Prolactin stimulates lactation in the postpartum period. Unlike the case with the other pituitary hormones, the hypothalamic control of prolactin secretion is predominantly inhibitory.

Melanocyte-Stimulating Hormone (MSH). MSH has an effect on the melanin granules in pigmented skin.

Hormones of the Neurohypophysis

Antidiuretic Hormone (ADH) or Vasopressin. During the normal activities of daily living, ADH is secreted in small amounts into the bloodstream to promote the reabsorption of water from the renal tubules, which leads to a decreased excretion of water by the kidneys. When ADH is secreted in large quantities, vasoconstriction of the smooth muscles occurs, which ultimately elevates the blood pressure. The pressor effects of ADH are produced only by large doses that are not in the usual physiologic range. The secretion of ADH is regulated by several feedback loops, one of which involves plasma osmolality. Within the hypothalamus are *osmo receptors* whose function is such that when plasma osmolality is increased, ADH is secreted. On the other hand, dilution of plasma inhibits ADH secretion. The second feedback loop or major stimulus of ADH secretion is the *volume* or *stretch receptors* located in the left atrium. These receptors are activated when the extracellular fluid (ECF) volume is increased, and, when this happens, ADH secretion is inhibited. The *baroreceptors*, which are located in the carotid sinus and aortic arch, are the receptors for the third feedback loop. A decrease in the arterial blood pressure will stimulate the baroreceptors, which in turn will stimulate a release of ADH. Both the stretch and the baroreceptors transmit their neuronal input to the brain via the vagus nerve.

Lack of antidiuretic hormone will lead to a condition called *diabetes insipidus*. This condition is characterized by the output of a large volume of dilute, sugar-free urine.

Oxytocin. This hormone causes the contraction of uterine muscle at the end of gestation and has a role in milk expulsion, i.e., in stimulating the contraction of the surrounding myoepithelial cells of the mammary glands.

Pituitary Dysfunction

Hyperfunction rarely involves more than one endocrine gland. On the other hand, hypofunction does usually involve more than one endocrine gland, although instances of isolated deficiencies have been reported. A common cause of pituitary hypofunction is compression of glandular cells by the expansion of a functional or non-

functional tumor, in which case an excess of one hormone may coexist with a deficiency of another.

The Pineal Gland

The pineal gland is situated in the diencephalon just above the roof of the midbrain. This gland is considered an intricate and highly sensitive biologic clock, as the secretory activity of the pineal gland is greatest at night. The pineal gland secretes melatonin, which affects the size and secretory activity of the ovaries and other organs. The production and release of melatonin are regulated by the sympathetic nervous system. In fact, the pineal gland is considered a neuroendocrine transducer because it converts nervous system input into a hormonal output.

The Thyroid Gland

The thyroid gland is located in the anterior middle portion of the neck immediately below the larynx. The gland consists of two lobes that are attached by a strip of tissue called the *isthmus*. Structurally, this gland is made up of tiny sacs called *follicles*. Each follicle is formed by a single layer of epithelial cells surrounding a cavity that contains a secretory product known as *colloid*. This colloid fluid consists mainly of a glycoprotein-iodine complex that is called *thyroglobulin*. Upon stimulation by the thyrotropin-stimulating hormone (TSH), the thyroid hormones are produced in the following steps: (1) iodide trapping, (2) oxidation and iodination, (3) storage of the hormones in the colloid as part of the thyroglobulin molecules, and (4) proteolysis (which can be inhibited by iodide) and release of the hormones. The two hormones released from the thyroid gland are triiodothyronine (T_3) and thyroxine (T_4). T_4 represents over 95 percent of the circulating thyroid hormone and is considered to be relatively inactive physiologically as compared with T_3. Consequently, although T_3 has a relatively low concentration, it passes out of the bloodstream faster than T_4, has a more rapid action, and is probably the major biologically active thyroid hormone. After these hormones are secreted by the thyroid gland, they are transported to all parts of the body via plasma proteins in the form of protein-bound iodinated compounds. Hence, the laboratory test for *protein-bound iodine (PBI)* is useful in determining the amount of circulating thyroid hormone in the blood.

Thyroxine and triiodothyronine regulate the metabolic activities of the body. More specifically, they regulate the rate of cellular oxidation. Along with this, they are essential for the normal growth and development of the body. Other metabolic activities that are influenced by T_3 and T_4 are the promotion of protein synthesis and breakdown, increase of glucose absorption and utilization, facilitation of gluconeogenesis, and maintenance of fluid and electrolyte balance. The thyroid hormones are also involved in a feedback mechanism. The concentration of T_3 and T_4 in the blood regulates the secretion of thyroid-stimulating hormone (TSH) by the anterior pituitary gland. TSH regulates the growth and secretory activity of the thyroid gland.

Another hormone secreted by the thyroid gland is *thyrocalcitonin* or *calcitonin*. This hormone helps to maintain the proper level of calcium in the blood. More specifically, calcitonin decreases the serum concentration of calcium by counteracting the effects of parathormone (PTH) and inhibiting the resorption of calcium from the bones.

Parathyroid Glands

The parathyroid glands are located on the posterior portion of the thyroid gland. In most cases there is one parathyroid gland on each of the four poles of the thyroid gland. The parathyroid glands release a polypeptide hormone called *parathormone (PTH)*. This hormone is the principal regulator of the calcium concentration in the body. Parathormone is released into the circulation by a negative feedback mechanism that is dependent on the serum concentration of calcium. Hence, a high serum concentration of calcium will suppress the synthesis and release of parathormone and a low serum calcium concentration will

stimulate the release of the hormone. Normal serum calcium concentrations depend on the regulatory mechanisms, which include parathormone, calcitonin, phosphorus, magnesium, and vitamin D. In fact, the serum calcium concentration is maintained by these regulatory mechanisms within narrow and constant limits. The normal serum calcium level is 9.0 to 10.3 mg per dl for men and 8.9 to 10.2 mg per dl for women. It should be noted that the serum levels of calcium expressed in milliequivalents per liter are one-half the value given in mg per dl.

Parathormone influences the rate at which calcium is transported across membranes in the bone, the gastrointestinal tract, and the kidneys. More specifically, calcium release from bone is facilitated by parathormone-induced stimulation of osteoclastic activity. The absorption of calcium by the gastrointestinal tract is enhanced by the parathormone-induced synthesis of vitamin D. Parathormone activates the synthesis of vitamin D, which leads to increased tubular reabsorption of calcium and enhanced renal tubular clearance of phosphorus. This results in more calcium entering the circulation.

The Adrenal Glands

The adrenal glands are located on the apex of each kidney. Each gland consists of an outer portion called the cortex and an inner portion called the medulla. The medulla is responsible for the secretion of catecholamines (see Chapter 5). The preganglionic fibers of the sympathetic nervous system provide the stimulation that facilitates the liberation of the catecholamines by the medullary cells. The cortex makes up the bulk of the adrenal gland and is responsible for the secretion of the *steroids*. The cortex is divided anatomically and physiologically into three zones: the *zona glomerulosa*, the *zona fasciculata*, and the inner *zona reticularis*. These are the sites of secretion of the three major steroid hormones: the *mineralocorticoids*, the *glucocorticoids*, and the *androgens*, respectively.

The mineralocorticoids are responsible for

the maintenance of fluid and electrolyte balance. Aldosterone is physiologically the most important mineralocorticoid. The basic action of aldosterone is to promote the reabsorption of sodium by stimulating cellular sodium pumps in the target tissue. Overall, aldosterone causes increased tubular reabsorption of sodium and excretion of potassium. This decreases urinary excretion of sodium and chloride and increases urinary secretion of potassium, consequently expanding the extracellular fluid compartment. Aldosterone secretion is increased by ACTH, a depletion of sodium, and an increase of potassium. The secretion of aldosterone is also regulated by the *renin-angiotensin system*. Thus, when the blood supply to the kidneys is low, the juxtaglomerular cells are stimulated to release *renin*. The renin, which is an enzyme, enters the blood and converts the plasma protein *angiotensinogen* to *angiotensin I*. In the lungs and elsewhere, angiotensin I is converted enzymatically to the physiologically active form, *angiotensin II*. One of the basic actions of angiotensin II is to stimulate the adrenal cortex to secrete aldosterone. Thus, aldosterone secretion is regulated by the blood pressure and volume, and, since it causes retention of sodium and a rise in blood pressure, aldosterone also acts as a feedback mechanism to shut off the further release of renin.

The glucocorticoids are secreted in the zona fasciculata. *Cortisol (hydrocortisone)* constitutes about 95 percent of the total glucocorticoid activity, with *corticosterone* and *cortisone* making up the remaining 5 percent. These hormones function to preserve the carbohydrate reserves of the body. They do this by promoting gluconeogenesis, glycogenesis, lipolysis, and oxidation of fat in the liver. Because they conserve carbohydrate, these hormones serve as functional antagonists to insulin. Finally, these hormones possess an excellent anti-inflammatory action. The major regulator of their secretion is ACTH, which is secreted by cells in the anterior pituitary gland. ACTH is, in turn, modulated by corticotropin-releasing hormone (CRH), which is secreted by the hypothalamus. Cortisol serves as a negative feedback mechanism to inhibit both ACTH and CRH production. Physical and mental stress will stimulate the release of CRH from the hypothalamus. Hence, in addition to the catecholamines, cortisol and ACTH are considered to be the major stress hormones.

The *androgens* or sex hormones are actively involved in the preadolescent growth spurt and in the appearance of axillary and pubic hair.

The Pancreas

Islet of Langerhans cells are scattered throughout the pancreas. There are three islet cell types, called *alpha, beta,* and *delta,* which secrete *glucagon, insulin,* and *somatostatin,* respectively. Glucagon has several functions that are diametrically opposed to those of insulin. Glucagon is commonly referred to as *hyperglycemic factor,* and its most important function is to increase the blood glucose level. This increased glucose level in the blood is due to the effects of glucagon on glucose metabolism, i.e., glycogenolysis (in the liver) and increased gluconeogenesis. When the blood glucose concentration falls below 70 mg per dl, the alpha cells will secrete glucagon to protect against hypoglycemia. Along with this, amino acids will enhance the secretion of glucagon. In this case, the glucagon will help to prevent the hypoglycemia that could result, since amino acids will stimulate insulin release, which tends to reduce the blood glucose concentration. The secretion of glucagon appears to be inhibited by the release of somatostatin from the delta cells of the pancreas, and, because it is a polypeptide, glucagon is rapidly destroyed by proteolytic enzymes.

Insulin is a protein secreted by the beta cells of the islets of Langerhans in response to elevated levels of blood sugar. Its secretion is inhibited by low blood sugar levels and somatostatin. In addition, insulin secretion can be inhibited by epinephrine, glucocorticoids, and thyroxine. When insulin is secreted by the beta cells, a metabolic state favoring the storage of nutrients is set into action. These physiologic actions include (1) retention of glucose by the liver, (2) slowing of hepatic glucose release, (3) increase in uptake of glucose by muscle (stored as glycogen) and adipose tissue (stored as triglycerides), (4) translocation of amino acids and neutral fats into muscle and adipose tissue, and (5) retardation of lipolysis and proteolysis. Hence, insulin seems to "open the door" of most of the cell membranes of the body to facilitate the movement of glucose, amino acids, and fatty acids into the cells. *Diabetes mellitus,* which is a disease involving the synthesis, storage, and release of insulin, is discussed in detail in Chapter 36.

The Gonads

The hormone *testosterone* is produced in the interstitial cells of the testes. The synthesis and secretion of this hormone are regulated by the luteinizing hormone (LH), which is secreted by the anterior pituitary gland. Testosterone regulates the development and maintenance of the male secondary sexual characteristics as well as having some metabolic effects on bone and skeletal muscle. Another action of this hormone is the modulation of male behavior by limbic system stimulation. *Estrogen,* another gonadal hormone, is secreted by the ovarian follicles in response to the follicle-stimulating hormone (FSH) and the luteinizing hormone (LH) of the anterior pituitary, and is responsible for the development and maintenance of the secondary sexual characteristics in the female. Estrogen, along with progesterone, which is produced by the cells of the corpus luteum, plays an important role in the menstrual cycle.

SELECTED SYNDROMES AND DISEASES ASSOCIATED WITH THE ENDOCRINE SYSTEM

Hypoadrenocorticism

A reduction in function of the hormones associated with the pituitary-adrenal axis can develop as a result of (1) the destruction of the adrenal cortex by degenerative disease, neoplastic growth, or hemorrhage; (2) a de-

ficiency of ACTH; or (3) a prolonged administration of corticosteroid drugs. *Primary adrenal insufficiency (Addison's disease)* results from destruction of the adrenal cortex. At present, the majority of cases of Addison's disease are caused by idiopathic atrophy that is probably due to an autoimmune disease. Other causes include tuberculosis, histoplasmosis, bilateral hemorrhage due to anticoagulation therapy, surgical removal of the adrenals, tumor chemotherapy, metastasis to the adrenals, and sepsis.

A deficiency of ACTH is associated with *panhypopituitarism.* Patients who have been administered frequent "bursts" of exogenous steroid preparations such as prednisone can experience a suppression of their output of endogenous corticosteroids because of the augmentation of the feedback mechanism to the anterior pituitary. Concern about the development of hypoadrenocorticism should be shown in the case of any patient who has received 20 mg of prednisone per day for more than two weeks in the preceding 12 months (although authors vary on dosage and length of time). The recovery of the normal function of the pituitary-adrenal axis may require as long as 12 months following the discontinuation of steroid therapy. Patients who are even remotely suspected of having hypoadrenocorticism are usually administered steroids preoperatively, intraoperatively, and postoperatively.

The reason for this perioperative steroid coverage is that infection, injury, operation, or other stressors activate the pituitary-adrenal axis. If this axis is suppressed (i.e., hypoadrenocorticism), *acute adrenal insufficiency (addisonian crisis)* can develop. This is a life-threatening situation requiring prompt action by the PACU nurse. Clinical manifestations of the addisonian crisis include dehydration, nausea and vomiting, muscular weakness, and hypotension, which are followed by fever, marked flaccidity of the extremities, hyponatremia, hyperkalemia, azotemia, and shock. Therefore, the PACU nurse should monitor patients who are even remotely likely to develop the addisonian crisis. If some of the signs and symptoms appear, the attending physician should be notified immediately. The severely ill patient must be treated while the diagnosis is being confirmed. Two to 4 mg of dexamethasone is usually administered intravenously along with IV therapy of 5 percent dextrose in normal saline. Dexamethasone is the drug of choice because it does not interfere with the diagnostic tests and yet does provide the needed glucocorticoid. If dexamethasone is not available, it would be advantageous to administer a single 100 mg dose of hydrocortisone intravenously to obtain both the glucocorticoid and the mineralocorticoid activity. This can be followed by 50 to 100 mg of hydrocortisone administered parenterally every 6 hours. During the administration of the treatment, the PACU nurse should monitor continuously the patient's cardiorespiratory status.

The Syndrome of Inappropriate Secretion of ADH (SIADH)

The syndrome of inappropriate secretion of antidiuretic hormone (SIADH) occurs when there is a continued secretion of antidiuretic hormone in the presence of serum hypo-osmolality. More specifically, there is a failure in the feedback loops that regulate ADH secretion and inhibition. Usually both dilution and expansion of the blood volume will serve to stimulate a suppression of the release of ADH. However, in SIADH, the feedback loops do not respond appropriately to the osmolar or volume change, and a pathologic positive feedback loop continues, resulting in continued production of ADH.

When hemorrhage and trauma occur during a surgical procedure, ADH secretion will be appropriately elevated, and in this situation SIADH can be induced as a result of overzealous fluid administration. Because of the urinary sodium loss occurring along with the water retention, the *syndrome of acute water intoxication* may be seen in the post anesthesia care unit. The symptoms of water intoxication derive from increased brain water, inoperative sodium pump, and hyponatremia. The symptoms begin with headache, muscular weakness, anorexia,

nausea, and vomiting, progressing to confusion, hostility, disorientation, uncooperativeness, drowsiness, and terminal convulsions or coma. These symptoms usually do not occur if the serum sodium is above 120 mEq per liter. Therefore, in patients who have experienced major vascular surgery, trauma, or hemorrhage, the PACU nurse should assess frequently for the symptoms of SIADH and notify the attending physician if the symptoms become evident. The focus of treatment for SIADH is fluid restriction, diuresis with mannitol or furosemide, and administration of sodium chloride. Along with this, the PACU nurse should frequently assess the neurologic signs and cardiorespiratory status of the patient with SIADH, and measure and record accurately the intake and output of all fluids.

PACU STRESS SYNDROME

The stress syndrome is basically a physiologic response by the endocrine system to external or internal psychologic stimuli (stressors). Although Chapter 2 of this text provides an introduction to the concepts of stress and burnout in the PACU, it is the intent of this section to describe the physiologic basis of stress as well as possible psychologic interventions necessary to return homeostasis to the endocrine system, with a special focus on methods PACU nurses can use to reduce stress resulting from their work.

In some ways, stress is purported to have a positive influence on the quality of life, while, on the other hand, if it is not controlled, it can become deleterious to an individual's health. Hans Selye, a Canadian physiologist, first introduced the concept that in response to various stressors the adrenal cortex is activated, producing an increase in cortisol secretion. As the body is stressed, secretions from the adrenal cortex will become elevated, and if the level of stress is not reduced, tissue changes can occur. For a stimulus to produce a stress reaction, harm does not actually need to occur, but need only be anticipated. One source of stress can be *cataclysmic events*, which are sudden and powerful events affecting large numbers of people, such as war, natural disasters, or economic depression. A second source is *personal failure*, or any personal loss, such as the death of a particular patient. The third category involves *"daily hassles"*, which are the ongoing chronic problems one encounters, such as interpersonal problems at work, living in a crowded environment, and driving in heavy automobile traffic to and from work.

The body's response to stress is an activation of both the pituitary-cortical and the pituitary-medullary axes. When a stressor is applied, the brain determines that the stimulus is a threat to the preservation of the organism, and the hypothalamus is activated, producing corticotropin-releasing hormone, which triggers the release of ACTH and beta-endorphin. The ACTH then activates the adrenal cortex to secrete cortisol and aldosterone, which influence blood sugar levels, metabolism, blood volume, and the immune system. The beta-endorphins affect mood, learning, and pain perception. This hypothalamic stimulus will also activate the adrenal medulla to secrete the catecholamines epinephrine and norepinephrine, which results in cardiovascular stimulation. This physiologic and behavioral response is sometimes referred to as the "fight-or-flight" response, and is, for the most part, physiologically identical to anxiety.

The Selye's general adaptation syndrome (GAS) is a three-stage biologic process in response to a stressor. In the first stage, called the *alarm reaction*, the body makes a biochemical response in an effort to mobilize defensive forces. During the alarm reaction, the body either becomes overwhelmed and dies or enters a second stage, called *resistance*, in which the body continues its biochemical response. If appropriate adjustments are not made, the person can enter the third stage, called *exhaustion*. It is at this stage that tissue damage can and does occur. The physiologic response continues, and disorders such as migraine, colitis, indigestion, insomnia, depression, hypersensitivity reactions, cardiac dysrhythmias and palpitations, and reactive hypoglycemia can occur. Stress over time equals *burnout*.

The essential requirement for stress reduction is *control*. Numerous studies support the idea that having control and perceiving oneself as having control over adverse outcomes has the effect of reducing stress. To facilitate this control, the nurse must use the problem-solving technique of first appraising the stressor and then developing some initial coping mechanisms to regulate response to the stressful event. The coping strategy may include exercising, going to a movie, or giving oneself a pep talk. Although these methods of coping will facilitate the individual's reevaluation of the stressor, they do not directly change the stressor itself. Finally, the nurse should develop an active or problem-focused method of coping, which can include talking with colleagues, head nurse, or supervisor about interpersonal problems, or moving to a new environment, or changing the work environment. After initiating such action, the nurse will probably receive feedback about the consequences. Positive feedback will facilitate control and the stress will decrease or cease. It is strongly suggested that one of the best ways to develop control over the stress syndrome is to "exercise" the stress response. Physical and emotional exercise will stimulate both the pituitary-cortical and the medullary axes. *This most needed exercise will facilitate control.* Physical exercise can involve any method to promote physical fitness. Emotional exercise for the PACU nurse could include developing positive relationships with physicians, peers, and difficult patients and families; providing PACU nursing care for challenging patients; and dealing with spouse and other significant persons in a constructive, positive manner.

Certainly, the patient in the post anesthesia care unit can also experience a stress reaction. Thus, the mechanisms suggested to reduce stress apply to the patient as well as to the PACU nurse. If a patient in the post anesthesia care unit experiences stress, it is important that the nurse appropriately assess the stressor, intervene, and provide positive feedback to facilitate control by the patient. Remember, when a person becomes a patient he loses some control; therefore, the nurse must develop interventions that return control to the patient. It cannot be overemphasized how important it is for the individual (nurse or patient) to assess and deal with the stress rapidly to prevent the occurrence of stress-related physiologic disorders.

REFERENCES

1. Brown, B.: Anesthesia and the Patient with Endocrine Disease. Philadelphia, F. A. Davis Co., 1980.
2. Chaffee, E., and Lytle, I.: Basic Physiology and Anatomy. 4th ed. Philadelphia, J. B. Lippincott Co., 1980.
3. Greenspan, F., and Forsham, P.: Basic and Clinical Endocrinology. Los Altos, Lange Medical Publications, 1983.
4. Guyton, A.: Textbook of Medical Physiology. 7th ed. Philadelphia, W. B. Saunders Company, 1986.
5. Kubo W., and Grant, M.: The syndrome of inappropriate secretion of antidiuretic hormone. Heart Lung 7(3):469–476, 1979.
6. Pender, J., and Basso, L.: Diseases of the endocrine system. In Katz, J., Benumof, J., and Kadis, L.: Anesthesia and Uncommon Diseases: Pathophysiologic and Clinical Correlations. 2nd ed. Philadelphia, W. B. Saunders Co., 1981.
7. Ramsey, J.: Basic Pathophysiology: Modern Stress and Disease Process. Menlo Park, Addison-Wesley Publishing Co., 1982.
8. Tasch, M.: Endocrine disease. In Stoelting, R., and Dierdorf, S.: Anesthesia and Co-Existing Disease. New York, Churchill Livingstone Inc., 1983.
9. Whitman, N., Spendlove, D., and Clark, C.: Student Stress: Effects and Solutions. ASHE-ERIC Higher Education Research Report No. 2., Washington, D.C., Association for the Study of Higher Education, 1984.

11

Immune System Physiology

Over the past two decades, there has been a virtual explosion of information about the immune system. Diseases whose causes were believed to be based in one of the other physiologic systems are now found, as a result of medical research, to have their basis in the immune system. For example, myasthenia gravis was once thought to be a neuromuscular disease; however, research has demonstrated the origin of the disease to be in the immune system. Today, post anesthesia care unit (PACU) nurses must deal with patients who are immunosuppressed, are experiencing a hypersensitivity reaction, or are suffering from immune diseases such as acquired immunodeficiency syndrome (AIDS). An informed appreciation of the physiology and pathophysiology of the immune system is essential for the appropriate PACU care of the surgical patient.

Definitions

Acquired immunity: the ability of the human body to develop an extremely powerful specific immunity against most invading agents.

Active acquired immunity: Immunity that develops when an individual comes into direct contact with a pathogen either by contracting the disease produced by the pathogen or by vaccination against the disease.

Antibody: a globulin molecule that can attack agents which are foreign to the host.

Antigen: protein, large polysaccharide, or large lipoprotein complex that stimulates the process of acquired immunity.

B lymphocytes or bursa-dependent cells: immunocompetent lymphocytes that are named for the preprocessing that occurs in the bursa of Fabricius of birds and is responsible for humoral immunity.

Cellular or cell-mediated immunity: a type of acquired immunity that utilizes sensitized lymphocytes as the primary defense.

Clone: a group of cells that originate from a single parent cell.

Hapten: a substance that has a low molecular weight, which combines with an antigenic substance to elicit an immune response.

Humoral immunity: a type of acquired immunity that utilizes antibodies as the primary defense.

Immunodeficiency disease: immunosuppression that results from a deficiency of a single humoral antibody group or from a combined deficiency of both the T- and the B-cell systems.

Immunosuppression: a state of nonresponsiveness of the immune system to antigenic challenge.

Immunity: the ability of the human body to resist almost all types of organisms or toxins that can damage tissues and organs.

Innate immunity: general processes in the human body, other than those of acquired immunity, that are responsible for protection against organisms and toxins.

Lymphopenia: decreased function of the lymphoid organs.

Passive acquired immunity: immunity resulting when an individual receives immune cells or immune serum produced by someone else.

Phagocytosis: the envelopment and digestion of bacteria or other foreign substances.

Sensitized lymphocytes: lymphocytes that are made competent by processing to facilitate their immunologic activity, such as their attachment to and destruction of a foreign agent.

Stem cells: an unspecialized cell that gives rise to specific specialized cells such as T and B lymphocytes.

T lymphocytes: sensitized lymphocytes that are responsible for cellular immunity.

PHYSICAL AND CHEMICAL BARRIERS

The body's *first* line of immunologic defense is the mechanical barriers provided by the epithelial surface. Some parts of the epithelium have extensions from their surface, such as the cilia and the mucus in the respiratory system. These extensions provide not only an additional physical barrier to the entrance of foreign substances but also an efficient removal system. In the stomach, hydrochloric acid, which is thought to have a bactericidal action, is secreted. As an additional defense, the skin produces chemicals that inactivate bacteria. The surfaces of the boundary tissues also have specific defenses in the form of secretory antibodies. Consequently, surgical incisions, intravenous cannulation, and many other invasive procedures can cause major breaks in the first line of defense. Hence, the PACU nurse should use good aseptic or sterile technique to prevent an overwhelming bacterial invasion through the boundary tissues.

INNATE IMMUNITY

Innate or nonspecific immunity is the body's *second* line of immunologic defense against foreign material. In this type of immunity, activation occurs during each exposure to an invading substance. Recognition does occur at the level of distinguishing between self and nonself; however, the mechanisms of innate immunity cannot identify the specific invader.

Phagocytosis is the primary mechanism of innate immunity. The cells in the body that carry out the phagocytotic functions of innate immunity are *monocytes*, which are *macrophages,* and *neutrophils (polymorphonuclear leukocytes)*, which are *microphages*. The phagocytes' overall immunologic functions are to localize the antigen and to destroy, inactivate, or process it for handling by other components of the immune system. The process of phagocytosis can be enhanced by the combination of an antigen with a plasma protein called *opsonin,* a substance associated with the immune system. Finally, phagocytosis gives transitory protection to the body so that it will not be overwhelmed by foreign materials before the immune system (acquired immunity) is activated.

ACQUIRED IMMUNITY

Acquired or adaptive immunity is the body's *third* line of immunologic defense. It is mediated by the capability of specific antibodies or sensitized lymphocytes to recognize and to react to antigens from the offending agent. Two closely allied types of acquired immune mechanisms occur in the body. They are *humoral immunity* and *cellular (cell-mediated) immunity.*

Humoral Immunity

Humoral immunity is conferred by circulating antibodies found in the globulin fraction of blood proteins and are therefore referred to as *immunoglobulins* (*Ig*). The processing that is involved to produce the immunoglobulin begins with the lymphocytic stem cells in the bone marrow. These stem cells, being incapable of forming antibodies, make pre-B lymphocytes that are taken up by the lymph nodes and processed in the as yet unidentified "bursa-equivalent" tissue to become mature immunocompetent B lymphocytes. These processed B lymphocytes are then released into the blood, where they become entrapped in the lymphoid tissue. Upon stimulation by an antigen, the B lymphocyte specific for that antigen will enlarge, divide, and differentiate into plasma cells having specificity for that antigen. The plasma cells then produce and secrete an antibody or sensitized lymphocyte. During their first exposure to the antigen, lymphocytes from one specific type of lymphoid tissue form *clones*. The clones are responsive only to the antigen responsible for their initial development. Upon their second stimulation by the same antigen, the clones proliferate rapidly, leading to the formation of a large amount of antibody. Some cells in this clone mature to form plasma cells, while other cells of the clone will become B lymphocyte memory cells. When the immune system responds to the first presentation of the antigen, the immune system will "remember" the antigen by means of the B lymphocyte memory cell. The immune system can remember the antigen for years. In other words, upon the first stimulation by an antigen, the plasma cells produce antibodies (immunoglobulins) as their *primary response*. The primary response is usually evident about 4 to 10 days after the initial exposure to the antigen. Upon the second stimulation by the same antigen, a *second response* occurs. This secondary response, in which a massive amount of antibody specific to the antigen is produced within 1 to 2 days, will last for months. The secondary response is more rapid, stronger, and more persistent than the primary response. This is because of the memory cells and clones that are produced by the initial exposure to the antigen. If the T lymphocytes are activated by the same antigen, the T lymphocyte helper cells will enhance the response of the B lymphocytes. Therefore, because of this cooperative effort, the total number of lymphocytes in the lymphoid tissue increases markedly. Upon second exposure to an antigen, the same plasma cell can produce the particular antibody needed and can convert from one type of antibody secretion to another as needed. Once the specific antibodies from the plasma cells are no longer needed, further production of the antibodies will be suppressed by the antibodies themselves or by *T lymphocyte suppressor cells* (Fig. 11–1).

The immunoglobulins are large proteins with specific structural arrangements of polypeptide chains with specific amino acid sequences. The immunoglobulins are divided into five primary classes based on structural arrangements: IgA, IgD, IgE, IgG, and IgM.

IgA is a small molecule that constitutes about 15 percent of the total immunoglobulins and is present in most body secretions. This antibody activates complement through the alternate properdin pathway. Along with this, secretory immunity is mediated by IgA. The secretory antibodies are found on the mucosal surfaces of the oral cavity, the lungs, and the intestinal and urogenital tracts, as well as in mammary secretions. This secretory IgA differs from other antibodies in that it has a protein molecule, called a secretory piece, attached to it. *Secretory IgA* (*SIgA*) is effective against viruses and some bacteria. *IgD* composes about 1 percent of the total immunoglobulins. The exact function of IgD is unknown. However, this immunoglobulin may be involved with the differentiation of the B lymphocytes, and a relationship has been suggested between IgD and antibody activity directed toward insulin, penicillin, milk proteins, diphtheria toxoid, thyroid antigens, and the products of abnormal tissue growth. *IgE* is present in very small quantities (about 0.002 percent of total serum immunoglobulins) and is associated with

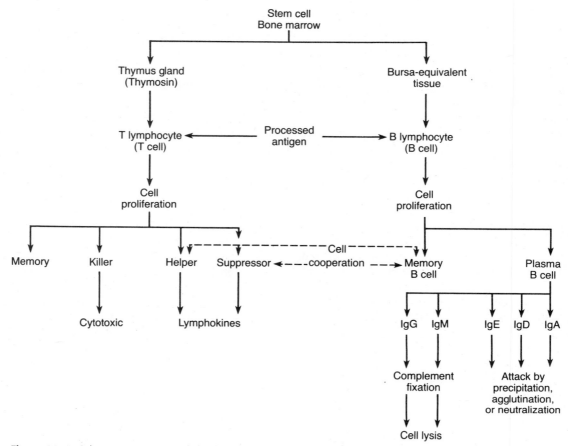

Figure 11–1. Schematic overview of the humoral and cellular immunologic pathways and the resulting effector substances or mechanisms of activity.

the Type I immediate hypersensitivity reaction. *IgG* is the smallest antibody, and it constitutes about 75 percent of the total plasma antibodies. It is the only antibody that can cross the placental barrier, thus conferring passive immunity to the fetus. IgG is the primary antibody involved in the secondary response. It is active against many blood-borne infecting agents such as bacteria, viruses, parasites, and some fungi. *IgM* is the largest antibody and it constitutes about 10 percent of plasma antibody. It is the main antibody involved in the primary antibody response, and IgM will fix complement.

Antibodies, once secreted by the plasma cells, protect the body against invading agents by three mechanisms of action: (1) attacking the antigen; (2) activating of the

complement system, which results in cell lysis; and (3) activating the immediate hypersensitivity reaction, which will localize the invader and may negate its virulence. More specifically, antibodies can inactivate the invading antigen by precipitation, agglutination, neutralization, or complement fixation. *Precipitation* occurs when an insoluble antibody forms a complex with a soluble antigen (such as tetanus toxin) and the resulting antigen-antibody complex becomes insoluble and precipitates. When antigens are bound together and react with an antibody, *agglutinated aggregates* occur. *Neutralization* is achieved when antibodies cover the toxic sites of an antigenic agent or when antibodies counteract toxins released by bacteria. Rarely are the very potent antibodies able to attack a cell membrane directly and cause lysis. However, one of the powerful effects of the binding of the antigen-antibody complex is the activation of *complement*, which serves to amplify this interaction. More specifically, when IgG or IgM binds to an antigen, the complement system is activated, and a cascade system of nine different enzyme precursors (C-1 through C-9) react sequentially. The final result of the activation of the complement system is puncture of the antigen's cell membrane (cell lysis), causing rupture of its cellular agents.

Cellular Immunity

Cellular immunity is the second type of specific immunity, and it utilizes *T lymphocytes* and *macrophages*. Some specific functions of the cellular immunity system are protection against most viruses, slow-acting bacteria, and fungal infections; mediation of cutaneous delayed hypersensitivity reactions; rejection of foreign grafts; and immunologic surveillance.

The T lymphocytes, like the B lymphocytes, originate from primitive stem cells and go through stages of maturation (Fig. 11–1). Once the immature lymphocyte leaves the bone marrow it migrates to the thymus gland, where it is acted upon by the hormone *thymosin*. The T lymphocyte then becomes mature and immunocompetent. Thus, they are thymus-dependent or T-lymphocytes. These mature T lymphocytes can circulate in the blood and lymph, or they may come to rest in the inner cortex of the lymph nodes, where they may form subgroups of T lymphocytes.

These T lymphocytes function overall in the immune system by serving in regulatory, effector, and cytotoxic capacities. The *regulatory T lymphocytes* are the *helper* or *suppressor T lymphocytes*. These lymphocytes amplify or suppress responses of other T lymphocytes or responses of B lymphocytes. The helper T lymphocytes produce a soluble factor that is required, in some cases, for antibody formation by B lymphocytes. This helper action is most important for IgE and IgG production. The under-

production of helper cells is associated with *acquired immunodeficiency syndrome (AIDS)*. The suppressor T lymphocytes appear to regulate or to suppress the activity of B lymphocytes in the production of antibodies. Evidence indicates that the suppressor T lymphocytes can become pathologically active against helper T lymphocytes and other aspects of cellular immunity. For this reason, these suppressor T lymphocytes may have a role in immune tolerance and in the development of autoimmune disease such as *myasthenia gravis*. *Effector T lymphocytes* are probably responsible for the delayed hypersensitivity reactions, the rejection of foreign tissue grafts and tumors, and the elimination of virus-infected cells. Effector T lymphocytes have antigen receptors on their surfaces that are significant in the initiation of cellular immunity. When an antigen enters the body, it undergoes processing by the phagocytes. The antigen then travels to the regional lymph node, which drains the area of antigen invasion. In this lymph node, the T lymphocyte recognizes the antigen, binds to the antigen, and proliferates. The T lymphocyte becomes sensitized when it comes into contact with the antigen. In addition, memory T lymphocytes result from this interaction. Hence, upon a second exposure to the antigen, a more intense, efficient, and rapid cellular immunity will result. This contact also results in the release of lymphokines by the T lymphocyte. Some of the lymphokines are (1) *chemotactic factor*, which recruits phagocytes into the area; (2) *migration inhibitory factor (MIF)*, which prevents the migration of phagocytes away from the area; (3) *transfer factor*, which induces noncommitted T lymphocytes to form T lymphocytes of the same antigen-specific clone as the original cells; (4) *lymphotoxin*, which is a nonspecific cellular toxin; and (5) *interferon*, which inhibits the replication of viruses.

The direct cellular cytotoxicity that is mediated by cellular immunity involves *cytotoxic lymphocytes*, or *killer cells*, and *macrophages*. The role of these cytotoxic T lymphocytes is not well established; however, they are believed to be involved in nonspecfic killing of viruses, rejection of allografts, and immune surveillance of malignant diseases.

HYPERSENSITIVITY REACTIONS

The immune system serves mainly to protect a person from harmful substances. However, in some cases, the activation of the immune system can cause many deleterious effects; this is termed allergic response or hypersensitivity reaction. Briefly, this response represents a magnified or inappropriate reaction by the host to an antigenic substance, and it can result in an immunologic disease. Hypersensitivity reactions are divided into four major categories and are called type I through type IV hypersensitivity reactions (Table 11–1).

Type I Hypersensitivity Reaction (Anaphylactic, Immediate)

Type I hypersensitivity reaction occurs in persons who were previously sensitized to a specific antigen. The antibodies formed against that antigen are of the IgE classification. The term *reagins* is used to describe these IgE antibodies. Reaginic antibodies bind to mast cells in tissues surrounding the blood vessels and to blood basophils. When the previously sensitized host is reexposed to the same antigen, the antigen reacts with the *reaginic antibody* that is attached to the cell, and there is an immediate swelling and then rupture of the basophil or mast cell, resulting in a release of chemical mediators into the local environment. These chemical mediators include (1) *histamine*, which causes local vasodilatation and increased permeability of the capillaries; (2) *slow-reacting substance of anaphylaxis (SRS-A)*, which causes prolonged contraction of some smooth muscle, such as that of the bronchi; (3) *chemotactic factor*, which draws neutrophils and macrophages into the area of the antigen-antibody reaction; and (4) *lysosomal enzymes*, which elicit a local inflammatory reaction. These chemical mediators act upon the "shock organs" such as the mucosa, skin, bronchi, and heart. The resulting clinical manifestations of the type I reaction include urticaria, allergic rhinitis, allergic asthma, and, in severe cases, systemic anaphylaxis.

Type II Hypersensitivity Reaction (Cytotoxic)

In this hypersensitivity reaction, the antigen and the antibody complex react, causing injury to the cell membrane or to a surface tissue by direct destruction by antibody of cellular elements. The antibodies involved in the type II reaction are either IgG or IgM, and the reaction is enhanced by complement. *Hemolytic anemia* is an example of a type II reaction that affects the

TABLE 11–1. Categories of Hypersensitivity Reactions

Type	Mechanism	Outcome	Reaction Time	Examples
I (Anaphylactic)	Antigen–IgE reaction at surface of mast cells and basophils	Release of mediators	Immediate	Asthma Hay fever Systemic anaphylaxis
II (Cytotoxic)	Binding of IgM or IgG with antigens on surface of cell. Enhanced by complement fixation	Cell lysis and tissue damage	Variable	Hemolytic anemia Goodpasture's disease
III (Arthus)	Microprecipitation of immune complex formed by antigen and IgM or IgG. Enhanced by complement fixation	Tissue damage and release of vasoactive substances	4–18 hr	Serum sickness Farmer's lung Allergic alveolitis Glomerulonephritis SLE
IV (Delayed)	Direct interaction of antigen with sensitized T lymphocytes	Release of mediators and tissue damage	24–48 hr	Contact dermatitis Tuberculosis

red blood cells. For example, when penicillin is absorbed on the red blood cell membrane, the interaction of antipenicillin antibody, penicillin, and complement causes a reaction that will result in the lysis of red blood cells.

Type III Hypersensitivity Reaction (Arthus)

The type III reaction involves the formation of immune complexes of antigen and antibody (IgG or IgM). These immune complexes precipitate in and around small vessels and damage the target tissue by activating complement. Also involved in this process is an inflammatory reaction that is initiated by the gathering of inflammatory cells and the release of vasoactive amines from platelets. As this process continues, polymorphonuclear leukocytes phagocytize the immune complexes, causing inflammation and necrosis of the blood vessels and surrounding tissue owing to the release of lysosomal enzymes. *Serum sickness* and *systemic lupus erythematosus* (*SLE*) are clinical examples of type III hypersensitivity reactions.

Type IV Hypersensitivity Reaction (Delayed or Cell-Mediated)

This is the only hypersensitivity reaction that does *not* involve antibodies. In the type IV reaction, the exposure to an antigen and the subsequent binding of the antigen with antigen-specific reactive T lymphocytes will initiate the production of lymphokines from the T lymphocytes, with tissue damage as the end result. The antigen responsible for the type IV reaction can be bacterial, fungal, protozoan, or viral. *Contact dermatitis, allograft rejection*, and *delayed response in tuberculin skin tests* are examples of delayed hypersensitivity reactions.

IMMUNOSUPPRESSION

With the advent of organ transplantation, patients can and do arrive in the post anesthesia care unit in an immunosuppressed state. Consequently, it is important for the PACU nurse to have a basic knowledge of the forms of immunosuppression and the appropriate nursing care measures that can be implemented for the immunosuppressed patient.

Forms of Immunosuppression

The nonresponsive state of the immune system may be due to a natural tolerance to self-antigens, to a pathologic state, or to induced immunosuppression. Researchers are attempting to understand immunosuppression by artificially manipulating the immune system to produce a natural tolerance to self-antigens. Pathologic states such as lymphoma and leukemia are examples of the second form of immunosuppression, in which the immune system becomes unresponsive owing to the pathology of the immunocompetent cells. Induced immunosuppression can be accomplished by the administration of an antigen, antisera or antibody, or hormones and cytotoxic drugs, by radiation, and by surgery. For the most part, induced immunosuppression is used for tissue and organ transplants.

For patients suffering from allergies, the administration of low-dose antigen will, in some cases, provide relief from the antigen-antibody reaction. This *desensitizing* process produces antibodies that block the interaction between the antigen and the antibody-producing cells. Another method of providing tolerance to self-antigens is by the administration of antisera or antibody in an attempt to coat the antigenic sites. The object is to prevent immunocompetent cells from combining with the antigen. This method of immunosuppression is 100 percent effective in preventing Rh sensitization and ultimately *erythroblastosis fetalis*. Corticosteroids produce immunosuppression by reducing the amount of T and B lymphocytes circulating in the blood, blocking lymphokine release, and decreasing the number of monocytes. Cytotoxic drugs are used in the treatment of cancer and autoimmune diseases. The most popular drugs are azathioprine and cyclophosphamide. These drugs suppress immune system function by killing unstimulated lymphocytes. X-irradiation suppresses most of the immunocompetent cells by the induction of a profound lymphopenia. Surgical removal of the thymus gland, spleen, or lymph nodes may alter the immune response by removing tissue needed for the maturation of both the cellular and the humoral immune systems.

PACU Care of the Immunosuppressed Patient

The major responsibilities of the PACU nurse caring for the immunosuppressed patient are prevention of and early diagnosis and treatment of infection. Views differ in regard to placement of the nonleukopenic patient in protective isolation. However, if the peripheral leukocyte count is less than 2000 cells/mm³, the patient probably will benefit from protective isolation. Before the patient is admitted to the post anesthesia care unit, sources of cross-contamination should be eliminated. Blood pressure cuffs and other equipment that are to be used directly on the patient should be cleaned and disinfected with appropriate solutions. Aseptic technique should be adhered to at all times. Additionally, needle puncture sites and surgical wounds should be cleaned and dressed with appropriate cleaners and ointments. If Foley catheters are used, those sites should be monitored closely for the beginning signs of infection. Immunosuppressed patients may not demonstrate the classic symptoms of infection. The temperature of the immunosuppressed patient should be closely monitored, and if it rises above 38°C the attending physician should be notified immediately. The use of rectal thermometers should be avoided because they can cause mucosal injury and contamination.

ACQUIRED IMMUNODEFICIENCY SYNDROME (AIDS)

Acquired immunodeficiency syndrome (AIDS) is a disease characterized by a marked deficiency of cellular immunity in the absence of any other cause of the immune defect with which opportunistic infections or unusual malignancy are associated; hence, AIDS is an immunodeficiency disease that produces immunosuppression in the infected individual. Since it was first reported in 1981, AIDS has begun to increase in epidemic fashion. At first, this syndrome was confined to specific risk groups and geographic areas; now, however, it is being reported in many subgroups throughout the United States. Persons suffering from AIDS are presenting themselves for surgical procedures such as node biopsy, intestinal exploration, abscess evacuation of the brain, and tracheostomy. Therefore, the PACU nurse should have a complete understanding of the pathophysiology and treatment of the disease as well as the precautions associated with the care of the AIDS patient.

Epidemiology

Persons in particular geographic areas or in specific risk groups have a significant chance of contracting AIDS. More specifically, the major risk groups for this syndrome in the United States are homosexual men; intravenous drug users; Haitian immigrants; recipients of blood transfusions, including hemophiliacs; and Africans or travelers to Africa.

Homosexual Men. In the United States, homosexuality or bisexuality is the major risk factor, as this factor is present in about 72 percent of cases occurring in the United States. Approximately 70 percent of the homosexual cases in the United States are reported from New York, Miami, San Francisco, and Los Angeles metropolitan areas, and about 95 percent of the individuals are between the ages of 20 and 49. It has been suggested that a sexually transmitted agent for AIDS is present in semen, and possibly other fluids whose entry is facilitated by a traumatized mucosal barrier. Studies indicate that the mean time from sexual contact to the development of AIDS is 10 months.

Intravenous Drug Users. This particular risk group represents about 20 percent of the total cases of AIDS in the United States, and only 15 percent of the cases have been reported outside the New York–New Jersey area. Most of these individuals present for medical care with *Pneumocystis* or other opportunistic infections. The common epidemiologic feature of persons in this risk group is the sharing of needles.

Haitians and Africans. About 5 percent of the AIDS cases are reported in Haitian immigrants or in persons who have recently traveled to Haiti. Although the prominent incidence of AIDS in Haitians has not been satisfactorily explained, it is believed that AIDS was transmitted to Haiti from elsewhere rather than imported from the United States. In regard to Africa, evidence suggests that AIDS originated there.

Recipients of Blood Transfusions and Hemophiliacs. Persons in these two groups represent 3 percent and 1 percent of the United States cases of AIDS, respectively. These persons have usually had multiple transfusions, and the median time from transfusion to the onset of the illness is 27 months. The mean age for the patients is 54 years, with an equal incidence in males and females.

Summary of Epidemiology of AIDS

Overall, the analysis of the clinical and epidemiologic data suggests that AIDS (1) is transmitted by a particular agent that is present in several body fluids; (2) has a latent period between time of infection and the appearance of clinical features of the syndrome of anywhere from 6 to 36 months; (3) is accompanied by a dramatic alteration in cellular immunity; and (4) can be transmitted, in the prenatal period, to infants born to high risk mothers and infants of mothers who have had sexual contact with persons in the high risk group.

Pathophysiology

The *human retrovirus* HIV (*human immunodeficiency virus*) is probably the agent that is responsible for AIDS. Retroviruses are an unusual group of viruses that carry their genetic information by means of RNA instead of DNA. Further studies are needed of the molecular organization and biochemical structure of HIV (also known as HTLV-III, LAV-I, or ARV-I) to facilitate an understanding of the biology of the virus and its pathophysiologic mechanisms in AIDS. Such studies should provide a basis for the diagnosis and treatment of the syndrome. Ultimately, it is hoped that the isolation of large quantities of the virus will lead to the development of a protective vaccine.

The hallmark of AIDS is a profound reduction in immune reactivity, with this immunodeficiency leading to infection and malignancy. The immunologic abnormality that has become synonymous with AIDS is a reversal in the ratio of helper ($T4^+$) to suppressor ($T8^+$) cells. The normal ratio ($T4^+/T8^+$) is 2, and in patients with AIDS it is less than 0.5. The reduction in the ratio is due to a decrease in the absolute number of circulating helper cells rather than to an increase in the number of suppressor cells. In patients with AIDS, there is a tenfold decrease in the number of helper cells. The production of soluble materials required for full cell-mediated reactivity, such as delayed hypersensitivity, is a main function of the helper T lymphocytes. Because of the diminution in the helper T lymphocytes, there is a reduction in the cooperation between the humoral and cellular immunity subsystems. Consequently, the humoral immunity activities are reduced in patients suffering from AIDS.

The immunologic functions affected by AIDS are listed in Table 11–2. Conclusions that can be drawn from a review of this table are that the reduced immunologic function leads to increased susceptibility to infections, and that the diminution in the killer cell activity accounts for the increased susceptibility to malignancy. Table 11–3 summarizes the pathophysiology that is associated with acquired immunodeficiency syndrome.

Treatment

At present, the therapeutic approaches are empirical. These approaches include the use of lymphocyte plasmapheresis, recom-

TABLE 11–2. Abnormalities in Immune Function Associated with AIDS

Cellular (Cell-Mediated) Immunity
↓ Reactivity to mitogens, soluble antigens, and alloantigens
↓ Reactivity to delayed hypersensitivity skin tests
↓ Production of the lymphokines
↓ Natural killer-cell activity
↓ Cytotoxicity of virus-infected cells

Humoral Immunity
↓ Circulating immunoglobins
↓ Circulating immune complexes
↓ Production of antibodies to antigenic challenge
↓ Helper T-lymphocyte activity

Adapted from Weiss, A., Hollander, H., and Stobo, J.: Acquired immunodeficiency syndrome: epidemiology, virology, and immunology. Annu. Rev. Med., 36: 545–562, 1985. Reproduced, with permission, from the Annual Review of Medicine, Vol. 36. © 1985 by Annual Reviews Inc.

binant interferon, identical-twin and allogeneic bone-marrow transplantation, and isoprinosine. The treatment of AIDS is basically symptomatic; *Pneumocystis carinii* infection is usually treated with pentamidine or trimethoprim-sulfamethoxazole (TMP-SMX), and the chemotherapeutic drugs are used to treat Kaposi's sarcoma. Public awareness of AIDS was accentuated by the death of actor Rock Hudson and has resulted in increased funding for ongoing research on AIDS. Research is focused on the development of possible antiviral drugs and vaccines and on the treatment of AIDS with interferon.

TABLE 11–3. Pathophysiology Associated with AIDS

Infections
Protozoan
  Pneumocystis
  Toxoplasma
  Cryptosporidium
Fungal
  Thrush
  Cryptococcus
Mycobacterial
Viral
  HSV (Herpes simplex)
  CMV (Cytomegalovirus)
  PML (Progressive multifocal leukoencephalopathy)

Tumors
Kaposi's sarcoma
Lymphoma (CNS)

Adapted from Conway, J.: AIDS: A practicing physician's perspective. J. La. State Med. Soc., *137*(9):37–40, 1985.

PACU Care of the AIDS Patient

Because the transmissible HIV virus has been identified as the cause of AIDS, certain general considerations should be reviewed before nursing care is rendered to these patients. These considerations are presented in Table 11–4. Table 11–5 suggests some formal precautions that should be instituted when nursing care is rendered to the AIDS patient.

The psychosocial impact of AIDS on the patient can be devastating. AIDS patients often exhibit extreme anxiety and severe depression with accompanying withdrawal. Because of the epidemiologic implications of AIDS, these patients often feel ostracized from society. In addition, they usually experience major changes in life, such as quitting their job, selling their business, dropping out of school, or leaving the community. In order to provide maximal support to these patients, all personnel in the post anesthesia care unit should view the disease of AIDS objectively. The patient with AIDS should be included with others and be treated with respect and empathy. Above all, the nurse should remain nonjudgmental. If possible, the nurse should

TABLE 11–4. General Considerations When Rendering PACU Nursing Care to the Patient with AIDS

1. AIDS appears to be transmitted by intimate sexual contact or by percutaneous inoculation of blood or blood products.
2. There has been no evidence of transmission by casual contact or by airborne organisms.
3. A serologic test is available that indicates exposure to HIV virus. A positive test indicates that a person has been *exposed* to the virus and has produced a response.
4. Accidental needle sticks represent the number one potential source of inoculation by health care personnel.
5. Suggested precautions should be instituted in the care of any patient who:
   a. possibly has AIDS,
   b. has chronic, generalized lymphadenopathy, unexplained weight loss, and/or prolonged unexplained fever, with a history suggestive of an epidemiologic risk for AIDS,
   c. has symptoms that meet Centers for Disease Control surveillance definition of AIDS—an opportunistic infection or malignancy predictive of cellular or immune deficiency in a person under age 60 who has no underlying immunosuppressive condition.

TABLE 11–5. Suggested Precautions to Be Taken When Rendering PACU Nursing Care to the Patient with AIDS

1. Use strict hand-washing technique before and after administering care, according to protocol for contaminated patients.
2. Wear gloves during blood drawing procedures.
3. Label all blood specimens from patients with AIDS.
4. Use a needle-locking (i.e., Luer-Lok) system when aspirating any of the body fluids to prevent further contamination.
5. Do not attempt to resheath or recover needles—drop needle and syringe into a puncture-resistant receptacle without touching the needle.
6. Gown and gloves are necessary when there will be contact with patient's blood, feces, or urine.
7. Use gown, gloves, and mask to avoid possible contact with the mucosal surfaces of the mouth, nares, and eyes.
8. Use disposable equipment when possible, e.g., oral airways, temperature probes, syringes, needles, etc.
9. If patient is incontinent, wear gown and gloves.
10. When removing linen from bed of AIDS patient, always hold the linen away from the body. If linen is soiled, wear protective clothing. To dispose of linen, use double bags, one of which is water-soluble, and label. AIDS patients' linen can be washed like linens of every other patient.
11. If patient is incontinent or immunosuppressed, establish isolation procedures in an effort to minimize the potential risk to patient and staff.
12. Contaminated materials that are to be reused can be disinfected with regular household 5.25% bleach that has been diluted to a 1:10 solution (to kill the HIV virus).

allow the patient the opportunity to verbalize his fears and feelings. Timely reassurance is also necessary to instill a feeling of security in the patient. These positive attitudes demonstrated by the PACU nurse should enhance the self-esteem, integrity, and basic security of the patient.

REFERENCES

1. Centers for Disease Control: Acquired immunodeficiency syndrome (AIDS): precautions for health-care workers and allied professionals. MMWR 32(34):450–451, 1983.
2. Chaffee, E., and Lytle, I.: Basic Physiology and Anatomy. 4th ed. Philadelphia, J. B. Lippincott Co., 1980.
3. Conway, J.: AIDS: A practicing physician's perspective. J. La. State Med. Soc. 137(9):37–40, 1985.
4. Fauci, A.: The acquired immunodeficiency syndrome: an update (NIH Conference). Ann. Intern. Med. 102:800–813, 1985.
5. Fruth, R.: Anaphylaxis and drug reactions: guidelines for detection and care. Heart Lung, 9(4):662–664, 1980.
6. Ganong, W.: Review of Medical Physiology. 12th ed. Los Altos, Lange Medical Publications, 1985.
7. Gorringe-Moore, R.: Immunology and the lung. In Traver, G. (ed.): Respiratory Nursing: The Science and the Art. New York, John Wiley & Sons, Inc., 1982.
8. Groenwald, S.: Physiology of the immune system. Heart Lung, 9(4):645–650, 1980.
9. Guyton, A.: Textbook of Medical Physiology. 7th ed. Philadelphia, W. B. Saunders Co., 1986.
10. Jocius, M.: Immunohematology and transfusion reaction. AANA J. 50(1):42–48, 1982.
11. Murray, J.: The Normal Lung. 2nd ed. Philadelphia, W. B. Saunders Co., 1986.
12. Rana, A., and Luskin, A.: Immunosuppression, autoimmunity, and hypersensitivity. Heart Lung, 9(4):651–657, 1980.
13. Silverman, M.: Definition, overview, and the "new" virus. J. La. State Med. Soc. 137(9):31–34, 1985.
14. Sophie, L.: Meeting the immunologic challenge of transplant nursing. Heart Lung, 9(4):690–694, 1980.
15. Stites, D., Stobo, J., Fudenberg, A., et al.: Basic and Clinical Immunology. Los Altos, Lange Medical Publications, 1984.
16. Summer, B.: An overview of acquired immunodeficiency syndrome (AIDS)—The disease and related anesthetic considerations. AANA J. 51(4):381–384, 1983.
17. Weiss, A., Hollander, H., and Stobo, J.: Acquired immunodeficiency syndrome: epidemiology, virology, and immunology. Annu. Rev. Medicine, 36:545–562, 1985.
18. Williams, W.: How does the medical profession protect itself? J. La. State Med. Soc. 137(9):53–55, 1985.

Concepts in Anesthetic Agents

12

Inhalation Anesthesia

BASIC CONCEPTS

In order to anticipate how a patient will react when emerging from an inhalation anesthetic, the post anesthesia care unit (PACU) nurse should have a good understanding of the pharmacologic concepts of inhalation anesthesia. Although the complexity of these agents, coupled with drug interactions and the various levels of physical health, makes it difficult to predict the exact nature of each patient's emergence from inhalation anesthesia, an understanding of some general principles will prepare the PACU nurse for the most commonly expected outcomes.

The Signs and Stages of Anesthesia

The standard signs and stages of anesthesia apply only to the rarely, if ever, used inhalational anesthetic diethyl ether; however, most anesthesia personnel still refer to the patient's level of anesthesia in terms of the ether signs and stages. Also, because of the long history of the use of ether (from 1846 to the 1960s), most of the newer anesthetic agents are still compared with it.

The ether signs and stages were devised to give some means of assessing the depth of anesthesia. The first three stages were described by Plomley in 1847, and a year later John Snow added a fourth stage, that of overdose. Guedel, during World War I, more accurately defined and described the signs and stages of anesthesia. A graphic representation of these signs and stages is provided in Figure 12–1.

Stage I begins with the initiation of anesthesia and ends with the loss of consciousness. It is commonly called the *stage of analgesia. Stage II* starts with the loss of consciousness and ends with the onset of a regular pattern of breathing and the disappearance of the lid reflex. This is also called the *stage of delirium.* It is characterized by excitement, and, because of this, many untoward responses such as vomiting, laryngospasm, and even cardiac arrest may take place during this stage. With the use of anesthetic agents that act much more rapidly than ether, this stage is passed rather quickly. In addition, the induction of anesthesia is usually facilitated by short-acting barbiturates, which expedite a short duration of stage II.

Stage III is the *stage of surgical anesthesia.* It is defined as lasting from the onset of a regular pattern of breathing to the cessation of respiration. Most surgical procedures are performed at this stage of anesthesia, which is divided into four planes. *Plane 1* is entered when the lid reflex is abolished and respiration becomes regular. It is during this plane that the vomiting reflex is gradually abolished. It is important for the nurse working in the post anesthesia care unit to

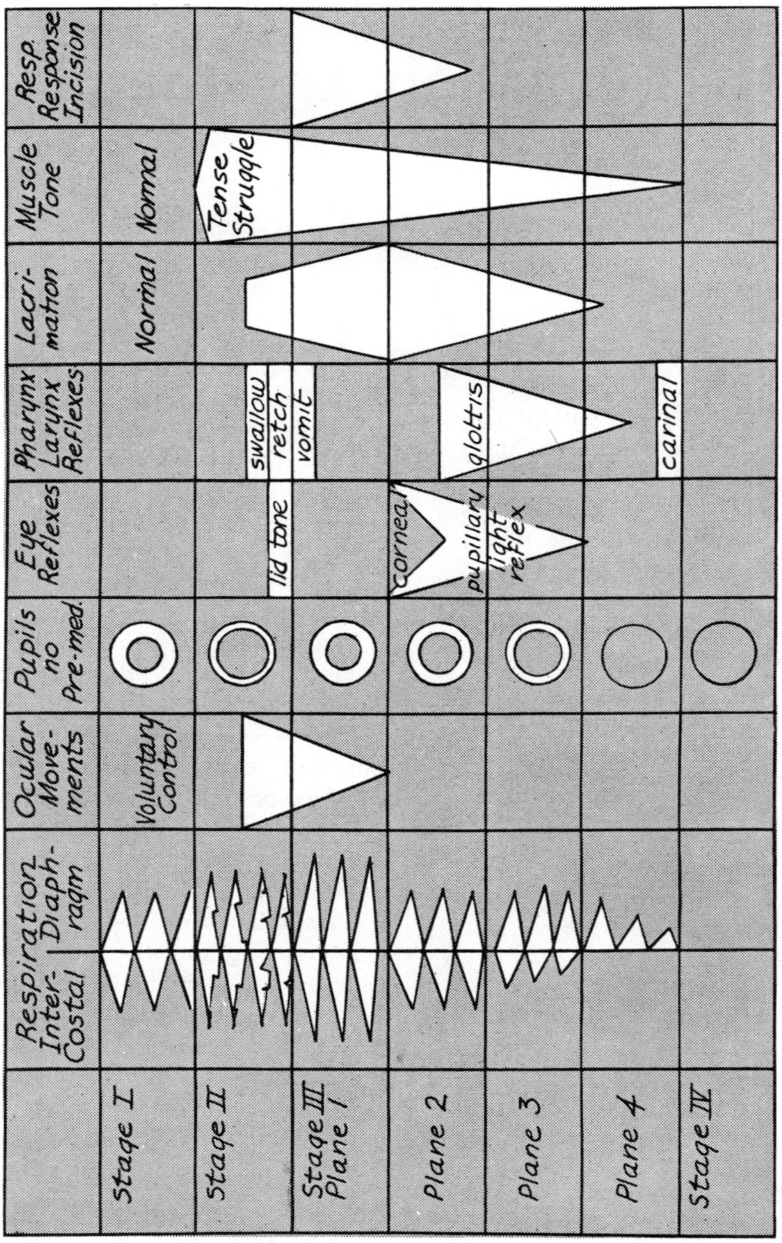

Figure 12–1. The signs and reflex reactions of the stages of anesthesia. (After Gillespie, N. A.: Anesth. Analg., 22:275, 1943, in Dripps, R. D., Eckenhoff, J. E., and Vandam, L. D.: Introduction to Anesthesia. 5th ed. Philadelphia, W. B. Saunders Co., 1977, p. 233.)

know that swallowing, retching, and vomiting reflexes tend to disappear in that order during induction and reappear in the same order during emergence from anesthesia.

Plane 2 lasts from the time the eyeballs cease to move and become concentrically fixed, to the beginning of a decrease of activity of the intercostal muscles, or thoracic respiration. The reflex of laryngospasm disappears during this plane. *Plane 3* is entered when intercostal activity begins to decrease. Complete intercostal paralysis occurs in lower plane 3, and respiration is carried on solely by the diaphragm. *Plane 4* lasts from the time of paralysis of the intercostal muscles to the cessation of spontaneous respiration.

Tracheal tug often appears in association with deep anesthesia and intercostal paralysis. This represents an unopposed action of the diaphragm, displacing the hilum of the lung and therefore increasing traction of the trachea.

Stage IV lasts from the time of cessation of respiration to failure of the circulatory system. This level of anesthesia is considered the stage of overdose.

These signs and stages will be seen in reverse order upon emergence from the anesthetic. No clinical sign can be considered a reliable indicator by itself of anesthetic depth. All clinical signs must be viewed in the context of the patient's status along with the particular characteristics of the individual anesthetic agent used.

Potency, Anesthetic Uptake, and Distribution

Three factors determine how rapidly an anesthetic agent will take a patient to surgical anesthesia: (1) the potency of the agent, (2) the partial pressure at which the agent is administered, and (3) the rate at which the anesthetic agent is taken up by the blood and tissues.

Potency. The potency of the anesthetic agent refers to its ability to take the patient through all the stages of anesthesia to respiratory and circulatory arrest without the occurrence of hypoxia or the use of pre-

anesthetic medication. Certainly, circulatory and respiratory arrest are not desired outcomes of the use of anesthetic agents; this feature is merely used to describe the potency of anesthetic agents that are used clinically. For example, halothane is 100 percent potent as compared with nitrous oxide, which is 15 percent potent. Halothane, when administered with oxygen to meet the patient's metabolic needs, and when given without premedication, will take the patient to circulatory and respiratory arrest, whereas nitrous oxide administered with oxygen will take the patient only to the first portion of surgical anesthesia and no farther.

Another way of determining potency is by the use of the MAC or *minimum alveolar concentration*. The MAC is found by determining the alveolar concentration (at one atmosphere of pressure) required to prevent gross muscular movement in response to painful stimuli in 50 percent of anesthetized patients. The lower the MAC value, the more anesthetic potency the inhalational anesthetic has. The minimum alveolar concentration of halothane in oxygen required to prevent patient movement in response to surgical incision is 0.75 percent. A geriatric patient might be administered 0.38 percent halothane in oxygen, which is commonly referred to as half MAC. MAC hours is the concentration in MAC units multiplied by the duration in hours of anesthetic administration. Consequently, the MAC hours for this patient would be 0.76 (0.38 × 2). When 70 percent nitrous oxide is added to the halothane, the MAC decreases to 0.29 percent. Thus, when halothane (or any 100 percent potent agent) is combined with a premedication and nitrous oxide, the MAC will decrease (Table 12–1). The MAC is reduced in patients who are hypothermic, elderly, or pregnant. Narcotics, diazepam, nitrous oxide, reserpine and alphamethyldopa will also decrease the MAC. On the other hand, amphetamines, which release catecholamines, will raise the MAC.

Partial Pressure. The partial pressure of an inhalation anesthetic in the brain will determine the depth of anesthesia. The more potent the anesthetic, the lower the

TABLE 12–1. Properties of Inhalant Anesthetic Agents

Agent	Flammability Range or Lower Limit (in O₂)	(in air)	Partition Coefficient (blood-gas)	(oil-gas)	Minimum Alveolar Concentration (% in Oxygen)	Minimum Alveolar Concentration (% in 70% N₂O)	Boiling Point at 760 mm Hg (°C)	Vapor Pressure (mm Hg) (at 20°C)	Appearance	Odor	Explosiveness
Diethyl ether	2.1 to 82.5%	1.8 to 48%	12.1	—	1.92	—	36.2	443	Clear, colorless liquid	Irritating, pungent	Yes
Trichloroethylene	Nonflammable		9.14	960.0	—	—	87.0	60	Clear, colorless liquid (blue dye added for identification)	Sweet	No
Halothane (Fluothane)	Nonflammable		2.37	224.0	0.75	0.29	50.2	243	Clear, colorless liquid	Pleasant, sweet	No
Chloroform	Nonflammable		10.3	265.0	—	—	61.0	166	Clear, colorless liquid	Sweet	No
Enflurane (Ethrane)	Nonflammable		1.9	98.5	1.68	0.57	56.5	175	Clear, colorless liquid	Pleasant, ethereal	No
Methoxyflurane (Penthrane)	Nonflammable in anesthetic concentration		13.0	930.0	0.16	0.07	104.70	25	Clear, colorless liquid	Pleasant, fruity	No
Fluroxene	4%	4.1%	1.37	56.8	3.4	—	42.70	286	Clear, colorless liquid	Pleasant, ethereal	Yes
Isoflurane (Forane)	Nonflammable		0.97	93.7	1.15	0.50	48.50	252	Clear, colorless liquid	Faint, ethereal	No
Nitrous oxide	Supports combustion		0.47	1.4	110.0	—	−88.44	52 atm.	Colorless gas	No odor or taste	No
Ethylene	2.9 to 79.9%	3 to 28.6%	0.14	1.28	—	—	−103.9	48 atm.	Colorless gas	Pleasant, ethereal	Yes
Cyclopropane	2.48 to 60%	2.4 to 10.3%	0.42	11.2	9.2	—	−34.0	5.6 atm.	Colorless gas	Pleasant, sweet	Yes

partial pressure of the agent required to produce a certain depth of anesthesia. Pulmonary ventilation plays the primary role in delivery of the anesthetic gas. If the minute volume ($\dot{V}_E$) is high, the anesthetic concentration increases quickly in the alveoli, as does the concentration in the arterial blood. This is an important concept to understand because the reverse also holds true. In the emergence phase of anesthesia it is important to have a good minute volume to ensure elimination of the anesthetic agent.

Distribution. The rate at which the anesthetic is taken up by the blood and tissues is governed in part by the solubility of the agent in blood. This is expressed as the *blood-gas partition coefficient* or the *Oswald solubility coefficient*. It is defined as the ratio of the concentration of an anesthetic in blood to that in a gas phase when the two are in equilibrium. This is a difficult concept to understand because the more soluble the anesthetic agent is, the slower the agent is in producing anesthesia. This is because the blood serves as a reservoir and a large volume of the agent must be introduced to attain an equilibrium between the blood partial pressure and the partial pressure in the lungs.

The blood conveys the anesthetic agent to the tissues. The partial pressure increases most rapidly in the tissues with the highest rates of blood flow. The tissue tensions increase and approach the arterial blood tension. When the administration of the anesthetic is terminated, a reverse gradient takes place. The partial pressure in the arterial blood declines first, followed by that in the tissues. The agent returns to the lungs and is then eliminated into the atmosphere. The factors that affect the rate of elimination of the agent are the same ones that determine how rapidly an anesthetic agent will take a patient to surgical anesthesia.

Of interest is the great variation in blood perfusion of certain tissues in the body. The body tissue compartments can be divided into four major groups: (1) The *vessel-rich group (VRG)*, which consists of the heart, brain, kidneys, hepatoportal system, and the endocrine glands; (2) muscle and skin, which are called the *intermediate group (IG)* of perfused tissues; (3) the *fat group (FG)*, which includes marrow and adipose tissue; and (4) the *vessel-poor group (VPG)*, which has the poorest circulation per unit volume and is composed of tendons, ligaments, connective tissue, teeth, bone, and other avascular tissue. The vessel-rich group of tissues receives 75 percent of the cardiac output; thus, the brain becomes saturated very rapidly with an anesthetic agent administered by inhalation. Upon termination of the anesthetic, the reverse takes place, and there is rapid removal of the agent from the brain.

The *oil-gas partition coefficient* is defined as the ratio of the concentration of the anesthetic agent in oil (adipose tissue) to that in a gaseous phase when the two are in equilibrium. Because some anesthetic agents are very fat soluble, they tend to be readily absorbed by the adipose tissue. This affects uptake of the anesthetic agent, but of more importance is the prolonged recovery phase that usually ensues with a high oil-gas partition coefficient such as in the case of halothane. Because adipose tissue is poorly perfused by blood, at the termination of the anesthesia the adipose tissue releases the agent slowly to the blood. Redistribution then takes place: Some of the agent is eliminated by the lungs, which are vessel rich, and some is distributed to the brain. The recovery period becomes significantly extended when the administration time of the anesthetic agent is prolonged in order to allow for complete saturation of the adipose tissue.

Halothane (Fluothane) has an oil-gas partition coefficient that is about double that of isoflurane (Forane) or enflurane (Ethrane). Consequently, some authors question the use of halothane in the ambulatory surgical setting. However, clinical observation indicates that patients who receive halothane appear to emerge from anesthesia at about the same rate as they do from isoflurane. Therefore, even with its relatively high oil-gas partition coefficient, halothane remains a popular inhalation anesthetic for use in the ambulatory surgical setting.

Other factors that influence the rate of uptake of an anesthetic agent administered by inhalation are diffusion of the anesthetic agent into the rubber tubing of the anesthesia machine; the small losses of anesthetic agent from the body by diffusion across skin and mucous membranes; and, to a lesser extent, the metabolism of the agents by the body.

TECHNIQUES OF ADMINISTRATION

The inhalation anesthetics are usually administered by means of an *anesthesia machine* (Fig. 12–2). The anesthesia machine is essentially a breathing circuit that conveys the agent and oxygen to the patient. It consists of a mask, corrugated tubing, an absorber to remove expired carbon dioxide, unidirectional valves, a reservoir bag, a pop-off valve, and vaporizers (Fig. 12–3).

Circle Systems

A variety of techniques can be used to deliver gaseous agents with the anesthesia machine by adding or removing certain features. The most common technique used is the *semiclosed circle method*, in which some rebreathing of expired gases occurs by opening the pop-off valve to vent some of the gas to the atmosphere. The *closed circle method* is used when explosive gases are being administered or when low gas flows are desired for nonexplosive agents. In this technique, the pop-off valve is completely closed and complete rebreathing of expired gases occurs. A carbon dioxide absorber is used in both the semiclosed and the closed techniques.

Insufflation Technique

The *insufflation technique* involves the delivery of large volumes of fresh gases administered continuously to the mouth by means of a hook made of hard plastic or metal. This technique permits the least rebreathing of expired gases, and, though not

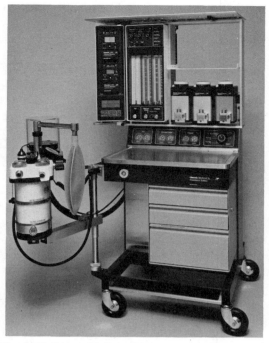

Figure 12–2. Anesthesia machine apparatus. (Courtesy of Ohmeda, a division of the BOC Group Inc., Madison, Wisconsin.)

often used today, has the advantages of posing little resistance to breathing and not requiring complex equipment.

Open Systems

The *open* or *nonrebreathing technique* ensures that the patient will inhale only the anesthetic mixture delivered by the anesthesia machine. Valves such as the Leigh, Fink, Rubin, or Stephen-Slater are used, and there is minimal rebreathing of the anesthetic gas.

Semiopen Systems

The *semiopen system* allows exhaled gases to pass into surrounding atmosphere, and some of the exhaled gases are rebreathed. Essentially, the semiopen method works without carbon dioxide absorption. The types of semiopen systems used are the open drop method, the Ayre T-piece, and the Magill attachment, and the Bain anesthesia circuit.

The *open drop method* was one of the first anesthesia methods ever used, and it re-

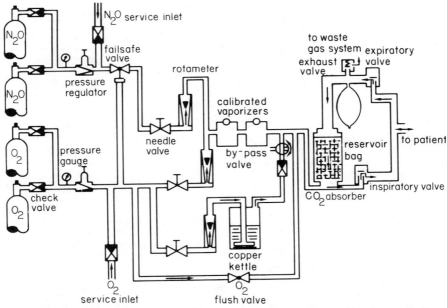

Figure 12–3. Anesthesia machine circuit. Oxygen and nitrous oxide enter the machine from cylinders, or from the hospital service supply. Pressure regulators reduce cylinder pressure to about 3 kg/cm². Check valves prevent transfilling of cylinders or gas flow from cylinders to service line. The fail-safe valve prevents flow of nitrous oxide if the oxygen supply fails. Needle valves control flows to rotameters. Calibrated vaporizers provide a preselected concentration of volatile anesthetics. The copper kettle delivers the saturated vapor of any agent; thus the effluent must be diluted. The bypass valve vents vapor from the kettle when it is not in service. Gases are delivered to the circle absorber, where unidirectional valves assure flow from patient through carbon dioxide absorber. Excess gas is vented through the exhaust valve into a waste gas scavenger system. The reservoir bag compensates for variations in respiratory demand. (From Dripps, R. D., Eckenhoff, J. E., and Vandam, L. D.: Introduction to Anesthesia. 5th ed. Philadelphia, W. B. Saunders Co., 1977, p. 60.)

quires the least equipment. A volatile anesthetic agent is dripped over a wire mask covered with gauze. Oxygen is usually administered by the insufflation technique to supply the metabolic needs of the patient. The open drop technique is not used in today's anesthesia practice because the anesthetic agents required in this technique are flammable and explosive.

The *Ayre T-piece* was devised to facilitate endotracheal anesthesia for infants and children (Fig. 12–4). One end of the T-piece is connected to the endotracheal tube, and the other end is open to the atmosphere. At the middle portion and at a right angle to the main limb a tube is attached, forming the T, through which the delivery of the anesthetic agent is accomplished. The modified Ayre T-piece consists of a rebreathing bag connected by corrugated tubing to the escape end of the T-piece. This gives the system more versatility and provides a

means of positive pressure to support ventilation. This method is simple and is used for children up to the age of 4.

The *Magill attachment* is similar to the modified Ayre T-piece, except that an expiratory valve is inserted into the circuit

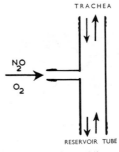

Figure 12–4. The Ayre T-piece. Nitrous oxide–oxygen supplemented with ether enters through the side tube. The tracheal end of the T-piece is connected to the endotracheal tube. The end marked "reservoir tube" is open to the air. (From Ayre, P.: Br. J. Anaesth., 28:520, 1956, in Dripps, R. D., et al.: Introduction to Anesthesia. 5th ed. Philadelphia, W. B. Saunders Co., 1977, p. 167.)

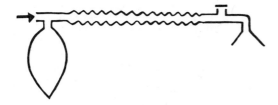

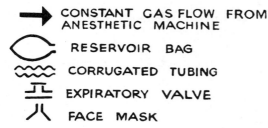

CONSTANT GAS FLOW FROM ANESTHETIC MACHINE

RESERVOIR BAG

CORRUGATED TUBING

EXPIRATORY VALVE

FACE MASK

Figure 12–5. The Magill attachment. (From Dripps, R. D., et al.: Introduction to Anesthesia. 5th ed. Philadelphia, W. B. Saunders Co., 1977, p. 169.)

close to the face mask and is separated from the reservoir bag by corrugated tubing (Fig. 12–5).

The *Bain anesthesia circuit* was introduced in 1972 and consists of a tube within a tube. The inner, noncorrugated tube, which provides fresh gases to the patient, is surrounded by a wider corrugated tube, which conveys exhaled gases away from the patient. The circuit attaches to a bag mount, which is attached to the anesthesia machine. The bag mount incorporates an exhaust valve and a bag port for attachment of an anesthesia bag or ventilator tubing (Fig. 12–6). The major advantage of this

circuit is its versatility: It may be used for both children and adults, has no directional valves, is especially useful in cases involving the head and neck, and does not require carbon dioxide absorption (no soda lime), yet patients may be maintained at a normal $PaCO_2$ and pH.

THE INHALATION AGENTS

Inhalant anesthetic substances may be divided into two groups: *volatile anesthetic agents* and *gaseous anesthetic* agents. Volatile anesthetic agents are chemicals in the liquid state at room temperature that have a boil-

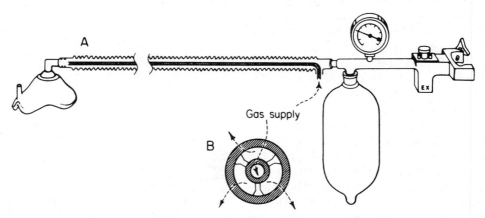

Figure 12–6. Bain system breathing circuit. *A*, Tube-within-tube design. *B*, Cross section of tubing. Arrows show air inflow and outflow. (From Chu, Y. K., Rah, K. H., and Boyan, C. P.: Is the Bain Breathing Circuit the future anesthesia system? Anesth. Analg., 56:84, 1977.)

ing point above 20°C. Ethyl chloride, which has a boiling point of 12°C, is also included in this class of anesthetic agents. The volatile inhalational anesthetic agents are divided into two major categories: the *halogenated hydrocarbons* and the *ethers*. Examples of the halogenated hydrocarbons are halothane, chloroform, and trichloroethylene. Enflurane, methoxyflurane, isoflurane, and diethyl ether are examples of the ethers. The gaseous anesthetic agents are those in the gaseous state at room temperature; nitrous oxide and cyclopropane are examples. The present-day anesthetic agents have evolved from the traditional inhalational anesthetics such as cyclopropane, chloroform, and diethyl ether. For that reason they will be described briefly before the present-day inhalational agents are presented in detail.

Traditional Inhalational Anesthetic Agents

Chloroform (Trichlormethane)

Chloroform was the most potent anesthetic agent available up to the 1970s. It offered many advantages, such as excellent muscle relaxation, no irritation of the respiratory tract, rapid induction and emergence, and nonflammability. However, the disadvantages of chloroform are clinically significant. Because deep anesthesia can be achieved rapidly with very small changes in concentration, it has a narrow margin of safety. The major problem with chloroform is that it is hepatotoxic and cardiotoxic and, therefore, is no longer administered to humans.

Being a hydrocarbon, chloroform has some excellent qualities that were preserved when researchers developed newer hydrocarbon inhalational anesthetic agents such as halothane. In this way, chloroform served as a model for the modern inhalational anesthetics.

Cyclopropane

Cyclopropane was introduced into clinical anesthesia in 1934. It is a colorless gas with the characteristic odor of petroleum ether. It is stored in orange metal cylinders as a liquid under pressure. The most notable property of this drug is its speed of induction and emergence. This is due to its blood-gas partition coefficient of 0.42. In fact, anesthesia can be induced in five or six deep tidal breaths in a premedicated patient.

The simplest of the cyclic hydrocarbons, cyclopropane is flammable and explosive in air and in oxygen. Like other explosive inhalation anesthetic agents, cyclopropane is no longer utilized in anesthesia practice.

Diethyl Ether

Ether, one of the first inhalational anesthetics administered in the United States, is rarely used today; therefore, it is presented to the reader for its historical significance only.

Ether has the relatively high blood-gas partition coefficient of 12.1. Consequently, when ether is administered alone, without any premedication, the induction time is long—usually 30 to 40 minutes. The same holds true for emergence. When the patient awakens he usually has some degree of analgesia. Because of its rather high blood-gas partition coefficient, ether has a built-in safety factor that provides a wide margin of safety for the patient. This consists in the fact that it is difficult to deepen the anesthesia rapidly; thus, the anesthetist has a reasonable length of time to appraise the patient's status and make corrections before a deeper anesthetic plane is induced.

Ether has other advantages: It improves the blood pressure and causes excellent muscle relaxation; in addition, it can be used with all techniques and is inexpensive. The disadvantages of ether are that it is flammable and explosive and has been implicated in the occurrence of convulsions, nausea, and vomiting.

Ethylene

Ethylene was discovered in 1923 and resembles nitrous oxide in its usage in anesthesia practice. The gas is about 25 percent potent and will take the patient to the lower border of plane 1 of stage III while supplying the metabolic oxygen requirement. A unique property of this agent is that it is lighter than air and will rise. Ethylene is a very rapid-acting agent because of its blood-gas partition coefficient of 0.14. This agent has been eliminated from use in anesthesia departments solely because of its flammability and explosive properties.

Fluroxene (Trifluoroethyl Vinyl Ether, Fluoromar)

Fluroxene was the first of the fluorine-containing hydrocarbons to be introduced into clinical practice. It is a mixed halogenated aliphatic ether. It is flammable, although less so than the nonfluorinated ethers. Because fluroxene is a derivative of ether, postanesthetic nausea and vomiting are not uncommon with its use. Since it is explosive and has strong emetic properties, it is not utilized today.

Methoxyflurane (Penthrane)

Methoxyflurane is a fluorinated alkyl ether that was introduced into anesthesia practice in 1959. It is nonflammable and nonexplosive in air, oxygen, or nitrous oxide mixtures at normal room temperature. Methoxyflurane can produce any desired depth of anesthesia in the absence of hypoxia and therefore meets the requirements for a 100 percent potent agent. The drug has a high blood-gas partition coefficient of 13 and thus features excellent controllability and analgesia, with good muscle relaxation.

Methoxyflurane was originally thought to be exhaled unchanged, but it is now known to be partially metabolized into several substances that contribute to renal dysfunction. The most important metabolite is free inorganic fluoride, which is nephrotoxic. The renal syndrome caused by methoxyflurane is called *vasopressin-resistant high-output renal failure*. Because methoxyflurane is nephrotoxic, it is no longer used in anesthesia practice.

Trichloroethylene (Trilene)

Like chloroform and ether, trichloroethylene is not utilized today in anesthesia practice. The drug is related chemically to chloroform and ethylene. Because the drug decomposes to dichloracetylene when it is exposed to soda lime, it was used only for its analgesic qualities in obstetrics, dentistry, and short surgical procedures. It was administered by techniques such as inhalers, insufflation, and blow-through vaporizers that did not have to incorporate soda lime in the circuit.

Modern Inhalational Anesthetic Agents

Enflurane (Ethrane)

Enflurane is a halogenated ether that is enjoying significant popularity in the practice of anesthesia. It is nonflammable, 100 percent potent, and very rapid acting. Enflurane promotes a fair amount of muscle relaxation and strongly potentiates any nondepolarizing skeletal muscle relaxant, such as d-tubocurarine and pancuronium.

Enflurane, like halothane, causes cerebral vasodilation, which results in a cerebral blood flow increase if the patient is normotensive. When the patient is hypotensive, enflurane can reduce the cerebral blood flow. This agent may cause no change or small and inconsistent increases in intracranial pressure in neurosurgical patients who are hyperventilated. The hemodynamic effects of enflurane are similar to those of halothane; however, it will depress arterial blood pressure, stroke volume, and systemic vascular resistance. The cardiac depression that enflurane produces appears to be due to direct negative inotropic effects on the heart, and it also produces a reduction in the peripheral vascular resistance. Enflurane tends to increase the heart rate or it may keep it normal, and bradycardia does not usually occur. Enflurane sensitizes the myocardium to the effects of endogenous and exogenous catecholamines. However, a lower incidence of dysrhythmias has been associated with enflurane as compared with halothane. In comparison with halothane, enflurane is a more potent respiratory depressant and will blunt a patient's response to hypercarbia.

Like methoxyflurane (another fluorinated ether), enflurane is metabolized to inorganic and organic fluoride. However, the maximum serum concentrations are not high enough to cause renal toxicity. There have been some isolated reports suggesting that enflurane causes slight hepatic dysfunction. Hence, enflurane may not be the anesthetic of choice for a patient with compromised hepatic function.

The patient regains consciousness from enflurane very quickly. This is due partially to its very low blood-gas partition coefficient of 1.37. There will usually be no residual analgesia, therefore, when the patient regains consciousness, it is important to assess his or her pain and administer a narcotic analgesic if indicated. It should be noted that some anesthetists administer a short-acting narcotic such as fentanyl at the end of the surgical procedure to reduce the amount of postoperative pain experienced by the patient in the post anesthesia care unit. Therefore, the PACU nurse should note at admission whether the patient has received any pain-relieving drugs during intraoperative period.

Incidence of nausea and vomiting has been minimal with enflurane. Some patients have exhibited shivering during emergence and recovery that is unrelated to body temperature. Because enflurane is a halogenated agent it continues to be studied as a possible cause of liver problems; however, it has yet to be linked with any hepatic syndrome.

Advantages of enflurane include marked cardiovascular stability, good operative analgesia, pleasant induction and emergence, and good patient acceptance. Enflurane is contraindicated in seizure disorders, in diabetes mellitus, with administration of catecholamines, in obstetric usage, especially in the first trimester of pregnancy, and in patients receiving enzyme inducers, particularly phenobarbital and dilantin.

Halothane (Fluothane)

Halothane is a saturated hydrocarbon. Unlike the traditional inhalation anesthetic agents, halothane was a product of planned research by chemists and pharmacologists, whose aim was to synthesize a volatile compound that combined the properties of anesthetic potency with nontoxicity and nonflammability. Halothane is 100 percent potent and a very rapid-acting drug. It is also very easily controlled, in that the depth of anesthesia can be changed quickly. Because it is such a potent agent, it is administered by finely calibrated vaporizers. Recovery to consciousness is rapid owing to the small amounts absorbed by the brain tissue and the low blood-gas partition coefficient of 2.37.

Halothane has demonstrated a low incidence of postanesthesia nausea and vomiting. It does, however, sensitize the heart to catecholamines. Therefore, epinephrine should be administered very cautiously to a patient in the PACU who has received halothane intraoperatively, as serious dysrhythmias could result. For the patient who is emerging from halothane (within 30 minutes of the termination of the intraoperative anesthetic), the following guidelines for the administration of epinephrine in the PACU will reduce the incidence of dysrhythmias: The epinephrine concentration should be no greater than 1:100,000 to 1:200,000, with a total adult dose not exceeding 10 ml of 1:100,000 solution in ten minutes, or a total dose of 30 ml of 1:100,000 solution in one hour.

When the position of a patient is being changed during emergence from halothane, the maneuver should be carried out slowly and gently because compensatory vasoconstrictor mechanisms are depressed. Bronchial dilatation, myocardial depression, peripheral vasodilatation, and nonirritation of respiratory tissues are other features of this agent.

The use of halothane anesthesia as a possible cause of hepatitis continues to be the subject of research studies. It is well known that postoperative jaundice and liver failure may be caused by factors other than the anesthetic. However, because of the possibility that halothane may cause hepatitis in certain sensitized individuals, it is usually not the anesthetic of choice when the patient has had recent exposure to halothane or has had any type of liver disease.

Halothane is widely used for all types of surgical procedures in patients of all age groups. The importance of maintaining the blood volume within reasonably normal limits should be stressed because of the peripheral vasodilating action of halothane. Diminution of the blood volume by preoperative fluid restriction, diuretic therapy, and hemorrhage will augment the hypotensive effect of halothane and should be corrected by intravenous infusions of the appropriate solutions.

Because the recovery phase of halothane is generally short, the *postoperative analgesic phase is also short.* Evaluation of postoperative pain should be thorough before a narcotic analgesic is administered to the patient, because the synergistic effect of halothane and a narcotic could result in marked respiratory depression.

Isoflurane (Forane)

Isoflurane, an analog of enflurane, is also a halogenated methyl ethyl ether. It produces a dose-related depression of the central nervous system. But, in contrast with enflurane, this anesthetic agent does not produce convulsive electroencephalographic abnormalities. Isoflurane will reduce the systemic arterial blood pressure and total peripheral resistance. However, during isoflurane anesthesia, the heart rate is usually increased and the cardiac output usually remains within normal limits. This agent will produce respiratory depression as well as skeletal muscular relaxation in a dose-related fashion, because isoflurane markedly potentiates the actions of the nondepolarizing muscle relaxants. Of interest to the PACU nurse is the fact that isoflurane does not sensitize the myocardium to catecholamines to the same extent as does halothane. Thus, the chance of dysrhythmias is reduced when the patient has received isoflurane anesthesia.

The recovery phase is rapid owing to isoflurane's low blood-gas partition coefficient of 0.97. The patient not only awakens promptly, but is also quite lucid within 15 to 30 minutes after termination of the anesthetic. However, clinical observation indicates that if the anesthesia time using isoflurane goes beyond 45 minutes to an hour, the patient will probably experience a slower emergence phase than would be expected given that the drug has such a low blood-gas partition coefficient.

The lung volumes and capacities, as measured by the Wright respirometer, return to normal in less than 30 minutes along with the ability to raise the head, protrude the tongue, cough on command and converse clearly. Blood pressure and pulse remain stable. Shivering is seen in 2 percent of patients, and nausea and vomiting occur only occasionally.

Isoflurane possesses some excellent qualities, i.e., a lack of sensitization of the heart to catecholamines, cardiovascular stability, limited biodegradation, good neuromuscular relaxation, and no central nervous system excitatory effects. Since its introduction into anesthesia practice, isoflurane has enjoyed continuing success among anesthesia practitioners and PACU nurses alike.

Nitrous Oxide

Nitrous oxide is the only inorganic gas used as an anesthetic agent. It is marketed in blue steel cylinders as a colorless liquid under a pressure of 30 atmospheres. As the pressure is released, nitrous oxide returns to the gaseous state. It is readily soluble in water and is heavier than air. Nitrous oxide was probably the first anesthetic agent to be used extensively. The fact that it is still being used indicates that, when used properly, it is a valuable and safe anesthetic agent.

Nitrous oxide supports combustion; that is, if a burning match is put into a jar containing nitrous oxide, it will continue to burn. However, this agent is not explosive. Although the nitrous oxide molecule contains oxygen, that oxygen is unavailable for respiration because nitrous oxide does not decompose in the body.

Nitrous oxide is a 15 percent potent agent; therefore, the maximum depth of anesthesia that can be produced while supplying the patient's metabolic need for oxygen is the middle of plane 1 of stage III. This agent has no real side effects unless hypoxia is present. It is nontoxic and nonirritating. Nitrous oxide is a rapid-acting agent owing, in part, to its blood-gas partition coefficient of 0.47. This agent does not combine with hemoglobin but is carried in physical solution in the blood. It is excreted for the most part unchanged by the lungs, although a small fraction is excreted through the skin. It does not sensitize the heart to epinephrine, and it provides a fair amount of analgesia. Even in subanesthetic concentrations it is analgesic to humans, and 20 percent concentrations of the gas have been claimed to be as effective as 15 mg of morphine sulfate. If this agent were more potent it would probably be considered an almost perfect anesthetic.

In anesthesia today, nitrous oxide serves an important role, as it is administered alone and in combination with various agents. Recently, the balanced technique of anesthesia has been favored, owing to the number of negative factors associated with some of the more potent volatile inhalation anesthetics. The *balanced technique* consists of the administration of narcotics that may or may not be in combination with a tranquilizer, a muscle relaxant, nitrous oxide, oxygen, and barbiturates. All the elements of anesthesia or nervous depression are met; sensory block (analgesia), motor block (muscle relaxation), block of reflexes, and mental block (narcosis). For short procedures, when only light anesthesia is desired, a *pent-nitrous technique* is sometimes used. This consists of nitrous oxide, oxygen, and sodium thiopental. This technique provides narcosis and limited analgesia for short, simple procedures.

When nitrous oxide is administered with a potent volatile inhalation anesthetic such as halothane, it acts as a carrier and also provides additional analgesic effect. The second gas effect occurs because of nitrous oxide's rapid uptake, after which the potent volatile agent takes the patient to the desired surgical plane. The reverse takes place at termination of the anesthetic.

The solubilities of nitrogen and nitrous oxide differ greatly. Nitrous oxide is 30 times more soluble than nitrogen. An enclosed gas-filled space in the body will expand if gas within it is more soluble than the gas respired. For this reason, any closed gas-filled cavity in the body will expand because of the slow exchange of nitrogen from the cavity for the rapid exchange of large volumes of nitrous oxide from the blood. This is why nitrous oxide is not advised in cases of intestinal obstruction or pneumothorax. Nitrous oxide has been shown to dislodge a tympanoplasty graft owing to the expansion of the air pocket in the middle ear.

Diffusion hypoxia following nitrous oxide anesthesia is another area of concern for the PACU nurse. This is sometimes referred to as the *Fink phenomenon*. It occurs when not enough nitrous oxide is removed from the lungs at the end of the surgical procedure. Normally, 100 percent oxygen is administered at the end of the procedure to remove the nitrous oxide. This is referred to as nitrous oxide washout. Diffusion hypoxia is directly related to the dilution of alveolar gas by the rapid diffusion of the nitrous oxide out of the blood. It is therefore highly advisable to administer oxygen per mask to all patients who are admitted to the PACU. This maneuver will forestall the development of severe hypoxia, should some unpredicted airway problem occur. Another measure for avoiding this complication is to provide adequate verbal and physical stimulation to the patient to promote good ventilatory effort. This should include a sigh every five minutes to ensure adequate removal of the anesthetic gases.

ASSESSING THE EFFECTS OF INHALANT DRUGS IN THE PACU

When assessing the patient's degree of emergence from inhalation anesthesia, it is important for the nurse to understand the pharmacologic effects of each anesthetic agent and of the preoperative medications used. Each anesthetic agent is, in essence, a depressant drug. Certain volatile agents, such as halothane, enflurane, and isoflurane, possess a high degree of myocardial and respiratory depressant properties. One parameter for monitoring the emergence phase when these agents have been administered is vital signs. Preanesthetic baseline vital sign readings are reliable indicators of the patient's cardiorespiratory status postoperatively and can be used to assess the patient's stage of recovery. When this assessment is being made, however, all other factors of the patient's condition must also be considered. Total assessment of the patient recovering from anesthesia is discussed in Chapter 17.

In order to understand the emergence phase of inhalation anesthesia, the nurse also needs a basic understanding of *blood-gas* and *oil-gas partition coefficients*. Anesthetic agents are usually administered in combinations, often with nitrous oxide as the carrier gas. The combination of agents usually consists of a 100 percent potent agent, a carrier agent, and oxygen to meet the metabolic needs of the patient. The agent with the highest blood-gas partition coefficient will take the longest time to be removed from the body. Therefore, if a halothane–nitrous oxide–oxygen combination were administered to a patient, the halothane, having the highest blood-gas partition coefficient, would be eliminated the most slowly.

Along with the factors due to the blood-gas partition coefficient, those due to the oil-gas partition coefficient should be considered in evaluation of length of time of emergence from the anesthetic. When the intraoperative phase is of long duration, an agent that has a high oil-gas partition coefficient will redistribute into the adipose tissue. As mentioned, because the vascular supply to adipose tissue is sparse, the release of the agent to the blood is slow and the emergence is prolonged. Both coefficients must be kept in mind when predicting the length of the emergence phase from an inhalation anesthetic agent. Halothane, for example, has the low blood-gas partition

coefficient of 2.37, and one would expect a rapid recovery from its administration. However, halothane has a high oil-gas partition coefficient of 224, so when it is administered for more than one hour, the adipose tissue will be saturated and emergence from the anesthetic agent prolonged. Nitrous oxide, enflurane, and isoflurane have low blood-gas and oil-gas partition coefficients.

Inhalation agents, because of their depressant effect on the hypothalamus, cause a disruption in the regulation of body heat that may be manifested by either a reduction or an elevation, depending on the environmental temperature. In the recovery phase, the emerging patient should be monitored for *hypothermia* or *hyperthermia*. Serious heat loss may occur in newborns, creating difficulties in reestablishment of adequate ventilatory effort after surgery. Body temperature should be monitored in patients who were febrile prior to surgery, and who received atropine before or during the operative procedure. Agents such as halothane, which have a direct vasodilatory effect on vascular smooth muscle, can cause a temperature drop of 1°C in esophageal temperature. Shivering and tremors have been reported during the postoperative period following use of halothane anesthesia, although this phenomenon has mostly been associated with a generalized loss of muscle tone during surgery and anesthesia.

Water and electrolyte balance is affected by inhalation anesthesia. Pituitary and adrenocortical systems appear to be affected in such a way that there is water and sodium retention and potassium loss following anesthesia. This balance is also affected in part by the stress of surgical trauma. Decreased glomerular filtration, increased tubular reabsorption, and varying degrees of oliguria exist in the recovery phase because of renal vasoconstriction. If renal blood flow is not impaired, glomerular function quickly returns to normal after the operation. The increased tubular reabsorption of water usually persists for 36 to 48 hours but may go on for several days in the elderly.

REFERENCES

1. Brown, B. (ed.): New Pharmacologic Vistas in Anesthesia. Philadelphia, F. A. Davis Co., 1983.
2. Chu, Y., Rah, K., and Boyan, C.: Is the Bain breathing circuit the future anesthesia system? An evaluation. Anesth. Analg., 56: 84–87, 1977.
3. Collins, V.: Principles of Anesthesiology. 2nd ed. Philadelphia, Lea & Febiger, 1976.
4. Dorsch, J., and Dorsch, S.: Understanding Anesthesia Equipment. Baltimore, Williams & Wilkins, 1975.
5. Dripps, R., Eckenhoff, J., and Vandam, L.: Introduction to Anesthesia. 6th ed. Philadelphia, W. B. Saunders Co., 1982.
6. Eger, E., Saidman, L., and Bradstater, B.: Minimum alveolar anesthetic concentration: a standard of anesthetic potency. Anesthesiology, 26:756, 1965.
7. Goodman, L., and Gilman, A.: The Pharmacological Basis of Therapeutics. 6th ed. New York, Macmillan Publishing Company, 1980.
8. Miller, R. (ed.): Anesthesia. 2nd ed. New York, Churchill Livingstone, Inc., 1986.
9. Wood, M., and Wood, A.: Drugs and Anesthesia: Pharmacology for the Anesthesiologist. Baltimore, Williams & Wilkins, 1982.

13

Intravenous Agents

The time-tested use of the inhalational anesthetic agents has proved that they have some definite disadvantages. Because of the biotransformation hazards that have been reported with the halogenated inhalation anesthetics, other techniques have been sought to provide general anesthesia. Along with the more commonly used barbiturates, neuroleptic, narcotic, and dissociative anesthesia are now finding their place in the improved anesthesia care of the surgical patient.

Intravenous anesthetics are generally grouped by primary pharmacologic action. The following groups will be discussed in this chapter: barbiturates, narcotics, neuroleptics, dissociative agents, tranquilizers, and other agents.

THE BARBITURATES

Intravenous anesthesia began with barbiturate anesthesia. The long-acting barbiturates were introduced clinically in 1927. It was not until 1934 that Tovell and Lundy began using thiopental in clinical anesthesia practice. Since then, barbiturate anesthesia has enjoyed great popularity and is still widely used in clinical anesthesia.

Thiopental (Sodium Pentothal)

Thiopental is most commonly injected intravenously to induce or sustain surgical anesthesia. It is usually used in conjunction with a potent inhalational anesthetic, and nitrous oxide–oxygen combinations. The main reason for the utilization of other anesthetic agents with thiopental is that thiopental is a very poor analgesic. For surgical procedures that are short and require minimal analgesia, thiopental and nitrous oxide–oxygen combinations can be utilized. This technique is commonly referred to as the pent-nitrous technique. Thiopental is also used (1) to maintain light sleep during regional analgesia, (2) to control convulsions, and (3) to quiet a patient rapidly who is too lightly anesthetized during a surgical procedure.

The mode of action of thiopental involves a phenomenon of redistribution. Thiopental has the ability to penetrate all tissues of the body without delay. Because the brain, as part of the vessel-rich group, is highly perfused, it receives approximately 10 percent of the administered intravenous dose within 40 seconds after injection. The patient usually becomes unconscious at this time. The thiopental then redistributes to relatively poorly perfused areas of the body. In the brain, the level of thiopental decreases to half its peak in five minutes and to one tenth in a half hour. Recovery of consciousness usually occurs during this period. Recovery may be prolonged if the induction dose was excessive or if circulatory depression occurs that would slow the redistribution phenomenon. Thiopental is metabolized in the body at a rate of 10 to 15 percent per hour.

Thiopental is a respiratory depressant. The chief effect is on the medullary and pontine respiratory centers. This depressant effect is dependent on the amount of thiopental administered, the rate at which it is injected, and the amount and type of premedication given to the patient. The response to carbon dioxide is depressed at all levels of anesthesia and is abolished at deep levels of thiopental anesthesia. Therefore, the drug can take a patient all the way to apnea.

Myocardial contractility is depressed and vascular resistance is increased after injection of thiopental, with the result that blood pressure is hardly affected, although it may be transiently reduced when the drug is first administered, when the vessel-rich group is highly saturated.

In addition to its being nonexplosive, the advantages of thiopental are (1) rapid and pleasant induction, (2) reduction of postanesthetic excitement and vomiting, (3) quiet respiration, (4) absence of salivation, and (5) speedy recovery after small doses. The disadvantages of the drug are adverse respiratory actions, including apnea, coughing, laryngospasm, and bronchospasm. Extravenous injection may result in tissue necrosis because of the high pH of the solution (10.5 to 11).

PACU Care. Because thiopental may have an antianalgesic effect at low concentrations, some patients who have pain may be irrational and hyperactive, and restless during the initial recovery phase. The patient may exhibit some shivering related to lowered body temperature, which may result from a cold operating suite. Of concern to the PACU nurse is the patient admitted with cold, clammy, cyanotic skin. This occasionally occurs with thiopental and is due, in part, to the peripheral vasoconstrictive action of the drug.

If the anesthesia time exceeds 1 hour, or if the total dose of thiopental exceeds 1 gram, patients may have a delayed awakening time owing to the redistribution of thiopental. This phenomenon is particularly common in obese patients, since the drug is very fat soluble. At present, no antagonist exists for the barbiturates. Therefore, airway management and monitoring of cardiovascular status are very important.

Methohexital (Brevital)

Methohexital is an ultra ultra short-acting barbiturate intravenous anesthetic agent. It is usually indicated for very short procedures in which rapid complete recovery of the patient is required. Methohexital is about three times as potent as thiopental, and the recovery time from anesthesia is very rapid (4 to 7 minutes) because the drug is redistributed from the central nervous system to the muscle and fat tissues, and a significant portion of the drug is metabolized in the liver. Consequently, the clearance of methohexital is about four times faster than that of thiopental. Methohexital causes about the same degree of cardiovascular and respiratory depression as does thiopental. It should be mentioned, however, that this drug can cause coughing and hiccoughs, and that, after injection, excitatory phenomena such as tremor and involuntary muscle movements may appear.

THE NARCOTICS

Narcotics or opioids are becoming very popular in today's anesthesia practice. They are usually utilized in the *nitrous-narcotic (balanced) techniques*, which involve the use of a narcotic, nitrous oxide, and oxygen, with or without a muscle relaxant, and thiopental for induction.

The effects of narcotics generally last well into the post anesthesia care unit phase, and every PACU nurse should have a good knowledge of the pharmacologic actions of each narcotic that is administered to the patient in the perioperative phase of the surgical experience.

Meperidine Hydrochloride (Demerol)

Meperidine was discovered in 1939 by Eisleb and Schauman. It was originally introduced as an antispasmodic agent and was not utilized as an anesthetic agent until 1947. The main action of this drug is subcortical with an analgesic effect. Its effect lasts for two to four hours. The onset of analgesia is prompt (10 minutes) after subcutaneous or intramuscular administration. All pain, especially visceral, gastrointestinal, and urinary tract, is satisfactorily relieved. It produces some sleepiness and causes little euphoria or amnesia. Meperidine increases the sensitivity of the labyrinthine apparatus of the ear, which explains the dizziness, nausea, and vomiting that sometimes occur in ambulatory patients.

This narcotic may slow the rate of respiration, but the rate generally returns to normal 15 minutes after intravenous injection. The tidal volume is not changed appreciably. In equianalgesic doses, meperidine depresses respiration to the same degree as does morphine. It has been noted by some authors that meperidine may release histamine from the tissues. Occasionally, one may notice urticarial wheals that have formed over the veins where meperidine has been injected. The usual treatment is to discontinue the use of meperidine and, if the reaction is severe, administer diphenhydramine (Benadryl). Diphenhydramine will further sedate the patient, however, and should be administered only if truly warranted.

Meperidine does not, in therapeutic doses, cause any significant untoward effects on the cardiovascular system. When this drug is administered intravenously, it usually causes an increase in heart rate that is usually transient. When administered intramuscularly, no significant change in heart rate will be observed.

Meperidine is generally metabolized in the liver; less than 5 percent is excreted unchanged by the kidneys.

Because of its spasmolytic effect, meperidine is the drug of choice for biliary duct, distal colon, and rectal surgery. It offers the following advantages: little interference with the physiologic compensatory mechanisms, low toxicity, smooth and rapid recovery, prolonged postoperative analgesia, excellent cardiac stability in elderly and poor-risk patients, and ease of detoxification and excretion.

Morphine

Morphine, one of the oldest known drugs, has only recently been utilized as an anesthetic agent. Alkaloid morphine is from the phenanthrene class of opium. The mechanism of action of morphine is not exactly known. In humans, it produces analgesia, drowsiness, changes in mood, and mental clouding. The analgesic effect can become profound before the other effects are severe and can persist after many of the side effects have nearly disappeared. By direct effect on the respiratory center, morphine depresses respiratory rate, tidal volume, and minute volume. Maximal respiratory depression occurs within seven minutes after intravenous injection of the drug and 30 minutes after intramuscular administration. Following therapeutic doses of morphine, the sensitivity of the respiratory center begins to return to normal in 2 to 3 hours, but the minute volume does not return to preinjection level until 4 to 5 hours have passed.

The greatest advantage of morphine is the remarkable cardiovascular stability that accompanies its use. It has no major effect on blood pressure, heart rate, or heart rhythm, even in toxic doses, when hypoxia is avoided. Of interest, morphine decreases the capacity of the cardiovascular system to adjust to gravitational shifts. This is important to remember since orthostatic hypotension and syncope may easily occur in a PACU patient whose care requires a position change. This phenomenon is primarily due to the peripheral vasodilatory effect of morphine. Therefore, a position change for a patient who has received morphine should be accomplished slowly, with constant monitoring of the patient's vital signs.

Morphine may cause nausea and vomiting, especially in ambulatory patients, by virtue of direct stimulation of the chemoreceptor trigger zone. The emetic effect of morphine can be counteracted by narcotic antagonists and phenothiazine derivatives such as chlorpromazine (Thorazine), prochlorperazine (Compazine) or benzquinamide (Emeticon). Histamine release has been noted with morphine, and morphine also causes profound constriction of the pupils, stimulation of the visceral smooth muscles, and spasm of the sphincter of Oddi.

Morphine is detoxified by conjugation with glucuronic acid. Ninety percent is excreted by the kidneys and 7 to 10 percent is excreted in the feces via the bile.

Morphine is utilized in the balanced or nitrous-narcotic technique with nitrous oxide, oxygen, and a muscle relaxant. This technique is useful for cardiovascular surgery along with other types of surgery in which cardiovascular stability is required. The patient may arrive in the PACU still narcotized from morphine with an endotracheal tube in place. Mechanical ventilation for a period of 24 to 48 hours is usually warranted. The morphine may or may not be supplemented during the time of ventilation. This type of recovery procedure facilitates a pain-free state and maximum ventilation of the patient during the critical phase of recovery. Morphine can also be utilized to provide basal narcosis when regional anesthesia is utilized.

Fentanyl (Sublimaze)

Fentanyl is a synthetic opiate related to the phenylpiperidines. It has a short duration of action and is 80 times as potent as morphine. This drug can be used alone in a nitrous-narcotic technique. It also is used in the PACU in the form of a low-dose intravenous drip for pain relief. Fentanyl is the narcotic portion of Innovar. Fentanyl will be discussed in detail in the section on neuroleptanalgesia.

Sufentanil (Sufenta) and Alfentanil

Two new analogs of fentanyl have been recently introduced into clinical anesthesia practice. These analogs, sufentanil and alfentanil, appear to have significant advantages over currently available opioid anesthetics. Sufentanil and alfentanil, like fentanyl, produce minimal hemodynamic effects and offer a high therapeutic index. In fact, the therapeutic index for the two drugs is higher than those of fentanyl and other opioids. A *therapeutic index* is the ratio of the lethal dose to the effective dose and the higher the therapeutic index, the farther away the lethal dose is from the dose used to get the desired effect. More specifically, the therapeutic index of fentanyl is 270, which is about four times safer than morphine. Alfentanil's therapeutic index is about 2.5 times more favorable than fentanyl's, and sufentanil's therapeutic index is 25,000 to 30,000.

Anesthesia with sufentanil can be induced more rapidly, using basically the same technique as that used for fentanyl, without increasing the incidence of chest wall rigidity. It should be noted that sufentanil can produce chest wall rigidity. Therefore, if it is administered in the PACU, equipment for administering oxygen by positive pressure and the skeletal muscle relaxant succinylcholine should be on hand. Sufentanil is approximately 5 to 7 times as potent as fentanyl, and the incidence of hypertension with sufentanil is lower than with comparable doses of fentanyl. Bradycardia is infrequently seen in patients who receive sufentanil, and when high-dose sufentanil is used in combination with nitrous oxide–oxygen, the mean arterial pressure and cardiac output may be decreased. The recovery time from the time of injection is no greater with sufentanil than with fentanyl and may actually be less. This is because the duration of action of sufentanil is about two-thirds that of fentanyl, and also it is very rapidly eliminated from tissue storage sites. Also, initial studies indicate that the incidence of postoperative hypertension, the need for vasoactive agents, and the requirements for postoperative analgesics are generally reduced in patients administered moderate or high doses of sufentanil as compared with patients given inhalation agents. Of particular interest to the PACU nurse is that sufentanil has an additive effect that will be exhibited in patients receiving barbiturates, tranquilizers, other opioids, general anesthetics, or other central nervous system depressants. Hence, when sufentanil is combined with any of these drugs, particular attention should be paid to any signs of decreased respiratory drive and increased airways resistance. Immediate countermeasures include maintaining a patent airway by proper positioning of the patient, by placement of an oral airway or endotracheal tube, and by the administration of oxygen. If indicated, naloxone should be employed as a specific antidote to manage the respiratory depression. The duration of respiratory depression following overdosage with sufentanil may be longer than the duration of action of the naloxone. Consequently, the patient should be constantly observed for the recurrence of respiratory depression, even after the initial successful treatment with naloxone.

Alfentanil, besides having a place in the operating room, may find a home in the PACU. Its rapid onset and very brief duration of action make it advantageous for the immediate pain relief needs of recovery room patients. The drug has about one-third the potency of fentanyl, but its onset of action is at least three times faster; its duration is one-third that of fentanyl, and it has a high therapeutic index. The drug produces few cardiovascular effects and thus should be of great value in the prevention of dangerous reflexes, such as tachycardia during intubation. It should also be stated that clinical observation indicates that the recovery time for this drug is extremely rapid. Hence, patients who receive this drug intraoperatively will most likely experience pain early in the *immediate* postoperative period, and the appropriate analgesic should be administered.

Pentazocine (Talwin)

Pentazocine, a narcotic antagonist analgesic, was first synthesized in 1959. The drug has significant activity and a low addiction potential. It is approximately one third as potent as morphine when given by the intramuscular route. It does have an advantage over morphine in that it can be given by the oral route. It can be used preoperatively as well as postoperatively for the relief of pain from abdominal, cardiac,

genitourinary, orthopedic, neurologic, and gynecologic surgery. The observed side effects of this drug include sedation, dizziness, nausea, and vomiting, but these occur infrequently.

Studies of the relative potency of this drug indicate that 30 mg of pentazocine is analgesically equivalent to 10 mg of morphine and 75 mg of meperidine. One study found the drug to be a significantly better analgesic than meperidine (20 mg pentazocine equals 100 mg of meperidine). It has been established that pentazocine can relieve severe pain and is approximately two to four times less potent than morphine when administered parenterally.

Pentazocine can be utilized in the nitrous-narcotic technique. The respiratory depression produced by pentazocine is potentiated when general anesthetics are used concomitantly. Pentazocine produces a rise in systolic pressure and does not appear to have depressant effects on the cardiac output. The drug should be used with caution in patients with renal or hepatic impairment. Pentazocine depresses the respiratory system in a manner comparable to morphine in equivalent analgesic doses. Tolerance to the analgesic effect of the drug does not appear to develop as it does with other narcotics. Since pentazocine is a narcotic antagonist, administration of this drug to a patient who is dependent on opiates might induce abrupt withdrawal symptoms.

The onset of analgesic activity of pentazocine is approximately two to three minutes when given intravenously and 15 to 20 minutes when given intramuscularly. The duration of action is about three hours. When given orally, the drug is about one third as potent as when given intramuscularly.

Butorphanol Tartrate (Stadol)

Butorphanol tartrate is a synthetic analgesic that is chemically related to the nalorphine-cyclazocine series with both narcotic and antagonist properties. In regard to its analgesic potency, it is about 5 times more potent than morphine, 30 times more than meperidine, and about 20 times more potent than pentazocine. Butorphanol can produce sedation, nausea, and respiratory depression. The respiratory depression is plateau-like in that 2 mg of butorphanol depresses respiration to a degree equal to 10 mg of morphine. The magnitude of respiratory depression with butorphanol is not appreciably increased at doses of 4 mg. The duration of the respiratory depression is dose related and is reversible by naloxone. Intravenous administration of butorphanol can produce an increased pulmonary artery pressure, pulmonary wedge pressure, left ventricular end-diastolic pressure, systemic arterial pressure, and pulmonary vascular resistance. Consequently, this drug increases the work of the heart, especially in the pulmonary circuit. Because of its antagonist properties, butorphanol is not recommended for patients physically dependent on narcotics, since butorphanol can precipitate withdrawal symptoms in those patients. See Table 13–1 for an overview of the clinical pharmacology of butorphanol.

Nalbuphine HCl (Nubain)

Nalbuphine is a potent analgesic with narcotic agonist and antagonist actions. It is chemically related to oxymorphone and naloxone. Nalbuphine is as potent as morphine and about three times as potent as pentazocine on a milligram basis. At a dose of 10 mg/kg nalbuphine will cause the same degree of respiratory depression as 10 mg of morphine. At higher doses, nalbuphine exhibits the same plateau effect as butorphanol, i.e., respiratory depression is not appreciably increased with higher doses. It should be stated that the respiratory depression that is produced by nalbuphine can be reversed by naloxone. Nalbuphine does not appear to increase the workload of the heart or to decrease cardiovascular stability. This drug has a lower abuse potential than morphine, but if it is given to a patient who is physically dependent on narcotics, withdrawal symptoms may appear. Signs of withdrawal include abdominal cramps, nausea and vomiting, lacrimation, rhinorrhea, anxiety, restlessness, elevation of temperature, and piloerection. Should these symptoms appear after the injection of nalbuphine, the administration of small amounts of morphine can relieve the objective effects of the syndrome. See Table 13–1 for an overview of the clinical pharmacology of nalbuphine.

TABLE 13–1. Comparison of Five Analgesics

	Morphine	Meperidine	Pentazocine	Butorphanol	Nalbuphine
Indication	Moderate to severe pain	Moderate to severe pain	Moderate to severe pain	Moderate to severe pain	Moderate to severe pain
Recommended IM Dose	10 mg	100 mg	30 mg	2 mg	10 mg
Recommended IV Dose	4–10 mg	100 mg	30 mg	1 mg	10 mg
Time Required for Onset of Analgesia	Rapid IV 30 min IM	Rapid IV 30 min IM	Rapid IV 20 min IM	Rapid IV 30 min IM	Rapid IV 15 min IM
Duration of Analgesia	4 hr	2–4 hr	3–4 hr	3–4 hr	3–6 hr
Respiratory Depression	High	High	Occurs, but less than morphine	Occurs, but less than morphine	Occurs, but less than morphine
Cardiovascular Effect	Decreases cardiac work	Decreases cardiac work	Increases cardiac work	Increases cardiac work	Good cardiac stability
Abuse Potential	High	High	Occurs; induces withdrawal syndrome	Occurs; induces withdrawal syndrome	Occurs; induces withdrawal syndrome

Adapted from Wood, M., and Wood, A.: Drugs and Anesthesia: Pharmacology for the Anesthesiologist. Baltimore, Williams & Wilkins, 1982.

Buprenorphine (Buprenex)

Buprenorphine is a parenteral opiate analgesic with agonist-antagonist properties, which is 30 times as potent as morphine sulfate. This drug is a derivative of the opium alkaloid thebaine and has a low abuse potential. It is proposed that the mechanism of action of buprenorphine involves the binding of the drug to the opiate receptors in the central nervous system. Buprenorphine at a dose of 0.3 mg has about the same respiratory depressant effect as 10 mg of morphine. This drug may cause a decrease or, rarely, an increase in pulse and blood pressure. Given by the intramuscular route of administration, the onset of analgesia is within 15 minutes, with a peak analgesic effect in 1 hour and a duration of 6 hours. When administered intravenously, the onset and peak times are shortened.

Of importance to the PACU nurse is the fact that the respiratory depressant effects of buprenorphine can be only partially reversed by naloxone. At present, there is no completely reliable specific antagonist available to reverse the respiratory depressant effects produced by buprenorphine. Consequently, patients who have been administered this drug should be assessed for respiratory depression for the next 6 hours. When a PACU patient is transferred, the nursing staff on the surgical units must be advised of the administration of and ramifications of the use of this drug.

The Narcotic Antagonists

Narcotic antagonists are used to reverse narcotic-induced respiratory depression. An opioid antagonist such as naloxone (Narcan) is a drug that completely antagonizes the effect of a narcotic. Drugs such as nalorphine (Nalline) and levallorphan (Lorfan) best typify the agonist-antagonists. These drugs partially reverse the effects of narcotics but also produce autonomic, endocrine, analgesic, and respiratory depressant effects similar to those of morphine.

Naloxone (Narcan)

Naloxone, a pure antagonist, reverses the depressant effects of narcotics. This drug also reverses the analgesic effect of the narcotic, which is important to remember when assessing the patient's respiratory effort. Naloxone should be titrated according to the patient's response. Usually 0.1 to 0.2 mg given slowly intravenously should be adequate for reversal. The onset of action of naloxone is one to two minutes, and if after three to five minutes inadequate reversal has been achieved, the naloxone may be repeated until reversal is complete. If the patient shows no sign of reversal, assessment of other pharmacologic agents administered is indicated. Drugs such as halothane, barbiturates, and muscle relaxants are not reversed by naloxone.

The duration of action of naloxone is 1 to 4 hours, depending on the route and amount of drug used. If long-acting narcotics were utilized, it is important to monitor the patient for respiratory embarrassment after the administration of naloxone, as the depressant activity of the narcotic may return. If this phenomenon occurs, supplemental doses of naloxone can be used. The intramuscular route of administration has been shown to produce a longer lasting effect.

One adverse effect to watch for when an excessive dosage of naloxone is used is an increase in blood pressure that may be seen as a response to pain. Too-rapid reversal may induce nausea, vomiting, diaphoresis, or tachycardia. During the reversal procedure, the vital signs should be monitored, and naloxone should be used with caution in patients with cardiac irritability.

Naloxone does not produce respiratory depression as do other narcotic antagonists. It also does not produce any significant side effects or pupillary constriction. Naloxone will reverse natural or synthetic narcotics, propoxyphene (Darvon) and the narcotic-antagonist analgesic pentazocine (Fortral, Talwin). Naloxone should be administered with great caution to patients who are physically dependent on opioids, since reversal may precipitate an acute withdrawal syndrome.

Levallorphan (Lorfan)

Levallorphan is an agonist-antagonist of narcotic depression. It has essentially been replaced by naloxone. It acts as a narcotic antagonist in the presence of a strong narcotic effect. If utilized when no narcotic is present, respiratory depression may occur. It does not counteract mild respiratory depression and may in fact intensify it. Repeated doses will decrease its effectiveness and it will eventually produce its own respiratory depression. Adverse reactions associated with levallorphan include dysphoria, miosis, drowsiness, nausea, and diaphoresis. It can also cause weird dreams, visual hallucinations, and disorientation.

THE NEUROLEPTANALGESICS

A *neuroleptic* drug is one that reduces motor activity, lessens anxiety, and effects a state of indifference in which the individual can still respond appropriately to commands. *Neuroleptanalgesia* is a state of profound tranquilization with little or no depressant effect on the cortical centers. Therefore, neuroleptanalgesia is achieved by the combination of the neuroleptic properties of the butyrophenone tranquilizers and a potent narcotic analgesic such as fentanyl. Going one step farther, *neuroleptanesthesia* is the combination of a neuroleptanalgesic (Innovar) and a skeletal muscle relaxant (nitrous oxide and oxygen). The main objective in developing neuroleptanesthesia was to provide a technique for all types of operations that would not depress the metabolic, circulatory, or central nervous system as severely as do conventional anesthetics.

Fentanyl (Sublimaze)

Janssen and associates introduced a series of highly potent meperidine derivatives that were found to render the patient free of pain without affecting certain areas of the central nervous system. Fentanyl appeared to be of special interest. It was found to be approximately 80 times as potent as morphine sulphate, and it had a rapid onset of action of 2 to 3 minutes, a peak effect within 5 to 15 minutes, with the analgesia lasting 20 to 40 minutes when administered intravenously. Via the intramuscular route, the onset of action was 7 to 15 minutes with analgesia usually lasting 1 to 2 hours. Intraoperatively, fentanyl is now being administered at three different dose ranges depending on the type of surgery and the desired effect. For example, the low dose range of 2 to 20 μg/kg will attenuate moderately stressful stimuli. The moderate dose range is 20 to 50 μg/kg and strongly obtunds the stress response, and the megadose range of up to 150 μg/kg blocks the stress response and is particularly valuable when protection of the myocardium is critical.

Fentanyl shares with most other narcotics a profound respiratory depressant effect, even to the point of apnea. Rapid intravenous injection could provoke bronchial constriction as well as resistance to ventilation caused by rigidity of the diaphragmatic and intercostal muscles. This is commonly referred to as the fixed chest syndrome and can occur when any potent narcotic analgesic is administered too rapidly by the intravenous route. Should this syndrome occur, intravenous succinylcholine (15 to 25 mg) will relieve the rigidity of the chest wall muscles. Along with this, once the succinylcholine is administered, the PACU nurse should be prepared to ventilate the patient until the skeletal muscle relaxant properties of succinylcholine subside.

Fentanyl, unlike most narcotics, has little or no hypotensive effects and usually does not cause nausea and vomiting. Because of its vagotonic effect, it may cause bradycardia, which can be relieved by atropine or glycopyrrolate. Fentanyl can be reversed by the narcotic antagonist naloxone, which, it should be noted, will also reverse analgesia. Should the fentanyl be reversed by naloxone in the post anesthesia care unit, the PACU nurse should continue to monitor the patient for the possible return of respiratory depression, because the duration of the respiratory depression produced by the fentanyl may be longer than the duration of action of the naloxone.

Droperidol (Inapsine)

Further investigation by Janssen and associates produced a new butyrophenone tranquilizer, droperidol. It produces a state of calm, disinclination to move, and disconnection from surroundings. It has an alpha-adrenergic blocking effect, which offers some protection against the vasoconstrictive components of shock, it leads to good peripheral perfusion, and it will unmask hypovolemia. More specifically, when a patient has compensated for a borderline hypovolemic state by activation of the alpha-vasoconstriction mechanisms, vital signs will be normal. When a drug such as droperidol is administered to this patient, by virtue of droperidol's alpha-blocking properties, the signs of hypovolemia will appear. Hence, the patient's hypovolemia is "unmasked." Droperidol also protects against epinephrine-induced arrhythmias and has an antiemetic effect. In fact, because of its excellent antiemetic properties, droperidol is sometimes administered toward the end of the surgical procedure or in the PACU to reduce the risk of vomiting and aspiration in anxious patients. Also, by virtue of its alpha-blocking properties, this drug may be administered in the PACU, on a short-term basis to reduce the afterload.

Droperidol is similar in its central nervous system effects to chlorpromazine (a tranquilizer); its mechanism of action, however, is different. Droperidol is more selective than chlorpromazine, as it provides more tranquility with less sedation and has less effect on the autonomic nervous system. Droperidol has been classified as a neuroleptic and is the main tranquilizing component of Innovar. Among its negative effects, droperidol may cause hypotension by virtue of its alpha-adrenergic blocking effect and peripheral vasodilation. It may cause extrapyramidal excitation, such as twitchiness, oculogyric seizures, stiff neck muscles, trembling hands, restlessness, and, occasionally, psychologic disturbances such as hallucinations. These can be reversed with atropine or antiparkinsonian drugs such as benztropine mesylate (Cogentin) or trihexyphenidyl hydrochloride (Artane). Clinically, patients who have received droperidol have reported the dichotomy of appearing calm on the exterior, while on the inside being terrified and unable to express it. Hence, the PACU nurse should provide emotional support to all patients who have received droperidol.

Droperidol is known to potentiate the action of barbiturates and narcotics. It has a high therapeutic margin of safety with a rapid onset of 10 minutes, and its activity is lessened in 2 to 4 hours, although some effects last as long as 10 to 12 hours.

Innovar

Droperidol and fentanyl, in combination as Innovar, provide tranquility and analgesia, that is, the *neuroleptic state*. Innovar can be used alone for some procedures, such as cast changes, or in combination with nitrous oxide and neuromuscular blocking agents. All the components of modern anesthesia are available through its use: analgesia, unconsciousness, and muscular relaxation. Droperidol and fentanyl are combined in 50 to 1 ratios by weight. Each milliliter of Innovar contains 0.05 mg of fentanyl and 2.5 mg of droperidol.

Some advantages of Innovar are: (1) maintenance of stable circulation during surgery, (2) fewer incidents of postoperative nausea and vomiting, (3) good acceptance by the patient, (4) possible prolonged assistance of respiration via endotracheal tube, and (5) low toxicity.

Innovar used as a premedication varies as to dose according to the personal preference of the anesthesiologist. Usually, it is given 30 to 60 minutes prior to the patient's arrival in the operating room. The usual dose is 0.5 to 2 ml, given intramuscularly, combined with atropine or scopolamine. When using Innovar as a premedication, the nurse must constantly observe the patient for respiratory depression, especially if the patient is suffering severe impairment of pulmonary function. Innovar should not be given when narcotic antagonists and facilities for assisted or controlled respiration are not readily available.

The nurse should also observe the patient for cardiovascular changes after Innovar is administered as a premedication. There is usually a drop in both systolic and diastolic blood pressure. This response usually starts about 10 minutes after the intramuscular injection, with effect progressing for approximately 30 to 40 minutes, after which time it is stabilized. The pulse rate tends to fall somewhat lower with Innovar than with meperidine when it is used as a premedication.

Innovar should probably not be given to patients having a history of Parkinson's disease, or to those with head injury, myasthenia gravis, or bronchospastic disease. It is also contraindicated in pregnant women, children under two years of age, and those taking large doses of narcotics or tranquilizers. Innovar should be administered only inside a health care facility, and should not be given on an outpatient basis.

PACU Care. In the immediate recovery period, the awakening from Innovar is rapid, extremely smooth, and usually uneventful. A striking feature is the extension of analgesia well into the postoperative period. It is difficult to explain the mechanism of such a prolonged pain-relieving effect with a drug such as fentanyl, in which the action is so rapid and the duration is so short.

Nursing personnel in the PACU should watch for respiratory depression. The use of narcotics with patients who have received Innovar should be avoided, or they should be given in minimal amounts. It is recommended that the dosage of narcotic drugs be as little as one-quarter to one-third the usual recommended dose owing to the additive potentiating effects of droperidol.

The patients should be encouraged to cough and perform the sustained maximal inspiration (SMI) maneuver (see Chapter 18) in the PACU. They will tend to drift back to sleep unless they are encouraged to move about. The nurse will find the patient who has received Innovar more willing to cough and perform the SMI, as the analgesia extends into the postoperative period. Innovar depresses both the respiratory rate and the tidal volume. The PACU nurse should be aware that if a patient arrives in the PACU depressed from Innovar, verbal stimulation is of utmost importance. If or-

dered, the patient will be able to take a deep breath, but otherwise respiration may remain slow and shallow. The patient may be apneic because the respiratory center is less responsive to the main respiratory stimulant, carbon dioxide. It is therefore essential that the PACU nurse remain with the patient until respiratory rate is adequate without the use of verbal stimuli.

The nurse should be alert for extrapyramidal symptoms; although rare, they have been detected up to 24 hours after a single administration of Innovar. Most of the reported extrapyramidal reactions occurred in children under 12 years of age. Because of the duration of action of Innovar, it is recommended that the PACU nurses provide information about the drug to the nursing personnel on the surgical units via hospital in-service education programs.

The nurse should alert all PACU personnel to be aware of patients who have received Innovar. Such patients should have a tag on their bed indicating that they have received Innovar and a reminder to reduce the dose of any narcotics or barbiturates given postoperatively. These visual reminders will aid nursing personnel in instituting a recovery regimen for these patients.

Innovar can be used in almost every type of surgical and diagnostic procedure, with the exception of those already mentioned. Neuroleptanalgesia is not a panacea, but it does provide an improved technique for certain types of patients. Coupled with good nursing care, the use of Innovar can be significantly beneficial to the patient who is undergoing the physical and emotional trauma of surgery.

THE DISSOCIATIVE ANESTHESTICS

Ketamine

Traditionally, general anesthetic agents achieved control of pain by depression of the central nervous system. An anesthetic agent, ketamine, has been introduced that has a totally different mode of action. It selectively blocks pain conduction and perception, leaving those parts of the central nervous system that do not participate in pain transmission and perception free from the depressant effects of the drug. Ketamine is termed *dissociative* because when the patient is totally analgesic he usually does not appear to be asleep or anesthetized but rather disassociated from his surroundings. The drug is nonbarbiturate and non-narcotic. It is administered parenterally and its effects are of a short duration. Early laboratory work using ketamine suggested that most of the drug's activity is centered in the frontal lobe of the cerebral cortex.

The clinical characteristics of ketamine consist of a state of profound analgesia combined with a state of unconsciousness. The patient will usually have marked horizontal and vertical nystagmus. The eyes will usually be open and shortly become centered and appear in a fixed gaze. The pupils will be moderately dilated and will react to light. Respiratory function is usually unimpaired, except after rapid intravenous injection, when it may become depressed for a short time. Ketamine is sympathomimetic in action and is beneficial to asthmatic patients because of its bronchodilating effect. When a patient receives ketamine, his pharyngeal and laryngeal reflexes remain intact. The tongue usually does not become relaxed, so the airway usually remains unobstructed. Ketamine accelerates the heart rate moderately and increases both the systolic and the diastolic pressures for several minutes, after which the pulse and blood pressure return to preinjection levels.

Ketamine can be administered intramuscularly or intravenously. The intramuscular dose is 4 to 6 mg per lb. The anesthesia lasts from 20 to 40 minutes. The intravenous dose is usually 0.5 to 2 mg per lb with anesthesia lasting 6 to 10 minutes. Complete recovery from ketamine varies according to the duration of surgery and the amount of ketamine used throughout the procedure. When a single dose of intravenous ketamine is used, recovery time is usually rapid and does not exceed 30 minutes. When supplemental intravenous doses need to be administered, more particularly when supplemental intramuscular doses are required, recovery is often markedly prolonged, sometimes up to 3 hours.

PACU Care. When patients are emerging from ketamine anesthesia, they may go through a phase of vivid dreaming, with or without psychomotor activity manifested by confusion, irrational behavior, and hallucinations. The PACU nurse should be aware that such psychic aberrations are usually transient and appear to be preventable by avoiding early verbal or tactile stimulation of the patient, which helps prevent fear and anxiety reactions. Short-acting barbiturates administered intravenously can effectively control the psychic responses sometimes seen after the administration of ketamine. Pediatric patients seem to be less prone to these psychic disturbances. Results of a study revealed that droperidol, the tranquilizer component of Innovar, may be effective in eliminating some of the adverse psychic emergence phenomena of ketamine. Other tranquilizers such as diazepam have also been found effective in suppressing these phenomena. Thus, the nurse should be aware of any tranquilizers the patient may have received when admitting him to the PACU.

Once the patient has arrived in the PACU, he or she should be secluded from auditory, visual, and tactile stimuli and be observed for any signs of respiratory depression. Mechanical airway obstruction, particularly when caused by marked salivation, accounts for most of the instances of respiratory insufficiency after ketamine anesthesia. When the patient does not have adequate respiratory exchange, oxygen should be administered by mask until it is restored. Other important signs to watch for are persistent blood pressure elevation, tachycardia, bradycardia, dreaming, delirium, hallucinations, euphoria, and increased muscle tone. It should be stressed to all PACU personnel that attempts to rouse the patient while he is still unable to see, hear, and orient himself may set off a chain of anxiety reactions that may ultimately lead to severe psychomotor responses and even more irrational behavior.

The widespread use of ketamine requires

an entirely new approach to anesthesia and PACU nursing care. Certainly, the agent has many deficiencies, but one fact frequently overlooked is that it is one of the safest anesthetics used. Its safety justifies its important place in the drugs used by the anesthesiologist. Ketamine appears to be an excellent anesthetic for pediatric patients, as the sole agent for short procedures, for inducing anesthesia in extremely poor-risk patients, and for patients suffering from burns that require surgical treatment. Certain adult orthopedic and diagnostic procedures have also been found suitable for the use of ketamine anesthesia.

Ketamine is the first of several drugs that will probably achieve clinical usage as dissociative agents. Its actions, therefore, should be well understood by the PACU staff to ensure good, informed care of the patient.

THE TRANQUILIZERS

The Benzodiazepines

The benzodiazepines, which are tranquilizers, have certainly enhanced the anesthesia outcomes of the surgical patient. They exert their activity by depressing the limbic system without causing cortical depression. Opiates and barbiturates enhance the hypnotic action of the benzodiazepines.

Diazepam. Diazepam is one of the most popular drugs used in anesthesia practice today. Because of its ability to allay apprehension, diazepam is indicated for use as a premedicant, as an adjunct to intravenous anesthesia, and as an induction agent. It should be stated that the recovery is usually not prolonged when diazepam is used for the induction of anesthesia. Diazepam can be used as the sole anesthetic agent for short diagnostic and surgical procedures and can also be used to provide sedation to make local anesthesia more acceptable to the patient.

Important actions of diazepam are its ability to produce anterograde amnesia for up to 48 hours postoperatively and its minimal cardiovascular depressant effects. Clinical doses of diazepam cause a slight degree of respiratory depression, although when combined with an opiate, the chance of respiratory depression, including apnea, is greatly increased.

Diazepam may possess some muscle relaxant properties. It has been reported that diazepam is antagonistic to depolarizing neuromuscular blocking agents such as succinylcholine, and that the action of the nondepolarizing neuromuscular blocking agents, such as d-tubocurare, pancuronium, and gallamine, are potentiated. Diazepam has been used clinically for psychomotor and petit mal seizures because of its anticonvulsant actions.

Because many patients who undergo cardioversion are debilitated, diazepam may be used to provide sedation for this procedure. Increments of 2.5 to 5 mg can be given at 30 second intervals until the speech of the patient is slurred or light sleep occurs. At the time of electrical discharge, there may be a brief muscle contraction and slight arousal of the patient. When this technique is employed, a significant number of the patients have complete amnesia regarding the event. Diazepam can also be used in endoscopic procedures, in dentistry, and to control behavior on emergence from ketamine.

Diazepam, when administered by the intramuscular route, can be quite painful to the patient. Along with this, the absorption is often very poor. Also, when diazepam is administered by the intravenous route, thrombophlebitis frequently occurs. When diazepam is administered intravenously, it should be injected slowly, directly into the vein. The drug should not be mixed with other drugs or diluted. The onset of action of diazepam intravenously is immediate, and the duration of action varies from 20 minutes to 1 hour. When administered intramuscularly, its onset of action is about 10 minutes and the duration of action may last up to 4 hours. Adverse reactions to diazepam include hiccoughs, nausea, phlebitis at the site of injection, and occasional acute hyperexcited states.

Lorazepam (Ativan). Lorazepam, a long-acting benzodiazepine, has recently been introduced into clinical anesthesia practice. This drug has actions very similar to those of diazepam but has a slow onset of action of 20 to 40 minutes; the pharmacologic activity may last up to 24 hours. Lorazepam produces profound anterograde amnesia, tranquilization, and a reduction of anxiety, and the drug has good cardiovascular and respiratory stability. Therapeutic plasma concentrations are achieved in about 3 hours when the drug is given orally. The drug is well absorbed via the intramuscular route; however, the patient will experience a significant amount of pain during the injection of the drug. Lorazepam can also be injected intravenously and the patient may experience some burning upon injection. Because of its slow onset and long duration, lorazepam is mainly used as a preanesthetic medication. If this drug has been administered in the preoperative period, because of its prolonged action, the effects of lorazepam may last well into the postoperative period. If a narcotic is administered in the PACU to a patient who received lorazepam preoperatively, the nurse should monitor for increased narcotic sedation and respiratory depression due to the potentiation of the narcotic by the lorazepam.

Midazolam. Midazolam is a new water-soluble benzodiazepine that may offer some real advantages over diazepam. This drug causes depression of the central nervous system by inducing sedation, drowsiness, and, finally, sleep with increasing doses. Midazolam, when compared with diazepam, is about three times as potent, has a shorter duration of action, produces less tissue trauma upon intravenous injection, and may have less of an effect on the cardiovascular system. Like diazepam, this drug also has good anticonvulsant properties and produces good retrograde amnesia.

OTHER AGENTS

Propanidid

Propanidid is a nonbarbiturate hypnotic/anesthetic agent. The drug may be used as an induction agent or to produce transient anesthesia. It exerts a biphasic effect upon respiration. After injection intravenously, an initial period of hyperventilation ensues that is caused by stimulation of the carotid chemoreceptors. This is followed by a short period of hypoventilation, periodic breathing, or apnea. When propanidid is administered, some degree of hypotension, usually due to cardiac depression, will be observed. Other side effects of propanidid are rigidity, coughing, hiccough, phonation, and uncontrollable movements.

The action of this drug is terminated by its being rapidly metabolized enzymatically by plasma pseudocholinesterase, whereas the ultrashort-acting barbiturates have their anesthetic action terminated by redistribution. Recovery from propanidid is usually more complete, and accumulation does not occur with repeated administration, in contrast to the barbiturates. Patients who receive propanidid usually have a smooth recovery with no hangover. During the recovery phase of this drug, headaches, nausea, and vomiting are more frequent than with thiopental. The patient may also complain of an unpleasant taste postoperatively. Propanidid is currently under investigation and is not available in the United States.

Steroid Anesthesia

Steroid anesthesia involves using steroids, administered intravenously, to produce an anesthetized state (loss of consciousness and immobility in response to stimuli). At present, the major use of steroid anesthestics is as a substitute for the commonly used intravenous barbiturates.

Althesin. Althesin, which is currently enjoying wide popularity in Great Britain, is a combination of two steroids: alphaxalone and alphadolone acetate. At present, this drug is not available in the United States. Used mainly as an induction agent, althesin has a similar onset and about a 5 to 10 minute longer duration of action when compared with thiopental. This drug does not seem to alter the cardiac output and often causes a short period of hyperventilation, which is sometimes followed by apnea. The major disadvantage of althesin is in the realm of hypersensitivity reactions. These reactions, which may be caused by histamine release, range from severe circulatory collapse, bronchospasm, and edema, to a generalized erythematous reaction.

Etomidate

Etomidate, which is a derivative of imidazole, is a new short-acting intravenous hypnotic that was synthesized in the laboratories of Janssen Pharmaceutica, in Beerse, Belgium. It is not related chemically to the commonly used hypnotic agents. This drug is a mere hypnotic and does not possess any analgesic actions. Etomidate is quite safe to administer to patients, as it has a high therapeutic index. Metabolism of this drug is accomplished by hydrolysis in the liver and by plasma esterases, with the final metabolite being pharmacologically inactive. The cardiovascular effects of etomidate are minimal; when the drug is injected in therapeutic doses, only a small blood pressure fall and a slight increase in heart rate may be observed. Studies have also shown that etomidate does cause a fall in the cardiac index and in the peripheral resistance. Although this drug does cause some pain at the site of injection, it does not appear to cause a release of histamine. Spontaneous involuntary movements have been observed after the injection of etomidate. These involuntary movements can be reduced by a meperidine premedication. This short-acting hypnotic is particularly well suited for the induction of neuroleptanalgesia and inhalation anesthesia. The induction dose ranges from 1 to 4.5 mg/kg, which produces sleep in 20 to 45 seconds after injection, with the patient awakening within 7 to 15 minutes after induction.

REFERENCES

1. Brown, B. (ed.): New Pharmacologic Vistas in Anesthesia. Philadelphia, F. A. Davis Co., 1983.
2. Collins, V.: Principles of Anesthesiology. 2nd ed. Philadelphia, Lea & Febiger, 1976.
3. Drain, C.: Innovar: a neuroleptic drug. Am. J. Nurs. 74:895–896, 1974.
4. Drain, C.: Recovery room care of the ketamine patient. RN Magazine. 36(11):OR1–2, 1973.
5. Goodman, L., and Gilman, A.: The Pharmacological Basis of Therapeutics. 6th ed. New York, Macmillan Publishing Company, 1980.
6. Katzung, B. (ed.): Basic and Clinical Pharmacology. 2nd ed. Los Altos, Lange Medical Publications, 1984.
7. Miller, R. (ed.): Anesthesia. 2nd ed. New York, Churchill Livingstone, Inc., 1986.
8. Wood, M., and Wood, A.: Drugs and Anesthesia: Pharmacology for the Anesthesiologist. Baltimore, Williams & Wilkins, 1982.
9. Wylie, W., and Churchill-Davidson, H.: A Practice of Anesthesia. 4th ed. Philadelphia, W. B. Saunders Co., 1978.

14

Muscle Relaxants

Neuromuscular blocking agents, or muscle relaxants, have been utilized in clinical anesthesia since the early 1940's. Significant advances have been made in both the physiology of neuromuscular transmission and the pharmacology of muscle relaxants, which have contributed greatly to clinical anesthesia as it is practiced today. Muscle relaxants are not used exclusively in the field of anesthesia; in post anesthesia and intensive care units and in emergency room settings, these drugs may be required to enhance patient care.

Muscle relaxants are used (1) to facilitate endotracheal intubation; (2) for procedures requiring muscle relaxation, such as intraperitoneal and thoracic surgery; (3) in ophthalmic surgery to relax the extraocular muscles; (4) to terminate laryngospasm and eliminate chest wall rigidity, which sometimes occur in rapid intravenous injection of a potent narcotic; and (5) to facilitate controlled respiration when mechanical ventilation is indicated, by producing total paralysis of the respiratory muscles.

The material presented in this chapter will help familiarize the practicing post anesthesia care unit (PACU) nurse with the physiologic and pharmacologic implications of the various neuromuscular blocking agents.

PHYSIOLOGY OF NEUROMUSCULAR TRANSMISSION

Because of the frequent and routine intra- and postoperative use of drugs that alter the patient's neuromuscular function, it is important to review the anatomy and physiology of the neuromuscular system, with emphasis on the chemical changes that occur at the receptor sites.

Activation of skeletal muscle is both an electrical and a biochemical event. The term *conduction* refers to the passage of an impulse along an axon to a muscle fiber. *Transmission* is a term that is applied to the passage of a neurotransmitter substance across a synaptic cleft (neuroeffector junction). The combined electrical and chemical event is called *neurohumoral transmission*.

As the fine terminal branch of a motor neuron approaches the muscle fiber, it loses its myelin sheath and forms an expanded terminal that lies close to a specialized area of muscle membrane called the *endplate* (Fig. 14–1). *Acetylcholine (ACh)*, which is the biochemical neurotransmitter involved in the initiation of muscle contraction, is formed in the body of the nerve cell and in the cytoplasm of the nerve terminal. Acetylcholine is stored in the small membrane-en-

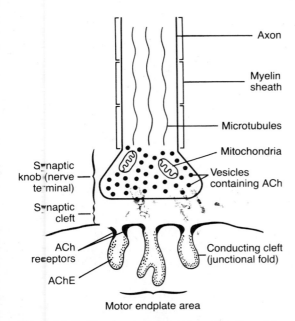

Figure 14–1. The myoneural junction at resting state (ACh = acetylcholine and AChE = acetylcholinesterase).

closed *vesicles* for subsequent release. A *quantum* is the amount of acetylcholine stored in each vesicle, or about 10,000 molecules of ACh. The presynaptic membrane contains discrete areas of specialization that are thought to be sites of release of the transmitter. The "active zones" lie directly opposite the acetylcholine receptors, which are located on the postsynaptic membrane. This alignment ensures that the ACh diffuses directly to the ACh receptors on the postsynaptic membrane quickly and in a high concentration. The acetylcholine receptor itself is a glycoprotein that exists as an integral part of the postsynaptic membrane of the neuromuscular junction (Fig. 14–1).

The initiation of skeletal muscle contraction occurs as a result of application of a *threshold stimulus*. An action potential travelling down the axon causes *depolarization* of the presynaptic membrane. As a result of this depolarization, the membrane permeability for calcium ions is increased and calcium enters or influxes into the presynaptic membrane. The calcium acts to unite the vesicle to the presynaptic membrane and causes the rupture of that coalesced

membrane, releasing ACh into the fluid of the synaptic cleft (Fig. 14–2).

The acetylcholine (ACh) molecules released from the nerve terminal into the synaptic cleft are subject to three main processes: (1) attachment to ACh receptors located on the postsynaptic membrane, leading to a change in ionic permeability of the muscle sarcolemma; (2) attachment to esterase molecules, which are enzymes secreted from the postsynaptic cleft that break down (hydrolyze) ACh; and (3) diffusional spread, leading to escape from the synapse. Within the conducting clefts of the postsynaptic membrane, competition exists between the ACh receptors and the acetylcholinesterase (AChE) molecules. The acetylcholinesterase will immediately destroy any acetylcholine that it comes in contact with, yet enough of the acetylcholine molecules (which bear a positive charge) must reach the ACh receptors (which bear a negative charge) to cause a change in the permeability of the muscle sarcolemma; the process of *excitation-contraction coupling (E-C coupling)* then takes place within that skeletal muscle cell. The physiologic outcome of E-C coupling is the contraction of the skeletal muscle.

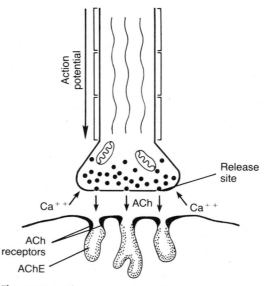

Figure 14–2. The myoneural junction when a threshold stimulus is applied (ACh = acetylcholine and AChE = acetylcholinesterase).

The strength of stimulus must be sufficient to cause the release of enough acetylcholine to bind to the ACh receptor. This process of competition between the ACh receptor and the acetylcholinesterase allows for a degree of regulation of the excitation process and for the recovery of the muscle cell membrane. The molecules of ACh either diffuse in a random fashion to the ACh receptor or are destroyed by the acetylcholinesterase. As the concentration gradient begins to decrease as a result of the destruction of the ACh by the acetylcholinesterase, the ACh receptor gives up its ACh, which is then destroyed, and the skeletal muscle relaxes. A small portion of the ACh can escape the acetylcholinesterase in the synaptic cleft and migrate into the extracellular fluid and from there into the plasma. The ACh within the plasma is then destroyed by plasma acetylcholinesterase or pseudocholinesterase, which is produced in the liver.

PHARMACOLOGIC OVERVIEW OF THE SKELETAL MUSCLE RELAXANTS

With the anatomy and physiology of neuromuscular transmission as a background, the principal pharmacologic actions of the nondepolarizing and depolarizing skeletal muscle relaxants will be presented. Table 14–1 presents a pharmacologic overview of the commonly used skeletal muscle relaxants.

The prototypical nondepolarizing skeletal muscle relaxants are pancuronium (Pavulon) and d-tubocurarine (curare). Pancuronium is an inhibitor of acetylcholine and is chemically viewed as two acetylcholine-like fragments, and has a bulky, inflexible nucleus. This drug attaches to the ACh receptors on the postsynaptic membrane and prevents depolarization. The skeletal muscle relaxant d-tubocurarine has the chemical structure of a monoquaternary compound. The principal pharmacologic action of this drug is to block the ACh receptor; in this way it stops acetylcholine from binding to the ACh receptor, resulting in a competitive neuromuscular blockade.

The pharmacologic actions of the nondepolarizing skeletal muscle relaxants can be reversed by anticholinesterase drugs such as neostigmine (Prostigmin). In effect, these drugs increase the quantum of acetycholine at the postsynaptic membrane by preventing destruction of the acetylcholine by the acetylcholinesterase. This promotes a more effective competition by the released acetylcholine with the nondepolarizing skeletal muscle relaxant that is occupying the ACh receptor. Because of the increased availability and mobilization of the acetylcholine, the concentration gradients favor acetylcholine and remove the nondepolarizing agents from the ACh receptor with the resultant return to normal contraction of the skeletal muscle.

The principal depolarizing skeletal muscle relaxant is succinylcholine (Anectine; Sucostrin). The molecular structure of this drug resembles two acetylcholine molecules back to back. Because of this structure, succinylcholine has the same effects as acetylcholine. Like acetylcholine, the succinylcholine molecule has a quaternary ammonium portion that is positively charged. This positively charged molecule is attracted by electrostatic action to the negatively charged ACh receptor. Once the ACh attaches to the receptor, a brief period of depolarization occurs, which is manifested by transient muscular fasciculations. After the depolarization of the ACh receptor takes place, succinylcholine promotes and maintains the receptor in a depolarized state and prevents repolarization. Succinylcholine has a brief duration of action. This is due to its rapid hydrolysis of the succinylcholine by the enzyme pseudocholinesterase, which is contained in the liver and plasma. The actions of succinylcholine cannot be pharmacologically reversed.

NONDEPOLARIZING NEUROMUSCULAR BLOCKING AGENTS

Tubocurarine Chloride (d-Tubocurarine Chloride, Curare)

d-Tubocurarine chloride (curare) was first known as an arrow poison used by the

TABLE 14–1. Pharmacologic Overview of the Commonly Used Skeletal Muscle Relaxants

	Atracurium Besylate (Tracrium)	Pancuronium (Pavulon)	d-Tubocurarine	Vecuronium (Norcuron)	Metocurine (Metubine)	Succinylcholine (Anectine)
Nondepolarizing	Yes	Yes	Yes	Yes	Yes	No
Depolarizing	No	No	No	No	No	Yes
Intubation dose (IV mg/kg)	0.4–0.5	0.06–0.1	0.6	0.08–0.1	0.25–0.4	0.5–1.0
Intubation time (injection to relaxation in minutes)	2.0–2.5	4.0	6.0–8.0 (rarely used for intubation)	2.5–3.0	4.0	<1.0
Muscle relaxation dose (IV mg/kg)	0.4–0.4	0.04–0.08	0.3	0.05–0.06	0.2–0.3	(IV drip) 0.1–0.2 mg/ml
Recovery time (in minutes)	30–45	84–114	74–87	25–40	94–117	4–6
Reversible? When ? (in minutes after initial dose)	Yes 20–35	Yes 40–60	Yes 40–60	Yes 25–30 (for 0.1 mg/kg) 40–80 (for 0.2 mg/kg)	Yes 45–60	No
Cumulative effects?	No	Yes	Yes	Slight	Yes	No
Fasciculations and muscle soreness	No	No	No	No	No	Yes
Risk of histamine release	Minimal	Slight to none	Significant	None	Moderate	Possible
Cardiovascular effects	Few	Slight ↑ in pulse and ↑ in BP	Hypotension	None	None	Slight ↓ in pulse

South American Indians. Curare blocks access of acetylcholine to the receptor at the neuromuscular junction of skeletal muscle. The action is a combination of electrical and chemical transmission, with d-tubocurarine preventing depolarization by impeding leakage of the sodium ions necessary for depolarization.

The peak action of d-tubocurarine occurs 30 to 60 minutes after intravenous injection. Fifty to 70 percent of injected d-tubocurarine is excreted unchanged in the urine in the course of 3 to 6 hours. In spite of this, the duration of action of d-tubocurarine is not unduly prolonged, even in the complete absence of renal function.

Certain side effects and variations of response to d-tubocurarine have been reported. A histamine-like reaction has been reported, as have hypotension, increased airway resistance, and skin erythema. Consequently, it is advisable to choose a relaxant other than d-tubocurarine for asthmatic patients and those with a history of allergic reactions. With d-tubocurarine's ganglionic blocking action coupled with its histamine-like actions, it can cause the blood pressure to fall in many patients.

Gallamine (Flaxedil)

Gallamine (Flaxedil), the first synthetic skeletal muscle relaxant, was introduced into clinical anesthesia six years after d-tubocurarine. This nondepolarizing skeletal muscle relaxant has been shown to be one fifth as potent as d-tubocurarine, with a 25 percent shorter duration of action. In clinical doses, gallamine will block the vagal ganglia in the heart, which will result in tachycardia. This property has been used to advantage when the drug is combined with halothane (Fluothane), which is normally a vagal stimulant. Gallamine is excreted entirely unchanged by the kidneys. This explains reports of prolonged action of the drug in patients with poor renal function.

Pancuronium Bromide (Pavulon)

Pancuronium bromide (Pavulon) was introduced into clinical anesthesia in 1972. This drug has demonstrated value particularly in terms of its safety, cardiovascular stability, and skeletal muscle relaxing properties. Because of these advantages, it is enjoying widespread clinical usage.

Chemically, pancuronium bromide is a biquaternary aminosteroid and is related to the androgens; however, it does not have any hormonal activities. Its action is similar to the action of d-tubocurarine, but it is five times more potent. Also, like d-tubocurarine, it is reversible by an anticholinesterase agent, such as neostigmine (Prostigmin), which is administered in combination with an anticholinergic, such as glycopyrrolate (Robinul) or atropine. It has been demonstrated clinically that this particular skeletal muscle relaxant is very difficult to reverse pharmacologically within the first 20 to 30 minutes after injection. In the PACU, should a skeletal muscle relaxant be required for a short duration, another reversible skeletal muscle relaxant, such as d-tubocurarine or atracurium, should be chosen. About 30 to 40 minutes after injection, pancuronium is easily reversed by the combination of an anticholinesterase and anticholinergic drug preparation. Pancuronium is best suited for surgical procedures lasting more than one hour. This drug is well suited for patients who require complete muscle relaxation when receiving continuous mechanical ventilation. The dosage for adults is approximately 0.08 to 0.10 mg per kg of body weight. Relaxation will last 60 to 85 minutes. If relaxation is required past this initial period, subsequent doses should be decreased to 0.02 to 0.04 mg per kg of body weight.

Pancuronium bromide does not produce ganglionic blockade, as evidenced by the fact that the systolic and diastolic blood pressure, pulse rate, and cardiac output are not lowered significantly while the drug is clinically active. Although some isolated cases of histamine release have been reported, pancuronium can probably be used in patients who have a marginal allergy history. Pancuronium bromide is compatible with anesthetic agents used clinically and is safe to use in most patients when a nondepolarizing skeletal muscle relaxant is indicated. However, pancuronium bromide is not indicated in situations in which a nondepolarizing muscle relaxant is to be used with caution.

Pancuronium bromide should be avoided in patients who have a history of myasthenia gravis. It is contraindicated in patients with true renal disease, since a major portion of the drug is excreted unchanged in the urine. This agent is contraindicated in patients known to be hypersensitive to it or to the bromide ion.

Alcuronium Chloride (Alloferin)

Alcuronium, which is chemically related to d-tubocurarine, is one of the newer nondepolarizing skeletal muscle relaxants that has been introduced into clinical anesthesia practice. This agent is about twice as potent as, and has a duration of action that is much shorter than, d-tubocurarine. Administration of 0.2 mg per kg of alcuronium can produce in 2 to 4 minutes muscular relaxation that lasts for about 20 minutes. It is also reversible by the combination of an anticholinesterase and an anticholinergic drug preparation. This drug produces about the same degree of hypotension as d-tubocurarine and causes about the same amount of histamine release as pancuronium. Because alcuronium is not metabolized and is excreted in an unchanged form by the kidneys, it should be used with caution in patients with any type of renal dysfunction.

Atracurium Besylate (Tracrium)

Atracurium is a new nondepolarizing skeletal muscle relaxant that offers an advantage over other skeletal muscle relaxants in that the drug does not depend on renal or hepatic mechanisms for its elimination. In fact, this quaternary ammonium compound actually breaks down in the absence of plasma enzymes through what is called Hofmann elimination and to a lesser extent ester hydrolysis. *Hofmann elimination* is a nonbiologic method of degradation that occurs at a physiologic temperature and pH.

This drug is less potent than pancuronium and has a rapid onset and duration of action that is about one third to one half that of pancuronium. Also, atracurium has little or no cumulative effect and is not influenced significantly by the specific general inhalational anesthetic dose or concentration. This drug has little or no cardiovascular effect and is easily antagonized by the combination of an anticholinesterase and an anticholinergic. Atracurium also has the distinct advantage of not having its neuromuscular blockade prolonged by renal failure or impaired hepatic function.

Fazadinium Bromide

Fazadinium is a nondepolarizing skeletal muscle relaxant that has a rapid onset and a short duration of action. This drug provides better skeletal muscle relaxation for endotracheal intubation than pancuronium during the first minute after its intravenous injection. The intubation dose is 1 mg/kg. However, it should be noted that this drug's onset of action is not as rapid as that of succinylcholine. Consequently, in an emergency situation in which endotracheal intubation must be performed, succinylcholine, owing to its very rapid onset of action, is the drug of choice. Because fazadinium produces minimal cardiovascular effects and has such a fast onset and short duration of action, its use is of value in intra- and postoperative periods.

Metocurine Iodide (Metubine)

Metocurine, which was originally introduced into clinical anesthesia practice in 1948 as dimethyltubocurarine, is now regaining popularity. Metocurine is a nondepolarizing neuromuscular blocking agent that is a trimethylated derivative of d-tubocurarine and, like d-tubocurarine, is quite

reversible by the drug combination of an anticholinesterase and an anticholinergic. The dosage for surgical relaxation is 0.2 mg per kg, and to facilitate endotracheal intubation, a dose of 0.3 to 0.4 mg per kg is required. It is about one to two times as potent as d-tubocurarine in neuromuscular blocking potency, and yet is less potent than d-tubocurarine in regard to its ability to inhibit autonomic responses and to release histamine. Consequently, the clinical cardiovascular and hemodynamic effects of metocurine seem to be much less than those of d-tubocurarine. Because metocurine produces minimal hemodynamic changes, it is useful for patients with hypertension and coronary artery disease.

Vecuronium Bromide (Norcuron)

Vecuronium is a new nondepolarizing skeletal muscle relaxant that has a more rapid onset of action and shorter duration of action than that of pancuronium. The potency of vecuronium is equal to, or slightly greater than, that of pancuronium. Vecuronium has little or no cumulative effect. Although a portion of vecuronium is metabolized, most of the drug is excreted in the urine and bile unchanged. However, the neuromuscular blockade produced by vecuronium is not prolonged by renal failure. The duration of neuromuscular blockade produced by vecuronium will be increased in patients with impaired hepatic function. Of clinical interest is that for unknown reasons vecuronium, like atracurium, when compared with pancuronium and d-tubocurarine, is less influenced by the various general inhalational anesthetics. This drug, in large part, has little or no cardiovascular effects and is easily reversed by the combination of an anticholinesterase and an anticholinergic drug.

Reversal of Nondepolarizing Neuromuscular Blocking Agents

To restore neuromuscular transmission, the antagonist must displace the competitive neuromuscular blocking agent from the

ACh receptor sites and open the way for depolarization of the postjunctional membrane. The antagonist is an antiacetylcholinesterase, which blocks the enzymatic action of the acetylcholinesterase located in the postsynaptic clefts so that acetylcholine is not hydrolyzed. The end result is a buildup of acetylcholine at the end-plate. The accumulated acetylcholine then displaces the competitive neuromuscular blocking agent, which then diffuses back into the plasma. Neuromuscular transmission is thus reestablished.

Neostigmine is usually the anticholinesterase of choice because its duration of action is long and it is a more reliable agent than edrophonium chloride (Tensilon). Atropine, an anticholinergic drug, is administered immediately before, or in conjunction with, the anticholinesterase in order to minimize the muscarinic effects of the anticholinesterase (bradycardia, hypotension, and bronchoconstriction). Generally, 2.5 mg of neostigmine is the maximum dose required for reversal; the suggested limit is 5 mg. The method is to give atropine, 0.4 mg intravenously, over a one-minute period, to observe for an increase in pulse rate, and then to administer 0.5 mg neostigmine intravenously and monitor the reversal. This procedure can then be repeated until reversal has been achieved or until the limit of neostigmine that can be given is reached.

Neostigmine should be administered cautiously. Cardiac monitoring is essential, especially in elderly or debilitated patients and those with cardiac disease. Atrioventricular dissociation and other dysrhythmias can be initiated by the anticholinesterases.

Pyridostigmine (Regonol) is an analog of neostigmine. It facilitates the transmission of impulses across the myoneural junction by inhibiting the destruction of acetylcholine by acetylcholinesterase. Clinical data indicate a lower incidence of muscarinic side effects with this drug as compared with neostigmine. As with neostigmine, pyridostigmine should be administered with caution to patients who suffer from bronchial asthma or cardiac problems. Signs of over-

TABLE 14–2. Observable Responses to Stimulation of Receptors

Nicotinic

Stimulation of autonomic ganglia—both sympathetic and parasympathetic

Stimulation of adrenal medulla, resulting in the release of both epinephrine and norepinephrine

Stimulation of skeletal muscles at the motor end-plate

Muscarinic

Stimulation or inhibition of smooth muscle in various organs or tissues

Stimulation of exocrine glands (i.e., salivary and sweat glands)

Slowing of cardiac conduction

Decrease in myocardial contractile force

dosage are related to muscarinic and nicotinic receptor stimulation (Table 14–2). The muscarinic side effects are blocked with atropine or glycopyrrolate. The nicotinic responses can be blocked by drugs such as ganglionic or neuromuscular blocking agents. The recommended dose for reversal is 0.15 mg per kg IV pyridostigmine, in combination with 0.007 mg per kg atropine IV. Full recovery occurs within 15 minutes in most patients; others may require 30 minutes or more.

Another parasympatholytic agent, glycopyrrolate (Robinul), has been substituted for atropine in the reversal technique by some clinicians. It offers advantages over atropine in that it has a longer duration of action; a lower incidence of arrhythmias; small, slow changes in heart rate; and does not cross the blood-brain barrier. The usual reversal dosage is 1 mg of neostigmine and 0.2 mg of glycopyrrolate in a 2 ml mixture. This dosage can be repeated if reversal is inadequate.

DEPOLARIZING NEUROMUSCULAR BLOCKING AGENTS

Succinylcholine (Anectine, Sucostrin)

Succinylcholine represents a valuable pharmacologic advance in modern anesthesia and in critical care, areas in which resuscitation of patients is required. This agent is usually included as one of the drugs available for emergency situations, especially those requiring endotracheal intubation. It is also used in areas outside the operating room for such procedures as amelioration of the impact of electroshock therapy; treatment of profound laryngospasm; control of the convulsive states of tetanus, of toxic reactions to local anesthetic drugs, and of status asthmaticus; in management of ventilation in the flail chest; and during reduction of fractures or dislocations.

Although succinylcholine is enjoying wide popularity in this country, it should be noted that this drug is not without definite side effects and complications, many of which can be avoided through a basic understanding of the pharmacology of the drug.

Succinylcholine acts at the myoneural junction by causing a persistent depolarization of the end-plate. It is a synthetic quaternary ammonium compound whose chemical structure closely resembles that of acetylcholine. The onset of action of succinylcholine is rapid upon initial injection. Its length of action is approximately 3 to 5 minutes. The drug is hydrolyzed rapidly by plasma pseudocholinesterase, an enzyme produced by the liver, to succinylmonocholine and choline. The succinylmonocholine is further hydrolyzed by pseudocholinesterase and true cholinesterase, found in the erythrocyte, to succinic acid and choline. (See equations at bottom of page.)

Untoward Reactions. Because the hydrolysis of succinylcholine is dependent upon enzymatic activity, it is important to understand the atypical responses that may occur. Pseudocholinesterase activity in the plasma may be elevated or reduced. Elevations are congenital and are extremely rare. These patients are very resistant to succinylcholine and do not relax well. The reductions in pseudocholinesterase activity may be acquired or congenital. The acquired deficiencies are more important to discuss because they are more common. They occur with liver disease, severe anemia, malnutrition, prolonged pyrexia, pregnancy, and recent renal dialysis. Drugs such as quinidine and propranolol (Inderal) inhibit pseudocholinesterase, as do echothiophate iodide eye drops (Phospholine). Patients with low pseudocholinesterase will exhibit a prolonged response to these drugs.

Atypical pseudocholinesterase occurs alone in about one in 2800 people; this atypical form is inherited. Patients with genetically induced deficiencies of pseudocholinesterase have remained apneic for as long as 48 hours after a usual dose of succinylcholine. These patients require mechanical ventilation and constant nursing care. Patients with a documented pseudocholinesterase deficiency should be advised to wear a MedicAlert bracelet. If needed, these patients should be administered nondepolarizing skeletal muscle relaxants, such as pancuronium, d-tubocurarine, or gallamine, if subsequent anesthetics are required, since such drugs can usually be reversed.

Disadvantages and Side Effects. Succinylcholine can be administered via single injection or by continuous infusion. These methods are not without their disadvantages. The single-injection method is utilized when neuromuscular relaxation is required for a short period of time, such as to facilitate endotracheal intubation. The usual intubation dose of succinylcholine is 1 mg per kg, intravenously. During the first intravenous injection, the cardiovascular status usually remains normal. If the injection must be repeated, the patient may exhibit profound bradycardia and various arrhythmias. Therefore, it is important to monitor the patient's cardiovascular status

Succinylcholine $\xrightarrow{\text{Pseudocholinesterase}}$ Succinylmonocholine and choline

Succinylmonocholine $\xrightarrow{\text{True and pseudocholinesterase}}$ Succinic acid and choline when succinylcholine is administered, especially if the dose is repeated.

It is also advisable to monitor pediatric patients completely because they are especially prone to bradycardia, even on the initial injection of succinylcholine. This complication can be easily overcome by prior administration of glycopyrrolate (Robinul) or atropine sulfate, either alone or mixed with succinylcholine. This appears to be the safest way of administering intravenous succinylcholine in the pediatric age group.

Another disadvantage of single-injection-succinylcholine is that this agent causes fasciculations of the muscles. These are a result of the initial depolarization of the skeletal muscle. These contractions frequently lead to muscle pain, which is usually noted by the patient the day after surgery. This is particularly true in patients who are ambulatory soon after surgery. In ambulatory patients, muscle pains occur in 60 to 70 percent of cases. This drops to 10 percent in those patients confined to bed. Some complaints of these patients include pain when blinking their eyes, pain when smiling, and generalized pain when ambulatory. These objective symptoms are usually noticed first by the nurse in the post anesthesia care unit. The pain usually does not require analgesics and subsides in a day or two. The fasciculations can be prevented by administering 3 to 6 mg of curare 3 minutes prior to the injection of succinylcholine.

Research indicates that when succinylcholine is administered to the patient with extensive burns, to the severely traumatized patient, or to the patient who has neurologic lesions, such as paraplegia or quadriplegia, a serious release of potassium from the damaged muscle and nerve cells can result. The elevation of the serum potassium, which can be as high as 10 to 15 mEq per liter, has been reported. The end result of this potassium elevation is cardiac dysrhythmias and cardiac arrest. The critical period for these reactions is between post-traumatic days 15 and 115, although if the neurologic trauma is at the cord level, suc-cinylcholine should not be administered for 48 hours after the injury.

Succinylcholine has been implicated as one of the trigger agents of *malignant hyperthermia (MH)*. Chapter 42 of this text contains a complete description of the pathophysiology and treatment of MH.

In pediatric and adult patients anesthetized with halothane, with succinylcholine as the muscle relaxant, there is an unusual incidence of plasma myoglobin. Myoglobin is an intracellular muscle protein and therefore should not be released into the plasma. If myoglobin is found in the plasma it can only mean that the muscle membrane has been injured. Further research is now being conducted on succinylcholine and complications related to it.

Succinylcholine can be administered in a drip infusion during a procedure that requires skeletal muscle relaxation for a longer period of time than a single injection could provide. It is usually administered in a 0.1 to 0.2 percent solution. If the infusion is administered for a prolonged period, the type of block can gradually undergo a change from a depolarizing block to a characteristic nondepolarizing block. The change is always from depolarization to nondepolarization, never in the reverse direction. This type of block is called a *dual block* or phase II block (see p. 210). The exact time relationship and the mechanism of action are still uncertain. Treatment is by mechanical ventilation and by careful monitoring of the patient until the dual block disappears.

Succinylcholine increases intraocular pressure by about 7.5 mm Hg in both children and adults, owing, in part, to the contraction of the extraocular muscles. d-Tubocurarine, when administered before the succinylcholine to prevent the contraction of the extraocular muscles, does not completely extinguish the rise in intraocular pressure. Therefore, even if succinylcholine is used in conjunction with d-tubocurarine, it is still contraindicated in patients in whom an increased intraocular pressure would be detrimental.

Advantages. Succinylcholine has some definite advantages that, in most cases, justify its clinical use. The very rapid onset of action coupled with its short duration of action has made this drug valuable when (1) rapid intubation is required, (2) laryngospasm is irreversible with positive pressure; (3) the skeletal muscles are rigid and prevent good ventilatory excursion; (4) procedures require short duration of skeletal muscle relaxation, such as reduction of dislocations and fractures; and (5) electroconvulsive therapy is utilized to decrease the negative effects of the convulsion. With continued use over a 30-year period, succinylcholine has been shown by studies to produce complications, which can, in most cases, be prevented if the basic pharmacodynamics of the drug are understood.

Hexafluorenium Bromide (Mylaxen)

Hexafluorenium bromide has both anticholinesterase and neuromuscular blocking effects. It is used clinically to potentiate the effects of succinylcholine and consequently reduces the total amount of succinylcholine used during the surgical procedure. This averts the accumulation of breakdown products of succinylcholine and also reduces muscular fasciculations and twitching when succinylcholine is initially administered. Hexafluorenium bromide is not used much in clinical anesthesia practice, because bronchospasm, tachycardia, hypotension, and cardiac dysrhythmias have been reported frequently after its use.

Decamethonium Bromide (Syncurine)

Decamethonium was first used clinically in 1949. This drug's action is similar to that of acetylcholine, in that it produces depolarization of the end-plate of the neuromuscular junction. It does liberate some histamine, but only about half as much as is released by use of d-tubocurarine. Decamethonium has no action on the myocardium and produces fasciculations, as does succinylcholine. This drug is not metabolized in the body and is excreted largely unchanged by the kidney. The intravenous route is the only satisfactory route of administration for this drug. The onset of action for decamethonium is about 30 to 40 seconds after injection, and its duration of action is about 15 to 20 minutes. Because of the difficulty in reversal, along with the problems of histamine release and fasciculations, decamethonium is rarely used in clinical anesthesia practice.

FACTORS INFLUENCING THE NEUROMUSCULAR BLOCKING AGENTS

Fluid Balance

Patients who are dehydrated are extremely sensitive to skeletal muscle relaxants. This is probably true because (1) dehydration decreases neuromuscular excitability, (2) the contracted extracellular fluid compartment permits an increase in the plasma concentration of the relaxant and thus intensifies the relaxant action, and (3) renal function is slowed and the elimination time of the relaxant and its metabolites is prolonged.

Sodium

A deficit of sodium may prolong the neuromuscular block. Experimental evidence indicates that a sodium deficiency itself may result in a partial neuromuscular block.

Potassium

Potassium deficiency appears to increase the blocking action of d-tubocurarine and other nondepolarizing neuromuscular blocking agents. On the other hand, depolarizing neuromuscular blocking agents are required in larger amounts when potassium deficiency exists. Depolarization is prevented to some extent, because a potassium deficiency appears to stabilize the muscle end-plate. A potassium depletion can occur from decreased intake or excessive loss, such as in chronic pyelonephritis, primary aldosteronism, chlorothiazide therapy, or chronic diarrhea.

Magnesium

An increase in magnesium concentration will cause a flaccid paralysis clinically similar to that caused by a nondepolarizing neuromuscular blocking agent. The principal action of magnesium is depression of the formation or release of acetylcholine, which reduces the end-plate potential and causes neuromuscular block.

Calcium

A deficiency in calcium prolongs the effects of nondepolarizing neuromuscular blocking agents by reducing the quantity of acetylcholine released and also by inhibiting neuromuscular transmission. The depolarizing neuromuscular blocking agents are also potentiated because a low calcium level will aid depolarization. Conversely, the administration of calcium chloride solution in calcium deficiency states will antagonize the nondepolarizing effects of agents such as d-tubocurarine. Experimental work also indicates that calcium chloride has a pronounced antagonism to the respiratory depressant effects of succinylcholine.

pH and Carbon Dioxide

The neuromuscular blocking effect of d-tubocurarine is enhanced in acidosis and in states of elevated carbon dioxide tension. In drugs such as gallamine and succinylcholine the neuromuscular blocking action is diminished. Alkalosis by itself decreased the effects of d-tubocurarine. Of interest is that hyperventilation has been thought to augment the abdominal muscle relaxation produced by d-tubocurarine. One explanation of this phenomenon is that changes in pH or plasma concentrations of d-tubocurarine reflect a change in binding to the receptor substance.

Catecholamines

Epinephrine and ephedrine have an anticurare effect on skeletal muscle. Clinically, an antagonism to d-tubocurarine has been demonstrated. This is caused by an increase in release of acetylcholine, the inhibition of acetylcholinesterase, a decreased excitability of muscle fibers, and the release of potassium when epinephrine and ephedrine are administered.

Mycins

A number of antibiotics exhibit a curariform neuromuscular blocking property. The clinical difficulties that result are related to a combination of factors, including large doses of antibiotics, parenteral administration into body cavities that represent a large surface area for absorption, and the concomitant use of a neuromuscular blocking agent. Neomycin and streptomycin have been most frequently implicated (Table 14–3).

Temperature

Hypothermia antagonizes the action of d-tubocurarine and potentiates the action of succinylcholine or decamethonium. During the recovery phase of an anesthetic, when

TABLE 14–3. Neuromuscular Blocking Properties of Various Antibiotics

Antibiotics that increase the action of the *nondepolarizing* agents include:

Neomycin	Polymyxin A
Streptomycin	Polymyxin B
Dihydrostreptomycin	Lincomycin
Kanamycin	Colistin
Gentamicin	Tetracycline

Antibiotics that increase the action of *succinylcholine* include:
Neomycin
Streptomycin
Kanamycin
Polymyxin B
Colistin

Antibiotics that do not exert any neuromuscular blocking activity include:
Penicillin
Chloramphenicol
Cephalosporins

a neuromuscular blocking agent has been administered, young infants should be specifically monitored for return of skeletal muscle tone. This is especially true when a nondepolarizing relaxant is administered to infants, who are prone to have some hypothermia by virtue of their immature heat-regulating system.

ASSESSMENT OF NEUROMUSCULAR BLOCKADE

Humans injected with d-tubocurarine first have motor weakness, and then their muscles become totally flaccid. The small, rapidly moving muscles, such as those of the fingers, toes, eyes, and ears, are involved before the long muscles of the limbs, neck, and trunk. The intercostal muscles, and finally the diaphragm, become paralyzed and then respiration ceases.

The PACU nurse should know the order of the return of muscle function after a patient has received a nondepolarizing muscle relaxant such as d-tubocurarine. The recovery of skeletal muscle function is usually in reverse order to that of paralysis; therefore, the diaphragm is ordinarily first to regain function. The order of appearance of paralysis after injection with a nondepolarizing neuromuscular blocking agent can be electromyographically assessed as follows:

1. *Small muscle groups:* oculomotor muscles, muscles of the eyelids; muscles of the mouth, facial muscles; small extensor muscles of the fingers, followed by the flexor muscles of the fingers.

2. *Medium-sized muscle groups:* muscles of the tongue and pharynx; muscles of mastication; extensor muscles of the limb, followed by flexor muscles of the limbs.

3. *Large muscle groups:* neck muscles; shoulder muscles; abdominal muscles; dorsal muscle mass.

4. *Special muscle groups:* intercostal muscles; larynx; diaphragm.

The order of paralysis is essentially the same after injection with a depolarizing neuromuscular agent, with the exception that the flexor muscles are paralyzed before the extensor muscles. Patients arriving in the post anesthesia care unit must be evaluated for residual effects from a neuromuscular blocking agent that was administered intraoperatively. In most instances the action of the nondepolarizing neuromuscular blocking agent will be pharmacologically reversed at the end of the operation, before the patient is admitted to the PACU; however, any patient who has received a neuromuscular blocking agent should be closely watched for signs of residual drug action. Table 14–4 describes the criteria for recovery from nondepolarizing neuromuscular blockade. It should be stated that the residual actions of the depolarizing muscle relaxants are similar to those of the nondepolarizing muscle relaxants, and the same nonrespiratory parameters and respiratory variables can be used to evaluate the neuromuscular blockade. The evoked responses differ between the depolarizing and nondepolarizing neuromuscular blocking agents.

The *peripheral nerve stimulator* (Figs. 14–3A and 14–3B) can be used in the PACU to assess the type and degree of a neuromuscular blockade. This electrical device can be used to stimulate the ulnar nerve at the

TABLE 14–4. Criteria for Recovery from Nondepolarizing Neuromuscular Blockade

Clinical Assessment of Neuromuscular Blockade
Nonrespiratory parameters
    Ability to open eyes wide
    Sustained protrusion of the tongue
    Sustained hand grip
    Sustained head lift for at least five seconds
    Ability to cough effectively
Respiratory variables
    Tidal volume of at least 5 ml/kg
    Vital capacity of at least 15–20 ml/kg
    Inspiratory force of 20–25 cm water, negative
      pressure

Evoked Responses
Return of the single twitch to control height
Sustained tetanic response to high-frequency stimulation
Recovery of the train-of-four to a ratio above 75%

Adapted from: Train-of-four technique facilitates assessment of NMB and correlation with recovery. Wellcome Trends in Anesthesiology/Symposium Perspectives, 3(6):8–10, 1985.

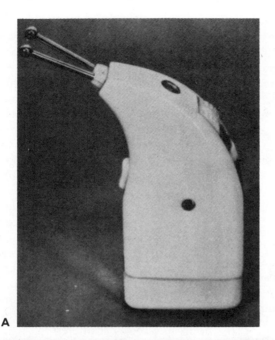

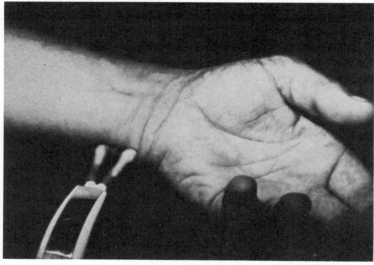

Figure 14–3. A, Peripheral nerve stimulator. B, Method of applying the peripheral nerve stimulator to the ulnar nerve at the wrist. (From Churchill-Davidson H. C., Wylie and Churchill-Davidson: A Practice of Anesthesia. 4th ed. Philadelphia, W. B. Saunders Co., 1978, p. 882.)

wrist or elbow, and, upon stimulation of the ulnar nerve, the nurse can observe the contraction of the fingers. The assessment of the depth of neuromuscular blockade using electrical stimulation is useful when greater than 70 percent of the acetylcholine receptors are blocked by a skeletal muscle relaxant. However, in most cases, if the patient in the PACU has a normal tidal volume, vital capacity, and maximal inspiratory force, and is able to lift the head for 5 seconds, the use of the peripheral nerve stimulator is not warranted. If one wishes

to identify the type of neuromuscular blockade used (depolarizing or nondepolarizing), or if some of the aforementioned parameters are marginal, the train-of-four or sustained tetanus utilizing the peripheral nerve stimulator (PNS) can be used to provide the objective data for assessment.

Although the mechanisms producing the nondepolarizing block are different, the diagnostic criteria using a peripheral nerve stimulator for assessing a nondepolarizing and phase II dual block are basically the same. Miller[8] points out that the hallmark of a nondepolarizing neuromuscular blockade is an inability to sustain contraction in response to a tetanic stimulus and post-tetanic facilitation. A *tetanic stimulus* is the usual 50 Hz of current for 5 seconds (sustained tetanus) produced by a peripheral nerve stimulator. *Post-tetanic facilitation* is a twitch after the response to tetanic stimuli higher than the twitch immediately before tetanus. It should also be stated that if a patient has a partial nondepolarizing neuromuscular block, *fade*, which is an unsustained contraction, will be seen after the initial tetanic stimulus (Fig. 14–4). The responses to electrical stimulation are due to the interaction of acetylcholine released and the number of acetylcholine receptors occupied by the relaxant. In patients with a partial nondepolarizing neuromuscular block, the first three single electrical stimuli will be of enough intensity to produce a twitch, but the twitch produced will not be of the same magnitude as a twitch produced in a subject who has not received a nondepolarizing skeletal muscle relaxant (Fig. 14–4). The three electrical stimuli will cause the normal quantum of acetylcholine to be released at the synaptic cleft; however, in this case, the reduction in twitch magnitude is due to the number of acetylcholine receptors being occupied by the nondepolarizing

relaxant. Consequently, if the patient had a complete nondepolarizing neuromuscular block in which all the cholinergic receptors were occupied, no twitch would be elicited from the three electrical stimuli.

In a normal subject, when a tetanic stimulus is applied for 5 seconds, the quantum of acetylcholine that is released decreases during the stimulus period. Along with this, only a fraction of acetylcholine receptors are activated at any one time to trigger an action potential. The excess in acetylcholine receptors is the safety margin of neuromuscular transmission. Consequently, in the normal subject who receives a tetanic stimulus, the magnitude of the twitch response will be maintained because of the large cholinergic receptor pool. However, if, for example, 75 percent of the acetylcholine receptors are occupied by a nondepolarizing neuromuscular relaxant, the twitch response will not be maintained and fade (unsustained contraction) will occur because the usual margin of safety of excess acetylcholine receptors has been abolished. Interestingly, in between the termination of a tetanic stimulus and the first single-twitch stimulus, a buildup of acetylcholine will occur in the presynaptic knob. Thus, after sustained tetanus, when the first electrical stimulus is administered, the height of the

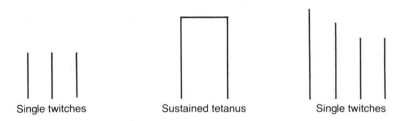

Single twitches   Sustained tetanus   Single twitches

Without nondepolarizing neuromuscular blockade

Decreased
magnitude   Fade   Post-tetanic
facilitation

Figure 14–4. Magnitude of post-tetanic facilitation without and with nondepolarizing neuromuscular blockade. Adapted from Miller, R. D., "Monitoring of neuromuscular blockade." In: Saidman, L. and Smith, (eds) *Monitoring in Anesthesia*, 2nd ed. Copyright 1984, Butterworth Publishers.

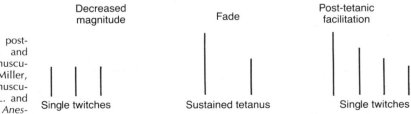

Single twitches   Sustained tetanus   Single twitches

With nondepolarizing neuromuscular blockade

first twitch will be greater than the pretetanus twitches. These large post-tetanic twitches (post-tetanic facilitation) will return to the pretetanus height as the acetylcholine mobilization also returns to the pretetanus level. Finally, it should be stated that greater than 70 percent of the acetylcholine receptors must be occupied before this tetanic stimulation test will be sensitive enough to detect neuromuscular blockade.

The major drawback to the delivery of a 50 Hz tetanic stimulus to an awake patient in the PACU is pain and general discomfort. For the patient who is awake and reacting, it would be more appropriate to use the *train-of-four stimulation* to assess the degree of neuromuscular blockade due to nondepolarizing skeletal muscle relaxants. In this test, the ulnar nerve is used, and four supramaximal electrical stimuli, 0.05 seconds apart, at 2 Hz, are administered via a peripheral nerve stimulator. This test, which produces minimal discomfort to the awake patient, is sensitive only when greater than 70 percent of the acetylcholine receptors are occupied. The index of neuromuscular blockade in this test is the ratio of the fourth to the first twitch amplitude. More specifically, when the fourth response is abolished, a 75 percent block exists (Fig. 14–5). When the third and second responses to stimulation are abolished, the respective reductions in neuromuscular blockade are 80 and 90 percent. Finally, when all four twitch responses are absent, a 100 percent or complete block exists.

The depolarizing neuromuscular blockade is characterized by an absence of posttetanic facilitation, a decreased response to a single impulse, a decreased amplitude (but sustained response to a tetanic stimulus), and, if present, a train-of-four ratio between the first and fourth stimulus that is greater than 70 percent.

SPECIAL PROBLEMS IN THE POST ANESTHESIA CARE UNIT

A prolonged response to succinylcholine sometimes occurs because a patient does not possess the proper blood level of pseu-

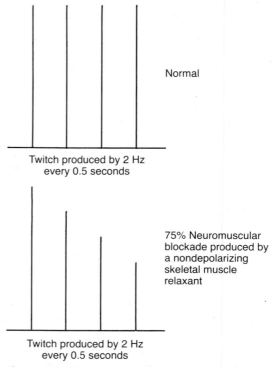

Normal

Twitch produced by 2 Hz every 0.5 seconds

75% Neuromuscular blockade produced by a nondepolarizing skeletal muscle relaxant

Twitch produced by 2 Hz every 0.5 seconds

Figure 14–5. Diagrammatic illustration of the train-of-four in normal response and 75 percent neuromuscular blockade produced by a nondepolarizing skeletal muscle relaxant.

docholinesterase. Other reasons for a prolonged response include (1) overdosage, (2) temperature changes, (3) acid-base imbalance, (4) carcinoma, (5) antitumor agents, (6) antibiotics, (7) myasthenia gravis, and (8) liver disease.

If a patient who arrives in the PACU is apneic, controlled respiration must be initiated and maintained as long as necessary. Careful monitoring of vital signs and evaluation of renal function are important. Identification of the neuromuscular block can be accomplished with the previously discussed peripheral nerve stimulator. If electrical stimulation results in vigorous contractions, it is unlikely that the apnea is the result of residual neuromuscular block. Consideration must then be given to other agents that might have caused the apneic state. The response of patients with neuromuscular disorders to muscle relaxants can include resistance, increased response, hyperkalemia, and even cardiac arrest; Table 14–5 is presented as a summary of the possible untoward responses in the clinical setting.

TABLE 14–5. Summary of the Response of Patients with Neuromuscular Disorders to Muscle Relaxants

Disorder	Pathophysiology	Response to Nondepolarizing Muscle Relaxant	Response to Depolarizing Muscle Relaxant
Hemiplegia	Sequelae of CVA; is caused by an upper motor neuron in the cerebral motor cortex	Resistance	Hyperkalemia can occur as early as 1 week and as late as 6 months post stroke
Parkinson's Disease	Extrapyramidal disorder	Normal	Hyperkalemia may occur
Multiple Sclerosis	Demyelinating disorder of the CNS	Normal	Hyperkalemia may occur
Diffuse Intracranial Lesions	No focal neurologic deficits or muscular denervation or paralysis (i.e., ruptured cerebral aneurysm)	Normal ?	Hyperkalemia and possible cardiac arrest
Tetanus	Acute infectious disease of the CNS caused by the endotoxin released by *Clostridium tetani*	Normal	Hyperkalemia and possible cardiac arrest
Paraplegia and Quadriplegia	Traumatic or pathologic transection of the spinal cord and interruption of pyramidal tracts	Increased response	Hyperkalemia as early as 3 weeks and as late as 85 days after spinal cord injury
Amyotrophic Lateral Sclerosis (ALS)	Degenerative disease of motor ganglia in the anterior horn of the spinal cord and of the spinal pyramidal tracts	Increased response	No reports of hyperkalemia in ALS; however, myotonia-like contracture may occur in ALS patients. Avoid succinylcholine in patients with significant muscular denervation
Muscular Denervation	Result of traumatic peripheral nerve damage—muscles undergo atrophy	Normal response	Muscular contracture and hyperkalemia
Myasthenia Gravis (MG)	Postsynaptic reduction in the number of ACh receptors caused by autoimmune disease	Increased response and prolongation of effects	Resistance and early appearance of phase II (dual) block
Myasthenic Syndrome	Differs clinically and electromyographically from MG. Associated with small cell carcinoma of the lung resulting in a presynaptic lesion at the neuromuscular junction	Exaggerated response	Exaggerated response
Myotonias	Lesion in the muscle fiber distal to the neuromuscular junction. Common symptom is delayed relaxation of skeletal muscles following voluntary contractions	Increased and prolonged. Some report normal response	Unpredictable. Many reports of increased rigidity
Muscular Dystrophies (MD)	Disorder of the muscle fiber proper that may be secondary to a neurogenic disorder	Normal to prolonged response. Ocular MD has a very high sensitivity to d-tubocurarine	Unpredictable. Best to avoid use of succinylcholine

Phase II Block

Various terms are used to describe the different types of blocks that succinylcholine is able to produce. The phase I block is synonymous with the depolarizing block the drug ordinarily produces. It is characterized by well sustained tetanus and no post-tetanic facilitation when the peripheral nerve stimulator is used.

Phase II block is also known as a dual block or a desensitization block. It is characterized by poorly sustained tetanus and post-tetanic facilitation. There are the same clinical features seen when d-tubocurarine is used; however, this does not mean that the two blocks are the same, as there is good evidence that the d-tubocurarine and succinylcholine phase II blocks differ in several respects. Some clinicians believe that the phase II block produced by succinylcholine can be reversed with anticholinesterases such as edrophonium (Tensilon), which has a shorter duration of action than neostigmine (Prostigmin). Edrophonium is used in this situation because it will either reverse or potentiate the block. If potentiation occurs, it will be of a shorter duration than if neostigmine were used. Most experts feel that routine reversal to antagonize the dual block is unwarranted. It is more advisable to ventilate the patient and wait for return of the normal neuromuscular transmission.

Recurarization

Recurarization is the reappearance postoperatively of the pharmacologic actions of a nondepolarizing skeletal muscle relaxant that was administered intraoperatively. The hazard of recurarization after the use of gallamine (Flaxedil) represents a significant problem that may be encountered in the post anesthesia care unit. This complication arises when renal insufficiency exists. The interesting facet of this complication is that even when the gallamine is reversed sufficiently at the end of the anesthetic, recurarization may still occur for a period up to eight hours. This reappearance may be partly due to the fading of the effect of the neostigmine (Prostigmin). Gallamine is normally excreted after two hours, but in renal insufficiency the excretion of the drug is poor and may take up to 30 hours. Therefore, in cases of renal insufficiency in which gallamine was utilized, signs of delayed excretion (weakness of the ocular muscles, difficulty in swallowing, or decrease in ventilation) should be sought. If symptoms appear, the required level of the reversal agent (neostigmine) must be kept up until that portion of the gallamine has been eliminated, so that symptoms do not reappear. If recurarization occurs, the postoperative use of morphine and similar narcotics should be avoided, as they will enhance a residual neuromuscular block sufficiently to make it clinically significant.

Recurarization from d-tubocurarine does not usually occur because only 20 to 40 percent of the drug is excreted through the kidneys. Recurarization owing to d-tubocurarine was caused by, in some reported cases, an increased sensitivity of the myoneural junction, associated with a fall in the plasma potassium concentration.

Bradycardia

Another problem occurring in the PACU is the appearance of bradycardia when a patient has received an atropine-neostigmine combination at the end of the anesthetic. The bradycardia is usually due to the longer duration of action of neostigmine as compared with that of the atropine. The treatment for this problem is glycopyrrolate (Robinul). Glycopyrrolate should not be administered, however, until other causes of bradycardia are eliminated, such as pain, hypoventilation, or a full bladder.

REFERENCES

1. Azar, I.: The response of patients with neuromuscular disorders to muscle relaxant: a review. Anesthesiology, *61*(2):173–187, 1984.
2. Bradshaw, H., Drain, C., and Dutton, M.: A review of skeletal muscle contraction

and neuromuscular function. AANAJ, *48*(4):334–343, 1980.

3. Churchill-Davidson, H. C.: Wylie and Churchill-Davidson: A Practice of Anaesthesia. 4th ed. Philadelphia, W. B. Saunders Co., 1978.

4. Collins, V.: Principles of Anesthesiology. 2nd ed. Philadelphia, Lea & Febiger, 1976.

5. Feldman, S.: Muscle Relaxants. 2nd ed. Philadelphia, W. B. Saunders Co., 1979.

6. Goodman, L., Gilman, A., Rall, T., and Murad, F.: The Pharmacological Basis of Therapeutics. 7th ed. New York, Macmillan Publishing Company, 1985.

7. Hooper, D.: Reversal agents in the postanesthetic state. JAANA, *44*(3):281–287, 1976.

8. Miller, R. (ed.): Anesthesia. 2nd ed. New York, Churchill Livingstone, Inc., 1986.

9. Miller, R., et al.: Clinical pharmacology of vecuronium and atracurium. Anesthesiology, *61*(4):444–453, 1984.

10. Oduro, K.: Glycopyrrolate methobromide comparison with atropine sulfate in anesthesia. Can. Anaesth. Soc. J., *22*(4):466–473, 1975.

11. Ostheimer, G.: A comparison of glycopyrrolate and atropine during reversal of nondepolarizing neuromuscular block with neostigmine. Anesth. Analg., *56*:182–186, 1977.

12. Reep, B.: Complications associated with the administration of succinylcholine. JAANA, *40*(3):193–203, 1972.

13. Savarese, J., Hassan, H., and Antonio, R.: The clinical pharmacology of Metocurine: dimethyltubocurarine revisited. Anesthesiology, *47*(3):277–284, 1977.

14. Wood, M., and Wood, A.: Drugs Used in Anesthesia: Pharmacology for the Anesthesiologist. Baltimore: Williams & Wilkins, 1982.

15

Regional Anesthesia

The term *regional anesthesia* refers to the various anesthetic techniques that use local anesthetic agents to block nerve conduction in an extremity or a region of the body.

Among the types of regional anesthesia are topical, infiltration, field block, and conductive. *Topical anesthesia* is produced when an anesthetic agent is applied to a surface, such as skin, mucous membrane, urethra, nose, or pharynx. *Infiltration anesthesia* is produced by injecting a local anesthetic into the tissue to be cut. *Field block anesthesia* is produced by injecting surrounding tissues of an area to be operated on with a local anesthetic agent. *Conduction anesthesia* is produced by depositing a local anesthetic agent into a nerve or nerves that supply a region of the body, in order to eliminate sensation or motor control or both. Epidural and subarachnoid blocks are conductive blocks.

The use of *regional anesthesia* has become popular in modern anesthesia practice because, when indicated, it offers many advantages over general inhalation anesthesia. To facilitate optimal recovery of the surgical patient from this type of anesthetic, the PACU nurse should have a complete knowledge of the pharmacology of local anesthetic agents and of the particular regional anesthetic technique employed.

LOCAL ANESTHESIA

Local anesthetic agents are defined as pharmacologic agents capable of producing a loss of sensation in an area of the body. They were first used in 1884, when cocaine was employed as a topical anesthetic agent by Köller. Local anesthetic agents act primarily on the inner aspect of the sodium channel to impede sodium conductance and thereby block nerve conduction.

In regard to their analgesic activity, local anesthetic agents can be divided into three groups according to potency. Procaine and chloroprocaine are the least potent of the commonly employed agents, while lidocaine, mepivacaine, and prilocaine are compounds of intermediate potency, i.e., they are twice as potent as procaine. Tetracaine, bupivacaine, and etidocaine are drugs of high potency that are approximately six to eight times more active than procaine (Table 15–1).

TABLE 15–1. Classification of Local Anesthetic Agents According to in vivo Potency and Duration of Action

Agent	Relative Potency	Duration (min)
Low Potency		
Procaine	1	60–90
Intermediate Potency		
Mepivacaine	2	120–240
Prilocaine	3	120–240
Lidocaine	4	90–200
Chloroprocaine	4	30–60
High Potency		
Tetracaine	16	180–600
Bupivacaine	16	180–600
Etidocaine	16	180–600

Adapted from Covino, B., and Vasallo, H.: Local Anesthetics: Mechanisms of Action and Clinical Use. New York: Grune & Stratton, Inc., 1976.

TAELE 15–2. Local Anesthetic Agents

Agent	Use	Discussion
The Esters		
Cocaine	*Topical*: 4–20% for use in nose and throat procedures; duration, 10–55 min; maximum dose, 3 mg/kg	Topical use only; vasoconstrictor; CNS stimulant in abuse
Procaine (Novocain)	*Topical*: 10–20% required; *infiltration*: 0.25–0.5%; *nerve block*: 1–2%; duration, 20–30 min plain, 45 min with epinephrine; maximum dose, 10 mg/kg plain and 14 mg/kg with epinephrine	Low potency, rapid hydrolysis in plasma, mild acetylcholine inhibition, poor stability
Chloroprocaine (Nesacaine)	*Infiltration*: 10 mg/ml solution; *peripheral nerve block*: 10 and 20 mg/ml solution; *epidural block*: 20–30 mg/ml solution	Not topically active; more potent but shorter duration of action than procaine. The safest local anesthetic in regard to systemic toxicity. The onset of action is 6–12 min, and the duration of anesthesia is from 30–60 min. Total dose should not exceed one gm with epinephrine and 800 mg without epinephrine
Tetracaine (Pontocaine)	*Topical*: 0.5–1%, duration, 55 min; *infiltration*: 0.1–0.25%; *nerve block*: 0.25%, duration, 3–4 hr plain, 5–7 hr with epinephrine; maximum dose, 1.5–2 mg/kg plain and 2–3 mg/kg with epinephrine	12 times as potent as procaine
The Amides		
Lidocaine (Xylocaine)	*Topical*: 2–4% onset, 2–4 min, maximum dose, 3 mg/kg; *nerve block*: 1–2%, maximum dose, 4–5 mg/kg plain or 7 mg/kg with epinephrine; duration, 1 hr plain, 2 hr with epinephrine; antiarrhythmic, 1 mg/kg bolus, then 1–2 mg/min IV drip	Rapid onset, intense analgesia, good penetration, stable. As antiarrhythmic, it depresses the automaticity of the Purkinje fibers and decreases their effective refractory period
Mepivacaine (Carbocaine)	*Infiltration*: 0.5–1%; *nerve block*: 1–2%, maximum dose, 5–6 mg/kg plain, and 7 mg/kg with epinephrine; duration, 1.5 hr plain, 2 hr with epinephrine	Derivative of lidocaine; less penetrance, slower metabolism; ineffective topically
Bupivacaine (Marcaine)	*Infiltration*: 0.1–0.25%; *nerve block*: 0.25–0.5%; long-acting, up to 12 hr	Less penetrance than other amides
Dibucaine (Nupercaine)	*Topical*: 2 mg/ml ointment, up to 15 ml; *spinal*: 2.5–5 mg/ml	Mainly used as a topical anesthesia; rarely used for spinal anesthesia owing to high systemic toxicity
Etidocaine (Duranest)	*Infiltration*: 2.5–5 mg/ml solution; *peripheral nerve block*: 5 and 10 mg/ml solution; *epidural block*: 5 and 10 mg/ml solution	Greater potency and longer duration of action than lidocaine. Maximum dose of a single injection should not exceed 400 mg in the adult

The ideal local anesthetic should have the following properties: selectivity of action, low toxicity, complete reversibility, nonirritation, short latency, good penetrance, sufficient duration, solubility in saline and water, stability, and compatibility with vasoconstrictors. Not all local anesthetic agents possess all these attributes. As new agents are discovered they are measured against these criteria.

Pharmacologic Classification

The local anesthetic agents are grouped pharmacologically into two categories, the amides and the esters (Table 15–2). The *amides* are metabolized in the liver, have no real history of documented allergic reactions, have good penetrance, and are stable. Drugs in this category are lidocaine, mepivacaine, prilocaine, etidocaine, and bupivacaine. The *esters*, except for cocaine, are hydrolyzed primarily in the plasma and are metabolized more rapidly than the amides. In general, the esters have poor penetrance, rare allergic reactions, and fair to poor stability. Epinephrine is added to some local anesthetic agents because it is a vasoconstrictor and therefore prolongs the activity of the local agent and decreases its toxicity by slowing its uptake.

Complications of Use

Allergic reactions to local anesthetic drugs can be divided into four types: (1) contact dermatitis; (2) serum sickness, which includes fever, lymphadenopathy, and urticaria 2 to 12 days after injection; (3) anaphylactic reaction, characterized by dyspnea, cyanosis, and death; and (4) atopic response, which includes bronchospasm, urticaria, and angioneurotic edema.

When the allergy is being evaluated, the first consideration is whether or not the reaction is caused by added epinephrine. Symptoms such as tachycardia, palpitations, restlessness, and anxiety would indicate epinephrine as the causative agent.

Overdosage of local anesthetic agents can occur because of inadvertent intravenous injection of the local anesthetic, variation in patient response, or injection of the local anesthetic into a highly vascular area. Table

15–3 summarizes the signs of overdosage of the local anesthetic agents.

The treatment and nursing care of a patient who has had an overdose of a local anesthetic agent begin with administration of 100 per cent oxygen. This should be followed by preparation for the management of convulsions, hypotension, and respiratory depression. Drugs such as short-acting barbiturates or diazepam are often utilized. Intubation and mechanical ventilation may be indicated. Vasopressors such as epinephrine may also be indicated.

SPINAL ANESTHESIA
Anatomy of the Spine

The vertebral column is made up of 33 vertebrae, including 7 cervical, 12 thoracic, 5 lumbar, 5 sacral, and 4 coccygeal vertebrae. The ligaments of the vertebral column, which bind it together and protect the spinal cord, are the supraspinous ligament, intraspinous ligament, ligamenta flava, posterior longitudinal ligament, and anterior longitudinal ligament (Fig. 15–1). When a midline spinal puncture is made, the needle will traverse the first three ligaments.

The spinal cord, which is a continuation of the medulla oblongata, occupies the upper two thirds of the vertebral canal. It is approximately 18 inches long and it ends at the lower border of the first lumbar vertebra. The lower portion of the spinal cord then becomes the filum terminale, which connects to the bone of the coccyx vertebra

TABLE 15–3. Signs of Overdosage of Local Anesthetic Agents

Central Nervous System
Stimulation of:
  Cortex: Excitement, disorientation, euphoria, dizziness, hallucinations, muscle twitching, numbness of fingers or lips, and convulsions
  Medulla: C-V center: Hypertension, tachycardia
         Respiratory center: Increased respiratory rate and variations in rhythm
         Vomiting center: Nausea and vomiting
Depression of:
  Cortex: unconsciousness
  Medulla: Vasomotor center: Hypotension
         Respiratory center: Apnea

Peripheral Nervous System
Heart: Bradycardia due to direct depression
Blood vessels: Vasodilatation from direct action

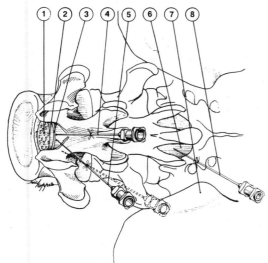

Figure 15–1. The dorsal view of the fourth and fifth lumbar vertebrae, their relationship to the sacrum and iliac bones, and the most frequently used approaches for needle puncture in subarachnoid and lumbar peridural techniques. Numerals represent the following: (1) the cauda equina; (2) the dura mater; (3) the ligamentum flavum at the L3-L4 interspace; (4) the midline approach for spinal and epidural techniques where the needle is introduced between the spines of L3 and L4 vertebrae, traversing the supraspinous and interspinous ligaments before piercing the ligamentum flavum; (5) the paramedian approach at this level where the needle puncture site is 1 to 2 cm lateral to the above midline approach; if the initial approach results in contacting the lamina of the vertebrae as shown in the dotted needle silhouette, then the needle is walked cephalad and medially until it slips off the lamina and contacts ligamentum flavum as shown; (6) the large interspace between S5 and L1, which is situated 2 cm medial and cephalad from (7) the posterior superior iliac spine; (8) the needle can be introduced at this site in the "Taylor" approach for either subarachnoid or epidural puncture. From Miller, R. (ed.): Anesthesia. 2nd ed. New York, Churchill Livingstone, Inc., 1986.

and holds the spinal cord in place. The spinal cord is encased by three membranes. The outermost membrane is the dura mater, which consists of two layers termed the periosteal and the dural layer, and ends at the second sacral vertebra. The arachnoid layer consists of a thin membranous sheath. The innermost layer is the pia mater and is separated from the arachnoid layer by a subarachnoid space filled with cerebrospinal fluid. This is where local anesthetic solutions are deposited.

There are 31 pairs of spinal nerves that travel from the spinal column through the layers of the cord and exit at the interver-

tebral foramina. There are 8 cervical, 12 thoracic, 5 lumbar, 5 sacral, and 1 coccygeal pairs of spinal nerves. It is these nerves that are blocked by the local anesthetic drug to produce anesthesia.

Action of Spinal Anesthetics

After the local anesthetic drug is injected into the subarachnoid space, a level of anesthesia will be achieved that is dependent upon the dosage of the agent used, the rate of injection, the specific gravity of the fluid injected, and the position of the patient

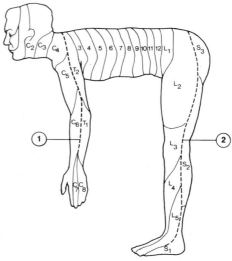

Figure 15–2. The dermatomes of the body show an orderly craniad to caudal sequence. By positioning the body as shown, the complex arrangement of dermatomes on the limbs is more readily understood. On the upper extremity, the limb dermatomes are distributed symmetrically about the axial line (1). Note that dermatomes C5 and C6 are distributed on the preaxial border of the limb and the postaxial dermatomes, C8, T1, and T2, are distributed on the postaxial part of the limb. C7, which is the central dermatome of the limb, is distributed more distally, that is, over the middle finger. There is an orderly sequence on the trunk from T3 to L1.

The dermatome distribution of the lower extremity is also arranged around the axial line (2). Large areas of skin, i.e., L2 and L3, have been borrowed from the trunk to supplement the true leg dermatomes of L4 through S3. Note as in the upper extremity, the craniad dermatomes, L4 and L5, are distributed on the preaxial border of the limb and the caudad dermatomes, S2 and S3, are distributed on the postaxial border of the limb. The central dermatome S1 is distributed over the lateral aspect of the plantar surface and lateral border of the foot. From Foerster I.: Brain 56:1, 1933. In Miller, R. (ed.): Anesthesia. 2nd ed. Churchill Livingstone, Inc., 1986.

TABLE 15–4. Sequence of Nerve Block

1. Vasomotor block—dilatation of skin vessels and increased cutaneous blood flow.
2. Block of cold temperature fibers.
3. Sensation of warmth by patient.
4. Temperature discrimination lost.
5. Slow and fast pain.
6. Tactile sense lost.
7. Motor paralysis.
8. Pressure sense abolished.
9. Proprioception (awareness of body or extremity position) lost.

From Collins, V. J.: Principles of Anesthesiology. Philadelphia, Lea & Febiger, 1970.

following injection. The level of anesthesia is referred to as the dermatome level (Fig. 15–2). Each dermatome is a cutaneous area that gets its nerve supply from a single nerve root. The order of blockage of the various nerve modalities is shown in Table 15–4.

During the recovery from a spinal anesthetic, the anesthesia will work its way back from the extremities toward the site where the anesthetic was administered. Therefore, the areas near the site of injection are the last to recover.

Complications of Spinal Anesthesia

The complications of spinal anesthesia are high or total spinal block, hypotension, nausea and vomiting, backache, palsies and paralysis, urinary retention, postspinal headache, and meningitis.

Total Spinal Block. The treatment of a total spinal block is initiated in the operating room. Treatment consists of efficient ventilation and oxygenation, and the maintenance of the blood pressure by vasopressors. This is a reversible complication; when the local anesthetic drug wears off, the patient will recover. The PACU care consists of maintaining the treatment initiated in the operating room. The patient will be intubated and probably placed on a ventilator. As the local anesthetic agent wears off, the patient may be unable to maintain tidal volume because of partial paralysis of the respiratory muscles. The ventilation of the patient should be assisted until an adequate tidal volume can be maintained.

Verbal contact should be established with the patient to decrease the anxiety and apprehension caused by being partially sedated and unable to breathe or move about.

In an effort to enhance the cardiac output, the patient's legs may be elevated, which will return the venous blood from the lower extremities back to the heart. If the vital signs still indicate neurogenic shock even after this maneuver has been performed, vasopressor therapy will usually be instituted. Vasopressors utilized in the treatment of this complication are usually of the alpha-adrenergic variety, as total spinal block produces a type of neurogenic shock. The alpha-adrenergic vasopressors produce peripheral vasoconstriction, which aids in getting the blood back to the heart, thereby improving the cardiac output.

Because of the height of the spinal block, the patient may also experience some bradycardia, which can be treated with atropine or glycopyrrolate (Robinul). Nausea and vomiting may also occur. Suction should be available, and antiemetics may have to be administered to the patient.

Hypotension. Hypotension produced by a sympathetic blockade from a high spinal block can best be treated by vasopressors. This problem is most likely to occur during the first 30 minutes in the PACU, and, if the patient is hypotensive, it is important to assess for bleeding, which may be causing the hypotension. If bleeding is not the cause, the anesthetist should be notified so that treatment can be instituted. If bleeding is the cause, the attending physician should be notified.

Nausea. Nausea and vomiting can be a result of hypotension, or of hypertension due to the vasopressors or to motion during change of positions, or to apprehension. If hypotension or hypertension is present, the anesthetist should be notified. It is important for the PACU nurse to assess the cause of the nausea and vomiting. Blood pressure should be taken and oxygen administered to the patient. Should vomiting occur, the patient should be placed in a Trendelenburg position with the head to the side, and a clear airway should be established and maintained. The anesthetist should be sum-moved if the patient experiences nausea and/or vomiting.

Paralysis. Palsies and paralysis usually occur postoperatively in the peripheral nerves. Of the cranial nerves, the sixth nerve is most often involved. In the post anesthesia care unit phase of the spinal anesthetic, the nurse should assess neurologic function of the extremities as the anesthetic wears off. If the patient has double vision or any other decreases in peripheral nerve function, the anesthetist and surgeon should be notified.

Urinary Retention. Urinary retention is usually caused by trauma to the bladder during surgery or a decrease in bladder tone due to the anesthesia. The patient will complain of severe pain and may become hypertensive or bradycardic. If the condition is not diagnosed and corrected, the patient may become incoherent and thrash about in bed. The PACU nurse should assess the patient for a distended bladder or hypoxia, as the symptoms are almost identical. If urinary retention is the problem, the patient should be encouraged to void. If the patient cannot void, the surgeon should be notified and an order for catheterization of the bladder obtained.

Headache. The true postspinal headache is caused by a persistent leak of cerebral spinal fluid (CSF) through the needle hole in the dura mater. Postspinal headache is usually transient but very annoying to the patient. The pain usually becomes severe when the patient is upright and lessens when he is in a supine position. As a prophylactic measure, most patients who have received a spinal anesthetic are encouraged to remain in the supine position for at least six to eight hours following surgery. It should be stated that some research indicates that the supine-bedrest prophylaxis is unnecessary and of no value in preventing postspinal headache. The advent of smaller-gauge needles has reduced the incidence of postspinal headache. Conservative treatment of the patient with this complication involves optimal hydration, analgesics, and reduction of environmental noise. However, if the postspinal headache becomes incapacitating or does not respond to conservative treatment within the first

two days after the administration of the spinal anesthetic, an *epidural blood patch procedure* may be performed. This procedure involves administering 5 to 10 ml of the patient's own venous blood into the epidural space at the site of the previous lumbar puncture. In essence, this procedure seals the hole in the dura mater, and prompt pain relief usually follows.

EPIDURAL ANESTHESIA

Epidural (peridural) block is produced by depositing an anesthetic agent in the epidural space. The location on the vertebral column or the segment where the epidural block is performed determines the type of epidural anesthesia the patient will receive. Thoracic epidural block, lumbar epidural block, and caudal epidural block or caudal anesthesia are the types of anesthesia possible.

Epidural block is usually performed with the patient lying on his side. The back is prepped and the needle inserted into the epidural space. After it has been determined that the needle is in the epidural space, the anesthetic solution is injected. The needle may be removed, or a catheter can be placed through the needle into the epidural space for the continuous (serial) epidural technique.

The epidural block is becoming the anesthetic technique of choice for caesarean section and is indicated in poor-risk patients and in those with cardiac, pulmonary, and metabolic diseases. It is contraindicated in patients being given anticoagulants, when hemorrhage or shock is present, when the patient has had previous surgery on the back, and when local inflammation exists.

PACU Care After Spinal or Epidural Anesthesia

After the patient's arrival in the PACU, care must be exercised when moving him or her, as the block's residual effects, such as lack of motor and sensory function, are still present. Care should be taken in positioning the patient, as good body alignment is important to reduce muscular soreness or injury. The joints of the body should not be hyperextended and bedclothes should not press upon the toes.

If a patient has any residual spinal anesthesia while in the PACU, care should be taken to avoid rapid position change, which causes severe decreases in blood pressure. This is because the circulatory system cannot compensate adequately for rapid position change when anesthesia is present.

If intravenous sedation was given during the operation, respiratory function should be monitored closely. Oxygen should be administered to all block patients until their motor and sensory functions return adequately. The patient should be encouraged to cough and breathe deeply every 15 minutes to reduce the incidence of atelectasis.

The patient should be checked for any signs of bladder distention. Catheterization may be required, especially in patients who have had pelvic or perineal surgery.

AXILLARY OR BRACHIAL PLEXUS BLOCK

Nerve blocks are employed to produce anesthesia in specific areas of the body. They are usually utilized for orthopedic procedures, obstetrics, and vascular surgery. Relatively safe, they usually have good patient acceptance.

The axillary or brachial plexus block is used to anesthetize the arm to facilitate surgery below the elbow. In performing this block, either the axillary or the supraclavicular approach is used.

PACU Care After Axillary or Brachial Plexus Block

PACU care of the patient who has received an axillary block centers on observation for complications. If the supraclavicular approach was utilized, pneumothorax is a possible complication. The first sign is a complaint by the patient of pain in the chest that is accentuated by deep breathing. Other signs of pneumothorax are increased resonance to percussion, absence of or decreased breath sounds, lag in expansion on the affected side in comparison with the

unaffected side, and difficulty in "getting breath."

PACU care involves administration of oxygen and advising the anesthetist of the complication. Analgesics are usually administered and, after a chest x-ray is taken, more definitive treatment may be instituted.

When the supraclavicular approach is used to perform the brachial plexus block, *Horner's syndrome* can result. This occurs when the anesthetic solution spreads so that it involves the stellate ganglion. Symptoms of this syndrome, which appear on the side where the block is performed, are flushing of the face, constricted pupils, ptosis, and stuffiness of the nose. Horner's syndrome clears as the block wears off.

Another complication caused by using the supraclavicular approach is *blockage of the phrenic nerve*. The incidence of this complication is related to the spread of anesthetic solution and is usually unilateral. Generally, there are no signs and symptoms, and the complication clears as the block dissipates itself.

Obliteration of the radial pulse is a possible complication of the axillary approach to the brachial plexus. It is caused by bleeding or the use of too great a volume of anesthetic solution. The radial pulse usually returns in two to four hours.

INTRAVENOUS REGIONAL ANESTHESIA

The intravenous regional or Bier block was named for August K. Bier, who originated it in 1908. It is very useful for emergency procedures on the forearm and hand, especially for a procedure such as Colles' fracture reduction, and is simple to administer. The Bier block involves starting an intravenous infusion in the hand, exsanguinating the arm with an Esmarch latex bandage, inflating a double pneumatic tourniquet above the elbow, and then removing the Esmarch bandage and injecting the local anesthetic agent (bupivacaine or lidocaine) while the tourniquet remains inflated. At the end of the surgical procedure, the tourniquet is released and the analgesia will cease within five to ten minutes. Usually there are no sequelae from the anesthetic agent; by the time the venous blood from the limb has passed through the lungs and becomes mixed with the rest of the venous return, the systemic arterial blood levels are, because of the dilution effect, not clinically significant. Should the blood levels of the local anesthetic remain high, the patient will experience cardiovascular depression, which is usually manifested by bradycardia. This cardiovascular depression is usually quite transient. Should this situation arise, vigilant monitoring coupled with appropriate interventions, such as oxygen and glycopyrrolate (Robinul) or atropine, will usually correct the problem.

The intravenous regional technique can also be used for surgery on the lower leg and foot. Although it requires a larger tourniquet and more local anesthetic agent, it is a good technique for this type of surgery.

PACU Care After Intravenous Regional Anesthesia

When the patient arrives in the post anesthesia care unit, all analgesia provided by the local anesthetic agent used in the intravenous regional anesthesia has usually dissipated. Medication for the relief of pain can be given very soon after the patient's arrival. The PACU nurse should assess the patient's level of sedation, including the amount of premedication and sedation during the surgical procedure, before administering the pain medication.

REFERENCES

1. Collins, V.: Principles of Anesthesiology. 2nd ed. Philadelphia, Lea & Febiger, 1976.
2. Covino, B.: Pharmacology, pharmacokinetics and metabolism of local anesthetics. Annual Refresher Course Lectures, American Society of Anesthesiologists, 1977.
3. Covino, B., and Vasallo, H.: Local Anesthetics: Mechanisms of Action and Clinical Use. New York, Grune & Stratton, Inc., 1976.
4. Dripps, R., Exkenhoff, J., and Vandam, L.: Introduction to Anesthesia: The Principles of Safe Practice. 6th ed. Philadelphia, W. B. Saunders Co., 1982.
5. Goodman, L., and Gilman, A.: The Pharmacological Basis of Therapeutics. 7th ed. New York, Macmillan Publishing Company, 1985.
6. Miller, R. (ed.): Anesthesia. 2nd ed. New York, Churchill Livingstone, Inc. 1986.
7. Moore, D.: Regional Block. 4th ed. Springfield, Ill., Charles C Thomas, Publisher, 1976.
8. Wood, M., and Wood, A.: Drugs and Anesthesia: Pharmacology for the Anesthesiologist. Baltimore, Williams & Wilkins, 1982.

16

Drug-Drug Interactions in the Post Anesthesia Care Unit

With the increasing use of new and more potent drugs administered in the perioperative period, drug interactions between anesthetic and nonanesthetic drugs has become an ever-intensifying area of interest to the post anesthesia care unit (PACU) nurse. With the growth of interest in the fields of drug interaction, drug surveillance, and clinical pharmacology, knowledge of drug-drug interactions in anesthesia and post anesthesia care could become an exceedingly meaningful and useful tool in the delivery of nursing care to the PACU patient.

DRUG TOXICITIES

Before considering drug interactions, the PACU nurse must become aware of the inherent toxicities of drugs to the biologic system. Hence, a review of the basic concepts of drug interactions will be presented, with particular emphasis on the patient in the post anesthesia care unit.

Hyperreactivity occurs when an individual reacts abnormally to an unusually low dose of a drug. Patients with Addison's disease, myxedema, and dystrophia myotonica ex-

hibit a hyperreactivity to unusually low doses of the barbiturates.

Hyporeactivity, or tolerance, indicates that an individual requires excessively large doses of a drug in order to obtain a therapeutic or desired effect. A prime example is an individual who has become addicted to narcotics and who requires larger than normal doses to elicit the desired therapeutic response.

In *metareactivity*, a drug produces unusual side effects unrelated to the dosage strength. Metareactivity is also referred to as an *idiosyncratic reaction*. An example of metareactivity is the occurrence of skeletal muscle pain and increased intraocular pressure when succinylcholine is administered. Another example of metareactivity is the response of an elderly patient or the child who responds to a dose of a barbiturate with excitation rather than sedation.

Hypersensitivity (anaphylaxis) refers to a drug-induced antigen-antibody reaction. The particular hypersensitivity reaction can be either a type I immediate (anaphylactic) or a type IV delayed reaction. Hypersensitivity reactions can occur with succinylcholine, with antibiotics, and with many other drugs that are administered in the post anesthesia care unit (see Chapter 11).

DRUG-DRUG INTERACTIONS

When a patient is simultaneously receiving two or more drugs, the drugs may or may not interact to cause a toxic reaction. Many patients are being given other drugs besides the ones that are associated with anesthesia and surgery. Hence, in these patients the potential for a drug-drug interaction is present. These interactions are divided into two broad categories: pharmacokinetic and pharmacodynamic (Table 16–1).

Pharmacokinetic Interactions

Interactions of a second drug that produce alterations in absorption, distribution, metabolism, or excretion of the first drug are known as pharmacokinetic interactions. Hence, when one drug alters any pharmacokinetic parameter of another, with a resultant alteration in the concentration of the drug at the receptor site, a pharmacokinetic interaction has taken place. In other words, the absorption, distribution, or elimination of the drug concentration at the receptor site is changed, which results in an altered pharmacologic response from the individual.

Absorption

Absorption of one drug may be enhanced or inhibited by another drug. With the addition of epinephrine to solutions of local anesthetics, the absorption of the anesthetic is prolonged through the vasoconstrictive action of epinephrine—the local vasoconstriction produced by the epinephrine delays the systemic absorption of the local anesthetic, and ultimately the effect of the local anesthetic is prolonged. When a patient has been administered a preoperative aluminum-containing antacid and then administered tetracycline in the late postoperative period, the absorption of the tetracycline will be reduced.

Distribution

Pharmaceutical incompatibility is one type of pharmacokinetic distribution interaction. This situation occurs, for example, when one drug reacts chemically with another. In this situation, when one drug (e.g., aspirin) displaces another drug (e.g., phenytoin) from plasma protein binding sites, the blood concentration of the free drug will be increased, which may result in toxic blood levels. Or, when a large dose of thiopental is administered to an obese patient who also receives halothane, the anesthetic action may be prolonged considerably, lasting well into the PACU phase. This is because of the prolonged retention of the thiopental in the adipose tissue due to the circulatory depressant action of halothane. Hence, at the end of the period of anesthesia, the redistribution and subsequent elimination of the thiopental will be delayed, resulting in a prolonged hypnotic effect.

Elimination

Biotransformation. When patients are administered enzyme-inducing agents, such as the barbiturates or the antibiotic rifampin, the activity of the enzyme systems of the liver will be increased. This results in a more rapid metabolism and excretion of drugs that are metabolized by a particular liver enzyme system. For example, if a barbiturate were administered to a patient who is on a stabilized dose of the anticoagulant warfarin, the warfarin blood level might be reduced, which would result in a lowered prothrombin time. Should this situation occur (stabilization by an anticoagulant and administration of an enzyme-inducing agent), and the barbiturate were to be discontinued, the nurse would have to monitor the patient for the potentially more serious problem of excessive anticoagulation and hemorrhage.

The drug cimetidine (Tagamet) is sometimes administered preoperatively to reduce the amount of gastric secretion and increase the gastric pH. This drug is a potent inhibitor of drug metabolism and can slow the elimination of antipyrine, warfarin, diaze-

TABLE 16–1. Drug-Drug or Drug-Induced Interactions in the Post Anesthesia Care Unit

Drug(s)	Interact(s) with	Result	Mechanism
Antihypertensive Drugs			
Reserpine	Inhalational anesthetics	Hypotension	Inhibits the synthesis and storage of norepinephrine in the sympathetic nerve endings
Diuretics	Halothane	Hypotension	Reduced extracellular sodium and water, which is compensated for by vasoconstriction. Halothane dilates the constricted vascular beds
Propranolol	Lidocaine	Enhanced negative inotropic effect	Propranolol reduces liver blood flow and lidocaine clearance
Lidocaine Procainamide Bretylium Phenytoin Digitalis Quinidine Disopyramide Propranolol	d-Tubocurarine	Increased duration of neuromuscular blockade	Synergistic effect
Digitalis	Succinylcholine	Arrhythmias	Direct effect, or due to the hyperkalemia that can be induced by succinylcholine
Quinidine	Digitalis (digoxin)	Can produce digitalis intoxication	Decreases digitalis clearance and increases concentration of digitalis
Propranolol	Heparin	Myocardial depression	Heparin increases free fatty acids, which displace propranolol from plasma protein binding sites leading to increased free propranolol
Quinidine	Myasthenia gravis plus skeletal muscle relaxants	Postoperative respiratory depression	Blockade of ACh receptors at neuromuscular postsynaptic membrane
Digitalis	Thiazide diuretics	Increased potassium excretion by the kidneys	Combined effect of the two drugs on the kidneys promotes potassium excretion
Antibiotics			
Neomycin Streptomycin Dihydrosteptomycin Polymyxin A Polymyxin B Colistin Viomycin Paromomycin Kanamycin Lincomycin Gentamicin Tetracycline	Nondepolarizing skeletal muscle relaxants	Potentiates nondepolarizing muscle relaxants, respiratory depression	Neuromuscular blockade due to a reduction in the amplitude of the end-plate potential
Narcotics			
Morphine Meperidine Sublimaze Sufentanil	Inhalation anesthetics	Potentiation, respiratory and cardiovascular depression	Depressant effects of inhalational anesthetics and the narcotics are additive
Meperidine	Enovid Norinyl	Birth control pill potentiates meperidine	Excess female sex hormones with oral contraceptive therapy, which may slow the metabolism of meperidine

TABLE 16–1. Drug-Drug or Drug-Induced Interactions in the Post Anesthesia Care Unit Continued

Drug(s)	Interact(s) with	Result	Mechanism
Sympathomimetic Amines			
Epinephrine	Halothane Enflurane	Cardiac arrhythmias	Anesthetic agents sensitize the myocardium to the endogenous and exogenous catecholamines
Electrolytes			
Elevated extracellular potassium	Skeletal muscle relaxants	Increased resistance to depolarization and greater sensitivity to nondepolarizing muscle relaxants	Acute increase in extracellular potassium will increase end-plate transmembrane potential, causing hyperpolarization
Reduced extracellular potassium	Skeletal muscle relaxants	Increased effects of depolarizing muscle relaxants, and increased resistance to nondepolarizing muscle relaxants	Acute decrease in extracellular potassium will lower the resting end-plate transmembrane potential
Increased calcium levels	Nondepolarizing skeletal muscle relaxants	Decreased response	Calcium increases the quantal release of ACh and enhances the E-C coupling mechanism
Magnesium ions	Muscle relaxants	Potentiation	Magnesium ions cause a partial muscle relaxation by blocking the release of ACh
Calcium chloride	Digitalis	Additive effect on the heart	High concentrations of calcium inhibit the positive inotropic actions of digitalis and potentiate digitalis toxicity
Miscellaneous			
Echothiopate iodide	Succinylcholine	Prolonged apnea	Echothiopate is a cholinesterase inhibitor, and succinylcholine is destroyed by pseudocholinesterase
Tolbutamide	Bishydroxycoumarin	Intensification of the effects of tolbutamide leading to hypoglycemia	Bishydroxycoumarin displaces tolbutamide from its binding site on plasma proteins and makes more tolbutamide available in the free form
Succinylcholine	d-Tubocurarine	Prolonged apnea	Both drugs act at the ACh receptor, causing a synergistic effect upon the myoneural junction
Procaine Nesacaine Pontocaine	Succinylcholine	Prolonged apnea	All these drugs are metabolized by the enzyme pseudocholinesterase. The concomitant use of these drugs may reduce the effective plasma concentration of the enzyme
Furosemide Thiazide Ethacrynic acid	Nondepolarizing skeletal muscle relaxants	Intensified neuromuscular block	Electrolyte imbalance (hypokalemia)
Aminophylline	d-Tubocurarine Pancuronium	Antagonized neuromuscular blockade	End-plate effect antagonized by the increase in neurotransmitter
Procaine Lidocaine	Nondepolarizing and depolarizing skeletal muscle relaxants	Enhanced neuromuscular blockade	Decreased end-plate potential
Lithium	Pancuronium Succinylcholine	Potentiated neuromuscular blockade	Lithium ions substituted for sodium ions at a presynaptic level

Table continued on following page

TABLE 16–1. Drug-Drug or Drug-Induced Interactions in the Post Anesthesia Care Unit *Continued*

Drug(s)	Interact(s) with	Result	Mechanism
Chlorpromazine	Nondepolarizing skeletal muscle relaxants	Enhanced neuromuscular blockade	Potentiation of neuromuscular blockade
All inhalational anesthetics	Nondepolarizing skeletal muscle relaxants	Augment block in a dose-dependent manner in the following decreasing order of potency: isoflurane and enflurane, halothane, nitrous oxide	CNS depression or presynaptic inhibition of ACh
Insulin	Corticosteroids, oral contraceptives, loop and thiazide diuretics	Reduction in effects	Insulin antagonizes effects
Diethylstilbestrol (Stilphostrol)	Succinylcholine	Prolonged neuromuscular blockade	Decreased plasma cholinesterase
Hydrocortisone Dexamethasone Prednisolone	Phenobarbital	Decreased effects of the steroids	Increased metabolism

pam, and propranolol. This will result in an increased drug concentration and enhanced pharmacologic effect of the latter drugs.

Excretion. The pharmacokinetic parameters of concern in excretion have to do with one drug either facilitating or hindering the excretion of another. An example of this occurs when probenicid is administered in conjunction with penicillin. The outcome of this interaction is that the pharmacologic actions of the penicillin are prolonged because of the slower elimination time produced by the probenicid. Certainly, this can be considered a desirable drug-drug interaction.

Pharmacodynamic Interactions

Pharmacodynamic interactions occur when one drug alters the pharmacologic effects of another drug. For example, when a patient is being treated with an antibiotic such as an aminoglycoside or polymyxin, and receives a skeletal muscle relaxant such as curare, a prolonged neuromuscular blockage may result. Another example would be the patient who is on thiazide diuretic therapy with resultant hypokalemia. If this patient is administered digitalis, digitalis toxicity may result. Also, if this patient who is on thiazide therapy is administered a nondepolarizing muscle relaxant, the neuromuscular blockade will be intensified.

DRUG-DRUG INTERACTIONS AND THE PACU

Antibiotics

Aminoglycoside and polymyxin antibiotics have been reported to interact with some anesthetic agents as well as skeletal muscle relaxants. Streptomycin and the other aminoglycoside antibiotics produce a partial neuromuscular blockade by inhibiting the release of acetylcholine from the presynaptic membrane and by stabilizing the postsynaptic membrane. The order of decreasing potency of aminoglycosides for causing a partial neuromuscular blockage is neomycin, kanamycin, amikacin, gentamicin, and tobramycin. When a nondepolarizing skeletal muscle relaxant, such as curare or pancuronium, is administered to a patient receiving an aminoglycoside antibiotic, the neuromuscular blockade will be intensified and difficult to reverse pharmacologically. Studies do indicate that the aminoglycoside neuromuscular blockade can sometimes be partially reversed by calcium and neostigmine, whereas the neuromuscular blockade produced by polymyxin B will be enhanced by neostigmine and not reversed by calcium. The antibiotics that have been cited as prolonging the actions of the nondepolarizing skeletal muscle relaxants are neomycin, streptomycin, dihydrostreptomycin, kanamycin, gentamicin, polymyxin A, polymyxin B, colistin, lincomycin, and tetracycline. The antibiotics that will enhance the pharmacologic actions of the depolarizing skeletal relaxant succinylcholine include neomycin, streptomycin, kanamycin, polymyxin B and colistin. These drugs must usually be given for at least two weeks before any clinically significant depression in the neuromuscular transmission will occur; such a depression may produce only slight muscle weakness in the patient. The antibiotics that do not have any skeletal muscle relaxant properties are penicillin, chloramphenicol, and the cephalosporins.

Sympathomimetic Amines

Halothane will sensitize the heart to sympathomimetic amines, such as epinephrine, producing cardiac arrhythmias. Patients who are recovering from halothane anesthesia in the PACU will still have a significant amount of halothane in their body. Consequently, epinephrine or other sympathomimetic amines should not be administered to these patients in the PACU. If epinephrine must be used for hemostasis or for vasoconstriction in a local anesthetic, the epinephrine concentration should not be greater than 1:100,000 to 1:200,000, and the total adult dose should not be greater than 10 ml of 1:100,000 solution in 10 minutes, or the total dose should not exceed 30 ml of 1:100,000 solution in one hour.

Antihypertensive Drugs

It is estimated that 1 to 2 million hypertensive individuals are anesthetized each year in the United States. Anesthetic agents have been reported to produce changes in cardiac output, peripheral resistance, and regional blood flow patterns in normotensive and hypertensive patients.

Treatment of hypertension is accomplished by lowering systemic vascular resistance or by the reduction of cardiac output, or both. Antihypertensive drugs alter the circulatory hemostasis and strongly influence the activity of pressor amines and may alter the response to muscle relaxants and narcotic analgesics. Antihypertensive drugs can produce systemic conditions that may result in a hypotensive crisis during anesthesia and in the immediate postoperative period. Hence, patients in the PACU who have been on long-term antihypertensive medication therapy and who have received a 100 percent potent inhalational anesthetic should be specifically monitored for cardiac dysrhythmias and hypotension. If a hypotensive crisis occurs in the PACU, the patient should have his legs elevated, and oxygen and, if necessary, vasopressors should be administered. The anesthesiologist and surgeon should be notified immediately, so that the specific treatment can be instituted.

Narcotics

Every PACU nurse has probably observed the drug-drug interaction between narcotics administered in the PACU and the inhalational anesthetic agents that were administered in the operating room. If the patient has not completely eliminated the anesthetic agent and is administered a narcotic, a synergistic effect between the two drugs will occur. The outcome of this interaction is usually respiratory depression, owing to the fact that both drugs are respiratory depressants.

If the two drugs have interacted in this way, a narcotic antagonist such as naloxone (Narcan) can be administered to reverse the respiratory depression produced by the narcotic. However, naloxone will not reverse respiratory depression produced by the inhalation anesthetic agents such as halothane (Fluothane), enflurane (Ethrane), or isoflurane (Forane).

Steroids

Although not truly an interaction of two drugs that alters one of the pharmacokinetic parameters, problems resulting from the administration of exogenous steroids to a steroid-dependent patient will be presented.

Patients suffering from adrenocortical insufficiency do not have the ability to withstand the stress of anesthesia and surgery. For example, if a patient with chronic obstructive pulmonary disease (COPD) has been treated with long-term steroids, there will usually be some degree of adrenocortical insufficiency. Hence, because of the alteration in the receptor site, the patient may react to surgery and anesthesia with hypotension, respiratory depression, or delayed recovery. To prevent a hypotensive crisis during the perioperative period, these patients are usually maintained on corticosteroids up to, through, and after the surgical procedure. Should these symptoms appear in a PACU patient who did not receive this steroid coverage, the first line of treatment would be hydrocortisone (see Chapter 10).

REFERENCES

1. Brown, B. (ed.): New Pharmcologic Vistas in Anesthesia. Philadelphia, F. A. Davis Co., 1983.
2. Churchill-Davidson, H. C.: Wylie and Churchill-Davidson: Practice of Anaesthesia. 4th ed. Philadelphia, W. B. Saunders Co., 1978.
3. Drain, C., and Campman, K.: Drug-drug interactions in general anesthesia. Anesth. Analg., 54:76–80, 1975.
4. Goodman, L., Gilman, A., Rall, T., and Murad, F.: The Pharmacological Basis of Therapeutics. 7th ed. New York, Macmillan Publishing Company, 1985.
5. Guyton, A.: Textbook of Medical Physiology. 7th ed. Philadelphia, W. B. Saunders Co., 1986.
   6. Katzung, B. (ed.): Basic and Clinical Pharmacology. 2nd ed. Los Altos, Lange Medical Publications, 1984.
7. Miller, R. (ed.): Anesthesia. 2nd ed. New York, Churchill Livingstone Inc., 1986.
8. Smith, N. T. (ed.): Drug Interactions in Anesthesia. Philadelphia, Lea & Febiger, 1981.
9. Wood, M., and Wood, A.: Drugs and Anesthesia: Pharmacology for the Anesthesiologist. Baltimore, Williams & Wilkins, 1982.

Postoperative Nursing Care in the Post Anesthesia Care Unit

17

Assessment of the Post Anesthesia Care Unit Patient

The primary purpose of the PACU is the critical evaluation of postoperative patients, with emphasis on anticipation and prevention of complications resulting from anesthesia or the operative procedure. It is, therefore, imperative that a knowledgeable, skillful nurse fully assess the condition of each patient not only at admission and at discharge but also at frequent intervals throughout the post anesthesia period. Assessment must be a continuous process, leading to sound nursing judgments and the implementation of therapeutic care. Assessment includes gathering information from direct observation of the patient (the primary source), from the physician and other health care personnel, and from the chart and the care plan.

In order to assess the post anesthesia patient and plan and implement appropriate care, it is imperative that preoperative information be available as a basis for comparison with postoperative data. Traditionally, PACU nurses have, with only limited information, performed the role of caring for the surgical patient in the vulnerable post anesthesia state.

The PACU nurse has a professional obli-

gation to review the patient's history, clinical status, and psychosocial state. This may be accomplished by chart review, personal preoperative visit, and consultation with other health care members providing care to the patient.

This chapter deals with the assessment of postoperative patients and their common needs. Specific assessments related to patient age, the type of surgical procedure, and problems resulting from complicated diagnoses are dealt with in following chapters. The assessment and management of postoperative pain are presented in Chapter 19.

Preoperative Assessments

Preoperative evaluation of both the physical and the emotional status of the surgical patient is extremely important, and nursing brings a unique perspective to this assessment. Nurses in a number of subspecialties, including PACU nurses, operating room nurses, and general unit nurses, have advocated making this assessment. Having each nurse who will care for the patient make a preoperative visit seems redundant and could be overwhelming for the patient. More appropriately, nurses should begin to treat each other as colleagues, communicating needs for specific information and documenting data to be used for planning care. Multidisciplinary care conferences can be instrumental in educating all those who will care for the surgical patient and in the development of communication patterns.

ADMISSION OBSERVATIONS

Physical assessment of the post anesthesia patient must begin immediately upon admission to the recovery room. Ideally, the patient is accompanied from the operating room to the recovery room by the anesthesiologist (or anesthetist) and by the surgeon who will report to the receiving nurse on the patient's general condition, the operation performed, and the type of anesthesia used for the surgery. In addition, the nurse should be informed of any problems or complications encountered during the surgery and anesthesia.

Since all anesthetics are depressants, postoperative assessment and care will generally be the same, regardless of the specific agent used. For special precautions required for certain agents, review the chapters on anesthesia (Chapters 12 through 16).

Rapid assessment of the life-sustaining cardiorespiratory system is of initial concern. Ensure that the airway is patent and that respirations are free and easy. Quickly inspect all dressings and drains for gross bleeding. Check and record the patient's blood pressure, pulse, and rate of respiration. The baseline observations, made immediately upon admission, should be reported to the anesthesiologist in attendance and recorded in the admission note.

Once these initial observations are made, it is essential to assess systematically the patient's total condition. This assessment may be made from head to toe or by systems, whichever the individual nurse prefers; the observations are essentially identical. Since our preference is for a systems approach, the following outline of post anesthesia assessment is presented. It should be noted that

each system of the body has an integral function, and therefore all observations are interrelated.

Respiratory Function

The postoperative patient has experienced some interference with his respiratory system; therefore, attention must be directed toward maintaining adequate gas exchange.

Respiratory function is assessed by observing the rate and character of the respirations and the patient's color. Coupled with these observations, assessment of the responses of the cardiovascular and neurologic systems in relation to adequacy of gas exchange is important in the total evaluation of ventilatory efficiency.

The resting rate of respiration in the normal adult is approximately 16 to 20 cycles per minute, regular in rate and rhythm. The respiratory rate is higher and the tidal volume is lower in infants and children than in adults (see Chapter 38). Respirations should be quiet, free, and easy. Any alteration in respiratory ability will affect the patient's recovery and must be detected early, and appropriate measures must be instituted to ensure adequate function. The most important respiratory problems encountered in the immediate postoperative period are hypoventilation, airway obstruction, aspiration, and atelectasis.

Inspection

The chest should move freely as a unit, and expansion should be equal bilaterally. Alterations in symmetry may be due to many factors, including pain that may cause splinting at the incisional site, consolidation, or pneumothorax. Note the character of the respirations. Intercostal retractions, bulging, nasal flaring, or use of the accessory respiratory muscles are signs of respiratory distress. The depth of respiration is as important as the rate. Shallow respiration is the cardinal sign of continuing depression from anesthesia or preoperative medications but may be due to numerous other factors, including incision pain, obesity, tight binders, or dressings that restrict movements of the thoracic cage or abdomen. Shallow respirations and the use of neck and diaphragmatic muscles may also indicate *recurarization* from the use of skeletal muscle relaxants such as succinylcholine chloride, tubocurarine chloride, or pancuronium (see Chapter 14).

Chest movements in themselves, however, are not adequate evidence that air exchange is occurring. The nurse should place a hand in front of the patient's airway (artificial or mouth and nose) and feel the amount of exhaled air. The duration of inspiration versus expiration is also important in determining whether or not there is airway obstruction. Check the patient's color. This is, at best, a difficult evaluation but may give some important clues to respiratory function. Cyanosis, when present, is a late sign indicative of severe tissue hypoxia, and immediate vigorous efforts must be made to determine the cause and correct it. Restlessness, confusion or anxiety, and apprehension are the earliest signs of hypoxemia and carbon dioxide retention and should receive immediate attention to determine their cause.

Note the presence of an artificial airway; airways are used primarily to maintain a patent air passage so that respiratory exchange is not hampered. Four types of airways commonly used are the balloon-cuffed endotracheal tube (extends from the mouth through the glottis to a point above the bifurcation of the trachea), the balloon-cuffed nasotracheal tube (extends from the nose to the trachea), the oropharyngeal airway (extends from the mouth to the pharynx and prevents the tongue from falling back and obstructing the trachea), and the nasopharyngeal airway (extends from the nose to the pharynx). The airway must be kept clear of secretions to serve its purpose and may need to be suctioned if gurgling occurs. The airway should not be removed until the laryngeal and pharyngeal reflexes return; these reflexes enable the patient to control the tongue, to cough, and to swallow. If the patient "reacts on the airway" (makes attempts to eject it) gagging may

occur that progresses to retching and vomiting. In this case the airway should be removed as soon as clinically possible.

An endotracheal tube can be removed as soon as the patient is able to maintain the airway without it or when the danger of aspiration is over. This may be difficult to determine; it is usually much easier to determine when a patient needs an airway than to decide when such an adjunct is not needed. Therefore, if policy permits removal of an airway, it should definitely cover insertion of an airway. Both procedures should, of course, be accompanied by appropriate education and skill training for the nurses who will perform them.

Palpation

Palpation and inspection of the chest may be carried out simultaneously to validate such observations as symmetry of expansion. In addition, crepitation may be heard or fremitus may be felt. The temperature, moisture, and general turgor of the skin, as well as the presence of any edema, should be noted.

Percussion

The normal sound over the lungs is resonance. Dullness heard where there should normally be resonance indicates consolidation or filling of the alveolar or pleural spaces by fluid.

Listening and Auscultation

First listen to the patient's respirations unaided. Normal respiration should be quiet; noisy breathing indicates a problem. Extraneous sounds always indicate some kind of obstruction; however, quiet breathing does not always indicate freedom from problems. The accumulation of mucus or other secretions evidenced by gurgling in any of the respiratory passages may cause airway obstruction and should be removed immediately. Purposeful coughing with good expiratory airflow is the most effective way of clearing secretions. If the patient is not yet reactive enough to do this alone, the secretions must be suctioned out orally and nasally. Nasotracheal suctioning may be useful to clear secretions and to stimulate cough, but the catheter is ineffective for reaching secretions distal to the carina. Obstruction may also occur from poor oropharyngeal muscle tone, resulting from the muscle relaxant effect of general anesthesia plus the rolling back of the tongue. To relieve this obstruction, provide support in the form of pressure anteriorly on the angle of the jaw to open the air passages.

Crowing may indicate *laryngospasm*, a sudden violent contraction of the vocal cords that may result in complete or partial closure of the trachea. If spasms continue, the airway must be maintained by the insertion of an endotracheal tube. Total blockage of the airway caused by laryngospasm produces no sound because of the absence of moving air.

Wheezing may indicate *bronchospasm* caused by a reflex from some irritating mechanism. Bronchospasm occurs most often in patients with preexisting pulmonary disease such as severe emphysema, pulmonary fibrosis, or radiation pneumonitis. Laryngeal edema following endotracheal intubation is not uncommon and can contribute significantly to airway obstruction. Acute changes in the patient's skin condition, cardiovascular status, and bronchospasm after regional anesthesia must alert the nurse to a possible allergic reaction, but this is rare.

Listen to the patient's chest with a stethoscope for quality and intensity of breath sounds. Locate, identify, and describe on the patient's chart any abnormality. Total absence of breath sounds on one side may signal the presence of a pneumothorax (collapsed lung), obstruction, or fluid or blood within the pleural space. Auscultation of breath sounds in the PACU is often difficult, since the patient frequently cannot sit up or respond to commands to breathe deeply with the mouth open. Positioning the patient on alternating sides during the stir-up regimen provides an opportunity for the nurse to examine the posterior lung field.

Cardiovascular Function and Perfusion

The three basic components of the circulatory system that must be evaluated are (1) the heart as a pump, (2) the blood, and (3) the arteriovenous system. The maintenance of good tissue perfusion is dependent upon a satisfactory cardiac output. Therefore, most assessment is aimed at evaluating cardiac output.

Inspection

Observe the overall condition of the patient, especially skin color and turgor. Peripheral cyanosis, edema, dilation of the neck veins, shortness of breath, and many other findings may be indicative of cardiovascular problems. In addition to checking all operative sites for blood loss, note the amount of blood lost during surgery.

Arterial Blood Pressure and Pulse

Arterial blood pressure and pulse are measurable indicators of cardiac output and should be noted, along with the rate and depth of respirations, at frequent intervals throughout the recovery period. Either an aneroid or mercury-type sphygmomanometer may be used to measure blood pressure, but it is essential that the correct cuff size be used. The inflatable bag encased in the cuff should be about 20 percent wider than the diameter of the limb on which it is to be used. If unable to obtain blood pressure measurements on either arm because of operative sites or other problems, the legs may be used. Center the bag of a wide cuff over the posterior surface on the lower third of the thigh and listen over the popliteal artery or at the ankle over the posterior tibial artery (just posterior to the medial malleolus). Systolic pressure in the legs is usually 20 to 30 mm of mercury higher than in the brachial artery.

A common course of error in blood pressure measurement is an auscultatory gap that may be present, especially in hypertensive patients. This gap is a silent interval between systolic and diastolic pressures.

During this gap, the pulse is palpable. Therefore, to avoid mistakenly low systolic readings, the cuff should be inflated until the pulse is obliterated. Blood pressure reading should be recorded completely, including the systolic pressure, the point at which the sounds become muffled and when they cease, and, if present, the range of the auscultatory gap.

Blood pressure readings in the postoperative period must be compared with baseline blood pressures taken before surgery to determine their significance. A low postoperative blood pressure may be due to a number of factors, including muscle relaxants, spinal anesthesia, preoperative medication, changes in the patient's position, blood loss, poor lung ventilation, and peripheral pooling of blood. The administration of oxygen to help eliminate anesthetic gases and to assist the patient in awakening sooner will cause an increase in blood pressure. Deep breathing, leg exercises, verbal stimulation, and conversation can be instituted to raise the blood pressure. A low fluid volume may be augmented by increasing the rate of intravenous fluids, which helps to maintain the arterial pressure, but this and all other methods designed to raise the pressure must be instituted with consideration for the patient's total condition.

An increase in blood pressure postoperatively is not uncommon, owing to the effects of anesthesia, respiratory insufficiency, or decreased respiratory rate and depth causing carbon dioxide retention. The surgical procedure, with its accompanying discomfort, also causes increased blood pressure. Emergence delirium, with its excitement, struggling, and pain, may also be a causative factor of a transient rise in blood pressure. Obviously, it is important to determine the cause before treatment is instituted. In patients with uncontrolled hypertension, continuous intravenous antihypertensive medications may be required. However, it is extremely important to diagnose the etiology of the hypertension so that rapid therapy may be employed.

The rate and character of all pulses should be assessed bilterally. Examine the pulses simultaneously to determine their equality and time of arrival. Peripheral arterial occlusion is not uncommon; if it is suspected, a Doppler instrument can be of great value in detecting the presence or absence of blood flow. Occlusion is an emergency and should be reported to the surgeon at once. If abnormalities are detected in the rate or rhythm of the pulse, they should be evaluated further with cardiac auscultation, electrical monitoring, or both. Arrhythmias of any type may occur during the postoperative period. Therefore, accurate electrocardiographic monitoring is a mandatory skill for the recovery room nurse.

Tachycardia in the postoperative patient may be due to numerous causes, including fever, pain, anxiety, hypotension, dehydration, overhydration, hypoxemia, or any combination of these factors. Tachycardia is a very important postoperative sign and should be fully evaluated before treatment is instituted. Increasing tachycardia is an early sign of shock and must be thoroughly investigated. Treatment of shock must be specific and directed toward the elimination of causative factors (see Chapter 43). The deleterious effects of tachycardias are generally related to diminished stroke volume and diminished cardiac output. In general, the patient with previously normal cardiac function can tolerate tachycardias up to 160 per minute without manifesting symptoms.

Other irregularities in pulse are most frequently caused by premature beats, generally premature ventricular contractions or premature atrial contractions. These irregular rhythms, like tachycardia, should be thoroughly investigated before therapy is administered (see Cardiac Monitoring in Chapter 23).

Pulse Pressure. Pulse pressure is an important determination in the evaluation of perfusion. Because of the pulsative nature of the heart, blood enters the arteries intermittently, causing pressure increases and decreases. The difference between the systolic pressure and the diastolic pressure equals the pulse pressure. The pulse pressure is affected by two major factors: the stroke volume output of the heart and the compliance (total distensibility) of the arterial tree. The pulse pressure is determined approximately by the ratio of stroke output to compliance. Therefore, any condition that affects either of these factors will also affect the pulse pressure.

To evaluate the patient's cardiovascular status accurately, all signs and symptoms must be evaluated individually as well as within the body system as a whole. For example, cool extremities, decreased urine output, and narrowed pulse pressure may be indicative of decreased cardiac output, even in the presence of normal blood pressure.

The Central Nervous System

All anesthetics affect the central nervous system (CNS), and it can be assumed for the present, even though we do not know exactly how narcosis occurs, that anesthetics are general, nonselective depressants. The complexity of the central nervous system, coupled with our incomplete knowledge of how it functions, makes it a most difficult system to evaluate.

Assessment of the central nervous system in the PACU generally involves only gross evaluation of behavior, consciousness, intellectual performance, and emotional status. A more detailed assessment of central nervous system function is necessary for patients who have undergone CNS surgery; this is discussed in Chapters 9 and 26.

Emergence from Anesthesia

Patients arrive in the PACU at all levels of consciousness, from fully awake to completely anesthetized. With modern anesthesia techniques, however, the majority of patients respond appropriately to verbal stimuli by the time they are established in the recovery room and become oriented very quickly when the sitr-up regimen is begun (see Chapter 18). In the past, about 25 percent of patients who underwent general anesthesia (especially when the anesthetic used was cyclopropane) had an agitated recovery, some with very marked delirium. However, with the use of fluorinated anesthetics, emergence is generally

quiet and uneventful. Occasionally, a patient will become agitated and thrash about; this seems to occur more often in teenagers and young adults than in other age groups. Emergence delirium also tends to occur more frequently in patients who have undergone intra-abdominal and intrathoracic procedures (see Emergence Excitement in Chapter 18). Additional information on emergence can be obtained by reviewing the chapters on specific anesthetic agents (Chapters 12 through 16).

If the PACU nurse tells the patient where he or she is, that the surgery is over, and what time it is as a part of the stir-up regimen, the patient will generally become oriented very rapidly. Reorientation occurs in reverse order from anesthesia: The patient first becomes oriented to person, then place, then time. This, of course, may not hold true for the patient who was somewhat confused or disoriented prior to surgery, which emphasizes the importance of recording accurate information concerning the mental status of the patient before anesthesia.

Alterations in cerebral function are often the first signs of impaired oxygen delivery to the tissues; therefore, an orderly and periodic assessment of mental function is necessary to detect early evidence of abnormal cerebral function. Unfortunately, restlessness, agitation, and disorientation occurring in the PACU may be ascribed to a number of other causes and are often difficult to evaluate.

TEMPERATURE

The measurement of temperature in the PACU is a particularly important but often neglected assessment. Normal body temperature may vary from 35.9°C to 38°C. In the normal healthy adult, body temperature remains fairly constant, owing to the balance between heat production and heat loss. Factors that will affect temperature in the PACU patient are listed in Table 17–1. Premedications, anesthesia, and the stress of surgery all interact in a complex fashion to disrupt normal thermoregulation. Both

TABLE 17–1. Factors Influencing Body Temperature of the PACU Patient

Anesthesia
Preoperative medications
Age of patient
Site and temperature of IV fluids
Vasoconstriction (secondary to blood loss or anesthetic agent)
Vasodilation (secondary to regional anesthesia or use of halothane)
Body surface exposure
Temperature of irrigations
Temperature of ambient air

hypothermia (temperature below 35°C) and *hyperthermia* (temperature above 39°C) are associated with physiologic alterations that may interfere with recovery (Table 17–2).

Patients at the age extremes and those who are extremely debilitated are at even greater risk for the development of temperature abnormalities postoperatively.

The accuracy of axillary, rectal, or oral measurement is frequently debated. Core temperature (approximate value of temperature of blood perfusing the major metabolically active organs) is only estimated by oral and rectal temperature readings. Invasive techniques that use the tympanic membrane or bladder as a site for monitoring temperature are more accurate. Cases of perforation of the tympanic membrane have been reported, and vigilance is necessary if this type of monitoring is used. Unless required during surgery or because of a specific problem, these temperature moni-

toring modalities are seldom used in the PACU.

Shell (skin) temperature may be measured at the axilla, forehead, or great toe with conventional thermometers or liquid crystal temperature strips. Shell temperature does not accurately reflect core temperature, although it may at least indicate gross trends that may otherwise be neglected if no temperature monitoring is implemented.

FLUID AND ELECTROLYTE BALANCE

Evaluation of a patient's fluid and electrolyte status involves total body assessment. Imbalances readily occur in the postoperative patient owing to a number of factors, including the restriction of food and fluids preoperatively, fluid loss during surgery, and stress (Table 17–3). The normal body response to stress of surgery is renal retention of water and sodium. In addition, patients often have abnormal avenues of fluid loss postoperatively.

Fluid Intake

Each patient must be evaluated to determine his baseline requirements and the

TABLE 17–2. Physiologic Alterations Associated with Hypothermia and Hyperthermia

Hypothermia	Hyperthermia
Bluish tint to skin (cyanosis)	Pale skin (mottled)
Increased metabolic rate with shivering, then decreased metabolic rate	Increased metabolic rate
Decreased oxygen consumption	Increased oxygen consumption
Decreased muscle tone	Decreased muscle tone
Decreased heart rate	Increased heart rate (rapid and bounding)
Dysrhythmias	Dysrhythmias
Decreased level of consciousness	Alterations in CNS (patient may be agitated)

TABLE 17–3. Common Clinical States Affecting Fluid and Electrolyte Balance in the Recovery Room

Clinical State	Effect on Fluid and Electrolyte Balance
Pain Anesthesia Fear Trauma	Heightened response to stress Water and sodium retention
Acute renal failure	Impaired acid-base regulatory mechanism
Blood loss Immobilization	Impaired fluid circulation
"-ostomies" Nasogastric suction Bleeding Vomiting	Excessive loss of fluid by abnormal routes Potassium and sodium deficit
Thyroidectomy Treatment of acidosis Excessive administration of citrated blood	Calcium deficit

fluid needed to replace abnormal losses. The normal adult, deprived of oral intake, requires 2000 to 2200 ml of water per day to make up for urinary output and insensible loss.

Intravenous Fluids

Most patients returning from the operating suite will be receiving intravenous fluids. The anesthetist must have an open intravenous line for the administration of necessary medications and replacement fluids intraoperatively, and postoperatively an open line is needed to supply necessary fluids and electrolytes. Since all efforts to substitute for normal oral intake of electrolytes and adequate volumes of water are, at best, temporary and inadequate, the first objective is to return the patient to adequate oral intake as soon as possible. Until this objective can be attained, an intravenous line must be maintained. The nurse should be aware of the type of fluid being administered and any medications that may have been added to it.

The intravenous site should be checked to ensure that the needle or cannula is still in the vein and that no extravasation has occurred. Watch for kinks or disconnected tubing and ensure that the rate of infusion is accurate. The arm should be positioned comfortably. It is not usually necessary to immobilize the arm; however, a short arm board may be helpful to maintain the intravenous site if the patient should become restless.

Pediatric patients may require a protective device over the site or soft restraints to prevent dislodging the needle or cannula. Small children are often delighted with the simple application of a Band-Aid over the site and will accept the nurse's explanation of the needle in his or her arm and the advice to leave it alone. A Band-Aid or bandage is particularly important for the pre-school–aged child who is concerned about body wholeness and would be upset by the sight of the needle or cannula through a clear plastic dressing.

A simple paper cup device can be invaluable in preventing dislodgment of the small needles used in the scalp veins of small babies. Snip the bottom out of the cup, thread the cup over the tubing, place the large opening over the intravenous site, and secure the cup to the baby's head with tape crisscrossed over the entire cup. In addition to providing protection for the intravenous site, this method allows the nurse to check the insertion site frequently.

After ensuring that the intravenous fluids are infusing correctly, check to see what fluids, if any, are to follow, or if the infusion is to be discontinued.

If the patient is on *hyperalimentation* or on total feeding by intravenous solutions, only feeding solutions should go through this line. Another intravenous pathway must be secured for other uses. The flow of these fluids should be maintained by an electronic device.

Oral Fluids

Oral intake must be prohibited after anesthesia until laryngeal and pharyngeal reflexes are fully regained, as evidenced by the patient's ability to gag and swallow effectively. If the patient is permitted oral intake, it is best to start with small amounts of ice chips, as these are less likely to cause nausea and subsequent vomiting. Some PACUs use *isotonic ice chips* that are made from a balanced electrolyte solution such as Lytren. If ice chips are well tolerated, the patient can progressively increase oral intake to include water and other clear liquids. Kool-aid and fruit-flavored popsicles are well tolerated and accepted by both children and adults. In addition, carbonated beverages may be soothing to a patient who feels slightly nauseated.

Fluid Output

Normal output in the average adult results from obligatory urinary output and insensible avenues of loss, including evaporation of water from the skin and exhalation during respiration. The amount of urine necessary for the normal renal system to excrete the waste products of a day's metabolism is approximately 600 ml. Optimally, 30 ml per hour or more of urine should be obtained from the catheterized adult to ensure proper hydration and kidney function. Urinary output should be closely monitored in the recovery phase; measurement of urinary output and urine specific gravity yields important clues to the overall status of the patient and may alert the nurse to overhydration, dehydration, or the development of shock.

A lower than normal urinary output can be expected in the postoperative patient as a result of the body's normal reaction to stress; however, an unduly small volume of urine (less than 500 ml in 24 hours) may indicate the presence of renal insufficiency, and the physician should be notified.

If a Foley catheter is in place, a more accurate observation of hourly output is available. If urine volume is low and specific gravity remains fixed at a low level, renal insufficiency is indicated. Small urine volume plus high specific gravity indicates dehydration. In addition to noting the volume and specific gravity of urinary output,

the nurse should observe closely for pus, blood, or casts in the urine.

The PACU nurse must evaluate abnormal as well as normal avenues of output. Abnormal losses include external losses from vomiting, nasogastric tubes, T tubes, or drainage from fistulas or wounds, and temporary functional losses from fluid shifting within the body, such as hemorrhage into soft tissues or the edema of surgical wounds.

The PACU nurse must take note immediately of the surgical site and check the dressing for drainage. The nurse must be aware of whether or not a drain is in place and how much drainage is expected.

Check all drainage tubes to ensure patency and observe the amount, color, and odor of any drainage. All tubes should be secure and either clamped shut or connected to drainage apparatus as the physician orders. A summary of imbalances that may occur with abnormal avenues of output is presented in Table 17–4. Any deviations

TABLE 17–4. Imbalances That May Occur with Abnormal Avenues of Output

Fluid	pH	Content (mEq/L)		Likely Imbalances with Significant Losses
Gastric juice (fasting) (NG suction)	1–3	Na^+ K^+ Cl^- HCO_3^-	60 10 85 0–15	Metabolic alkalosis Potassium deficit Sodium deficit Fluid volume deficit
Small intestine (suction) Jejunum	7–8	Na^+ K^+ Cl^- HCO_3^-	111 4.6 104 31	Metabolic acidosis Potassium deficit Sodium deficit
Ileum		Na^+ K^+ Cl^-	117 5.0 105	Fluid volume deficit
New ileostomy		Na^+ K^+ Cl^-	129 11 116	Potassium deficit Sodium deficit Fluid volume deficit Metabolic acidosis
Biliary tract fistula	7.8	Na^+ K^+ Cl^- HCO_3^-	148 5.0 101 40	Metabolic acidosis Sodium deficit Fluid volume deficit
Pancreatic fistula	8.0–8.3	Na^+ K^+ Cl^- HCO_3^-	141 4.6 76 121	Metabolic acidosis Sodium deficit Fluid volume deficit

From Bland, J.: Clinical Metabolism of Body Water and Electrolytes. Philadelphia, W. B. Saunders Co., 1963; and Guyton, A. C.: Textbook of Medical Physiology. 7th ed. Philadelphia, W. B. Saunders Co., 1986.

TABLE 17–5. 24-Hour Intake/Output Worksheet

TWENTY-FOUR HOUR PATIENT INTAKE AND OUTPUT WORKSHEET				FROM _____ HOURS TO _____ HOURS		TOTAL HOURS COVERED			DATE

INTAKE

ORAL				INTRAVENOUS					
TIME	TYPE	AMOUNT	ACCUM TOTAL	TIME STARTED	AMOUNT	TYPE (Include Medications)	AMOUNT RECD	TIME COMPL	ACCUM TOTAL

				IRRIGATIONS (N/G, Bladder, etc.)			
				TIME	TYPE	AMOUNT	ACCUMULATIVE TOTAL

BLOOD/BLOOD DERIVATIVES								
TIME STARTED	PRODUCT (i.e. B1, Alb, P. cells, etc.)	TIME COMPL	AMOUNT	ACCUM TOTAL	OTHER INTAKE			
					TIME	TYPE	AMOUNT	ACCUMULATIVE TOTAL
					GRAND TOTAL INTAKE			

TABLE 17–5. 24-Hour Intake/Output Worksheet *Continued*

								OUTPUT	
URINE						NASOGASTRIC			
TIME	AMOUNT	ACCUM TOTAL	TIME	AMOUNT	ACCUM TOTAL	TIME	AMOUNT	TYPE	ACCUM TOTAL
CHEST						EMESIS			
TIME	AMOUNT	ACCUM TOTAL	TIME	AMOUNT	ACCUM TOTAL	TIME	AMOUNT	TYPE	ACCUM TOTAL
STOOLS						OTHER OUTPUT			
TIME	COLOR	CHARACTER		AMOUNT	ACCUM TOTAL	TIME	AMOUNT	TYPE	ACCUM TOTAL
						GRAND TOTAL OUTPUT			

PATIENT'S IDENTIFICATION

TABLE 17–6. Signs and Symptoms of Acute Fluid and Electrolyte Imbalance

Imbalance	Symptoms and Findings

Hyperosmolarity
  Water excess
  Sodium deficit
	Polyuria (if kidneys are healthy), twitching, hyperirritability, disorientation, nausea, vomiting, weakness, serum Na^+ ↑ 120 mEq/L

Isotonic disturbances
  Dehydration
  Circulatory collapse
  Volume excess
	Weakness, nausea, vomiting, oliguria, postural drop in systolic blood pressure, elevated hematocrit, normal serum Na^+ → SHOCK
	Dyspnea, cough, sweating, edema

Hydrogen ion imbalances Metabolic acidosis	Apathy, disorientation, increased rate and depth of respiration → Kussmaul's respiration, symptoms of K^+ excess, ABG pH ↓ 7.35, HCO_3 ↓ 25, acid urine with pH ↓ 6.0
Metabolic alkalosis	Increased irritability, disorientation, shallow, slow respirations, periods of apnea, irregular pulse, muscle twitch, ABG pH ↑ 7.45, HCO_3 ↑ 29, alkaline urine with pH ↑ 7.0
Respiratory acidosis (CO_2 retention)	Increased rate and depth of breathing, tachycardia and other arrhythmias, drowsiness, ABG pH ↓ 7.4, Pco_2 ↑ 40, HCO_3^- 25–35
Potassium imbalances Deficit (hypokalemia)	Weakness, mental confusion, shallow respirations, hypotension, arrhythmias, serum K^+ ↓ 3.5 (this is a measurement of extracellular K^+ and only gives a vague reflection of intracellular balance)
Excess (hyperkalemia)	Intestinal colic, oliguria, bradycardia, cardiac arrest, serum K^+ ↑ 5 mEq/L
Calcium imbalances Deficit (hypocalcemia)	Tingling of the fingers, laryngospasm, facial spasms, painful muscle spasms, positive Trousseau's sign, positive Chvostek's sign, convulsions, palpitations, cardiac arrhythmias, serum Ca^{++} ↓ 4.5 mEq/L
Excess (hypercalcemia)	Not usually seen in the recovery room. Usually due to pathology involving the parathyroid glands

from the normally expected drainage in a specific route should be reported promptly to the surgeon.

Obviously, the accurate measurement and recording of all intake and output are vital to the assessment of each patient's fluid and electrolyte status. Keeping a running total on the tally sheet is invaluable for saving time when quick evaluations are needed. An example of a useful intake and output worksheet is shown in Table 17–5.

In addition to observing and assessing avenues of intake and output, the astute PACU nurse will be alert to symptoms of fluid and electrolyte imbalance, which are summarized in Table 17–6.

PSYCHOSOCIAL ASSESSMENT

Assessment of the patient's psychologic/emotional well-being is an important component of post anesthesia nursing. As with any other assessment, this must be made in the context of the whole patient. Illness,

hospitalization, surgery, and pain all take on a variety of values depending upon the individual experiencing them. The meaning of surgery to the individual must necessarily be explored preoperatively and will probably have been accomplished by other health care providers; this information should be communicated to the PACU nurse who will care for the patient. Likewise, the PACU nurse must ensure that additional assessment information and psychosocial care instituted in the PACU are shared with those who will care for the patient upon his or her transfer.

Almost all surgical patients experience a degree of anxiety about anesthesia and the surgical procedure, and fear of postoperative pain. The physical signs and symptoms of anxiety are the same as those produced by any stressor. Reactions are mediated by the sympathetic nervous system and are listed in Table 17–7.

The PACU nurse must carefully differentiate symptoms of anxiety from those of

TABLE 17–7. Signs and Symptoms of Anxiety

Tachycardia
Increased blood pressure
Pale cool skin
Increased respiratory rate
Hyperventilation
Increased muscle tone
Restlessness/agitation
Dilated pupils

other causes. Differentiation is particularly difficult while the effects of anesthesia are still present.

A quiet, calm environment is important to the post anesthesia recovery of the surgical patient. A calm, confident nurse can do much to allay anxiety for the recovery room patient through both verbal reassurance and communication through touch. Hearing is the first sense to return; it is not necessary to yell at the patient—he may not respond even though he hears you. In fact, yelling at the patient may increase anxiety early in the PACU period, since the patient may believe he is not recovering as quickly as he should.

Attention to comfort and the reassuring presence of the nurse are calming. Once the patient has fully regained consciousness, simply talking to him may significantly allay anxiety. Simple, factual statements repeated frequently are best. At this point, the nurse may be able to explore further with the patient the cause of distress.

For the patient in acute distress due to anxiety, a mild tranquilizer, such as diazepam (Valium), may be indicated; however, tranquilizers must be used judiciously. An added advantage of their use is that it will often allow a reduction of the narcotic analgesia dosage necessary to control pain.

Attention to the psychosocial ramifications of specific surgical interventions is addressed in each of the following chapters on postoperative care. In keeping with our philosophy that attention to psychosocial assessment and care is an integral component of nursing, these comments are generally not highlighted with subtitles but are incorporated into the overall text wherever deemed appropriate. For further discussion of the relationship between pain and anxiety see Chapter 19.

SUMMARY

Obviously, the PACU nurse must be an expert in assessment. Not only must he or she understand the normal physiologic functioning of the human body, but the nurse must also be able to differentiate and evaluate the variety of pathologic symptoms that may arise in the postanesthesia patient. The PACU nurse must be aware of the interrelationships between mind and body and must be sensitive to the psychosocial factors influencing the patient's reactions. Knowledgeable assessment of the patient determines the basis upon which all medical treatment and nursing care for the PACU patient will be provided.

REFERENCES

1. Aldrete, J. A.: The preoperative visit by the recovery room nurse. Curr. Rev. Recov. Room Nurses, 4(4):27–29, 1981.
2. Beeman, T. A.: Augmenting nursing assessment with arterial blood gas analysis. Today's OR Nurse, 1:14–19, 1979.
3. Borchardt, A. C., and Fraulini, K. E.: Hypothermia in the post anesthetic patient. AORN J., 36(4): 648–669, 1984.
4. Cook, K. G.: Assessment and management of anxiety in recovery room patients. Curr. Rev. Recov. Room Nurses, 7(5):51–55, 1983.
5. Croushore, T. M.: Postoperative assessment: the key to avoiding the most common nursing mistakes. Nursing '79, 9(4):47–51, 1979.
6. Cullop, M. E.: Hypertension: A postoperative complication in the recovery room. Today's OR Nurse, 1:20–23, 1979.
7. Durbin, N.: The application of Doppler techniques in critical care. Focus Crit. Care, 10(3):44–46, 1983.
8. Eckenhoff, J. E., Kneale, D. H., and Dripps, R. D.: The incidence and etiology of postanesthetic excitement. Anesthesiology, 22: 667–669, 1961.
9. Fraulini, K. E.: Coping mechanisms and recovery from surgery. AORN J., 37(6):1198–1208, 1983.
10. Geelhoed, G. W.: Pulmonary physiology and the anesthetist. Part 2. AANA J., 48:133–138, 1980.
11. Jackson, B. S.: How post-op complications

can burgeon into crisis. RN, *44*:26–32, 1981.

12. Kneedler, J.: Perioperative Patient Care. St. Louis, C. V. Mosby Co., 1983.

13. Kruse, D. H.: Postoperative hypothermia. Focus Crit. Care, *10*(2):48–50, 1983.

14. Lewis, K. P., and Cressey, I.: Nursing care for postanesthesia shivering. AORN J., *30*(2):357–366, 1979.

15. McConnell, E.: Toward complication-free recoveries for your surgical patients. RN, *43*(6):31–33, 82–90, 1980.

16. Ozuna, J. M., and Foster, C.: Hypothermia and the surgical patient . . . inadvertent hypothermia. Am. J. Nurs., *79*:646–648, 1979.

17. Shields, J. R.: A comparison of physostigmine and meperidine in treating emergence excitement. MCN, *5*:(3)170–175, 1980.

18. Shipley, S. B.: Response to "The preoperative visit by the recovery room nurse." Curr. Rev. Recov. Room Nurses, *4*(4):29–31, 1981.

19. Vaughn, M. S.: Shivering in the recovery room. Curr. Rev. Recov. Room Nurses, *6*(1):3–7, 1984.

18

Care of the Post Anesthesia Patient

This chapter deals with the nursing care of postoperative patients in relation to emergence from anesthesia including the stir-up regimen, intravenous therapy, blood transfusions, oxygen therapy, control of infection, and general comfort measures.

THE STIR-UP REGIMEN

The stir-up regimen is probably the most important aspect of postanesthesia nursing care. Like most other PACU activities, the basics of the stir-up regimen are aimed at prevention of complications, primarily atelectasis and venous stasis. It can be divided into five major activities: (1) deep breathing exercises, (2) coughing, (3) positioning, (4) mobilization, and (5) pain relief.

Deep Breathing Exercises

The primary factor contributing to postoperative pulmonary complications is decreased lung volumes. The major factor contributing to low lung volumes in the post anesthesia patient is a shallow, monotonous, sighless breathing pattern caused by general anesthesia, pain, and narcotics. Full inflation of the lungs prevents small areas of patchy atelectasis from developing and assists in the elimination of inhalational anesthetics, thus hastening the awakening process. Intravenous anesthesia differs from inhalational anesthesia in that, once injected, there is practically nothing that can be done to expedite removal of the drug; however, the prevention of atelectasis by deep breathing remains just as important.

The patient must be stimulated to take three to four deep breaths every 5 to 10 minutes. Full expansion is important. This may be impeded by a number of factors discussed in the previous chapter. Every effort must be made to enhance the patient's ability to expand his lungs. Many gadgets and maneuvers have been proposed to improve postoperative lung expansion, but they have had limited success. One of the problems for the post anesthesia patient is the inability to achieve a tight fit on the mouthpiece of the mechanical devices. In addition, these are fairly expensive.

The sustained maximal inspiration (SMI) maneuver has been introduced recently as a method to enhance the lung volumes of postoperative patients. The SMI maneuver consists of the patient inhaling as close to total lung capacity as possible and, at the peak of inspiration, holding that volume of air in the lungs for 3 to 5 seconds before

243

exhaling it. The SMI maneuver produces maximal alveolar inflating pressure, time, and volume. In controlled studies, the SMI maneuver has been more effective than simple deep breathing in preventing a reduction in lung volumes in the immediate postanesthesia period.

Ideally, the patient will receive instruction and coaching in the use of this maneuver preoperatively. During the immediate postoperative period, the patient must be coached with verbal and tactile (hands on the chest) cues to perform the SMI maneuver.

If the patient's vital capacity is inadequate or respiratory depression due to anesthesia is prolonged, deep breathing and the SMI maneuver may be augmented with a self-inflating bag connected to any oxygen source or with an IPPB (intermittent positive-pressure breathing) apparatus.

Coughing

The patient must be instructed to cough along with performing SMIs. The best way to clear the air passages of obstructive secretions is a purposeful cough. The effectiveness of a cough depends upon the inspired tidal volume and the velocity of expired air flow.

For the patient recovering from anesthesia, the cascade cough is the most effective cough maneuver. The patient should be taught to take a rapid, deep inspiration to increase the volume of air in the lungs, which will in turn dilate the airways, allowing air to pass beyond the retained secretions. Upon exhalation, the patient should perform multiple coughs at succeedingly lower lung volumes. With each cough during exhalation, the length of the airways undergoing dynamic compression will increase, enhancing cough effectiveness.

Coughing is most effective with the patient sitting up. Splinting of incisions and adequate analgesia facilitate a good cough. If the patient is supine, having him bend his knees to decrease abdominal tension and allow maximal movement of the diaphragm may improve the cough.

Between cascade cough maneuvers, the patient should be encouraged to inhale and close his glottis. This dilates the airways and, by increasing the pleural pressure, further compresses the airways so as to "milk" the secretions toward the larger airways, where they can be removed in succeeding cough maneuvers.

If an effective cough cannot be produced, secretions from the respiratory passages must be suctioned manually. If the patient cannot or will not cough effectively it may be necessary to stimulate cough by means of tracheal suctioning or cricothyroid cannulation with a fine sterile polyethylene catheter. A cough may also be stimulated by finger pressure against the trachea just above the manubrial notch. This may also produce retching and vomiting, however, and should be used cautiously.

Preoperative teaching of postoperative breathing exercises and cough and of their importance is very effective and should be included in the preoperative regimen whenever possible. Some institutions arrange for each scheduled surgical patient to have a formal teaching session before surgery. These programs have been very successful.

Positioning

When possible, patients in the recovery room should be maintained in a semiprone, side-lying position. The semiprone position promotes maintenance of a patent airway, prevents aspiration of vomitus into the trachea, and permits optimal ventilation of the lower lung lobes. Frequent repositioning of patients (at least every hour) is essential for the prevention of atelectasis and peripheral stasis. The patient's position should be changed from side to side. Care must be taken to ensure that all drainage tubes and intravenous catheters remain in place and patent, and that no tension on any of these lines is created. As soon as he or she is able, the patient should be encouraged to turn and change positions alone.

Mobilization

To prevent venous stasis the patient must be encouraged to move his legs and arms in a rhythmic fashion. Have the patient flex and unflex his extremities. Mobilization and flexion of the muscles aids venous return, automatically causes deep breathing, and improves cardiac function.

Pain Relief

The provision of adequate pain relief is included in the stir-up regimen because without it the first four activities are very difficult to achieve. Narcotics depress the cough reflex and ciliary activity and may lower alveolar ventilation by direct depression of the respiratory center; they must not be used indiscriminately. If breathing is painful and splinting occurs, however, or if the patient refuses to cough or move because of pain, nothing is gained. Pain relief is discussed in detail in Chapter 19.

Modifications of the Stir-up Regimen

Some modifications of the stir-up regimen may need to be made in accordance with the type of anesthesia used and the operative procedure performed. When ketamine is the anesthetic used, the stir-up regimen is eliminated from routine PACU care and verbal and tactile stimulation of the patient are avoided as much as possible. Cough must be eliminated after eye surgery and other delicate plastic procedures. Positioning is probably the activity most often modified in the stir-up regimen. Positioning of the patient and modifications of the stir-up regimen after specific surgical procedures and anesthetics are discussed in related chapters.

RECOVERY ROOM EXCITEMENT

It is hoped that most patients will emerge from general anesthetic in a calm, tranquilized manner. Some patients, however, will emerge in a state of "excitement," a condition characterized by restlessness, disorientation, crying, moaning, or irrational talking. In the extreme form of excitement, which is referred to as *emergence delirium*, the patient will scream, shout, and thrash about wildly.

The incidence of emergence excitement is high among children and is most common in healthy patients. As age increases, the incidence increases. Barbiturate and scopolamine premedication seem to increase its occurrence. Factors such as fear of disfigurement, fear of cancer, and a feeling of suffocation also increase the likelihood of emergence excitement. The PACU nurse should assess the patient's status if emergence excitement is encountered. Respiratory function should be checked first because restlessness is also a well-known manifestation of hypoxia. Other situations for concern include the patient with a full bladder, the patient who has cramped muscles and joints, owing to prolonged maintenance of an abnormal position on the operating table, and the patient with postoperative pain.

The restless patient requires constant, careful observation. Restraining straps may be required to prevent injury. If hypoxia, pain, and full bladder are ruled out, a change in position may have a quieting effect. The most effective treatment is the injection of a narcotic such as morphine. Use of meperidine (Demerol) should be avoided because it may cause nausea and vomiting. If narcotic treatment is instituted, the patient should then be monitored for hypotension, respiratory depression, or renarcotic action.

INTRAVENOUS THERAPY

Postoperative parenteral fluid requirements vary with the patient's preoperative status and with the surgical procedure. For a discussion of fluid and electrolyte balance see Chapter 17.

BLOOD TRANSFUSIONS

The administration of whole blood or blood components (serum, plasma, red cells, platelets) is a common, often lifesaving modality of treatment for the postoperative patient. However, the inherent dangers are numerous and recovery room nurses must be well aware of the principles of safe administration of blood and blood components.

Whole Blood

The only indication for whole blood transfusion in the PACU is hypovolemic shock, to restore and maintain circulating blood volume that has been depleted, owing to hemorrhage or trauma. The nurse may anticipate this need in patients who have required emergency surgery and in patients who have been subjected to extensive dissection. The only other indications for whole blood transfusions are exchange transfusions to remove toxic substances from the blood or to prime the oxygenating pump for cardiac surgery. These are rare occurrences in the PACU. Most other clinical situations requiring replacement therapy can be handled with blood components.

Every possible safeguard must be exercised to prevent the administration of incompatible blood to the patient in need of replacement. Before any blood or blood component is administered, typing and crossmatching of the donor and the recipient blood must be done. Whether it is known in advance that the patient will need blood replacement for major surgery or only that the patient might need blood replacement (e.g., for a breast biopsy that develops into a radical dissection for malignancy), this typing and crossmatching should be carried out before the start of surgery, and compatible blood should be available for administration.

Great care must be taken in the identification of the recipient and the unit of blood prepared for him or her. An information form listing the donor's and recipient's types, crossmatches done and identification number, the recipient's name, and the date prepared must be cross-checked with the label on the unit of blood to be administered and with the patient's identification bracelet. At least two persons should be involved in the identification of the recipient, preferably a physician and a nurse, or two nurses. Since post anesthesia patients are often not well known by the nurse and are frequently only partially conscious owing to anesthesia, scrupulous attention must be directed toward positive identification of the recipient. If any discrepancy at all exists,

do not give the blood until clarification is obtained.

Once positive identification of the recipient and the unit of blood to be transfused is established, the blood must be inspected for hemolysis and abnormal cloudiness or color. Red cells settle to the bottom of whole blood and plasma rises to the top. Before beginning the transfusion and from time to time during the transfusion, whole blood should be gently and thoroughly mixed by tilting the bag back and forth.

Blood and blood components should be administered via large-bore intravenous needles or by plastic cannulae in a large vein of the forearm. Only blood administration sets designed for use with any plug-in type of blood, plasma, or serum container should be used for transfusion. The drip chamber must be filled enough to just cover the filter before the infusion is started. If the filter becomes clogged during the infusion, it may be cleared by squeezing the flexible drip chamber above the filter after the clamp has been completely closed. The level is then reset by squeezing the chamber. Squeezing the plastic drip chamber above the filter assures that particulate matter will not be forced into the filter and that the filter will not be bent.

The solution of choice to start an infusion before beginning blood replacement is sodium chloride (isotonic) injection, U.S.P. It is completely compatible with blood. If the patient's sodium intake must be restricted, a suitable solution would be 5 percent dextrose in quarter-strength saline. Small clumps or globules of red cells may form when blood is administered with dextrose in water, and many of the "balanced" solutions (e.g., Ringer's injection, U.S.P.; lactated Ringer's injection, U.S.P.) contain calcium, which may cause citrated blood to clot. Solutions containing calcium or a potent drug (e.g., any anesthetic or muscle relaxant) should never be used in the primary bottle when blood is administered by secondary or "piggyback" hookup.

Be sure that you have baseline vital signs, including temperature, before beginning the administration of blood. Untoward reactions to blood generally occur during the first 15 minutes of administration, so begin the transfusion slowly (20 to 40 drops per min) for the first quarter hour. If no symptoms of reaction develop, the rate of administration may be increased to 80 to 100 drops per min or the rate ordered by the physician.

A unit of blood is usually administered over a period of 1½ to 2 hours; however, in emergency situations, such as shock or hemorrhage, a unit of blood can be infused within 10 minutes under pressure. A pressure cuff similar to a blood pressure cuff is slipped over the collapsible plastic blood container and pumped up to compress the bag and literally push the blood into the patient's veins. When pressure transfusion equipment is used, every precaution must be exercised to prevent air from entering the system and causing air embolization. All tubing and the blood container itself must be checked for leaks. The infusion site must be monitored very carefully for signs of infiltration to prevent the infusion of blood into subcutaneous tissue.

Once the blood infusion is started, the flow rate should be checked frequently. Remember that changing the height of the intravenous stand or the bed may alter the rate of the infusion, as will repositioning of the patient, changes in location of the needle in the vein, or changes in the tone of the vein.

Transfusion Reactions

The incidence of transfusion reactions is not exactly known. Reports of their incidence vary from 0.2 to 10 percent, and some reactions are undoubtedly not recognized and go unreported.

Nurses in the PACU must be especially adept at assessing the patient receiving blood, since many of the signs and symptoms of an adverse reaction to blood may be difficult to separate from those caused by other variables such as the patient's illness, surgery, or medications (including anesthesia). In addition, the patient who is not fully conscious may not complain of symptoms. Blood transfusion reactions may be either immediate or delayed. Immediate reactions include hemolytic, febrile, bacterial contamination, and allergic reactions.

Hemolytic Reactions. Fifty to 75 ml of ABO incompatible blood can precipitate a hemolytic reaction resulting in agglutination, or clumping, of red cells, which block the patient's capillaries, obstructing the flow of blood and oxygen to vital organs. In time, hemolysis of the red cells occurs, releasing free hemoglobin into the plasma. Free hemoglobin may plug the renal tubules and disrupt the work of the nephrons, resulting in renal failure. Improper storage, overheating, or freezing of blood may also cause hemolysis of the cells and release of free hemoglobin.

The clinical signs of the hemolytic reaction occur quickly and include sudden hypotension; tachycardia; substernal chest pain; abdominal, leg, and back pain; dyspnea; and sensorium changes, most often anxiety. Headache may be one of the patient's first complaints if he is conscious. Pain may occur along the vein path. Fever and chills develop later, along with hemoglobinuria, which leads to oliguria. Many of these symptoms may be significantly masked under the influence of anesthesia. Bleeding from the wound is strongly suggestive that the patient has received incompatible blood; it is also a poor prognostic sign.

Febrile Reactions. Febrile reactions are most often due to sensitivity to leukocytes and platelets and are seen most frequently in patients who have received multiple transfusions. A febrile reaction may also be attributed to bacterial contamination. In febrile or bacterial contamination reactions the patient may complain of headache and chills, followed by a rapid rise in temperature. Backache, nausea, vomiting, diarrhea, and abdominal pain follow. Hypotension and tachycardia develop quickly. Pyrogenic reactions caused by the polysaccharide products of bacterial metabolism are manifested by the same symptoms, except that blood pressure does not drop, and the temperature usually returns to normal within 12 hours.

Allergic Reactions. Allergic reactions occur in about 1 percent of all transfusions and are most often seen in patients who have a history of allergy. Symptoms include mild edema and hives, sometimes accompanied by itching, occasionally by fever and chills, and bronchial wheezing. More severe reactions include symptoms of asthma, bronchospasm, severe dyspnea, laryngeal edema, and finally, anaphylactic shock.

Treatment of Immediate Reactions

At the first sign of a reaction, the transfusion must be stopped and the physician notified. The donor blood and the intravenous tubing, along with a sample of the recipient's blood, should be returned to the laboratory for type and crossmatch, and for culture and sensitivity tests. The first voided specimen should be sent to the laboratory and tested for hemoglobin and urobilinogen. Urine output must be monitored carefully. Ideally, a Foley catheter should be inserted and hourly output recorded. Vital signs must be monitored and the patient treated according to his symptoms. The intravenous line should be kept open with 5 percent dextrose in quarter-strength saline to counteract shock and promote diuresis. Blood transfusion with properly matched blood should be used to correct blood volume deficits and control shock. Vasoconstricting drugs may be required to control blood pressure but must be used with caution since they may contribute to renal damage, especially if blood volume has not been restored. Oxygen and epinephrine may be used to treat dyspnea and wheezing. Steroids and broad-spectrum antibiotics may be necessary to treat reactions caused by bacterial contamination. Antihistamines and antipyretics are given to the patient suffering from an allergic reaction.

Delayed Reactions

Delayed reactions include the transmission of disease (hepatitis, malaria, AIDS), transfusion siderosis, circulatory overload, citrate intoxication, cardiac dysrhythmias, and bleeding due to depleted coagulation factors.

Circulatory overload results when fluid is infused into the circulatory system either too rapidly or in too great a quantity. Elderly patients and those with minimal cardiac reserve are particularly susceptible. The use of packed red cells in these patients should be considered carefully. Symptoms of circulatory overload include cough, dyspnea, edema, tachycardia, hemoptysis, and frothy pink-tinged sputum. If the patient is conscious, he may complain of a pounding headache, a feeling of constriction around his chest, back pain, and chills. If these symptoms develop, the transfusion should be stopped and the physician notified.

When large amounts of banked blood are transfused, *citrate intoxication* may occur. If the blood is infused rapidly, the liver cannot metabolize the citrate ions, which combine with the calcium in the blood, causing calcium deficit symptoms, such as tingling of the fingers, muscular cramps, and nervousness. If the calcium deficit is not corrected, cardiac dysrhythmias, including ventricular fibrillation, may occur. Treatment consists of slow intravenous administration of calcium gluconate, 1 gm for every 1000 ml of blood the patient received. If calcium gluconate is not available, calcium chloride may be used, but this is more irritating to the veins.

The rapid infusion of cold blood may result in *cardiac dysrhythmias*. Blood should be warmed to room temperature or passed through a warming coil, taking care not to overheat it, which would cause hemolysis of the red blood cells.

In cases of massive blood replacement, *bleeding from dilution of coagulation factors and platelets* can occur. If massive transfusions are required, it is suggested that several fresh blood infusions (less than four hours old) be used along with banked blood.

Blood must be properly stored and refrigerated at 5°C. In most instances blood should be stored in the blood bank until required. If blood is to be kept in the PACU, proper storage requirements must be met. When units of blood prepared for a given recipient are not used, they should be promptly returned to the blood bank.

Blood Component Transfusions

Packed Red Cells

The use of packed red blood cells can eliminate many of the problems associated with whole blood transfusion. Packed cells are prepared by drawing off about two thirds of the plasma, either through the natural settling-out process or by centrifugation. Patients who require red blood cells to improve the oxygen-carrying capacity of the blood should be treated with packed cells to minimize volume increase and the risks of circulatory overload or cardiovascular failure. In addition, a better balance of sodium, potassium, and ammonium ions is maintained, and citrate intoxication is prevented. When plasma is removed, the antibody content of blood is markedly reduced and hence minimizes reactions to plasma factors.

Platelets and Plasma Proteins

Other blood components that may be used in the PACU include platelets and the plasma proteins. Transfusion of platelets is the treatment of choice when bleeding occurs and the platelet count is less than 10,000/cu mm. Platelets are very cohesive and must therefore be administered with a nonwettable infusion set that includes an 80 μ mesh nonwettable filter and a nonwettable needle. This equipment is usually kept in the blood bank.

Plasma proteins may be used to treat specific deficits. *Albumin* is used to treat shock due to hemorrhage, trauma, or infection. It is prepared in concentrations of 5 percent in buffered saline and of 25 percent in salt-poor diluent. It is administered with a large-bore needle and may be infused through standard intravenous tubing.

Fibrinogen may be used when there is a fibrinogen deficit, but it carries a very high risk of transmitting hepatitis and must be used with extreme caution. All those who handle fibrinogen products must avoid exposure via needle scratches or small cuts, and, if exposure occurs, a prophylactic dose of gamma globulin is recommended.

Dextran is a synthetic plasma substitute that may be used in acute hemorrhage until more specific blood components can be given. It is inexpensive, readily available, and carries no risk of disease transmission. It does not interfere with crossmatch tests and is rarely antigenic. Dextran may interfere, to some extent, with platelet function and may be associated with a transient prolongation of bleeding time. Dextran is administered through standard intravenous tubing.

MAINTENANCE OF RESPIRATORY FUNCTION

Oxygen Therapy

The optimal use of the oxygen-carrying capacity of arterial blood is the goal of oxygen therapy. All anesthetized patients have experienced some interference with their respiratory process, and it is for this reason that most experts suggest routine oxygen administration to all postanesthesia patients in the PACU. However, oxygen is a drug and should be treated as such, with full prescription information provided by the anesthetist or physician. This information may be contained in standard orders that are individualized for each patient.

Low-flow oxygen administration assists the patient in maintaining adequate oxygenation of all tissues. Optimal arterial oxygen tension should be between 70 and 100 mm Hg. Patients with chronic lung disease may be maintained with low-flow oxygen administration which keeps the oxygen tension in the range of 50 to 70 mm Hg. Pulmonary processes should be monitored carefully in the PACU, and nurses should never be reluctant to draw arterial blood gases to aid in assessment of a patient's status. For discussion of arterial blood gases and the method for obtaining their measurement, see Chapter 4.

Complications of oxygen therapy do occur, and nurses should be aware of them. Respiratory depression, atelectasis, substernal chest pain, and pulmonary oxygen toxicity may occur when high concentrations are administered over prolonged periods. For more detailed discussions of these complications, the reader is referred to the respiratory references at the end of this chapter.

Methods of Administration

Routine oxygen administration in the recovery room can be accomplished with nasal catheters, nasal cannulae (prongs), or face masks (Fig. 18–1). The nasal catheter is inserted into one of the nares until the tip reaches the oropharnyx just below the soft palate and is then retracted slightly until it cannot be seen when the patient's mouth is opened and the tongue is depressed. Nasal catheters deliver an oxygen concentration between 30 and 50 percent when a 6 to 8 liter flow per min is used.

Method	Max Per Cent Oxygen	Flow (L/min)	Comments	Method	Max Per Cent Oxygen	Flow (L/min)	Comments
A. *Nasal catheter*	30–40%	6–8	Comfortable. Higher flows provide up to 40% oxygen, but can cause respiratory depression and drying of mucosa.	F. *Mask without bag*	35–45% 45–55% 55–65%	6–8 10 10–12	Poorly tolerated. Significant CO_2 rebreathing possible at low flows. Highest percentage requires tight mask fit.
B. *Nasal prongs*	30–40%	6–8	Comfortable. Higher flows provide up to 40% oxygen, but can cause respiratory depression and drying of mucosa.	G. *Mask with bag* 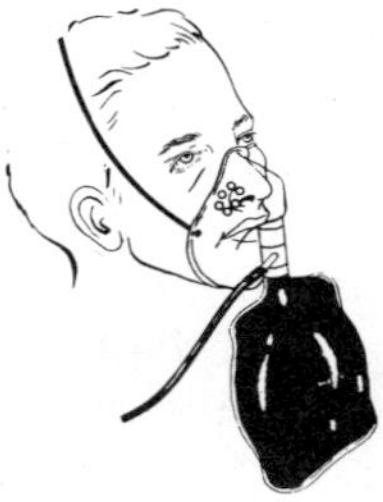	40–55% 50–60% 90 + %	6 8 8–12	Poorly tolerated. Significant CO_2 rebreathing possible at low flows. Highest percentage requires tight mask fit and a large bag.
C. *T-piece*	40–60%	4–12	Provides enriched oxygen mixtures and humidification. Used most often in weaning patients from ventilator assistance before endotracheal tube is removed.	H. *Pressure-regulated ventilator* 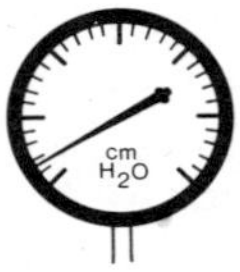	40–100%	Direct from supply	Oxygen per cent unpredictable
D. *Face tent*	30–55%	4–8	Well tolerated. Good for supplying extra humidity.	I. *Volume-regulated ventilator* 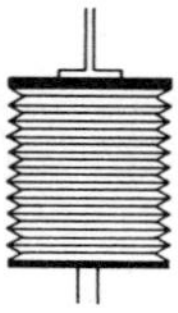	20–100%	Direct from fupply	Bennett MA1, Ohio 560 can be set to any desired per cent.
E. *Venturi mask*	25–35%	4–8	Mask well tolerated. Accurate concentrations delivered.				

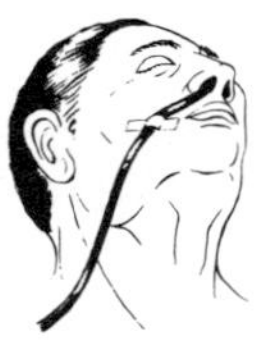

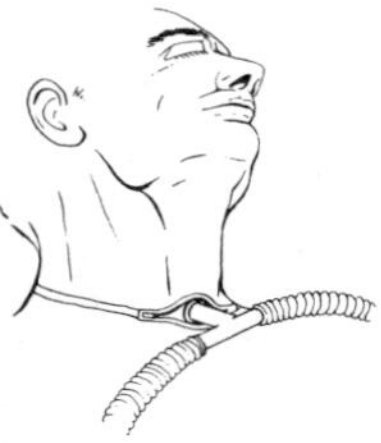

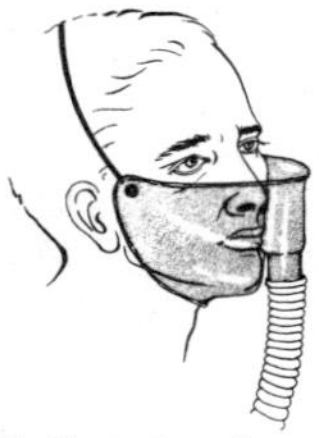

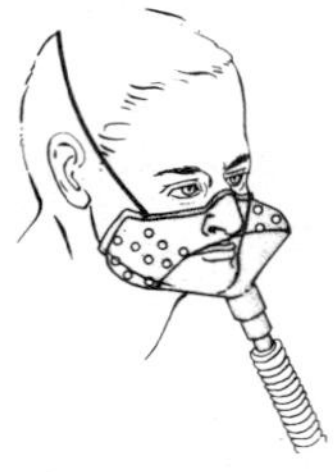

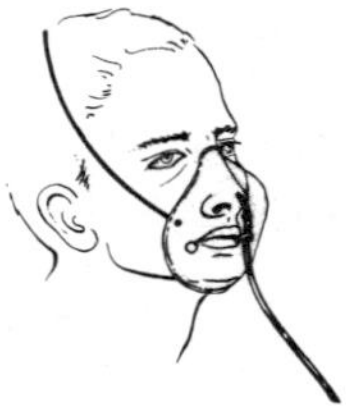

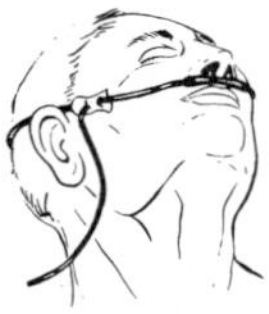

Figure 18–1. Methods of oxygen administration. (From Sanderson, R. G. [ed.]: The Cardiac Patient. Philadelphia, W. B. Saunders Co., 1972, p. 310.)

Nasal catheters are not generally used in the PACU, since they are difficult to place properly in an unconscious patient, proper humidification of the oxygen is impossible, and the loss of epiglottal reflexes in unconscious and semiconscious patients may lead to abdominal distention due to accumulation of air.

Nasal cannulae are advantageous for routine short-term oxygen administration in the PACU. The cannula is made of plastic tubing with two soft plastic tips that insert into the nostrils for about 1.5 cm. The prongs will deliver an oxygen concentration of 30 to 40 percent when a 4 to 6 liter per min flow is used. The prongs are easily inserted, comfortable, inexpensive, and disposable. Simple, clear plastic disposable face masks may be used for oxygen administration in the PACU. They are also easy to apply and comfortable. The oxygen concentration delivered depends upon the mask fit and the patient's inspiratory flow rate however, an oxygen flow rate of 6 to 8 liters per min will yield an inspired oxygen concentration of approximately 30 to 45 percent. Face masks in the PACU must be clear to provide adequate observation of the patient's nose and mouth. The mask should be removed intermittently to dry the face.

Humidity

Surgery and anesthesia often interrupt the normal functioning of the nose in heating and humidification of inspired air. It is, therefore, frequently necessary to augment these functions temporarily in the recovery room. A number of devices may be used for these purposes. Humidifiers convert water from the liquid to the gaseous state, whereas nebulizers produce tiny water particles. Both devices require heat to produce a high relative humidity. The nurse must observe these mechanical devices frequently and ensure that the water containers never run dry, because hot dry air is damaging to the respiratory mucosa.

Mechanical Ventilation

Fortunately it rarely occurs, but some patients recovering from anesthesia may

TABLE 18–1. Terminology: Common Ventilatory Modes

Mechanical ventilation with positive airway pressure:
MV	= mechanical ventilation
CV	= controlled ventilation
AV	= assisted ventilation
IPPB	= intermittent positive-pressure breathing
IPPV	= intermittent positive-pressure ventilation
CPPB	= continuous positive-pressure breathing
CPPV	= continuous positive-pressure ventilation
PEEP	= positive end-expiratory pressure
ZEEP	= zero end-expiratory pressure
NEEP	= negative end-expiratory pressure
CMV	= controlled mechanical ventilation
IMV	= intermittent mandatory ventilation
SIMV	= synchronized intermittent mandatory ventilation
IAV	= intermittent assisted ventilation
IDV	= intermittent demand ventilation

Spontaneous breathing (SB) with positive airway pressure:
CPAP	= continuous positive airway pressure
EPAP	= expiratory positive airway pressure
IPAP	= inspiratory positive airway pressure

require some form of mechanical ventilation in the PACU. Recently, various techniques such as PEEP, CPAP, and IMV have been developed to improve the respiratory status of the patient. Table 18–1 gives the terminology of the common ventilatory modes.

Positive End-Expiratory Pressure (PEEP)

PEEP is a technique that can be utilized to help prevent collapse of the alveoli during the expiratory phase of ventilation and to increase the lung's functional residual capacity (FRC) and reduce the amount of physiologic shunting. PEEP will also increase the P_aO_2, which will usually enable the fractional inspired oxygen concentration (FiO_2) to be reduced, thus lessening the chances of oxygen toxicity. In patients with preexisting obstructive lung disease, PEEP should probably be used cautiously, as it may overexpand relatively normal alveoli. When it is used under such circumstances, the dead space will increase and occasionally cause a decrease in the P_aO_2 and an increase in the $PaCO_2$.

When a patient is placed on PEEP, hemodynamic status should be monitored because this ventilatory technique retards venous return and may cause a fall in cardiac output, especially in the hypovolemic patient. In some instances the reduced cardiac output can cause a fall in systolic blood pressure. Other parameters to be monitored are vital signs, skin perfusion, and urine output.

Continuous Positive Airway Pressure (CPAP)

CPAP helps to keep the lungs expanded. The patient breathes out against increased pressure of up to 10 to 20 cm H_2O, but the mechanics of ventilation do not change. The lung performs at a larger, more inflated volume, thereby increasing the functional residual capacity and decreasing the tendency to atelectasis. CPAP is a technique that can be utilized for weaning a patient from a ventilator. When CPAP is being utilized, the patient should be monitored for tachypnea, tachycardia, increase in blood pressure, arrhythmias, or generalized distress, which should be reported to the physician, if detected.

Intermittent Mandatory Ventilation (IMV)

IMV was originally devised to facilitate the weaning process from mechanical ventilation. It is currently used when a patient is first given mechanical ventilation. This technique allows the patient to breathe on his own as often and as deeply as he would like; it also ensures that every minute a set tidal volume will be delivered at a predetermined back-up rate. IMV allows gradual progression from complete ventilatory support by the respirator to spontaneous provision of ventilation by the patient.

Nursing Responsibilities

All PACU nurses must be familiar with the specific types and mode of operation of ventilators used in their area (Figs. 18–2 to 18–4). There are, however, nursing responsibilities that remain the same regardless of the type of mechanical ventilator used.

1. Ascertain that the patient is being ventilated by frequently observing the chest for bilateral synchronous and equal expansion and by listening for bilaterally present and equal breath sounds.

2. Check the airway frequently for complete patency. See that the patient ventilator system is free of significant leaks by listening for air gurgling in the upper airway during ventilation and by comparing the exhaled volume with the tidal volume set on the ventilator.

3. Ensure that the cuff is *never* overinflated. Inflate the cuff until there is no leak on tidal ventilation and a small, barely audible leak on sigh volume.

4. Empty the ventilatory hoses frequently of excess water from condensation.

5. Be sure that proper humidification is being delivered to the patient by the presence of water droplets in the ventilator hoses.

6. The humidifier should be checked and filled frequently to ensure proper humidification.

7. The temperature gauge should be between 90° and 98°F, and the ventilator hoses and the humidifier should be warm to the touch, never cold or hot.

8. There must *never* be any pull on the patient's endotracheal or tracheostomy tube.

9. Tracheostomy wound care should be performed as needed during the PACU phase.

10. Suction the mouth and the pharynx, then deflate the cuff as positive pressure is being held on the airway with the anesthesia bag; then suction the secretions that are blown up into the throat.

11. Ascertain frequently that all alarms on the ventilator are **on** and **functioning properly.**

The observations and checks of mechanical devices often seem simple and routine but are an important part of nursing the mechanically ventilated patient. Ideally, all these checks, along with measured parameters of the patient's respiratory status, should be recorded on a flow sheet attached to the patient's bed or to the ventilator. Such a flow sheet is vital for clinical evaluation of the patient's response to therapy. A sample flow sheet is shown in Figure 18–5.

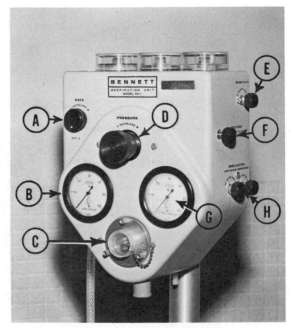

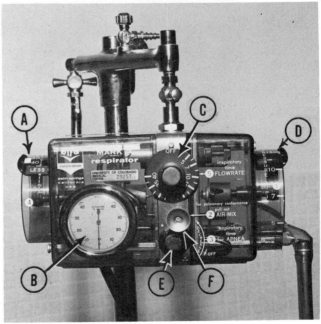

Figure 18–2. Mechanical ventilators. *Top*, The Bennett PR-1 has the following features: A, rate control; B, airway pressure indicator; C, flow-sensitive valve; D, pressure control; E, sensitivity control; F, oxygen diluter; G, machine pressure indicator; H, humidifier controls. *Bottom*, The Bird Mark 7 has: A, sensitivity control; E, airway pressure indicator; C, flow control; D, pressure control; E, rate control; F, oxygen diluter. (From Nett, L.: Nursing Clin. N. Am., 9:128, 1974.)

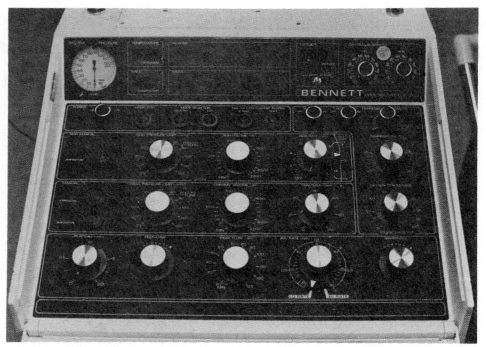

Figure 18–3. Photograph of the front panel of the Bennett MA–II ventilator. The top upright panel consists of the system pressure gauge, with digital indicators for temperature, rate, alarm, mode, and delivered oxygen percentage, followed by oxygen high- and low-percentage dials. The front panel indicates the power control, with testing apparatus for lamp, mode selection, cycle, and audio alarms (*left to right*). The second row consists of the sigh panel for manual sigh, pressure limit, and volume and rate setting, including a multiple sigh control. The inspiration/expiration panel allows manual inspiration and expiration. This panel is followed by pressure limit, volume, and rate dials. The bottom panel contains the plateau dial, which holds the inspiration for a set number of seconds, and the PEEP/CPAP dial. The rate of maximal inspiratory flow (peak flow) and the IMV rate are indicated here. There is also a setting for patient sensitivity. The right column has controls for nebulization, humidity, and temperature, and a setting for oxygen percentage. (From Sanderson, R. G., and Kurth, C. L.: The Cardiac Patient. 2nd ed. Philadelphia, W. B. Saunders Co., 1983.)

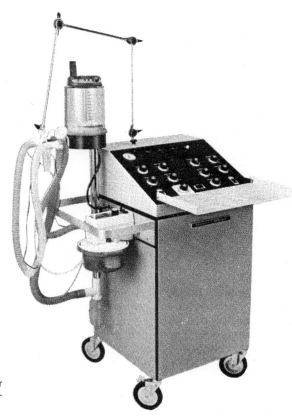

Figure 18–4. A volume ventilator used either to assist or to control a patient's respirations. (Courtesy of Puritan-Bennett Corp., Kansas City, Mo.)

SUCTIONING

When large amounts of secretions accumulate that cannot be handled effectively by coughing, suctioning must be instituted to assist the patient in clearing air passages.

Oral and Nasal Suctioning

Suctioning the nose and mouth is simple and safe. This procedure is commonly used to assist the patient in eliminating secretions before he or she has regained full consciousness and cannot spit out secretions. The catheter used should be soft and pliable. Technique should be clean but need not be strictly sterile.

Tracheal Suctioning

Tracheal suctioning may be performed through the mouth or nose, via endotracheal tube, or through a tracheostomy tube (Fig. 18–6). Tracheal suctioning must be accomplished atraumatically using strict sterile technique. A selection of sterile suctioning catheters in a variety of sizes should be kept at the bedside of every patient in the PACU along with sterile gloves and sterile water or normal saline. The catheter chosen for suctioning should not have an external diameter that exceeds by one third the internal diameter of the tube to be suctioned. Most commonly, a number 14 or 16 (Fr) is used for adult patients. The catheter must not completely occlude the trachea or endotracheal tube.

The procedure should be explained to the patient even if apparently totally unconscious. Explaining the procedure alleviates fear and also helps to gain cooperation from the patient to the extent that he or she is able.

Before suctioning the patient, ensure proper ventilation. In most patients, suctioning lowers the arterial pressure of oxy-

Date/ Time	F$_i$O$_2$	PO$_2$/% Satn	PCO$_2$	$\frac{pH}{BE}$	Hct	$\frac{VC}{IF}$	V$_T$/PAP	On/Off Resp	RR	Wt.	24 hr. Intake-Output	Comments and Signature

Figure 18–5. Sample respiratory flow sheet.

Date and Time—It is critical to know when certain measurements were made and under what clinical settings.

F$_i$O$_2$—The fractional inspired oxygen concentration.

PO$_2$ and Percentage of Saturation—The partial pressure of oxygen in the arterial blood as measured by the arterial blood gases and the percentage of hemoglobin saturated with oxygen.

PCO$_2$—The partial pressure of carbon dioxide in the arterial blood.

$\frac{pH}{BE}$ —Hydrogen ion concentration expressed as a logarithm and the base excess. Used to determine the acid-base status of the patient.

Hct—The hematocrit.

VC—The vital capacity.

IF—Inspiratory force.

V$_T$—Tidal volume.

PAP—Peak airway pressure.

On or Off Respiratory—This is a simple notation to aid in evaluation of other parameters.

RR—The respiratory rate.

Wt.–Weight. Absolute values are not critical but changes are.

Previous 24 hours intake and output.

Comments and Signature—In this area the patient's progress or lack of progress, changes in ventilator settings, such as the addition of PEEP, time off the ventilator, culture and sensitivity results, and evidence of GI bleeding may be recorded.

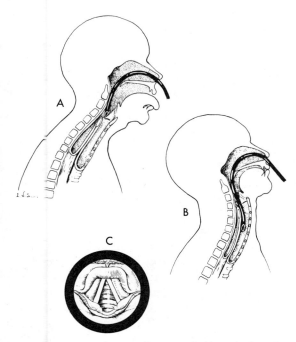

Figure 18–6. Technique of nasotracheal suctioning. *A,* Optimal position of head in order to direct catheter tip anteriorly into the trachea. The neck is flexed and the head is extended. The tongue is protruded (and held there by a gauze 4 × 4). *B,* After the catheter has been advanced into the trachea, the tongue is released and the patient's head may be more comfortably positioned. *C,* View of the vocal cords from above. The cords are most widely separated during inspiration. (From Sanderson, R. G. [ed.]: The Cardiac Patient. Philadelphia, W. B. Saunders Co., 1972, p. 304.)

gen 30 to 35 mm Hg. Since suctioning removes oxygen, which may in turn initiate cardiac dysrhythmias, the nurse should, before beginning the procedure, assess the total physiologic condition of the patient. Is he restless, agitated, or disoriented? While these conditions can be caused by other factors, they often indicate inadequate oxygenation. If the patient is conscious, ask him to take four or five deep inspirations. If the patient cannot cooperate, hyperventilation must be done with an Ambu or anesthesia bag. The nurse can deliver 1000 ml volume with two hands. If the patient has an endotracheal airway in place and is on a respirator, several sigh volumes can be delivered at an increased FiO_2 before suctioning.

To suction the patient with no airway adjunct, have him stick out his tongue. Grasp the tongue with a gauze pad and apply gentle traction to make the glottis open and move in line with the trachea. Gently insert the catheter into the nostril. A slight curvature in the tubing may facilitate intubation of the larynx. Advance the catheter until intubation of the trachea is accomplished. Listen through the catheter or feel for air movement against your cheek through the proximal end of the catheter. An increasing intensity of breath sounds or more air against the cheek indicates nearness to the larynx. If the breath sounds decrease or the patient begins to gag, you are in the hypopharynx. Draw back and advance again. A sudden cough indicates presence of the catheter in the larynx; advance quickly with the next breath.

Once the catheter is positioned in the trachea, apply intermittent suction by occluding and opening the vent of the Y-connector with your thumb and withdraw the catheter in a spiral motion. If an airway adjunct is present, suctioning may be accomplished through it.

Never apply suction until the catheter is in the trachea, and never apply suction longer than 15 seconds. One useful trick is to hold your breath while suctioning the patient to remind yourself of the time limits. Monitor the patient carefully during all suctioning procedures. Any form of suctioning can lead to dysrhythmias, and prolonged suctioning may produce hypoxia, asphyxia, and cardiac arrest. Remember that suctioning removes oxygen as well as secretions, so hyperventilate the patient after the procedure as well as before.

Tracheostomy care is discussed in Chapter 20.

INFECTION CONTROL

Infection control in the PACU is always a problem. All postoperative patients are exceedingly vulnerable to infection since their body defenses are down. Prevention of the spread of infection involves blocking infectious agents from the three major avenues of transmission in the recovery room: (1) air, (2) human carriers, and (3) inanimate objects used in the care of patients, particularly instruments.

When a patient is received in the PACU for whom air may reasonably be expected to act as a vector, that patient should be isolated in a single room and the hospital's standard isolation techniques carried out. Ideally, a separate isolation room with glass partitions should be planned for the PACU to allow for separation of contaminated cases. Ease of observation of a patient placed in the isolation room is essential. If the patient in isolation cannot be fully observed, he or she should be attended until complete recovery from anesthesia.

Good handwashing technique cannot be overemphasized in the control of infection. All personnel should wash their hands thoroughly after caring for each patient, and there should be no deviation from this practice except in extreme emergencies. Handwashing facilities must be easily accessible to the observation area.

Disposable patient care items such as thermometers, drinking glasses, catheter sets, and irrigation sets have contributed immensely to infection control programs. As many of these products as possible should be utilized in the PACU; they must be used as specified and then discarded and must not be resterilized for reuse. All items that are not disposable should be cleaned and sterilized appropriately after use before contact with a new patient.

Personnel must be scrupulous in their personal hygiene. Personnel should never work in the recovery room if they know or suspect that they suffer from any infectious disease, especially an upper respiratory infection. Open cuts or sores should disqualify a person from working with postoperative patients.

The wearing of scrub attire in the PACU has in recent years come into question. While recommendations for its use continue, no definitive studies exist to indicate that scrub suits should be mandatory.

Every hospital has its own physical limitations, and modifications in isolation techniques must be made to fit the circumstances; however, good practice dictates utilizing scientific principles and knowledge when making plans to prevent the spread of infection.

GENERAL COMFORT AND SAFETY MEASURES

General comfort and safety measures are important parts of PACU care. For safety, there should always be at least two nursing attendants present in the recovery area whenever patients are present. An unconscious patient should never be left alone, and side rails should be raised on the bed whenever direct patient care is not being provided. The wheels of the bed should be locked to prevent sliding when care is being rendered.

General physical measures such as cleanliness should not be overlooked in the PACU. Often, in the hustle of caring for postanesthesia patients, we forget just how important these comfort measures are to the total well-being of the patient. As soon as the patient is settled into the unit and assessment has been accomplished, all excess skin preparations, electrodes, and electrode paste should be removed; in addition to providing comfort, washing off excess skin preparations gives the nurse an excellent opportunity for further assessment of the patient's general condition. A good back rub at this time may prevent later complaints of discomfort from being in one position in the operating suite for a long time. This is also a good time to change the patient's position, assist with range of motion exercises, and encourage deep breathing. Frequent changes of position are very important to prevent atelectasis, promote circulation, and prevent pressure from developing on the skin surfaces.

Mouth care with lemon-glycerin swabs is usually very comforting to the patient who has not only had nothing by mouth, but who has also received preoperative medication for drying up secretions. When the patient is fully conscious and his laryngeal reflexes have returned, he can rinse his mouth with mouthwash and water. An exceptionally pleasant and well-liked mouthwash is plain cola. Ice chips and small sips of water or juice may be offered to the patient who has not been ordered to have nothing by mouth. A petrolatum-base ointment should be applied to the lips after mouth care to prevent further drying and consequent cracking.

Patients often complain of being cold when returning from the operating suite. This is due in part to the effects of general anesthesia and premedications and in part to the cool atmosphere of the operating suite and the PACU. This must be explained to the patient. Warm cotton blankets should be provided, and the patient must be protected from drafts. Blankets should not, however, obscure the intravenous lines, arterial lines, or other monitoring apparatuses from the direct view of the attending nurse.

Some units have warming lights to assist in rewarming the patient after surgery. These may be useful; however, there is no evidence that they are more efficient than warm blankets, and they make the environment less comfortable for the nursing personnel. If warming lights are used, the patient's temperature should be monitored closely and overheating avoided. Keep in mind that the disruption of the patient's temperature-regulating mechanism may increase vulnerability to heat as well as to cold, and that there is a carry-through effect from warming; for these reasons the lights should be discontinued prior to achieving the desired patient temperature.

In addition to physical comfort measures, remember to provide psychologic comfort. Reorientation, especially to time and place, is important to the postanesthesia patient, as is constant reassurance that the surgery is completed and that all went well.

TRANSFER OF THE PATIENT FROM THE PACU

When the patient has recovered from the effects of anesthesia, vital signs will have stabilized; if no surgical complications have arisen, the patient is ready for transfer to the parent unit. The patient's PAR score, if this system is used, should be 10, unless criteria for exception are noted. The patient should have regained a satisfactory level of consciousness to the point of being oriented and able to call for assistance, if necessary, and should be clean and dry and dressed in appropriate hospital garb. All dressings should be dry and intact and all drainage receptacles emptied.

No patient should be discharged immediately after receiving narcotic medications. In such cases discharge should be delayed at least 30 minutes to allow for close monitoring while restabilization occurs.

A summarizing PACU discharge note should be written on the patient's progress record indicating condition and time of transfer. The nurse should alert the parent unit that the patient is being transferred and request the preparation of any specialized equipment for care and the assignment of a receiving nurse.

The patient may be transferred in the recovery room bed, if feasible, or on a stretcher. In either case, safety precautions must be strictly followed. Do not attempt to transfer a patient by yourself; always use at least two people. A third person may be necessary to assist with the transfer of the patient if a great deal of extra equipment or many drainage tubes are present. Ensure that all drainage tubes and catheters are safely transferred, that no kinking occurs, and that they do not become tangled underneath the patient. All drainage receptacles should remain below the level of the patient. Intravenous tubing and solution must be carefully transferred to the portable stand attached to the stretcher.

Stabilize both the bed and the stretcher by locking the wheels when transferring the patient from one to the other. Ensure that the patient is adequately covered with bed linens, including a warmed blanket if hallways of the hospital are kept cool. Lock the side rails of the stretcher in place, and secure the safety straps comfortably around the patient. Two persons should be used to wheel the stretcher to the receiving unit: The person in back pushes, the person in front steers, both moving at a reasonable speed.

A receiving nurse should meet the patient upon arrival at the parent unit and direct the transfer to the patient's room. The patient is transferred to the bed along with all apparatuses. Drainage tubes should be connected to suction or gravity drainage as indicated and their proper functioning checked.

Ensure that the patient's call light is properly positioned so that he can reach it and that other items he may need are within easy reach. Check the intravenous infusion rate and adjust as necessary. Side rails on the bed should be raised.

The PACU nurse should then give a complete report to the receiving nurse, including pertinent facts about the following:

1. The operative procedure performed.

2. The anesthesia used.

3. The patient's general condition and PACU recovery course.

4. The incision, any drains placed, and the dressing.

5. Any drainage tubes or catheters.

6. Intake and output. The flow sheet should be reviewed.

7. Any medications given in the recovery room, especially narcotic analgesics.

REFERENCES

1. Association of Operating Room Nurses: Standards for infection control in recovery room nursing. AORN J., *29*(7):1305–1312, 1979.

2. Beeman, T. A.: Augmenting nursing assessment with arterial blood gas analysis. Today's OR Nurse, *1*:14–19, 1979.

3. Borchardt, A. C., and Fraulini, K. E.: Hypothermia in the post anesthetic patient. AORN J., *36*(4):648–669, 1984.

4. Chalikian, J., and Weaver, T.: Mechanical ventilation. Am. J. Nurs., *84*(11):1373–1379, 1984.

5. Cook, K. G.: Assessment and management of anxiety in recovery room patients. Curr. Rev. Recov. Room Nurses, *7*(5):51–55, 1983.

6. Cramer, C.: The postanesthetic record. Curr. Rev. Recov Room Nurses, *21*(6):166–171, 1984.

7. Croushore, T. M.: Postoperative assessment: the key to avoiding the most common nursing mistakes. Nursing '79, 47–51, 1979.

8. Drain, C. B.: Postanesthesia lung volumes in surgical patients. AANA J., *49*(3):261–268, 1981.

9. Geelhoed, G. W.: Pulmonary physiology and the anesthetist. Part 2. AANA J., *48*:133–138, 1980.

10. Kneedler, J.: Perioperative Patient Care. St. Louis, C. V. Mosby Co., 1983.

11. McConnell, E.: Toward complication-free recoveries for your surgical patients. RN, *43*(6):31–33, 82–90, 1980.

12. Risser, N. L.: Preoperative and postoperative care to prevent pulmonary complications. Heart Lung, *9*:57–67, 1980.

13. Schneider, M.: Meeting the criteria for discharge. Curr. Rev. Recov. Room Nurses, *6*(4):43–47, 1982.

14. Smith, L. G.: Reactions to blood transfusions. Am. J. Nurs., *84*(9):1096–1101, 1984.

CHAPTER
19

Assessment and Management of Postoperative Pain

The postoperative pain experience is so common that it is an expected consequence of surgical intervention. Pain can be a frightening experience and, in fact, the fear of postoperative pain ranks second only to the fear of death for surgical patients.

Pain is an extremely complex phenomenon and may well be the most difficult symptom to assess. Postoperative pain perception is a subjective phenomenon influenced by the tissue damage caused by incision, manipulation, retraction, and excision; in addition, responses to pain are influenced by myriad other factors including age, personality, mood, culture, and emotional state.

It is clear that pain is more than just a physiologic experience; it is a psychologic experience as well. Emotional and psychologic factors not only modify pain, but may even cause pain. Anxiety has been commonly recognized as a component of the pain experience as well as a modifier of pain perception.

For the surgical patient, a variety of factors may influence the level of anxiety, including fear of surgery, fear of pain, or fear of the unknown. The exact relationship between anxiety and pain perception remains elusive, owing to the multiplicity of uncontrollable intervening variables. It is, however, generally accepted that a positive relationship exists between the two.

Feelings of helplessness or lack of control may also contribute to anxiety and fear and hence influence the perception of pain (Fig. 19-1). These feelings may be enhanced by the constraints of postoperative care, i.e., lying flat in the bed, the presence of casts and dressings, and other apparatus needed for care.

ASSESSMENT

The very nature of pain makes it a most difficult symptom to assess. The patient is the only expert on what he is feeling. There are no reliable invariable signs or symptoms of pain; however, there are some indications that a person is suffering.

The assessment of pain is based on a variety of observable behavior and physiologic manifestations. Increased blood pressure, increased pulse and respiratory rate, pallor, dilated pupils, increased muscle tension, cold perspiration, and nausea are

261

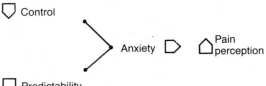

Figure 19–1. Wire diagram of direct relationships between control, predictability, anxiety, and pain perception.

physical indicators of pain. Restlessness is a common manifestation of pain and, when present, must be very carefully evaluated to differentiate it from restlessness due to hypoxemia. The patient's vocalizations, including groaning, grunting, and crying, as well as statements about having pain, must be carefully evaluated.

The patient's responses to pain will vary according to the extent to which his level of consciousness is altered. As the patient emerges from the second stage of anesthesia, there may be a period of excitement and overreaction to all stimuli, including pain. As the patient emerges from the first stage of anesthesia (analgesia), there may be enough pain-relieving effect left from the anesthetic so that he awakens, complains of pain, and then falls asleep again.

Postoperative pain, although certainly influenced by many factors, is largely governed by the site and the nature of the operation. Patients who have undergone abdominal and intrathoracic operations generally experience the most pain, and this may be the reason that postanesthesia delirium and excitement are most common after these procedures. Surgery on the joints, back, and anorectal area is also generally quite painful.

Communication with the postanesthesia patient may be difficult owing to a clouded sensorium and the presence of apparatuses such as NG tubes, artificial airways, and so forth. However, the nurse must collaborate with the patient to identify the location, intensity, and quality of pain being experienced.

Complaints of pain or discomfort by the postoperative patient may not be brought on by incisional pain, as might be assumed, but rather by headache or sore throat as a result of anesthesia technique, by discomfort at the site of intravenous infusion, or by irritation from other associated apparatuses, such as nasogastric tubes. Each would require a very different intervention.

Pain may arise from other causes such as angina pectoris, and this must be differentiated from surgical pain. A very common source of postoperative pain and restlessness is a distended bladder, and this possibility must not be overlooked. Other common sources of pain or discomfort in the PACU that may be easily corrected by removing their source are open safety pains on dressings, improper positioning so that stress is placed on a suture line, and dressings and casts that are too tight and are restricting circulation or creating friction.

Several tools have been developed to assist with the assessment of pain intensity. Although not in common use in the PACU, the verbal rating scale and the visual analog scale are simple to use, easily explained, even to the patient in the postanesthesia state, and can greatly improve the consistency of pain assessment. These tools depend upon anchors at either end of a scale upon which the patient rates his pain. The anchors are arbitrary. The verbal rating scales ask the patient to rate pain on a scale ranging from 0 to 10 or 0 to 100. The pain score is the patient's chosen number and can be recorded for comparison with later complaints of pain or to evaluate the effectiveness of relief measures.

The visual analog scale (VAS) is a 10 cm line with anchors of "no pain" at the left end and "severe pain" or "pain as bad as it can be" at the right end. The distance in centimeters from the left end of the line to the point marked by the patient on the line constitutes the measurement (Fig. 19–2). With the VAS, there are an infinite number of points between the extremes, which allows sensitivity for many grades of pain as

Please make a mark on the line (_____|_____) that best describes the pain you are experiencing right now.

NO PAIN _____ SEVERE PAIN

Figure 19–2. Visual analogue scale.

experienced by the patient without forcing the patient to translate a feeling into words.

In addition to assessing the location and severity of pain experienced, the patient's general condition and the premedications and anesthetics received must be evaluated.

PAIN MANAGEMENT

Prevention

The prevention of pain and the promotion of comfort should be a major goal in the care of the post anesthesia patient. Positioning to avoid stress on incisions and to promote adequate ventilation is especially important in the PACU. Injured tissue must be handled carefully and further trauma avoided whenever possible. Postoperative patients should have been taught preoperatively how to splint abdominal and thoracic incisions externally to minimize noxious stimuli during ventilatory exercises, but they will probably need assistance during the post anesthesia period.

Reassurance that surgery is over and the patient is doing well, as well as explanations of what is going on and what sensations will be experienced, do much to allay anxiety.

Attention to details that promote patient comfort (see Chapter 17) can do much to reduce suffering from pain. In addition, sensory stimulation, including noise and bright lights, should be reduced as much as possible, as sensory overload reduces pain tolerance.

Analgesics

A large number of pharmacologic agents have been incorporated into the list of medications for pain relief. The more commonly used analgesics are listed in Table 19–1. Just as there are no objective indicators for pain, there are no reliable indicators of analgesic requirement. Drugs are often prescribed based on weight, but weight does not seem to be a reliable predictor of the amount of analgesic needed.

The analgesics are categorized as non-narcotic and narcotic. The non-narcotic an-

TABLE 19–1. Common Analgesics for Use in the PACU

Generic Name	Brand Name
Non-Narcotics	
Aspirin	
Acetaminophen	Tylenol, Tempra, Datril, Panadol
Ibuprofen	Motrin, Nuprin
Fenoprofen	Nalfon
Phenacetin	
Narcotics	
Codeine	Codeine
Oxycodone	Percocet
Pentazocine	Talwin
Meperidine, Pethidine	Demerol
Morphine	Morphine
Hydromorphone	Dilaudid
Methadone	Dolophine
Levorphanol	Levo-Dromoran Levorphan
Fentanyl	Sublimaze

algesics are generally administered orally, and are fairly weak. They have few side effects, however, and may be very useful in conjunction with other modalities to provide relief of mild to moderate pain states for the patient who can tolerate oral medications and fluids.

Concern for the side effects of narcotic analgesia (Table 19–2) has drastically limited treatment with narcotics that could be effective if used properly. While it is true that the narcotics eventually cause addiction, this has never been a significant problem when they are used to treat acute pain. Respiratory depression occurs with the use of narcotics, and the patient should be monitored carefully for adequacy of ventilation. This should be standard practice within the controlled environment of the PACU, and the possibility of respiratory depression should not preclude the use of narcotic analgesia when it is needed. In fact, narcotics can be titrated to produce appropriate analgesia by observing for normalcy of res-

TABLE 19–2. Side Effects of Narcotic Analgesia

Respiratory depression
Cardiovascular depression
Nausea
Vomiting
Clouding of sensorium
Drowsiness

piratory pattern, i.e., the presence of expiratory pause versus the shortening or absence of expiratory pause in the respirations of a patient in pain.[18]

The patient should be evaluated for previous narcotic use, for this will influence the doses of narcotics necessary to control pain. Patients who are physically dependent on narcotics, including those persons who have been in drug rehabilitation programs and are on a methadone maintenance schedule, will require larger doses of narcotics to prevent the symptoms of withdrawal during this vulnerable time.

Age Considerations

The elderly patient is often undermedicated for severe acute pain because it is assumed that the elderly have a higher pain threshold or tolerate pain better. This is not necessarily so. The elderly patient should be assessed for concomitant physical problems, such as decreased circulation or decreased kidney and liver function, which would affect both uptake and clearance of analgesic drugs and therefore prolong the duration of action of these drugs. This does not change the amount of drug per administration needed to control pain for these patients. The nurse should also be alert to an increased likelihood of drug interactions if other medications are being administered for associated disease processes.

Children are also undermedicated for postoperative pain, mainly owing to lack of knowledge about pain and how it is expressed in children. Children do experience pain but have very different ways of expressing it. The small child may be able to express pain only by crying. Comfort and reassurance may be provided for infants and small children by holding and rocking them. Codeine is the narcotic of choice for severe pain in infants and children with its wide margin of safety due to limited respiratory or cardiovascular depression. Dosages, of course, must be adjusted for the individual child.

Austin[2] relates that the plethora of new analgesics in the drug cabinet is not an indication that good analgesics have not

been found, but rather that we are still not using appropriate methods of drug delivery. For the post anesthesia patient, the intramuscular route of administration is clearly inferior. The peak levels of serum drug concentration are variable, partially owing to the variable absorption rates from muscle. Administration of postoperative analgesia should be via the intravenous route because of the inability of most post anesthesia patients to tolerate anything orally. An added advantage to the intravenous route is the assurance of accurate dosage and absorption and more prompt action and, thus, relief. Small amounts of a narcotic administered frequently to maintain serum drug concentrations via the intravenous route control pain more effectively.

The patient-controlled analgesic (PCA) device (Fig. 19–3) is an electronically controlled infusion device that includes a timer and a mechanism for presetting doses of analgesics. This device allows the patient to self-administer analgesia as necessary. A lockout mechanism can be set to preclude inadvertent overdoses, but initial evidence indicates that patients do a much better job of assessing the dosage of analgesics needed to relieve pain without deleterious side effects than do either nurses or physicians. Blood serum concentrations are maintained at a more stable level, preventing the development of severe pain which is more difficult to abate without producing drowsiness (Fig. 19–4). The beneficial aspects of this device are obvious; it combines individualized analgesic therapy, based on each patient's subjective appreciation of pain, with the reassurance and sense of control that patients derive from knowing that pain relief is at hand.

An interesting sidelight of trials of this device is that data indicate that patients need far more analgesia in the immediate postoperative period to relieve pain than was previously supposed, but that patients taper off their use of narcotic usage more quickly when they regulate administration themselves.

Use of this device in the PACU has been limited so far; however, it would appear to hold great promise.

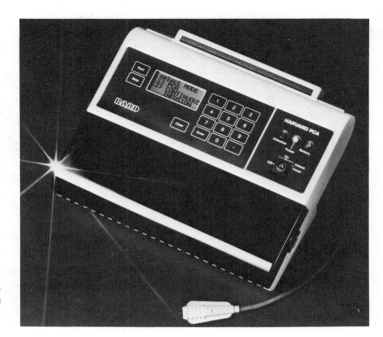

Figure 19–3. The patient-controlled analgesia device (PCA). (With permission from Bard Electro Medical Systems, Inc., Englewood, Colo.).

Analgesic Adjuncts

Retching and vomiting aggravate the effects of noxious stimuli, and alleviation of these symptoms may significantly reduce the pain experience. Often an antiemetic, such as promethazine hydrochloride (Phenergan) or chlorpromazine (Compazine), may be ordered and may be given concurrently with an analgesic. Droperidol (Inapsine) has been used very successfully in the PACU as an antiemetic. Anxiety may be alleviated by the administration of a mild tranquilizer such as diazepam (Valium). The narcotics are potentiated by most phenothiazines, and the nurse must be alert for an exaggeration of respiratory depression when these are administered in the postanesthesia period.

Transcutaneous Electrical Nerve Stimulation

Transcutaneous electrical nerve stimulation (TENS) involves external stimulation of nerves through electrodes placed over the skin. The stimulation is produced by electrical current activated by a battery-powered device (Fig. 19–5). The electrical current

produces a mild tingling or vibrating sensation over the area of application.

Controlled studies have demonstrated TENS to be particularly effective for the alleviation of acute incisional pain. It is not satisfactory as the sole modality, but can

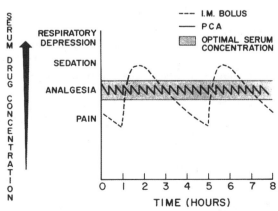

Figure 19–4. Narcotic analgesics exhibit a "hierarchy of response" to increasing serum drug concentrations. Typically there exists an optimal concentration where the patient is both analgesic and unsedated. Intermittent intramuscular injections of narcotics produce much wider swings in serum drug concentrations than do smaller, more frequently administered intravenous boluses. (From Bennett, R. L., and Griffen, W. O.: Patient controlled analgesia. Contemp. Surg., 1983, vol. *23*, with permission.)

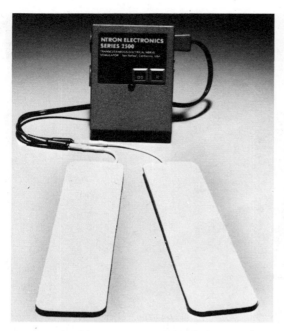

Figure 19–5. The transcutaneous electrical nerve stimulation device (TENS). (With permission of NTRON International Sales Co., San Rafael, California.)

significantly reduce the dosages of narcotic analgesia needed to provide comfort. It seems to work better when the patient is drug-naive. Patients report that it potentiates relief from analgesics and gives them a sense of control over pain.

A number of different units are on the market. Most are simple to use. Generally, electrodes, similar to those used for cardiac monitoring, are applied to the area to be stimulated and the current flow adjusted until the patient reports discomfort. The current flow is then reduced until stimulation is felt but is a comfortable sensation. Each patient must make this determination.

In the event a patient does not identify the stimulation as uncomfortable but a muscle response becomes apparent, the current flow should be reduced until the muscle response is obliterated. On many models, pulse rate and pulse width may be adjusted in a similar manner.

Since there are no deleterious side effects with TENS, it is an excellent adjunct for pain relief in the PACU. It has been particularly effective for relieving the incisional pain associated with large thoracic and ab-

dominal incisions. It may also be effective for relieving pain associated with chest tubes and sternal pain following open heart surgery. Initially, the use of TENS for patients scheduled for cardiac surgery or who had either internal or external pacemakers was contraindicated. Recent evidence indicates that it is safe for these patients to use TENS, although it should be used with caution and the patient observed closely for any adverse effects. TENS may interfere with electrical monitoring equipment, and this should be observed. Caution should also be exercised when using TENS for patients who are taking anticoagulant medications, for those who are pregnant, and for those who have a diagnosis of myasthenia gravis.

Relaxation

Relaxation has been studied repeatedly as a pain relief adjunct with demonstrated effectiveness for increasing tolerance to pain and reducing narcotic analgesia necessary to control pain. Learning the techniques and practicing take time, which is seen by some as a disadvantage. However, there are major advantages in that relaxation is fairly simple to learn, is noninvasive, and has no known deleterious effects; furthermore, the patient can easily transfer the technique from one situation to another.

The effective use of cognitive relaxation techniques appears to be dependent upon coaching, and this may be another means by which the patient's family can contribute to care.

Relaxation is usually not effective when used as the sole pain relief modality but can be very useful to augment analgesics and increase tolerance by providing a sense of control over pain, which reduces anxiety.

Not to be overlooked are alternative methods for inducing relaxation, including back rubs or massage, light stroking, application of heat, and the reassurance of personal attention.

Pain management is often neglected in the PACU and the patient relegated to the parent ward prior to pain assessment and institution of comfort measures. For humanitarian reasons as well as for promoting physical well-being, pain management should be a priority for the patient in the PACU, for pain is known to decrease lung volumes, increase oxygen consumption, and deplete patient energy. Pain involved with specific procedures and its management are also discussed in each of the individual chapters.

REFERENCES

1. Anderson, R., and Krogh, R.: Pain as a major cause of postoperative nausea. Can. Anaesth. Soc. J., 23:366–369, 1976.
2. Austin, K. L., Stapleton, J. V., and Mather, L. E.: Multiple intramuscular injections— a major source of variability in analgesic response to meperidine. *Pain, 8:47–62,* 1980.
3. Bakker, S. B. C., Wong, C. C., Wong, P. C., et al.: Transcutaneous electrostimulation in the management of postoperative pain: initial report. Can. Anaesth. Soc. J., 27(2):150–155, 1980.
4. Cristoph, S. B.: A comparison of patient-controlled transcutaneous electrical nerve stimulation with traditional analgesics for relief of postoperative pain. Doctoral Dissertation, Washington, D.C., The Catholic University of America, University Microfilms, 1985.
5. Drain, C. B., and Cain, R. S.: The nursing implications of postoperative pain. Milit. Med., 146:127–130, 1981.
6. Flaherty, G. G., and Fitzpatrick, J. J.: Relaxation techniques increase comfort level of postoperative patients: a preliminary study. Nurs. Res., 27:352–355, 1978.
7. Lim, A. T., Edis, G., Kranz, H., et al.: Postoperative pain control: contribution of psychological factors and transcutaneous electrical stimulation. Pain, 17:179–188, 1983.
8. Locsin, R. G. R.: The effect of music on the pain of selected post-operative patients. J. Adv. Nurs., 6:19–25, 1981.
9. McCaffery, M.: Nursing Management of the Patient with Pain. 2nd ed. Philadelphia, J. B. Lippincott Co., 1979.
10. McGuire, L.: Managing pain . . . in the young patient. Nursing '82, 12(8):52–55, 1982.
11. Meinhart, N. T., and McCaffery, M.: Pain: A Nursing Approach to Assessment and Analysis. Norwalk, Appleton-Century-Crofts, 1983.
12. Panayotoff, K.: Managing pain . . . in the elderly patient. Nursing '82, 12(8):53–57, 1982.
13. Patient-controlled analgesia. Lancet, 1(8163): 289–290, 1980.
14. Scott, L. E., Clum, G. A., and Peoples, J. B.: Preoperative predictors of postoperative pain. Pain, 15:283–293, 1983.
15. Siang-Yang Tan: Cognitive and cognitive-behavioral methods for pain control: a selective review. Pain, 12:201–228, 1982.
16. Steward, D. J.: Postoperative pain relief in children. Curr. Rev. Recov. Room Nurses, 17(7):135–138, 1985.
17. Sweeney, S. S.: OR observations: Key to postop pain. AORN J., 32:391–400, 1980.
18. Tamsen, A., Hartvig, P., Dahlstrom, D., et al.: Patient-controlled analgesic therapy in the early postoperative period. Acta Anesthesiol. Scand., 23:462–470, 1979.
19. Van Poznak, A.: Role of respiratory patterns in the treatment of pain and anxiety. In Luczun, M. E. (ed.): Postanesthesia Nursing. Rockville, Aspen Systems Corp., 1984.
20. Weisenberg, M.: Pain and pain control. Psychol. Bull., 84(5):1008–1044, 1977.
21. Wells, N.: The effect of relaxation on postoperative muscle tension and pain. Nurs. Res. 31940: 236–238, 1982.
22. White, P. F.: Use of parenteral narcotics in the postoperative period. Curr. Rev. Recov. Room Nurses, 15(7):118–123, 1985.

Postoperative Care After Ear, Nose, Throat, Neck, and Maxillofacial Surgery

SURGERY ON THE EAR

Otologic surgery has been revolutionized in recent years by antibiotics, the operating microscope, new and more delicate instruments, and an increased understanding of the anatomic structures involved (Fig. 20–1). New methods have been devised to treat hearing loss surgically by correcting conduction apparatus abnormalities, and selected patients can now be surgically relieved of the disabling symptoms of sensory-neural hearing loss.

Definitions

Fenestration: reconstruction of the outer and middle parts of the ear by means of a new drum or skin flap; creation of a new window into the internal ear mechanism by a newly established drum or skin flap.

Labyrinthectomy: opening of the labyrinth in order to destroy the inner ear in an attempt to relieve medically uncontrollable symptoms of unilateral Menière's syndrome.

Mastoidectomy: removal of mastoid air cells and of the tympanic membrane. Radical mastoidectomy also involves removing the malleus, incus, chorda tympani, and mucoperiosteal lining.

Myringotomy: incision of the tympanic membrane under direct vision.

Stapedectomy: removal of the stapes (Fig. 20–2A) followed by the placement of a prosthesis (Fig. 20–2B).

Tympanoplasty (myringoplasty): reconstruction of the tympanic membrane.

The immediate postoperative care for patients who have undergone surgery on the ear is generally the same, no matter what the procedure. Immediate postoperative complications are rare. Occasionally, excessive bleeding may occur, especially if a large blood vessel has been entered during the operation. If bleeding has occurred, it should be reported to the nurse who is to care for the patient when he or she is brought from the operating suite. Recovery assessment should follow the same format as for any patient undergoing general anesthesia. In addition, postoperative assessment should include testing for function of the facial nerve. Have the patient frown, smile, wrinkle the forehead, close the eyes, bare the teeth, and pucker the lips. Inability

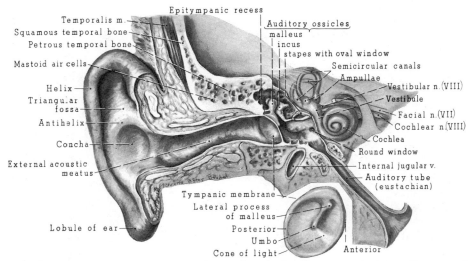

Figure 20–1. Frontal section through the outer, middle, and internal ear. (From Jacob, S. W., Francone, C. A., and Lossow, W. J.: Structure and Function in Man. 4th ed. Philadelphia, W. B. Saunders Co., 1978, p. 320.)

to perform these actions indicates injury to the facial nerve and should be appropriately indicated in the patient's chart and reported to the surgeon.

Aseptic techniques for all dressings and protection from infection are especially important for the patient who has undergone surgery on the ears, since infection could easily be transmitted to the meninges and the brain.

Postoperative positioning for the patient who has undergone ear surgery should be indicated by the surgeon. If position is un-

important, the patient should be allowed to assume a position of comfort, usually whichever side causes less vertigo. Generally, lying on the unoperated side is the most comfortable for the patient.

Since nausea and vertigo commonly occur in patients following ear surgery, side rails should remain raised on the bed. The patient may minimize discomfort by remaining in the position ordered, moving slowly, and avoiding quick, jerky movements. Advise the patient to take slow deep breaths through the mouth to minimize nausea.

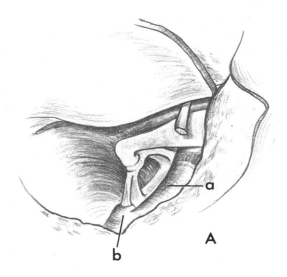

Figure 20–2. *A*, Stapedectomy. Adequate footplate exposure is achieved when (a) facial canal and (b) pyramidal process are seen.

Illustration continued on following page

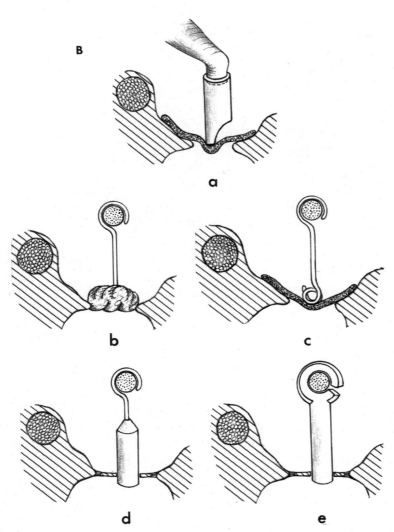

Figure 20–2 *Continued B,* Stapedectomy prostheses: (a) vein/polyethylene strut (Shea); (b) wire/fat (Schuknecht) (connective tissue preferred by author); (c) wire on compressed Gelfoam (House); (d) wire/Teflon piston; (e) Teflon piston (Shea). (From Paparella, M. M.: *In* Paparella, M. M., and Shumrick, D. A.: *Otolaryngology.* Vol. II. Philadelphia, W. B. Saunders Co., 1973, p. 165.)

Antimotion drugs and sedatives such as dimenhydrinate (Dramamine), diazepam (Valium), or chlorpromazine (Thorazine) may be ordered to prevent or treat nausea and vertigo. Avoid jarring the bed; when approaching the patient, place your hand on top of his or her head as a reminder not to turn toward you suddenly when you speak.

Special Considerations

Myringotomy. Position the patient so as to promote drainage from the ear. A small piece of sterile cotton may be placed loosely in the external ear to absorb the drainage that commonly occurs. This should be changed frequently to avoid contamination.

Mastoidectomy. A firm, bulky dressing is placed over the ear and held in place with a circular head bandage after mastoidectomy. This dressing may be reinforced, if necessary, but should be changed only by the physician. Minimal serosanguineous drainage may be expected, but bright bloody drainage should be reported to the surgeon.

The patient should be placed in a position of comfort, usually on the unoperated side. Grafts are often taken from the arm or leg for radical mastoidectomy and the donor sites should be assessed for drainage and treated according to local policy. Dizziness and vertigo are common following mastoidectomy and may be treated with the previously mentioned measures.

Tympanoplasty. Patients are usually positioned on the unoperated side after tympanoplasty. Care must be taken to keep bandages and grafts in place. The patient should be instructed not to blow the nose or cough in order to avoid disrupting grafts.

Fenestration. Fenestration is not commonly performed any longer; however, it may occasionally be the procedure of choice for patients who have lost effective hearing in both ears. It is a major surgical procedure and is usually performed under general anesthesia. Nausea, vertigo, and pain upon moving the jaws can be expected following fenestration. The patient is usually placed on the operated side to keep drainage from the operative site from entering the ear. The patient may be allowed to change position from the operated side to the back for nursing care and comfort.

Stapedectomy. Patients who have undergone stapedectomy usually return to the recovery room with ear packing in place, and this should not be disturbed. Occasionally, patients complain of vertigo postoperatively. Patients should be advised not to blow their noses.

SURGERY ON THE NOSE AND SINUSES

Nasal and sinus surgery is generally accomplished under local anesthesia, and many patients are returned directly to their rooms. Occasionally, however, this type of surgery is performed under general anesthesia, and in some institutions patients who have received local anesthesia for nasal and sinus surgery are returned to the recovery room for a short period of close observation.

The anatomy of the nasal cavity is shown in Figure 20–3.

Definitions

Intranasal antrostomy (antral window): creation of an opening in the lateral wall of the nose under the middle turbinate and the removal of the anterior end of the inferior turbinate.

Radical antrostomy (Caldwell-Luc operation): use of an incision into the canine fossa of the upper jaw and exposure of the antrum for removal of bony, diseased portions of the antral wall and contents of the sinus; establishment of drainage by means of a counteropening into the nose through the inferior meatus to establish a large opening in the nasoantral wall of the inferior meatus, which will ensure adequate gravity drainage and aeration and will permit removal of all diseased tissue in the sinus under direct vision.

SMR (submucosal resection): removal of either cartilaginous or osseous portions of the septum that lie between the flaps

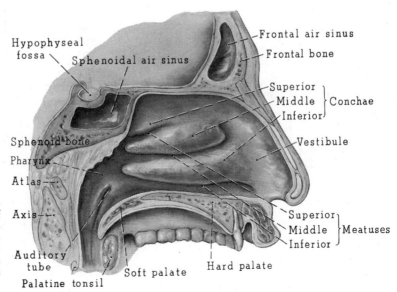

Figure 20–3. Nasal septum removed, showing lateral aspect of nasal cavity with conchae (turbinates). (From Jacob, S. W., Francone, C. A., and Lossow, W. J.: Structure and Function in Man. 4th ed. Philadelphia, W. B. Saunders Co., 1978, p. 422.)

of the mucous membrane and the perichondrium to establish an adequate partition between the left and right nasal cavities, thereby providing a clear airway for both the internal and external cavity and the parts of the nose.

Nasal Surgery

Conscious patients who return to the PACU after nasal surgery should be placed in a semi-Fowler position to promote drainage, reduce local edema, minimize discomfort, and facilitate respiration. Some postoperative serosanguineous drainage is expected; however, the nurse should observe closely for gross bleeding. The patient usually returns with one or both nostrils packed and a "mustache dressing" in place to catch any drainage from the packing (Figs. 20–4 and 20–5). The position of the nasal packs and the amount of drainage should be checked frequently. The mustache dressing may be changed as necessary; it is not unusual for it to be changed two to three times within four hours.

The back of the patient's throat should be checked frequently for blood. Frequent belching (from the accumulation of blood in the stomach) and frequent swallowing as well as the classic signs of hemorrhage, such as tachycardia, are additional signs of unusual bleeding. The patient should be instructed not to blow his or her nose and not to swallow secretions but rather to spit

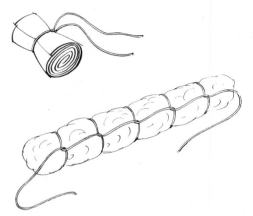

Figure 20–5. Postnasal packs. (From Sutton, A. L.: Bedside Nursing Techniques in Medicine and Surgery. 2nd ed. Philadelphia, W. B. Saunders Co., 1969.)

them into a basin. An ample supply of disposable tissues along with an emesis basin should be placed within easy reach of the patient.

Airway obstruction may occur if a postnasal pack accidentally slips out of place. A scissors, flashlight, and hemostat for emergency removal of nasal packing must be kept readily available at the patient's bedside.

Since nasal packing forces the patient to breathe through the mouth, rectal temperatures should be taken.

Fluids are usually withheld for two to four hours postoperatively to prevent development of nausea and vomiting. Occasionally, an antiemetic may be ordered to alleviate nausea and vomiting. Nasal packs make swallowing difficult and, therefore, only liquids are usually allowed until the packing is removed.

Mouth breathing, bleeding, and postnasal drainage create a dry offensive taste and odor in the patient's mouth, so once the gag reflex has returned, oral hygiene is a priority. Lemon-glycerine swabs or mouthwash may be used for mouth care and to make the patient more comfortable. A petrolatum-base ointment may be applied to the lips to prevent drying and cracking.

Ice packs across the nose may be ordered to minimize the pain, edema, discoloration, and bleeding. These ice packs should be small and lightweight and can be most easily made by filling a rubber glove par-

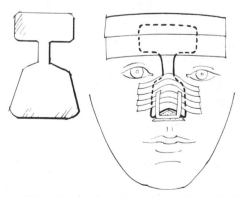

Figure 20–4. Nasal splint. (From Sutton, A. L.: Bedside Nursing Techniques in Medicine and Surgery. 2nd ed. Philadelphia, W. B. Saunders Co., 1969.)

tially with chipped ice. One advantage to using glove ice packs is that they can be fitted over the area of the face where needed.

Sinus Surgery

Following surgery on the sinuses, the patient usually returns with packing in place. It is not unusual for the upper lip and teeth to feel numb. Following general anesthesia, the patient should be positioned well on one side to prevent aspiration of drainage. The conscious patient should be placed in a semi-Fowler position, with the head elevated 45 degrees to promote drainage and minimize edema. The same general care, including oral hygiene and instructing the patient not to blow his or her nose, should be followed as for the patient with nasal surgery.

SURGERY ON THE TONGUE

Definitions
Ankyloglossia ("tongue-tie"): a short lingual frenulum that may cause difficult suckling in the infant and subsequent speech impairment. It is treated surgically by clipping of the frenulum.
Glossectomy: removal of the tongue.

The tongue occupies a large portion of the floor of the mouth. Surgery on the tongue generally involves excision of benign or malignant lesions, correction of congenital anomalies, or repair of traumatic lacerations. Lesions may be excised without associated neck dissection; however, when the lesion is malignant, surgical treatment usually involves a combined operation that may include radical neck dissection and resection of both the mandible and the tongue.

Local anesthesia is used for minor surgical procedures such as incision and longitudinal closure of the frenulum in ankyloglossia. Local infiltration is also used when repairing lacerations due to trauma. More extensive surgical procedures on the tongue require endotracheal anesthesia.

Postoperatively, the patient must be placed in a side-lying position with the head slightly dependent to allow for the drainage of secretions out of the mouth. When protective reflexes have returned, the patient should be placed in a sitting position to promote venous and lymphatic drainage.

Maintenance of the airway is the most crucial nursing concern. Suctioning equipment with soft-tipped catheters must be immediately available at the bedside. The patient should be instructed to allow saliva to run out of the mouth. A wick of gauze may be placed in the patient's mouth to assist in the elimination of secretions (Fig. 20–6). Swelling of the tongue may occur, causing obstruction of the airway. Therefore, an intubation tray should be handy.

Because of the vascular nature of the tongue and oral cavity, postoperative bleeding may be a problem. If excessive bleeding occurs, local pressure should be applied until the surgeon can be notified and repair effected in the operating room.

THROAT SURGERY

Definitions
Laryngectomy: removal of the larynx.
Total laryngectomy: complete removal of the cartilaginous larynx, the hyoid bone, and the strap muscles connected to the

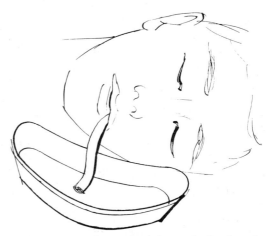

Figure 20–6. A wick to assist drainage of saliva from the mouth. (From Sutton, A. L.: Bedside Nursing Techniques in Medicine and Surgery. 2nd ed. Philadelphia, W. B. Saunders Co., 1969, p. 362.)

larynx and possible removal of the pre-epiglottic space along with the lesion (Fig. 20–7 and Table 20–1).

Laryngofissure: opening of the larynx for exploratory, excisional, or reconstructive procedures.

Laryngoscopy: direct examination of the interior of the larynx with a laryngoscope.

Tonsillectomy and adenoidectomy (T&A): surgical removal of the tonsils and adenoids (Fig. 20–8).

Tracheostomy: opening of the trachea and insertion of a cannula through a midline incision in the neck below the cricoid cartilage.

Surgery on the throat and neck is generally accomplished under general anesthesia. Aside from routine care and assessment, specific recovery room care for the patient who has undergone surgery on the throat revolves around (1) close observation for bleeding from the surgical site, (2) maintenance of a patent airway, (3) prevention of aspiration of secretions, and (4) awareness of possible cerebral complications that may develop.

The most common procedures are tonsillectomy, either alone or in combination with adenoidectomy, and tracheostomy.

Tonsillectomy and Adenoidectomy (T&A)

A great majority of patients undergoing T&A are children and young adults. Patients who have undergone T&A with local anesthesia or who return to the recovery room fully conscious may be positioned on the back with the head elevated 45 degrees. Patients who return following general anesthesia and who are unconscious or semiconscious must be placed in the tonsillar position—well over on the side with the face partially down. This may be accomplished by positioning a pillow under the patient's shoulder. In this position secretions are easily drained from the mouth. An oral airway should be left in place until the swallowing reflex has returned and the patient can handle secretions. The patient

should be advised to spit out secretions as much as possible and to try not to cough, clear the throat, blow the nose, or talk excessively. An ice collar may be applied to minimize pain and postoperative bleeding. The administration of cool, humidified air to the T&A patient provides comfort, helps minimize swelling, and supplies oxygen.

The most common complication of T&A is postoperative bleeding. Frequent swallowing, clearing of the throat, and vomiting of dark blood are indications of possible bleeding. The nurse should frequently check the back of the throat with a flashlight for trickling blood. If any of the cardinal symptoms of hemorrhage occurs, such as decreased blood pressure, tachycardia, pallor, or restlessness, the surgeon should be notified. Since the surgeon may wish to treat a bleeding episode in the recovery room, a tonsil tray should be available, containing the following equipment:

tongue depressors
1 Hurd retractor
2 mouth gags
1 Allis clamp
2 tonsil hemostats
1 short sponge forceps
1 pair scissors
sterile towels
epinephrine hydrochloride
   (Adrenalin) 1:1000
1 set tonsil suture needles
1 needle holder
1 glass medicine cup
1 sterile basin
cotton balls
tonsil tampons
1 soft rubber catheter
petrolatum

Appropriate illumination with a gooseneck lamp and a head mirror should be available, along with suction equipment. Postoperative bleeding after T&A can often be controlled by the application of vasoconstrictors via nasal packing with pressure. If significant bleeding occurs, however, the patient may have to return to the operating room for suturing or cauterizing of blood vessels.

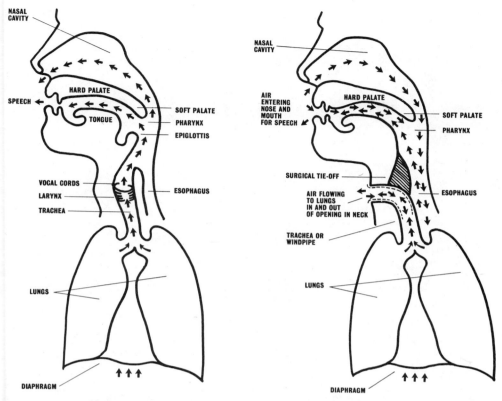

Figure 20–7. Total laryngectomy. (From Rehabilitating Laryngectomies. © 1960, American Cancer Society, Inc., 4R-50M-2/69-No. 4506-PS. *In* Luckmann, J., and Sorensen, K. C.: Medical-Surgical Nursing. 2nd ed. Philadelphia, W. B. Saunders Co., 1980, p. 2099.)

TABLE 20–1. Laryngectomy

Structures Removed	Structures Remaining	Postoperative Conditions
	Total Laryngectomy	
Hyoid bone Entire larynx (epiglottis, false cords, true cords) Cricoid cartilage Two or three rings of trachea	Tongue Pharyngeal walls Lower trachea	Loses voice; breathes through tracheostomy; no problem swallowing .
	Supraglottic or Horizontal Laryngectomy	
Hyoid bone Epiglottis False vocal cords	True vocal cords Cricoid cartilage Trachea	Normal voice; may aspirate occasionally, especially liquids; normal airway
	Vertical (or Hemi-) Laryngectomy	
One true vocal cord False cord Arytenoid One-half thyroid cartilage	Epiglottis One false cord One true vocal cord Cricoid	Hoarse but serviceable voice; normal airway; no problem swallowing
	Laryngofissure and Partial Laryngectomy	
One vocal cord	All other structures	Hoarse but serviceable voice; occasionally almost normal voice; no airway problem; no swallowing problem
	Endoscopic Removal of Early Carcinoma	
Part of one vocal cord	All other structures	May have a normal voice; no other problems

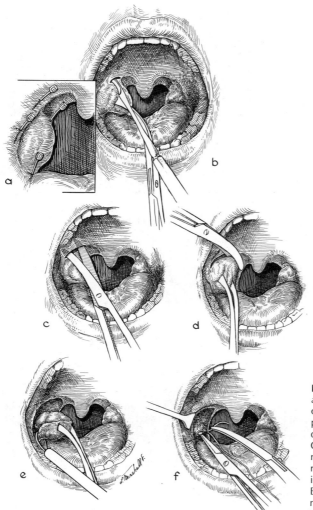

Figure 20–8. A method of dissection tonsillectomy. a, Points of infiltration for local anesthesia. b, Start of incision with tonsil knife at attachment of anterior pillar to the tonsil superiorly. c, Separation by scissor dissection of the superior pole of the tonsil. d, Continuation of dissection of tonsil from its attachment to pillars and bed of tonsillar fossa. e, Separation of the tonsil by snare at the lower pole, including the plica triangularis. f, Hemostasis. (From Boies, L. R., Hilger, J. A., and Priest, R. E.: Fundamentals of Otolaryngology. 4th ed. Philadelphia, W. B. Saunders Co., 1964.)

Once the patient is conscious and the reflexes have returned, ice chips and fluids may be offered. Large swallows of lukewarm fluids seem to cause the least discomfort to these patients. Sucking may precipitate bleeding, so a straw should not be offered to the patient. Oral hygiene, including alkaline mouthwash, may provide comfort. Apply petrolatum ointment to the lips to prevent drying and cracking.

Patients who have undergone T&A are especially prone to laryngeal spasms and must be observed very closely for patency of the airway. Airway obstruction may be created by swelling of the palate or nasopharynx, swelling in the retropharyngeal space, or swelling of the tongue and nose.

Laryngoscopy

Laryngoscopy is generally accomplished with only local anesthesia and appropriate sedation; however, occasionally general anesthesia must be used, especially in children. Since the gag and cough reflexes are obliterated with both types of anesthesia, these patients should be sent to the recovery room for a period of close observation. The patient should not be given anything orally until these reflexes have fully returned. The conscious patient may be placed in a semi-Fowler position, lying on either side. If unconscious, the patient should be placed in the tonsillar position to avoid aspiration.

These patients are especially susceptible to the development of laryngospasm, and the most important observations in the postlaryngoscopy patient are aimed at ascertaining the patency of the airway. Laryngeal stridor, dyspnea, or shortness of breath should alert the nurse to respiratory impairment, and the physician should be notified. Equipment for endotracheal intubation and emergency tracheostomy should be immediately available at the bedside should laryngeal edema or laryngospasm develop (see Table 20–2).

A certain amount of throat discomfort can be expected and may be relieved by the use of an ice collar. High humidity oxygen by mask will decrease throat irritation. After the cough and gag reflexes have returned, the patient may be allowed sips of warm normal saline, which is very soothing to irritated tissues. If severe pain occurs in either the throat or the chest, the physician should be notified. Watch for signs of hemorrhage, including coughing or regurgitation of blood, apprehension, and the classic signs of tachycardia and lowered blood pressure.

TABLE 20–2. Contents of Tracheostomy Tray

#3 knife handle with #15 blade
#11 blade
1 Metzenbaum scissors
1 one-point sharp scissors
1 curved tenotomy scissors
1 Collier needle holder
1 6-inch needle holder
2 Acson forceps
1 tissue forceps
1 dressing forceps
4 curved mosquito forceps
2 straight mosquito forceps
2 Allis clamps
4 small towel clips
1 sponge stick (or forceps)
1 probe
1 grooved director
1 Acson or Poole suction (without guard)
1 goiter right-angle retractor
1 tracheostomy hook
2 vein retractors
2 Army-Navy retractors
1 tonsil suction with tip screwed on
1 10-ml, 3-ring syringe
1 25-gauge × ⅝-inch needle
1 prep cup
1 medicine glass
Tracheostomy tubes, 1 ea, sizes 00–8
4 hand towels

In patients who have had a laryngoscopy and biopsy, or removal of polyps, vocal rest is very important. Coughing should be avoided if possible, and paper and pencil or "magic slate" should be made available so the patient can communicate without talking.

Tracheostomy

A tracheostomy, the making of an incision into the trachea and the insertion of a cannula, may be done as either an emergency or an elective procedure. Ideally, a tracheostomy is performed in the operating suite under controlled conditions. Tracheostomies are done to improve the airway and to provide access for suctioning of secretions from the trachea and bronchi. The recovery room nurse should know what condition necessitated the tracheostomy.

Recovery room personnel should anticipate the arrival of a tracheostomized patient and have the following items at the bedside: suction equipment; respirator; Ambu or anesthesia bag; extra sterile tracheostomy tray, including tracheostomy tubes of proper size, sterile forceps, tracheal hook, and Troussea tracheal dilator; sterile gauze squares; sterile scissors; tracheostomy ties; cleaning solutions for the tracheostomy tube and the incision; syringe; and hemostat for inflating the cuff of the tracheostomy tube (see Table 20–2).

A great variety of tracheostomy tubes are available, and the nurse should be familiar with those used in the particular institution. Several common varieties are shown in Figure 20–9.

Immediate postoperative care of the newly tracheostomized patient includes complete assessment of the patient's general condition as well as detailed attention to respiratory status and tracheostomy wound care. Because of the many nursing needs and the necessity of intensive ongoing respiratory assessment, the newly tracheostomized patient requires constant attendance.

Assessment of respiratory function should include all parameters mentioned in

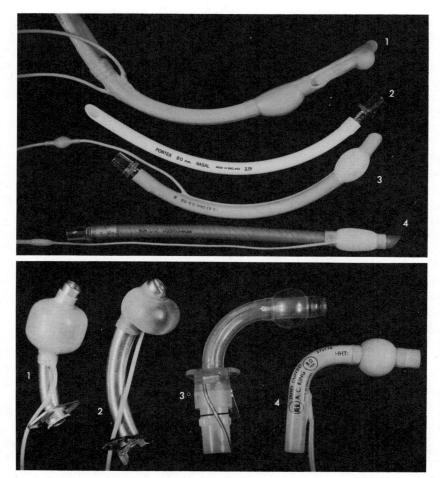

Figure 20–9. *Top,* Endotracheal tubes: (1) the Robert-Shaw double-lumen tube to isolate the flow to each lung. Note the individual inflatable cuffs for the trachea and the left bronchus; (2) the Portex nasotracheal tube, without attached cuff; (3) an orotracheal tube with attached inflatable cuff (very commonly used); and (4) the LA (Latex-Armored) tube. Note the spiral winding to prevent kinking.

Bottom, Tracheostomy tubes: (1) the Hollinger-tracheostomy tube with separately attached "Soft-Cuf" cuff. Note the relatively shallow curve of the tube and the evenly inflated (low-pressure) cuff; (2) the Jackson tracheostomy tube with separately attached cuff. Note the relatively sharp angle of the tube and the eccentrically inflated (high-pressure) cuff; (3) the Portex plastic tracheostomy tube with attached cuff which inflates evenly at relatively high pressure; and (4) the James tracheostomy tube with attached cuff which inflates evenly; this tube is occasionally used in short-necked patients. (From Sanderson, R. G. [ed.]: The Cardiac Patient. Philadelphia, W. B. Saunders Co., 1972.)

previous chapters. The nurse should auscultate the patient's chest frequently for normal bilateral breath sounds and report any adventitious sounds or indications of pulmonary congestion.

Suctioning and Tracheostomy Care. Patency of the newly created airway is vital, and frequent suctioning is necessary owing to increased secretions from the tracheobronchial tree as a result of trauma. Suctioning the tracheostomy must be sterile and atraumatic—a sterile disposable catheter and glove should be used for each procedure. A suction catheter in a plastic sleeve provides a means of suctioning without the use of gloves and is most convenient for use in the recovery room. Catheters should be smooth and small enough to pass easily into the lumen of the tracheostomy tube without obstructing it.

As with any suctioning technique, the patient should be hyperventilated with increased FiO_2 both before and after the procedure. To suction, insert the catheter 6 to

8 inches into the tracheostomy tube. Do not apply suction during insertion. Apply suction intermittently by occluding the Y connector with the thumb, at the same time slowly withdrawing the catheter in a twisting motion. Suctioning should not continue for longer than 5 seconds. Time should be allotted between each suctioning for adequate oxygenation of the patient. Suctioning often stimulates forceful coughing, which is effective in bringing up secretions, so the nurse should be prepared to wipe expelled secretions away from the tracheostomy tube orifice with plain gauze squares. To determine the effectiveness of the suctioning, the chest should be auscultated immediately afterward.

If deep suctioning is indicated, a coudé-tip catheter should be used. Insert the catheter with the tip pointing in the direction of the mainstem bronchus to be suctioned. Recent evidence indicates that positioning the patient's head to the left or the right has little effect, if any, on which bronchus will be entered.

If the patient's secretions are exceptionally thick, the physician may order instillation of 3 to 5 ml of normal saline (sterile) into the tracheostomy tube to help loosen secretions and promote cough. Although this is a common procedure, it is questionable whether or not it is actually effective, and if the normal saline is not immediately removed by suctioning, it may produce the effects of any inhaled fluid as well as acting as a contaminant. More effective measures to ensure liquefaction of secretions include providing inspired air that is well humidified and making sure that the patient is well hydrated.

Immediate postoperative care of the newly tracheostomized patient also includes care and cleaning of the tracheostomy tube, which may be necessary as often as every hour. A variety of methods may be used to clean the inner cannula of the tracheostomy tube, including normal saline and hydrogen peroxide or 2 percent sodium bicarbonate solution. A small test tube brush or pipe cleaners may be used to scrub off sticky crusts of mucus. Whatever the method used, it must be a sterile procedure and no supplies should be used that may leave lint or other debris, which might be inhaled by the patient, on the cannula.

Wound drainage from the tracheostomy is generally minimal. Soiling of the tracheostomy dressing occurs, however, from secretions and sweating. The dressings should be changed as often as necessary and the skin kept clean and dry to prevent maceration and infection. The skin around the stoma should be cleansed with hydrogen peroxide and normal saline and dried with sterile gauze pads, and an antibiotic ointment such as bacitracin applied. The tracheostomy dressing should be plain gauze with the edges bound and should have no cotton filling or loose strings. Special tracheostomy "pants" that fit over the tracheostomy tube and have all edges sewn make the best dressing. Sterile gauze may be cut halfway to the center and fitted over the tube; however, this has the disadvantage of cut edges that may fray and allow bits of gauze to enter the wound or the trachea (Fig. 20–10).

Fabric tapes or ties are used to secure the tracheostomy tube in place. These should be checked frequently to ensure the proper tension. If they are too tight they will be uncomfortable for the patient and may compress the external jugular veins. If they are too loose, the cannula will slide up and down in the trachea or even be expelled. When the tapes are tied so that one finger

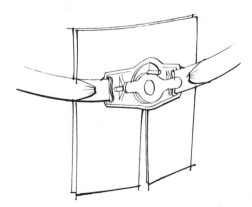

Figure 20–10. Gauze square cut to serve as tracheostomy dressing. (From Sutton A. L.: Bedside Nursing Techniques in Medicine and Surgery. 2nd ed. Philadelphia, W. B. Saunders Co., 1969.)

can easily slip underneath, the tension is right.

Complications. Complications of a tracheostomy do occur, and recovery room nurses should be especially astute in observing symptoms of danger. The most common complication is respiratory obstruction due to external pressure, foreign bodies, tracheal edema, or excessive secretions. If suctioning does not relieve airway obstruction, the tracheostomy tube may be removed immediately, the tracheal stoma held open with a tracheal dilator and hook or forceps (Fig. 20–11), and the surgeon or anesthesiologist summoned.

Occasionally, a tube is coughed out either because the ties are not sufficiently tight or because the tube is too short. If a tube is accidentally expelled, it must be reinserted by persons qualified to do so. In some institutions, nurses practice changing tracheostomy tubes under the supervision of physicians so that, if accidental expulsion should occur in the PACU, the nurse will be skilled in replacement. If the tube cannot be inserted easily, the stoma should be held open and the surgeon called. Misplacement or displacement of the tube is a common complication and must be corrected immediately (Fig. 20–12).

Respiratory insufficiency may also occur owing to obstruction below the tracheostomy tube. Respiratory adventitious sounds, unequal lung expansion, and marked respiratory efforts, including supraclavicular, intercostal, and substernal retractions, should alert the nurse to this problem and the physician should be notified.

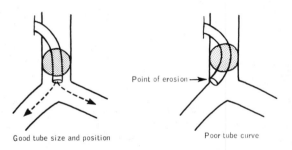
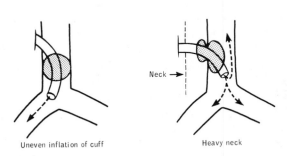
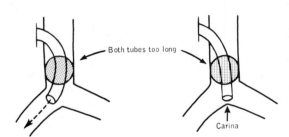

Good tube size and position

Point of erosion →   Poor tube curve

Neck →   Uneven inflation of cuff   Heavy neck

← Both tubes too long

Carina

Figure 20–12. Tracheostomy tube positions and factors affecting them. (From Murphy, E. R.: Intensive nursing care in a respiratory unit. Nursing Clin. N. Am. 3:433, 1968.)

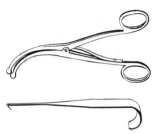

Figure 20–11. Tracheal dilator and hook. (From Sutton, A. L.: Bedside Nursing Techniques in Medicine and Surgery. 2nd ed. Philadelphia, W. B. Saunders Co., 1969.)

Some bloody secretions from the tracheal stoma may be expected in the immediate postoperative period, but frank bleeding is abnormal and the surgeon should be notified. Sometimes there is bleeding from a thyroid vein or other neck vessel next to the tube, and blood, which runs down into the trachea, is sprayed about with every cough. This is usually not serious and can often be controlled with local packing with petrolatum gauze. Occasionally, however, serious bleeding does occur and the patient must be taken back to the operating room where the wound is reopened and the bleeding vessel ligated.

Subcutaneous emphysema may occur as a

complication of tracheostomy if the wound is sutured too tightly about the tracheostomy tube and air can enter the subcutaneous tissues, or it may be the result of an overly large incision or a partially obstructed tube. Although subcutaneous emphysema is annoying, it is usually not serious and generally clears after several days. If the nurse notices a crackling sensation under the skin of the neck, chest, or face of the patient, it should be reported to the surgeon since removal of a suture or two may readily correct this problem.

It should be noted that the complications of tracheostomy in infants and children are almost always more serious, since the relative size of the airway is smaller and there is very little tolerance for any obstruction.

Laryngectomy

Partial laryngectomy is the surgical treatment of choice for patients with a limited malignant process of the vocal cords. It is commonly performed through a laryngofissure, and tracheostomy is usually performed concomitantly to assure a good airway during the immediate postoperative period. Postoperative nursing care is essentially the same as that for a post-tracheostomy patient.

Subcutaneous emphysema is not uncommon postoperatively and should be reported to the surgeon. Laryngectomy patients have trouble swallowing and need frequent suctioning and reassurance.

Supraglottic laryngectomy is done for carcinoma of the epiglottis and adjacent structures above the level of the true vocal cords. A tracheostomy is mandatory for these patients; they also have a great deal of difficulty swallowing and require close observation and assistance with elimination of saliva and other secretions.

Total laryngectomy is reserved for patients with advanced carcinoma of the true cords. Tracheostomy is always performed. Some means of communication should be established preoperatively for postoperative use.

The primary nursing concern after laryngectomy is maintenance of an adequate airway. Tracheostomy care, as previously dis-

cussed, should be deftly carried out and the air well humidified. The patient will need frequent suctioning in the immediate postoperative period, not only of the tracheostomy but also of the nose and mouth, since he cannot blow his nose and may have difficulty spitting. Frequent mouth care will provide additional comfort, and a petrolatum ointment should be applied to the lips to prevent drying and cracking.

Postoperatively, the patient should be positioned on the side until full consciousness is regained. When conscious, the patient may be positioned in a low semi-Fowler position with the head elevated about 30 degrees. This position will promote drainage, minimize edema, prevent uncomfortable pressure on suture lines, and facilitate respirations.

Postoperative pain should be minimal and can be alleviated with analgesics such as rectal aspirin or acetaminophen. Narcotics should be avoided, since they depress respirations and the cough reflex.

Dressings should be checked frequently for excessive drainage and reinforced or changed as necessary. Sometimes drainage catheters are placed under the wound flaps to remove fluid from the potential dead space left after removal of the larynx and related structures. Drainage catheters must be connected to a constant vacuum source at 40 to 60 mm Hg, and free drainage must be maintained within the system. Excessive bloody drainage should be reported to the surgeon. The most common site for hemorrhage is the base of the tongue.

Laryngectomy patients are frequently very apprehensive upon awakening and should have someone in close attendance at all times. Although prepared for their loss of voice preoperatively, the first experiences of being voiceless and unable to call for help are always very frightening. A bell to ring or other noisemaker is more assuring in this case than the routine pencil-and-paper communication system.

RADICAL NECK SURGERY

The radical neck operation itself is a relatively simple procedure involving removal of all the subcutaneous fat, lymphatic channels, and some of the superficial muscles within a prescribed area of the neck (Fig. 20–13). Generally, the procedure involves the removal of the sternocleidomastoid muscle, omohyoid muscle, internal and external jugular veins, and all lymphatic tissue on one side of the neck. It is the purposeful resection of the eleventh cranial nerve (spinal accessory nerve) that causes atrophy of the large trapezius muscle. In the modified neck dissection, the accessory nerve and the internal jugular vein are spared.

Postoperative nursing care after radical neck surgery is somewhat less demanding than after laryngectomy, since these patients do not have a tracheostomy and can talk and eat normally. The patient should be placed in a low semi-Fowler position with the head elevated 30 to 45 degrees to improve venous return. Pillows must be used cautiously when positioning patients to avoid restricting venous return or compressing the bases of pedicle flaps. Venous

congestion, when present, gives the patient's face a purplish hue. This can be differentiated from cyanosis due to inadequate ventilation by observing the color of the extremities to confirm good circulation. Postoperative pain is usually minimal after radical neck dissection and can be managed with analgesics such as aspirin or propoxyphene (Darvon). Occasionally, a stronger analgesic such as pentazocine and hydrochloride (Talwin) may be used.

Dressings are minimal. Skin flaps are secured over drainage tubes, which should be connected to constant suction at 40 to 60 mm Hg. The suction catheters constantly working under the skin flaps suck them firmly against the neck. Approximately 70 to 120 ml of serosanguineous drainage can be expected the day of operation. This is drastically reduced the second day and becomes minimal (below 30 ml) the third day. If the dressing soaks through with blood, notify the surgeon at once.

Edema of the recurrent laryngeal nerve

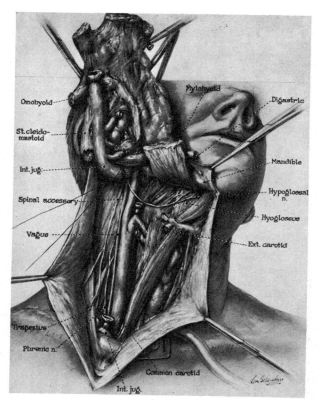

Figure 20–13. Drawing showing the extent of the usual radical neck dissection. The specimen is retracted superiorly. As is shown, resection of the posterior belly of the digastric muscle permits high ligation of the internal jugular vein and also facilitates dissection around the hypoglossal nerve. (From Edgerton, M. T., and DeVito, R. T. In Converse, J. M. [ed.]: Reconstructive Plastic Surgery. Volume III. Philadelphia, W. B. Saunders Co., 1964.)

and of the nerves to the pharynx may cause difficulty in swallowing and in expectorating secretions; therefore, frequent gentle suctioning of oral secretions may be needed. Extreme care must be taken to avoid any trauma to the internal suture lines. A gauze wick placed in the corner of the patient's mouth can alleviate the annoyance of constant dribbling of mucus and saliva. Mouth care is important for the comfort of this patient and can be accomplished by any of the conventional methods.

Complications. Edema of the lower part of the face on the same side as the surgery is to be expected. Lower facial paralysis may occur, owing to injury of the facial nerve during dissection. The most common complication following radical neck dissection is hemorrhage. This is most often due to inadequate hemostasis in the immediate postoperative period. The most serious complication is rupture of the carotid artery ("carotid blowout"). Fortunately, this is not common and occurs almost exclusively when radical neck dissection is combined with total laryngectomy. It is more likely to occur in a patient who has had a course of radiation therapy preoperatively or who has a fistula that bathes the carotid artery in secretions. If the danger of a blowout of the carotid is present, all personnel should be aware of it and know what to do if it occurs.

If a carotid blowout occurs, digital pressure with gauze pads, bath towels, or anything available should be applied immediately and help summoned. Intravenous fluids must be started immediately if they are not already infusing. Fluids should be administered at an increased rate to replace loss and combat shock. Inflate the cuff on the tracheostomy tube and perform tracheal suctioning to prevent aspiration of blood. Most importantly, maintain a patent airway and administer oxygen. Patients on "carotid precautions," i.e., those who may suffer this complication, should be typed and cross-matched for whole blood, and appropriate emergency equipment, including gauze pads, vascular clips, and suture ties, should be immediately available at the bedside.

Reconstruction in Head and Neck Cancer

Any of a large variety of reconstructive procedures may be employed to re-establish both contour and function after the removal of large areas of the head and neck for malignant disease. Skin grafts have largely been replaced with skin flaps or muscle-skin combined flaps which can cover extensive areas both inside and outside the neck. These flaps provide lining of the throat or mouth and can also replace excised skin on the external surfaces. The commonly used flaps are the pectoralis major muscle-skin unit and the deltopectoral flap, both from the anterior chest area. In rare instances, a "free flap" may be used. This flap is usually a skin-muscle flap which is moved a long distance from one area of the body to another. To be successful, this type of flap requires the microsurgical repair of its tiny artery and vein with an artery and vein in its new location. In general, these reconstructive flaps must be free of any pressure or dressings. A light coat of antibacterial ointment is usually applied along the suture lines and the area is frequently observed for color, warmth, and bleeding. Since these flaps depend on a single small artery and vein, any kinking or external pressure may result in death of the flap.

MAXILLOFACIAL SURGERY

The care of patients with extensive maxillofacial surgery follows the principles outlined above for tracheostomy care, care after laryngectomy, and care following radical neck dissection. Care of these patients is very demanding, and attention to detail is the basis for the prevention of complications.

Maxillofacial surgery may be required to correct trauma and fractures or to correct congenital skeletal deformities. Following this type of surgery the patient will be in intermaxillary fixation (IMF) with the jaws wired shut. Care revolves around protection of the airway.

Some additional emergency equipment is

required at the bedside of patients who are admitted with IMF, including wire cutters, a suture set, additional nasal airways, small suction catheters, and gauze pads. Upon admission of the patient, the surgeon should review placement of the IMF wires with the nurse. A line drawing of these wires indicating which ones to cut in case of extreme emergency (e.g., cardiac or respiratory arrest) should be posted at the head of the bed.

Preoperative preparation of the patient undergoing IMF is particularly important and should include instructions on how to clear secretions or remove vomitus while remaining in IMF. The patient should also be taught how to use the suction catheter. These instructions will have to be repeated frequently in the PACU as the patient recovers. Having the jaws wired closed is a frightening experience for any patient, no matter how well prepared. Blood, emesis, lingual and pharyngeal edema, hematoma formation, or laryngospasm may further compromise the oral airway, which is already obstructed up to 90 percent by fixation of the jaws. Reassurance is provided by maintaining proximity to the patient, ensuring a means to attract attention, and explaining fully all treatments and procedures.

The patient will arrive in the PACU with a nasotracheal tube in place. Extubation should not be considered until the patient is fully awake and reflexes have returned sufficiently to allow handling of secretions. A soft nasal airway may be inserted following extubation to assist in maintaining a patent airway.

Observe closely for bleeding. Some oozing of blood is normal but excessive amounts should be reported to the surgeon. Frequent gentle suctioning with a small catheter will assist in keeping the airway clear by removing blood and saliva. The patient may be more comfortable doing this alone when able. It is reassuring to these patients to have a suction catheter in hand for use as necessary.

Vomiting and subsequent aspiration is a significant risk for this patient. A nasogastric tube is frequently used to reduce the likelihood of nausea and vomiting. Ensure that it is correctly positioned and patent. Antiemetics should be administered as necessary, and pain should be treated promptly to prevent the development of nausea and vomiting.

Despite all efforts to prevent it, vomiting may occur. If the patient is still drowsy, he should be turned immediately to the lateral or semiprone position and the emesis suctioned out via the nose or mouth. If the patient is awake, assist him to sit up, lean over, and allow emesis to flow out of the mouth and nose. Retract the cheeks by holding them out with the fingers. Most importantly, repeat instructions and reassurances quietly but confidently to keep the patient calm. It is rarely necessary to cut the wires.

The patient should be positioned with the head of the bed elevated 30 degrees to assist in maintaining the airway by controlling edema. Ice packs are usually ordered postoperatively to assist in controlling edema and promote comfort. A surgical glove partially filled with cracked ice can be used, or ice collars can be molded to the jaws, chin, or nose. Iced saline gauze pads may be applied to the eyes.

Petrolatum ointment or other emollient cream should be applied to the lips and corners of the mouth to relieve tenderness and prevent drying and cracking. Dental wax can be molded and applied to protruding wires which are quite irritating to the oral mucosa.

When the patient is fully awake and protective reflexes have sufficiently returned, rinsing the mouth with warm saline will provide additional comfort. The patient may then also have small sips of liquids.

REFERENCES

1. Arnet, G., and Basehore, L. M.: Dentofacial reconstruction. Am. J. Nurs., *84*(12):1488–1490, 1984.
2. Burke, S.: Tracheostomy: Common contemporary application of an ancient surgical technique. Lamp, *36*:38–43, 1979.
3. Darvich-Kodjouri, C.: Nursing care of the

patient with a new tracheostomy. Curr. Rev. Recov. Room Nurses, 3(7):18–23, 1985.
4. Frost, C. M., and Frost, D. E.: Nursing care of patients in intermaxillary fixation. Heart Lung, 12(5):524–528, 1983.
5. Lyons, R. J., and Coren, D. A.: The head and neck patient. AORN J., 40(5):751–760, 1984.
6. Saunders, W. H., Havener, W. H., Keith, C. F., et al.: Nursing Care in Eye, Ear, Nose, and Throat Disorders. St. Louis, C. V. Mosby Co., 1979.
7. Tedesco, M. B.: Total nursing care of the vestibular nerve section patient . . . Meniere's disease. J. Neurosurg. Nurs., 12:2–6, 1980.

21

Postoperative Care Following Eye Surgery

The assessment and care of patients who have had surgery on their eyes are always a challenge for the PACU nurse. As with all other types of patients, the PACU nurse must consider not only the elements of surgery performed, but the whole patient. Eye surgery is performed on patients of all ages. The special precautions that apply to specific age groups must therefore be taken into account. For the elderly patient, it is wise to keep in mind that those who need an operation on the eyes may also have hypertension, cancer, diabetes, emphysema, or congestive heart failure. In addition, the PACU nurse's assessment and care of the ophthalmic patient will be greatly influenced by the type of anesthesia used intraoperatively.

Many eye surgeries are performed under local anesthesia and more and more often are being performed as day surgery. Cataract surgery, after which few restrictions are necessary, is often performed on an outpatient basis. Postoperative care instructions should be discussed with the patient and a significant other both preoperatively and postoperatively. Instructions should also be written so that they may be reviewed as necessary after discharge. Special care of the patient undergoing day surgery is outlined in Chapter 34.

The anatomy of the normal eye is shown in Figure 21–1.

Definitions

Blepharoplasty: surgical removal of a segment of skin from the eyelid.

Cataract: an opacity of the lens. Surgical treatment consists of removal of the lens.

Chalazion: a chronic granulomatous inflammation of one or more of the meibomian glands in the tarsal plate of the eyelid. Surgical treatment consists of incision and curettage.

Dacryocystitis: infection of the lacrimal sac.

Dacryocystorhinostomy: creation of a new pathway from the lacrimal sac to the nasal cavity.

Dermatochalasis: relaxation of the skin of the eyelid due to atrophy. Surgical treatment is blepharoplasty.

Epiphora: Excess tearing. May be caused by blocked lacrimal drainage system. Surgical treatment for epiphora and dacryocystitis caused by blockage is probing of the lacrimal duct.

Ectropion: eversion of the margin of the eyelid. Surgical treatment is to shorten the lower lid in a horizontal direction.

Entropion: inversion of the margin of the eyelid; usually affects the lower lid, but may affect the upper lid. Surgical treat-

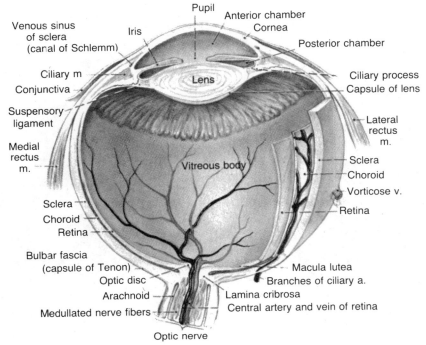

Figure 21–1. Anatomy of the normal eye. Midsagittal section through the eyeball showing layers of retina and blood supply. (After Lederle.) (From Jacob, S. W., et al.: Structure and Function in Man. 6th ed. Philadelphia, W. B. Saunders Co., 1982.)

ment involves either removing a base triangle of skin, muscle, and tarsus, and suturing the edges together to evert the lid margin, or exposing the orbicular muscle, dividing it, and suturing it to the lower border of the tarsus.

Enucleation: removal of the entire eyeball after the eye muscles and optic nerve have been severed.

Evisceration of the eye: removal of the contents of the eye, leaving the sclera intact and the muscles attached to the sclera.

Exenteration of the eye: removal of all orbital contents.

Glaucoma: a disease of the eye characterized by increased intraocular pressure. Surgical treatment is aimed at establishing an evacuation route for outflow of aqueous fluid.

Goniotomy: surgery for congenital glaucoma wherein the trabecular meshwork is incised.

Iridectomy: removal of a section of iris tissue (Fig. 21–2).

IOL implant: intraocular lens implant (Fig. 21–3).

Keratoplasty: corneal transplant (Figs. 21–4 and 21–5).

Pterygium: a fleshy triangular encroachment on the cornea. Surgical treatment is by excision.

Ptosis: drooping of the upper eyelid. Surgical treatment involves either elevating the lid with a sling or shortening the levator muscle of the lid (levator resection).

Retinopexy: surgical correction of retinal detachment (Fig. 21–6) by sealing the hole. Sealing is accomplished by causing scar formation by heat, electrical current, or cold.

Scleral buckle: surgical correction of a retinal detachment by compressing the sclera in order to rejoin the underlying retinal pigment epithelium to the detached sensory retina. Used in conjunction with retinopexy.

Strabismus: condition in which the eyes are not simultaneously directed toward the

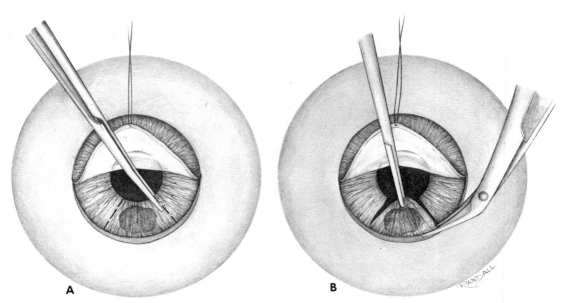

Figure 21–2. Technique of sector iridectomy for iris tumor. *A*, A limbal incision has been made for 180°, and two radial cuts are made from the pupillary margin to the iris root (dotted lines). *B*, After the radial incisions are done, the iris is cut at its base to free it from the anterior portion of the ciliary body. (From Spaeth, G. L.: Ophthalmic Surgery: Principles and Practice. Philadelphia, W. B. Saunders Co., 1982.)

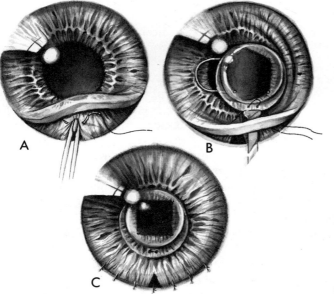

Figure 21–3. Implantation of medallion intra-ocular lens, illustrating (*A*) placement of iris suture, (*B*) insertion of implant, and (*C*) appearance of implant after closure of incision. (From Spaeth, G. L.: Ophthalmic Surgery: Principles and Practice. Philadelphia, W. B. Saunders Co., 1982.)

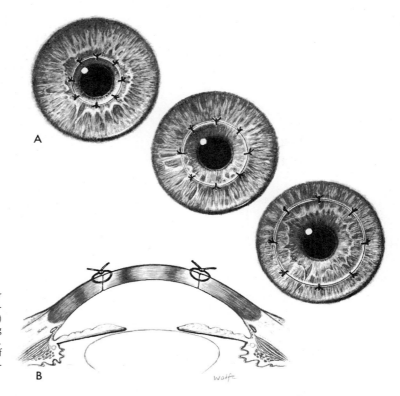

Figure 21–4. Corneal transplant or keratoplasty. (*A*) Grafts of three different sizes. Interrupted sutures. (*B*) Sagittal section of cornea showing full-thickness graft. (From Scheie, H. G. and Albert, D. M.: Textbook of Ophthalmology. 9th ed. Philadelphia, W. B. Saunders Co., 1977.)

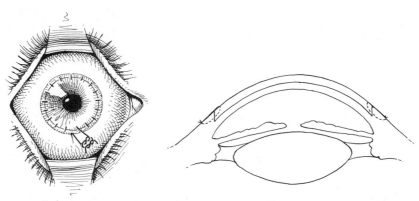

Figure 21–5. Suturing of graft. (From Spaeth, G. L.: Ophthalmic Surgery: Principles and Practice. Philadelphia, W. B. Saunders Co., 1982.)

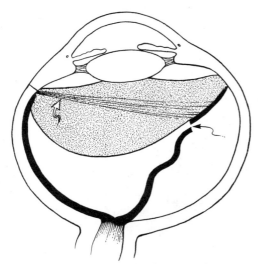

Figure 21–6. Retinal detachment following penetrating injury. The break (thin arrow) is caused by contraction of fibrovascular tissue that has proliferated from the entry wound (open arrow). (From Spaeth, G. L.: Ophthalmic Surgery: Principles and Practice. Philadelphia, W. B. Saunders Co., 1982.)

same object. *Esotropia* is inward deviation of the eyes, and *exotropia* is outward deviation. Surgical treatment involves changing the relative strength of individual muscles either by resection (the shortening of a muscle by removal of part of the tendon) or by recession (the surgical

transfer of a muscle insertion backward from the original attachment on the eye).

Trabeculectomy: creation of a drainage channel from the anterior chamber to the subconjunctival space; used to treat intractable glaucoma.

Vitrectomy: surgical removal of vitreous from the eye, usually to clear opacified vitreous for better visualization or to sever vitreous traction bands (Fig. 21–7).

ANESTHESIA

Ophthalmic procedures are often performed under local anesthesia, and many patients are treated in the day care or ambulatory surgery center. For cooperative adult patients, local anesthesia is generally preferred in order to avert the restlessness and nausea or vomiting that may occur after general anesthesia. Infants, children, uncooperative or particularly anxious patients, and psychotic persons usually require general anesthesia. General anesthesia is also indicated when a local anesthetic might accentuate an eye problem, when surgery is to be performed on extraocular muscles, or when the surgery planned is extensive, as in enucleation or evisceration. The ophthalmic patient who has undergone

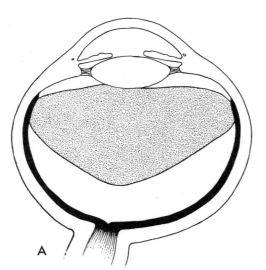
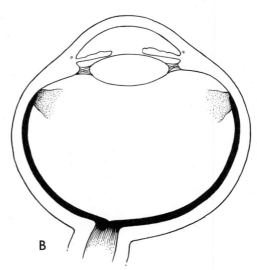

Figure 21–7. *A*, Simple vitreous hemorrhage with complete posterior vitreous detachment. *B*, Central vitreous removed by vitrectomy. (From Spaeth, G. L.: Ophthalmic Surgery: Principles and Practice. Philadelphia, W. B. Saunders Co., 1982.)

general anesthesia must be assessed and cared for as previously described for any general anesthesia patient. The special precaution for these patients is that modifications in care must be made to prevent stress on the eyes and surrounding musculature (see Fig. 21–1).

NURSING CARE
Positioning

The patient will usually arrive in the PACU awake. The nurse should begin to orient the patient as soon as he or she enters the PACU. It is particularly important to alert the patient when about to be moved and to prepare the patient for being touched in order to avoid any startle reflexes. Every caution should be observed when transferring the patient from stretcher to bed to avoid bumping and jarring. Movement should be kept to a minimum and should be slow and smooth.

To prevent pressure on the operated eye, the patient should be positioned on his or her back or on the unaffected side. The patient who has had surgical correction of a detached retina may require special positioning of the head to allow proper approximation and healing of the retinal hold. The surgeon should provide explicit positioning instructions for all special cases.

If the patient has had only one eye operated on or has only one eye bandaged, it is important to determine just how much sight exists in the unaffected eye before formulating a plan of care. It is not safe to assume that the patient can see with the unoperated eye. The nurse should tell the patient exactly what to expect and what will be expected of him or her. The patient is instructed not to move the head or eyes and to remain as quiet as possible.

Cardiorespiratory Assessment and Care

Assessment of the cardiorespiratory system should proceed as previously described. Vital signs should be assessed and the stir-up regimen begun. The real challenge here is keeping the patient's lungs clear without increasing intraocular pressure. Deep rhythmic breaths at frequent intervals will assist in the prevention of atelectasis. The nurse should spend more time than usual coaching this type of patient in deep inspirations since coughing must be avoided. If the patient feels the urge to cough, help him concentrate on his breathing, which may help dispel that feeling. Sucking on ice chips, throat lozenges, or hard candy may soothe the throat and prevent coughing. In some cases codeine or meperidine may be administered to control coughs. If coughing does occur and cannot be controlled, the surgeon must be notified.

Vomiting, sneezing, straining, or any exertion on the part of the patient may increase intraocular pressure which may be damaging to the affected eye. These reactions must therefore be avoided, if at all possible. As a precaution against the development of nausea and vomiting after general anesthesia, oral fluids and diet are routinely delayed for a short time. Some ophthalmologists routinely order an antiemetic drug for the first 24 postoperative hours to allay nausea and subsequent vomiting. The patient should be instructed to alert the nurse immediately if he or she begins to feel nauseated so that an antiemetic such as prochlorperazine (Compazine), trimethobenzamide (Tigan), or dimenhydrinate (Dramamine) can be administered without delay. In addition, deep breathing and sucking on ice chips or hard candy may help alleviate nausea. If vomiting occurs in spite of these interventions, the surgeon should be notified. Pain, along with nausea and vomiting, may indicate intraocular hemorrhage which requires immediate intervention by the ophthalmologist.

The exertion of hard crying, often a problem with children and infants, must be prevented. Some children will respond well to being held by the nurse. If this is not successful, it may be necessary to ignore the usual "no visitors" policy of the PACU and to allow the mother or father to hold the child.

No patient should be restrained, since exertion against the restraints will increase intraocular pressure. If a child cannot be persuaded to leave the eyes alone, straight elbow splints may be applied. This allows the child to move his or her arms about but not to reach the eyes (Fig. 21–8). In some cases, in both children and adults, tranquilizers may be required to ensure patient cooperation and a smooth recovery course.

Pain

Pain is not common after most eye surgery. The eye is usually quite comfortable, owing to the intraoperative use of topical steroids and cholinergic blockers, such as atropine, which paralyze the ciliary muscle. In addition, medications in ointment form are often applied to the eye prior to patching. These ointments soothe the eye and promote comfort.

Complaints of itching, scratchy or grating feelings, or a "pins and needles" sensation should be interpreted as pain and treated as such. Eye discomfort that may occur with more common ophthalmic procedures can usually be controlled with acetaminophen (Tylenol), propoxyphene hydrochloride (Darvon), and similar analgesics. Patients undergoing posterior vitrectomy may experience significant pain. The administration of narcotic analgesia as well as the

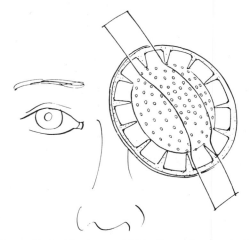

Figure 21–9. Metal eye shield. (From Sutton, A. L.: Bedside Nursing Techniques in Medicine and Surgery. 2nd ed. Philadelphia, W. B. Saunders Co., 1969.)

application of ice packs to the operative site should control the pain. If meperidine (Demerol), codeine phosphate, or other opiates are necessary for pain relief, they should be used in conjunction with an antiemetic, since they frequently cause nausea and subsequent vomiting when used alone. Significant pain that is not relieved with the prescribed analgesics is so unusual that investigation by the surgeon is warranted.

Dressings

Dressings are often not required, especially after relatively minor procedures or plastic ophthalmic surgery. Hemorrhage or excessive discharge is uncommon. A slight, blood-tinged, watery discharge from the eyes is not unusual and may be gently wiped from the face, taking care not to apply pressure to the eye. Although an infrequent occurrence, hemorrhage may be a problem after enucleation, exenteration, or orbital surgery. If bleeding occurs in the PACU the surgeon may be able to control it with pressure, but in some cases the patient may have to return to the operating room.

Frequently, one or both of the eyes are bandaged. If bandages are present, these should not be disturbed. The patient must be prevented from disturbing the bandage or inadvertently rubbing the eyes.

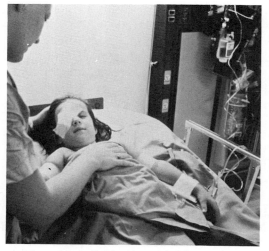

Figure 21–8. Child with straight elbow splints.

Following enucleation, a firm pressure dressing is applied for 48 to 72 hours. After surgical correction of a retinal detachment, both eyes are bandaged to prevent quick eye movements. Whenever both eyes are bandaged, extra care must be taken to orient the patient and to provide reassurance. Frequently metal eye shields (Fig. 21–9) are placed over the dressing as an additional protection for the eye. Dressings should not be changed unless ordered by the surgeon, and if accidentally dislodged, they should be replaced and the physician notified. The tape used to hold eye patches or shields in place should not extend to the maxilla, or movement of the jaw may cause disruption of the dressing.

Psychological/Emotional Assessment and Care

Caring for the patient who has undergone ophthalmic surgery requires not only finely honed physical assessment skills, but also a great deal of sensitivity to the meaning of sight, and a creative approach to promoting comfort and preventing complications.

Postoperative care for the patient who has undergone eye surgery involves a great deal of empathy and reassurance. Our eyes and the sense of sight are very precious—when sight is threatened by disease or surgery, the patient is understandably anxious and apprehensive. Injuries, particularly those produced by imbedded foreign bodies, may provoke even greater anxiety for the patient who often goes to surgery with the prognosis for visual acuity completely unknown. It is important that the PACU nurse be armed with factual information from the surgeon about expectations for the patient so that reassurances offered are realistic. In addition, the PACU nurse must be prepared to provide significant support through both verbal communication and touch.

REFERENCES

1. Duane, T. D.: Ophthalmic Surgery, vol. 5. *In* Clinical Ophthalmology. Hagerstown, Md., Harper & Row Publishers, Inc., 1980.
2. Hill, B. J.: Sensory information, behavioral instructions and coping with sensory alteration surgery. Nurs. Res., 31(1):17–21, 1982.
3. Hirschman, H.: Intraocular lens implantation: Faster, more complete rehabilitation of the cataract patient. J. Am. Geriatr. Soc., 25(1):35–38, 1977.
4. Kornzweig, A. L.: New ideas for old eyes. J. Am. Geriatr. Soc., 28(4):145–152, 1980.
5. Marta, M.: A guide to the posterior vitrectomy. Today's OR Nurse, 5(1):26–29, 69, 1983.
6. Moore, C. R.: Scleral buckling for retinal detachment. AORN J., 36(3):495–506, 1982.
7. Murphy, S. B., and Donderi, D. C.: Predicting the success of cataract surgery. J. Behav. Med., 3(1):1–14, 1980.
8. Saunders, W. H., Havener, W. H., Keith, C. F., and Prescott, A. W.: Nursing Care in Eye, Ear, Nose, and Throat Disorders. 4th ed. St. Louis, C. V. Mosby Co., 1979.
9. Shipley, S. B.: Patient teaching and day care anesthesia. Focus, 9(4):14–16, 1982.
10. Smith, J. F., and Nachazel, D. P.: Ophthalmic Nursing. Boston, Little, Brown & Co., 1980.
11. Whitton, S.: Penetrating keratoplasty: the gift of sight. Today's OR Nurse, 5(1):20–24, 72, 1983.
12. Zack, P. L., and Smirnow, I. H.: IOL implantation. Today's OR Nurse, 5(1):12–18, 68, 1983.

22

Postoperative Care After Thoracic Surgery

Gayle Whitman, R.N., M.S.N., C.C.R.N.

Thoracic surgery involves procedures on the structures contained within the chest cavity, including the lungs, heart, great vessels, and esophagus. In this chapter, discussion will primarily center on surgical procedures performed on the lungs and give detailed instructions on the care of the patient following the insertion of chest tubes, since any time the thoracic cavity is entered, chest tubes are required to reexpand the lungs and allow healing of the chest wall to occur. Specific postoperative care following cardiac surgery is discussed in Chapter 23; care following surgery of the great vessels is discussed in Chapter 24; and care following surgery of the esophagus is discussed in Chapter 28.

Surgical procedures on the lungs involve diagnostic procedures as well as the removal of tumors or diseased parts or all of the lung. In addition, thoracic surgery may be performed to correct congenital or acquired chest wall injuries and to repair traumatic damage to the lung.

Definitions

Atelectasis: collapse of part of the lung, caused primarily by obstruction of the lower airway, resulting in collapse of the alveoli due to the extraction of gas from them. Obstruction is most commonly caused by the accumulation of respiratory secretions, although it may be caused by tumors, bronchospasm, foreign bodies, or any other form of obstruction.

Bronchoscopy: visualization of the tracheobronchial tree by use of a lighted scope (Figs. 22–1 to 22–3).

Chylothorax: collection of lymph in the pleural space. Although a rare occurrence, this can develop following chest trauma or from surgical procedures performed through the pleural space on mediastinal structures.

Decortication (of the lung): removal of fibrinous deposits or restrictive membranes on the pleural lining that interfere with ventilatory action.

Hemothorax: a collection of blood or serosanguineous fluid, or both, within the pleural cavity (Fig. 22–4).

Lobectomy: removal of one or more lobes of the lung.

Mediastinoscopy: visualization of lymph nodes or tumors at the tracheobronchial junction, subcarina, or upper lobe bron-

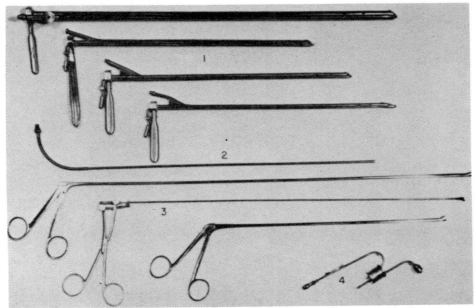

Figure 22–1. Rigid bronchoscope. (From DeWeese, D. D., and Saunders, W. H.: Textbook of Otolaryngology. St. Louis, The C. V. Mosby Co., 1968.)

chi via a lighted scope. This is done by passing the mediastinoscope through a small incision at the suprasternal area and then down along the anterior course of the trachea.

Pectus excavatum: (trichterbrust or chone- chondrosternon): a structural defect, usually congenital, of the anterior thoracic wall, characterized by a posterior depression of the sternum; also called a funnel chest.

Pneumonectomy: removal of the lung.

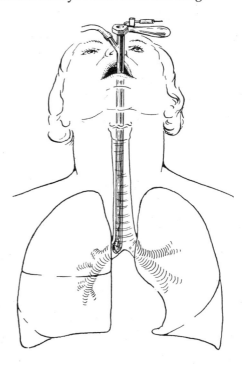

Figure 22–2. Diagram of a bronchoscope in place. Note: During bronchoscopy the patient's hair and eyes would be covered. (From DeWeese, D. D., and Saunders, W. H.: Textbook of Otolaryngology. St. Louis, C. V. Mosby Co., 1968.)

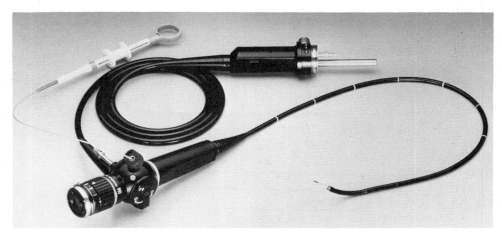

Figure 22–3. Flexible fiberoptic bronchoscope. (Courtesy of The Olympus Corporation, New Hyde Park, New York.)

Pneumothorax: collection of air or gas within the pleural cavity (Fig. 22–4).

Segmental resection of the lung: excision of individual bronchovascular segments of the lobe of the lung with ligation of segmental branches of the pulmonary artery and vein and division of the segmental bronchus.

Sternotomy: incision through the sternum.

Thoracentesis: insertion of a needle through the chest wall into the pleural space to remove either fluid or air.

Thoracoplasty: removal of ribs or portions of the ribs to reduce the size of the thoracic space and to collapse a diseased lung.

Thoracotomy: incision into the chest cavity. Closed thoracotomy (intercostal drainage) is the insertion of a drain (i.e., catheter, chest tube, or thoracotomy tube) through the intercostal space in order to establish drainage of accumulated air or fluid from the pleural cavity and to restore the normal negative pressure of the pleural space.

Wedge resection: the excision of a small, wedge-shaped section from the peripheral portion of a lobe of the lung.

INVASIVE DIAGNOSTIC PROCEDURES

Invasive diagnostic procedures involving the thoracic cavity include bronchoscopy, mediastinoscopy, thoracentesis, and needle biopsy. Besides being diagnostic, these procedures may be therapeutic. They may be performed at the bedside, in a special procedures room, or in the operating suite, depending on the urgency of the procedure, the reason it is being performed, and the condition of the patient.

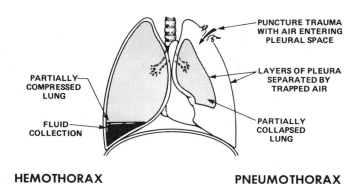

HEMOTHORAX   **PNEUMOTHORAX**

Figure 22–4. Schematic representation of a hemothorax vs. a pneumothorax.

Bronchoscopy

Bronchoscopy is performed to visualize the structures of the tracheobronchial tree; to remove secretions, washings, mucus plugs, or foreign bodies; to biopsy tissue; or to apply medication. Bronchoscopy may also be performed to accomplish bronchography, which involves the instillation of a radiopaque medium into the tracheobronchial tree, making it visible on x-ray. In recent years, laser therapy has also begun to be used with bronchoscopy. Ablation of tracheal and bronchial obstructions can be accomplished by using a laser beam in conjunction with a bronchoscope. Carbon dioxide and neodymium YAG lasers are the laser sources most frequently used in these techniques.

Bronchoscopy can be performed with either a topical or a general anesthetic. The choice is determined by the patient's condition and the anesthesiologist's preference. Prior to the procedure, the patient is required to abstain from liquids for at least 6 hours. Premedication generally consists of sodium pentobarbital and meperidine. Preprocedure patient education and instructions should include these routines as well as a brief description of and rationale for the procedure itself.

If a topical anesthetic is used, a 4 percent lidocaine hydrochloride solution is sprayed or instilled into the pharyngeal and laryngeal areas. Other agents that can be used include tetracaine hydrochloride and hexylcaine hydrochloride. Toxic reactions can occur with any of these agents, and emergency equipment should be available. If a general anesthetic is used, thiopental sodium and a muscle relaxant are the preferred agents.

Upon return to the PACU, the patient is placed flat in the side-lying position or on his side with the head of the bed raised 20 to 30 degrees. Nursing observations and care are directed toward maintenance of a patent airway. The patient must be carefully observed for the development of laryngeal edema or laryngospasm, either of which requires prompt action to restore an open airway. Intubation equipment, along with an emergency tracheostomy tray, must be immediately available. The application of a light crushed ice collar and administration of warmed, humidified oxygen help prevent the development of edema and promote comfort.

The patient must be given nothing by mouth until the pharyngeal and laryngeal reflexes have returned (after two to eight hours). Once the gag reflex has fully returned, the patient may gargle with warmed saline or suck on anesthetic throat lozenges to relieve the sore throat that is inevitable following bronchoscopy. The patient should be advised to rest the voice and to avoid coughing or clearing the throat. After the gag reflex has returned, the patient is allowed fluids and soft foods as desired and tolerated.

If a needle biopsy was also performed, the patient must be observed for bleeding. Sputum that is pink-tinged or streaked with blood can be expected following this procedure; however, grossly bloody sputum or coughing up of frank blood should be reported. Subcutaneous emphysema or dyspnea indicates perforation of the trachea or bronchus. Pain experienced in this area may be mistaken by the patient for "heartburn." If any of these symptoms is present, the patient must be given nothing by mouth and the physician notified immediately.

Mediastinoscopy

Care following mediastinoscopy is similar to that after bronchoscopy, although general anesthesia is almost always used for this procedure. A small dressing is placed over the stab wound and should be inspected for any drainage.

Thoracentesis

Thoracentesis is performed to remove air or fluid from the pleural space in order to relieve lung compression or for diagnostic purposes. Fluid removed is evaluated for chemical, bacteriologic, and cellular composition. Thoracentesis is almost always performed at the bedside with only local anesthesia.

Post-thoracentesis care includes positioning the patient in the side-lying position on the unoperated side and observing for complications, which, fortunately, are rare. The thoracentesis site is sealed with a small piece of Vaseline-impregnated gauze, and a sterile dressing is applied. The site should be checked for drainage.

A decreasing blood pressure along with an increasing pulse rate may indicate the development of shock due to hemorrhage from a damaged blood vessel and should be reported. This is most likely to occur when large amounts of fluid are removed; the patient must also be observed for symptoms indicating mediastinal shift, including pallor or cyanosis, dyspnea, increased respiratory and pulse rates, and a deviation of the larynx and trachea from their normal midline position in the neck. This is a serious complication and must be reported at once. Compression of the great vessels and decreased blood return to the heart compromise the cardiorespiratory system quickly, so mediastinal shift must be corrected without delay.

Hemoptysis, vertigo, syncope, decreased blood pressure, increased pulse rate, uncontrollable or persistent cough, dyspnea, cyanosis, tightness in the chest, and subcutaneous emphysema alone or in combination are danger signs and indicate damage to the lung that could result in pneumothorax, tension pneumothorax, or the reaccumulation of fluid in the intrapleural space. If any of these distress symptoms develops, the physician should be notified immediately and preparations made for the insertion of thoracotomy tubes and the institution of closed chest drainage.

Needle Biopsy

Needle biopsy may be performed to remove tissue specimens from the pleura or lungs for diagnostic purposes. Needle biopsy is generally performed with only local anesthesia, and care is essentially the same as that following thoracentesis. Complications are infrequent, but the patient should be observed closely over several hours for signs and symptoms of damage to the lungs.

CHEST TUBES AND CLOSED CHEST DRAINAGE

Surgery on the structures of the chest involves entrance into the thoracic cavity and the creation of a pneumothorax (atmospheric air admitted into the pleural cavity and collapse of the lung) under controlled conditions. General endotracheal anesthesia is required. Endotracheal anesthesia allows the anesthetist to control fully both inspiration and expiration as the lung is ventilated on the unoperated side.

The surgical approach to the chest cavity may be made through a median incision in the sternum (sternotomy) or through variously placed lateral thoracic incisions through the bed of a rib or between two ribs (Fig. 22–5). Resective surgery on the lung is approached by way of a posterolateral parascapular incision through the

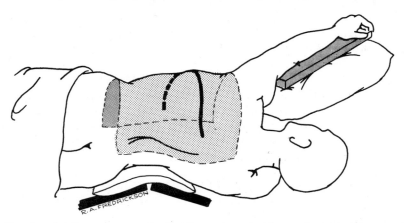

Figure 22–5. Position for a left thoracotomy, a standard thoracotomy incision, and extent of the prep. (From LeMaitie, G. D., and Finnegan, J. A.: The Patient in Surgery. 3rd ed. Philadelphia, W. B. Saunders Co., 1975, p. 406.)

fourth, fifth, sixth, or seventh intercostal space or an anterior incision through the third, fourth, or fifth intercostal space. Generally, less pain and disability result from the anterior approach.

Indications and Methodology

Following thoracotomy (except after pneumonectomy), the surgeon strategically places large chest tubes in the intrapleural space to remove air and blood or other accumulated fluid, to restore the normal negative pressure, and to allow reexpansion of the lung on the operative side. Contrary to popular belief, care of the patient with chest tubes is logical and follows very simple principles. The reader is advised to review the principles of normal ventilatory mechanics (see Chapter 4) if necessary.

Chest tubes are placed after thoracic surgery to remove both air and fluid. Since blood or other fluids are heavier than air, they tend to accumulate in the lower portion of the pleural space, with air tending to accumulate in the upper portion. Therefore, usually two chest tubes are placed through the chest wall through stab wounds or through the incision—one for fluid and one for air. An upper or anterior chest tube is placed anteriorly in the second intercostal space to allow for air removal. A lower or posterior chest tube is positioned in the eighth or ninth intercostal space just anterior to the postaxillary line to allow for drainage of fluid from the pleural space (Fig. 22–6). Occasionally, two lower or posterior chest tubes are used to drain fluid. The two posterior chest tubes are positioned in the same intercostal space approximately 4 cm apart. This decreases postoperative pain for the patient and minimizes intercostal damage.

As the surgeon places the chest tubes and closes the chest, the anesthesiologist mechanically expands the lung of the operated side as fully as possible. The chest tubes are sutured to the patient's skin and also securely taped with regular cloth adhesive to prevent accidental removal (Fig. 22–7). Since regular cloth adhesive can cause skin breakdown, it is advisable to place Stom-

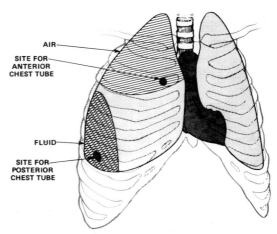

Figure 22–6. Since air rises to the top of the cavity, chest tube placement for treatment of a pneumothorax is at the second intercostal space, close to the sternum. Chest tube placement for fluid removal is generally at the level of the 6–8 lateral intercostal space, as this is where fluid will collect.

adhesive on the skin around the chest tube site and then to place the tape over the Stomadhesive. Since the chest tube is inserted between two ribs, any movement back and forth of the tube against the insertion site can be painful. Making sure that the tube is anchored with an appropriate dressing is therefore essential to minimize the patient's discomfort. Each chest tube is then connected to its appropriate drainage system. These systems are sterile and must remain so until the tubes are removed.

Types of Drainage Systems

The purpose of chest tube drainage systems is to provide a means by which air and fluid can be removed from the intrapleural space. Once this air and fluid are removed, the visceral and parietal pleurae are brought back together and the pressure in the intrapleural space becomes negative once again. Evacuation of air and fluid is

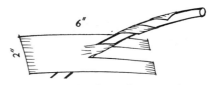

Figure 22–7. Taping the chest tube. (From Sutton, A. L.: Bedside Nursing Techniques in Medicine and Surgery. 2nd ed. Philadelphia, W. B. Saunders Co., 1969, p. 226.)

facilitated by three forces: positive pressure, gravity, and suction. The trapped air itself in the intrapleural space creates the positive pressure. As long as it is present it facilitates the functioning of the chest tube system by helping to draw air into the system. Gravity assists primarily in fluid evacuation; suction, when applied, assists in removing both air and fluid. All systems use these three forces to varying degrees to assist in reexpanding the lung.

One-way drainage systems depend primarily upon the forces of positive pressure and gravity. Figure 22–8 illustrates a one-bottle water seal drainage system. Air and fluid pushed from the patient's chest by positive pressure facilitated by gravity drainage enter the water-sealed tube. The tube is generally immersed in 1 to 2 cm of water. The force of the patient's exhalation pushes air out through the bottom of the tube. The air then bubbles to the surface and can escape into the atmosphere via the other outlet. During inhalation, air is prevented from entering the tube by the water sealing it. During inhalation water will rise in the water-sealed tube, owing to the suction that inhalation produces. How deeply the tube is submerged plays a role in how difficult it is for the patient to push air through the water seal; the more deeply the tube is submerged, the more difficult it is.

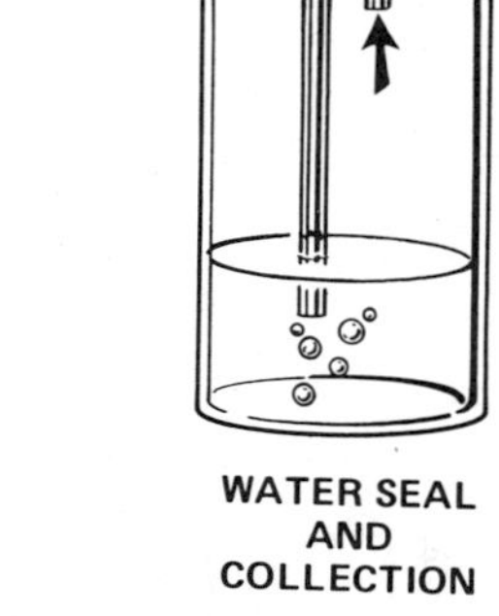

FROM PATIENT

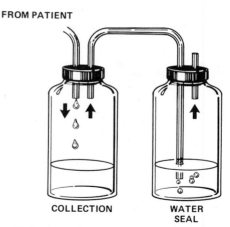

COLLECTION   WATER SEAL

Figure 22–9. A two-bottle system in which one bottle collects fluid and the other serves as a water seal.

This, then, is perhaps not the best system to utilize if the patient has significant fluid accumulation, as this will increase the level of submersion of the tube. If this occurs, the bottle needs to be emptied at frequent intervals, or a second bottle can be attached (Fig. 22–9). With this setup, the water-sealed tube is in the second bottle. This system is particularly useful for fluid collection. Again, both of these systems work owing to the forces of positive pressure and gravity. Another one-way system is the B-P Heimlich Chest Drainage Valve (Fig. 22–10). This is a sterile plastic disposable device that employs a rubber diaphragm to act as a one-way valve. This device is not commonly used in the recovery room but rather replaces the water seal system two or three

FROM PATIENT

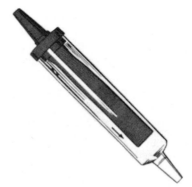

**WATER SEAL
AND
COLLECTION**

Figure 22–8. A one-bottle water seal drainage system.

Figure 22–10. B. P. Heimlich Chest Drainage Valve. (Courtesy of Becton, Dickinson and Co., Rutherford, N. J. From Luckmann, J., and Sorensen, K. C.: Medical-Surgical Nursing. Philadelphia, W. B. Saunders Co., 1974, p. 1036.)

days postoperatively, when patient activity is increased and mobility is hampered by the cumbersome water seal system. The valve is not gravity-dependent and functions in any position.

Suction

Suction is the third force that can facilitate fluid and air removal and can be added to both the one- and the two-bottle systems. The purpose of the suction is to lower the pressure over the surface of the fluid in the water seal system. By doing this, the pressure of the water that the patient must displace to force air out through the water seal is decreased. Suction requires adding another bottle for suction control to the current system (Fig. 22–11). The suction-control bottle is attached to the water-seal bottle via the air vents. The suction-control bottle will also have one outlet that is at-

tached to the suction source and another inlet for air, called the manometer tube. When the suction is applied, bubbles are created at the bottom of the manometer tube. When the manometer tube is pushed up close to the surface of the fluid, the suction exerted against the patient's pleural space decreases, since most of the suction can pull in atmospheric air through the tube. In this instance it is harder for the patient to exhale. As the manometer tube is submerged to a greater depth, the suction exerted on the patient's pleural space increases and exhalation is easier. Orders will usually request that 20 cm of negative pressure be applied to the system. In this instance the manometer tube should be submerged 20 cm below the water level in the control bottle. The suction machine or wall vacuum outlet is, of course, also set to produce 20 cm of negative pressure. If a

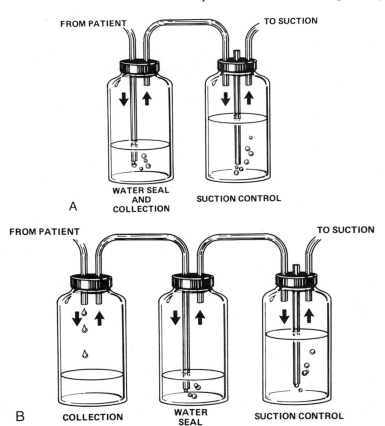

Figure 22–11. Two methods to establish a suction control. (a) This system is primarily designed for controlling the amount of suction and removing air from the chest cavity. (b) This system facilitates fluid collection, maintains the water seal and allows for the application of suction.

wall vacuum outlet is used, a valve and meter must be connected between the outlet and the water-seal bottle to control the suction.

Immediate PACU Care

As soon as the patient is returned to the PACU, the chest tubes are attached to water-seal drainage if this has not already been accomplished in the operating room. All connections are inspected to ensure that they are secure and airtight. All connections must be airtight in order for the system to work properly. The connections should be wrapped with adhesive tape as double protection against air leaks and accidental disconnections. All tubing and receptacles must be kept below the level of the patient's chest to maintain gravitational flow. If they are raised above the patient's chest, fluid and air may return to the pleural space.

The bottles of the apparatus should be securely fastened at the patient's bedside in a special rack designed for this purpose, or they should be placed on a large-rimmed, wheeled cart at the bedside.

Monitoring Volume of Drainage

The drainage water-seal bottles (these are the same in the single-bottle system) are marked with a strip of adhesive tape if they are not already marked by the manufacturer, and the level of water in the water-seal bottle is indicated. Usually 100 ml of sterile water or saline is used initially. As drainage collects, the time and volume are marked on the tape at the fluid level. In the two- or three-bottle system, a separate drainage bottle is provided, and the water-seal fluid and drainage do not mix. The advantage of this system is that the volume and character of the chest drainage can be more accurately assessed. Marking the bottle at 2 to 4 hour intervals, depending on how fast the drainage is accumulating, allows personnel to evaluate the volume of chest drainage and its rate of accumulation. If a one-bottle system is used, the water seal tube must be elevated as drainage accumulates, so that it remains only 1 to 2 cm below the fluid level.

If the drainage bottle becomes more than two-thirds full, it should be replaced. Under no circumstances should the drainage be allowed to accumulate to the point that openings to the air vent or tubing to the control bottle or suction machine are occluded. A full drainage bottle will not allow the system to function properly and may, in fact, be dangerous to the patient. If replacement of the drainage bottle becomes necessary, a person who is thoroughly familiar with the apparatus should perform this procedure. All necessary equipment must be gathered and arranged, ready to making the replacement. Remember that the entire system must remain sterile. The chest tube of the system that needs to be replaced (usually only the lower or posterior tube) is clamped at the end close to the patient's chest wall to prevent air from entering the pleural cavity, and the full bottle is replaced with the new setup and the clamps removed. This should be accomplished swiftly and deftly so that the chest tube is clamped only momentarily. Prolonged clamping of the chest tube may produce tension in the cavity, allowing air or fluid or both to accumulate within the pleural space.

Most institutions currently use prefabricated disposable chest drainage units such as the Pleur-evac (Fig. 22–12) and the Argyle Double Seal System (Fig. 22–13). The principles of positive pressure, gravity, and suction apply equally to these systems. The Pleur-evac system consists of a collection chamber, a water seal chamber, and a suction control chamber. The Argyle Double Seal System is a four-chambered system with a collection and suction control chamber and two water seal chambers. The second water seal chamber serves as a safety vent for the patient.

Ensuring Patency of Tubing

The flexible drainage tubing that connects the chest catheters to the drainage apparatus must be long enough to allow the patient to turn fully and to sit up in bed but not so long that dependent loops of tubing are formed. The tubing must be draped and secured in such a way that it forms a

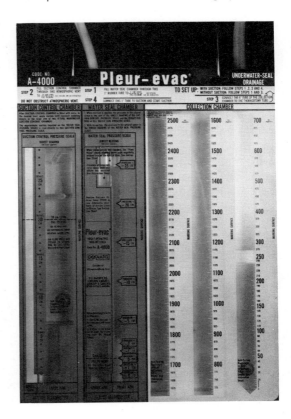

Figure 22–12. Disposable Pleur-evac A-4000 unit. (Courtesy Krale Laboratories, a Division of Deknatel, Inc., New York.)

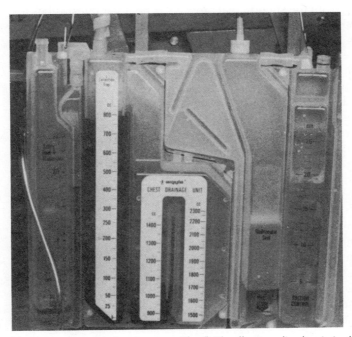

Figure 22–13. Disposable plastic pleural drainage system. The fluid collection chamber is in the center, the suction control is on the right, and the water-seal chamber is on the left. (Courtesy of Argyle, Division of Sherwood Medical, St. Louis, Missouri.)

straight line to the receptacles to allow unobstructed gravitational flow. The tubing can be secured to the bed linen by wrapping a rubber band or a piece of adhesive tape around it and then pinning the tape or rubber band to the sheet. Excess tubing should be coiled flat on the bed. If more than two loops of tubing are present, a length of tubing should be removed to make the connection shorter. Excess tubing gets in the way of patient care, obstructs smooth flow of drainage, is likely to fall off the bed into dependent loops, and is more likely to become kinked, tangled, or constricted.

Patency of the system and proper functioning should be checked frequently. In the first 2 or 3 hours postoperatively, this should be checked every 30 minutes or so along with the vital signs. If straight gravitational closed chest drainage is used, proper functioning is evidenced by fluctuation of the fluid in the water-seal tubing in response to the patient's respiration. If mechanical suction is being used with a two- or three-bottle system, the apparatus must be changed to the setup of the simple water-seal system to check the patency of the system. This is accomplished by disconnecting the tubing from the suction machine or outlet and leaving it open to atmospheric air to provide an air vent.

The fluid moves up the tubing approximately 2 to 6 cm as the patient inhales, owing to decreased intrapleural pressure, and then moves back down the tubing as the patient exhales, owing to increased intrapleural pressure. If fluctuation does not occur, check the tubing for obstruction due to kinking, compression, or the presence of blood clots. Ensure that the tubing has not become obstructed by the patient lying on it.

During pressure ventilation, the opposite occurs: With positive pressure inspiration, intrapleural pressure approaches or exceeds atmospheric pressure, and therefore the drainage tube fluid is forced downward.

"Milking" or "stripping" the chest tubing may dislodge clots of blood blocking the tubing (Fig. 22–14). Start close to the chest wall and work toward the drainage bottle. Never work toward the patient, as fluid or

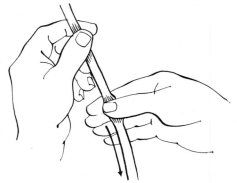

Figure 22–14. Milking the chest tube. (From Sutton, A. L.: Bedside Nursing Techniques in Medicine and Surgery. 2nd ed. Philadelphia, W. B. Saunders Co., 1969, p. 226.)

clots may be forced into the pleural space. Gently compress the tubing inch by inch down its entire length. This may be done by holding an alcohol swab in the hand stripping the tube, while the other hand holds the tube firmly in place and prevents traction on the insertion site. The hand-over-hand method may also be used: Gently squeeze the tubing with one hand and then the other, working in this fashion down its entire length. Some chest tubes are provided with chest tube strippers (Fig. 22–15). Whenever chest tubes are stripped, the procedure should be carried out gently, as it

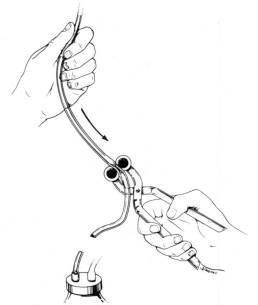

Figure 22–15. Technique for stripping the chest tube using "chest tube strippers."

changes intrapleural pressure in the patient's chest cavity and may produce pain. Recently, some studies have indicated that stripping chest tubes can create negative pressures considerably higher than the normally prescribed suction pressures of -15 to -20 cm H_2O. Therefore, each clinical situation should be evaulated individually before routine stripping is initiated. If large amounts of clotted blood appear in the chest tube, it seems reasonable to attempt to strip the tube. A chest tube draining only air does not require routine stripping.

Having the patient turn, cough, and breathe deeply may improve patency of the chest tube. If fluctuation does not occur after these measures, the surgeon should be notified, and an x-ray will probably be ordered. The cessation of fluctuation may indicate full reexpansion of the lung, but this is a most unusual occurrence in the relatively short period of time the patient resides in the PACU. Most commonly, the system is blocked somewhere. If the tubing appears patent and milking has not improved the system's functioning, the physician may try irrigating the chest tube with a small amount of sterile saline.

Maintaining Proper Functioning

Intermittent bubbling in the water-seal bottle as the patient exhales or coughs indicates that the system is working properly and that air is being removed from the pleural space. Continuous bubbling in the water-seal bottle, however, indicates an air leak in the system that should be remedied immediately. Check all connections to ensure that they are snug. Check the entire length of the tubing for small leaks that can be corrected by taping. Check the dressing and the catheter at the insertion site on the patient's chest. If the catheter appears loose at the insertion site, gather skin around it and apply sterile Vaseline gauze around the skin and catheter to form an airtight seal. Cover with gauze and tape firmly. If no leak can be found and corrected and bubbling continues, the physician must be notified, as this may indicate an incision or tear in lung tissue that is allowing a large amount of air leakage from the lung.

In the closed chest drainage apparatus attached to suction, continuous bubbling should occur and indicates proper functioning. Proper functioning can be determined by examining the suction control tube. This tube should be emptied periodically of fluid and then refilled. If continuous bubbling does not occur, check all the connections and the suction machine. Check for air leaks as described earlier.

Do not clamp chest tubes unless specifically ordered. Clamping chest tubes, which may allow the development of a tension pneumothorax, is considerably more dangerous than allowing an open pneumothorax to occur. If something disrupts the system, correct the problem. If the water-seal bottle is tipped and the seal is disrupted, return the bottle to the upright position to reestablish the seal. If the water-seal bottle is inadvertently raised above the level of the patient's chest, lower the bottle at once to reestablish drainage. If the water-seal bottle is broken, or if the tubing becomes disconnected, sterilize the end of the tubing with antiseptic solution and reconnect it, or connect another sterile water-seal bottle. Make sure to retape all connections after they are fit snugly together.

Once the problem is remedied, have the patient breathe deeply and cough to assist in forcing out any air or fluid that may have entered or accumulated within the pleural space during disruption of the system. If a large pneumothorax was precipitated by the event, as evidenced by asymmetric chest expansion, chest pain, and difficult breathing, a chest x-ray should be ordered and the physician notified.

GENERAL CARE FOLLOWING THORACIC SURGERY

As previously stated, the anesthesia used for surgery on the lung is always general inhalational anesthesia.

Positioning

Positioning following chest surgery varies. *Check the surgeon's orders.* Generally, the patient is kept in the supine position until reflexes begin to return. The supine position reduces the threat of hypoventilation by preventing restriction of thoracic expansion, and the abdominal organs do not impinge upon the diaphragm or cause pressure on the mediastinal structures. The Trendelenburg position is contraindicated after chest surgery, even in the presence of shock, because it causes the abdominal organs to press against the diaphragm, thus restricting movement and creating pressure on the mediastinal contents, which decreases venous return and cardiac output. If hypotension develops owing to venous pooling of blood in the legs, apply elastic stockings or raise the legs.

Once the patient's reflexes have started to return and vital signs are stabilized, the head of the bed is raised 30 to 45 degrees to allow the diaphragm to drop to normal position, thus enhancing lung expansion and facilitating chest tube drainage. The specific surgical procedure will determine what changes in position can be made during the first 24 to 48 hours postoperatively. Surgeons differ in the theory of positioning, but several guidelines may be generally followed. After pulmonary resection (lobectomy, segmentectomy, wedge resection), the patient may be turned to a full lateral position on either side to allow full expansion of lung tissue on both the operated and the unoperated sides. Occasionally, a surgeon does not want the patient turned onto the operated side in order to enhance full expansion of remaining lung parenchyma on that side; however, this ignores the necessity for full ventilation on the unoperated side, the lack of which may be just as detrimental. After median sternotomy the patient may be positioned on the back, which is the most comfortable position, or on either side. The patient with a pneumonectomy may be positioned on the back or turned on the operative side. Extreme lateral positioning on the unoperative side is contraindicated after pneumonectomy, because the mediastinum is no longer confined by lung tissue and may move freely and cause compression of the remaining lung or create traction or torsion phenomena on the vena cava. Additionally, if the bronchial stump is ruptured while in this position, the unaffected lung would be drowned with secretions from the pneumonectomy site.

Position changes are an important part of the stir-up regimen. During the first 4 to 6 hours, the patient should be turned every hour, then every 2 hours until ambulatory. Ambulation is started as soon as possible after recovery from anesthesia and stabilization of vital signs. Mobilization, through position change, exercise, and ambulation, is important to promote drainage of secretions and chest tube drainage of fluid and air, to prevent venous stasis, and to promote comfort. When turning the patient or helping him or her to sit or slide up in the bed, support the back of the head and assist from the unoperated side. The patient can help in turning by grasping the side rail and pulling. A draw sheet may be kept under the patient for the first 4 to 6 hours to assist in turning the patient comfortably. When changing the patient's position, ensure that chest tubes remain free, that they remain patent (i.e., no kinking or compression), and that no dependent loops are formed. Active and passive arm exercises are initiated within the first postoperative day. Simple exercises, such as arm circles and lifting the arm out to the side on the affected side, are encouraged.

Chest Tubes

Thoracotomy tubes are connected to a sterile, closed chest drainage system with or without suction, as the surgeon specifies, if this has not already been accomplished in the operating room. Chest drains are not usually placed after pneumonectomy because serous fluid accumulation, which eventually consolidates and fills the empty thoracic space left by removal of the lung, is desirable to prevent mediastinal movement of the heart and remaining lung. Occasionally, a clamped chest tube is placed as a monitoring device to check bleeding and for measuring and regulating pressure in the thoracic space. The chest tubes are cared for as previously described.

Chest tube drainage must be checked

frequently for character, volume, and rate of formation. The drainage is usually grossly bloody for the first 3 to 4 postoperative hours, after which it becomes more serous and only pink-tinged. Approximately 100 to 300 ml of drainage can be expected in the first 2 hours, after which it should slow to 50 to 100 ml per hour. Total drainage in the first 24 hours postoperatively will be 500 to 1000 ml. If drainage of more than 50 ml of grossly bloody fluid per hour persists 3 hours after surgery, hemorrhage should be suspected and the surgeon notified. These figures must be interpreted in light of patient activity, since a sudden gush of 50 ml of drainage at one time would not be unusual after turning the patient to the operated side or having him cough and breathe deeply. Check the patient's vital signs and urine output for interrelated features of developing shock.

Vital Signs

All vital signs are measured and recorded every 15 minutes for the first 2 hours and then every 30 minutes until stable. A CVP line, Swan-Ganz catheter, or arterial line may be present to assist in monitoring the patient. They must be correctly connected to monitoring devices and maintained with flushing solution. All flushing solutions must be included in the parenteral intake computations.

Nursing assessment and intervention are aimed at maintaining adequate respiratory and circulatory function and at preventing complications from hypoxia, hypoxemia, and circulatory insufficiency.

SPECIFIC ASPECTS OF POSTOPERATIVE CARE

Respiratory Functions

Maintenance of a Patent Airway

Maintaining a patent airway depends primarily upon assessment and initiation of the stir-up regimen as outlined in Chapter 18. Assess air movement: Stridor, wheezing, gurgling, decreased chest expansion, and decreased breath sounds upon auscul-

tation may indicate airway obstruction. If obstruction is not relieved by repositioning of the head and jaw or suctioning the airway, notify the anesthesiologist. Emergency equipment, including laryngoscope, endotracheal tubes, Ambu or anesthesia bag, and tracheostomy sets, must be immediately available.

Assessment of Respiratory Function

Vital signs are taken every 15 minutes for the first 2 hours (at least until reflexes are returning), then every 30 minutes to an hour until stable. The frequency of vital sign measurement will be determined by the discrepancies between preoperative, intraoperative, and postoperative levels. Observe respiratory rate, rhythm, and depth, and auscultate for adventitious or diminished breath sounds. Observe the quality of respirations: Labored breathing, dyspnea, stridor, chest retraction, nasal flaring, and asymmetry of chest expansion may indicate obstruction. Intrapleural air or fluid (blood) or both may compress lung tissue and decrease ventilation quantitatively.

Paradoxic respiration (Fig. 22–16), which may occur after thoracoplasty, is very deleterious. Paradoxic respiration results not only in hypoventilation but also in obstruction due to accumulation of secretions that the patient cannot effectively remove by coughing. Tight dressings, binders, or abdominal distention may also restrict chest

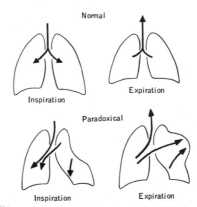

Figure 22–16. Paradoxical motion of the flail chest. (From Sutton, A. L.: Bedside Nursing Techniques in Medicine and Surgery. 2nd ed. Philadelphia, W. B. Saunders Co., 1969, p. 217.)

excursion. Restlessness, irritability, disorientation, inappropriate behavior, and other cerebral symptoms offer significant evidence of hypoxia. Although these symptoms may be difficult to assess and may be attributable to pain and other causes, inadequate oxygenation should be the first possibility that comes to mind.

Quantitative measurements, including arterial blood gases and spirometry (the measurement of tidal volume, minute volume, and vital capacity), are also used to assess respiratory function. An arterial line should be present so that frequent arterial samples may easily be obtained. Blood gas measurements are extremely important in guiding oxygen therapy. (For information on analysis of blood gases see Chapter 4).

Institution of Oxygen Therapy

All patients should receive supplemental humidified oxygen in the PACU. Some degree of hypoxemia while breathing room air is usually present for 5 to 7 days following thoracic surgery. As stated previously, oxygen should be viewed and treated as a drug, and the physician should individualize dosage and administration route for each patient. Preferably, oxygen is administered via catheter or cannula, since the patient needs to cough up secretions at frequent intervals. Oxygen administration, humidification, and airway adjuncts are discussed in more detail in Chapter 15.

Initiation of the Stir-Up Regimen

The stir-up regimen, including positioning, mobilization, deep breathing, cascade coughing, and pain relief, is especially important for this patient. Positioning and mobilization have already been discussed. Deep breathing and coughing exercises are the easiest ways to maintain a patent airway after the patient is reactive to verbal command. Preoperative teaching is extremely important; the patient who has been well educated and knows what is expected of him postoperatively can cooperate by breathing deeply and coughing effectively even if not fully reactive.

Once the patient is fully conscious, rigorous deep breathing and coughing are con-

tinued every hour. This regimen is most effective with the patient sitting up to allow full lung expansion. If the patient cannot sit up, raise the head of the bed and have him or her bend the knees to relax the abdominal muscles. The patient is instructed to take a deep inspiration to expand the lungs and relax the abdominal muscles so that the belly pouches out. Four to five deep breaths are taken, and then the patient is instructed to give a full forceful cough to clear the tracheobronchial tree of accumulated secretions. The most forceful and effective cough is produced if the patient takes a full breath of air and then bears down in the Valsalva maneuver before opening the glottis and letting the air fairly "explode" out of the airway, carrying with it the secretions. Endotracheal secretions are usually excessive after thoracic surgery, owing to trauma to the tracheobronchial tree during the operation and intubation, to decreased lung ventilation, and to decreased cough reflex. Pain or fear or both may interfere with the patient's ability to breathe deeply and cough.

Pain Relief

The thoracic surgery patient should be told preoperatively to expect a fair amount of incisional pain postoperatively but that breathing deeply and coughing are essential. The patient should be assured that the nurses will assist in this, and that medications will be provided to alleviate pain.

Postoperatively, the nurse must provide adequate analgesia to allow the patient to cooperate effectively with the stir-up regimen. Post-thoracic surgery patients generally experience a great deal of incisional pain and pain caused by the chest tubes. Posterolateral incisions tend to be more painful than anterolateral ones. Narcotic analgesics such as morphine sulfate or meperidine hydrochloride are usually the agents of choice for pain control. Naloxone HCl (Narcan), a narcotic antagonist, is usually kept readily available to reverse the effects of the analgesics if they begin to depress respiratory functioning; since both morphine and meperidine depress respiration and cough reflex, they must be administered judiciously. Meperidine may be preferred to morphine, since it seems to be somewhat less of a depressant and acts as a bronchodilator. The opiates, such as codeine, are generally contraindicated, since they severely depress the cough reflex, stimulate bronchospasm, and produce thickened secretions. Frequently, a potentiating drug such as hydroxyzine (Atarax, Vistaril) or promethazine hydrochloride (Phenergan) is added to the narcotic so that the dosage of the narcotic can be reduced, yet pain is adequately relieved.

The smallest dose of narcotic that will give adequate pain relief should be administered. Small doses given frequently decrease their tendency to depress respiratory centers. An order such as "Demerol 15 to 25 mg IV every 1 to 2 hr as necessary for pain" is advantageous, since the nurse can use discretion and give the minimal dose necessary to provide adequate analgesia.

The patient should be observed closely after the administration of narcotics for indications of depression. The administration of analgesics 15 to 30 minutes prior to deep breathing, coughing, and mobilization will assist the patient in cooperative efforts and decrease physiologic splinting and restriction of chest movement.

Pain can also be reduced and fear lessened by providing proper manual support for the incision during coughing (Fig. 22–17). Patients often fear that they may tear the incision or that a lung may protrude through the incision if they breathe too deeply or cough too vigorously. They should be reassured verbally that this will not occur, and the nurse can support the incision with the hands to reassure the patient physically and prevent pain. Manual support decreases stretching of the incision, thereby decreasing pain, and assists in depressing the thoracic cage during expiration.

To splint the incision correctly, stand to the side of the patient with the face posterior to the patient's head for protection from the cough and to be able to listen to the chest. Apply firm, even pressure with the open palms placed anteriorly and posteriorly over the incision. Do not squeeze

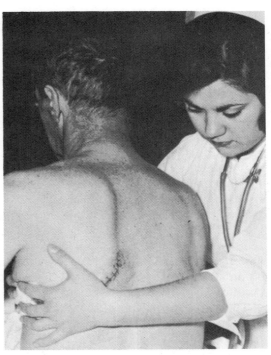

Figure 22–17. Correct position for "splinting" a patient's chest. (From MacVicar, J., and Mendelsohn, H. J.: *In* Meltzer, L. E., Abdellah, T., and Kitchell, J. R. (eds.): Concepts and Practices of Intensive Care for Nurse Specialists. Philadelphia, The Charles Press, 1969.)

across the chest, depress the sternum, or restrict movement of the lower rib cage. The diaphragm contributes more than 50 percent to the ventilatory process and must not be restricted. The thoracic incision may also be splinted by applying firm pressure upward underneath the incision and exerting pressure on the shoulder of the affected side with the other hand.

Auscultate the chest after deep breathing and coughing. If the lungs are not clear, allow the patient to rest for a short time and repeat the deep breathing and coughing. If the chest does not clear, other methods of mobilizing and removing secretions and fully inflating the lungs may have to be instituted. Syncope may occur while the patient is performing deep breathing and coughing but recovery is usually quick, since syncope is self-limiting. Syncope during these exercises is probably caused by (1) impeded venous return from the increase in intrathoracic pressure with subsequent reduced cardiac output and cerebral ischemia, and (2) the sudden reduction of carbon dioxide in the blood, owing to hyperventilation, which, if not reversed, can result in loss of consciousness.

The best way to clear the tracheobronchial tree of secretions is by an effective cough. If the patient cannot clear the airway of secretions effectively with deep breathing and coughing, other methods must be instituted, e.g., respiratory therapy adjuncts may be ordered to assist the patient.

Other pain-control methods that can be used include single-dose intercostal nerve blocks, continuous intercostal nerve blocks via indwelling intercostal analgesic catheters, or the use of transcutaneous electrical stimulation (TENS). In this last method, stimulation of large myelinated fibers is accomplished by the placement of small electrodes on either side of the thoracotomy incision. Stimulation via these electrodes inhibits the pain response of the small unmyelinated fibers.

Tracheal Suctioning

Tracheal suctioning of the post-thoracic surgery patient may be necessary to assist in removing accumulated secretions. Suctioning technique has been described in Chapter 15.

The patient should be in the sitting position. The catheter is introduced into the nares and the pharynx is suctioned. This removes secretions and also stimulates a good cough, which may be all that is necessary to mobilize secretions from the lower airway. Tracheal suctioning must be accomplished carefully, especially after pneumonectomy, when a suture line may be interrupted by introduction of the catheter. If the catheter is difficult to pass, pull the tongue forward. Do not force the catheter. There is no evidence that turning the patient's head or neck will help pass the catheter to the left mainstem bronchus, although this is a frequently advocated procedure. If, after suctioning, the airway does not clear, the physician may have to perform a bronchoscopy to remove secretions. Remember that suctioning removes oxygen

as well as secretions, and the patient must be hyperventilated before and after suctioning.

Incentive Spirometry, Intermittent Positive Pressure Breathing (IPPB), and Blow Bottles

Incentive spirometry, IPPB, and blow bottles may be used to promote lung expansion and effective coughing but should not replace the patient's efforts. These treatments may conveniently be started in the PACU.

Humidification

Reservoir nebulizers and humidifiers with aerosol masks, face tents, continuous positive airway pressure (CPAP) masks, and T tubes can provide both supplemental oxygen and dense water vapor or medicated mist. These are all effective methods of thinning tracheobronchial secretions, thus permitting the ciliary mechanism and coughing to clear the airway.

The most effective therapy device is the ultrasonic nebulizer, which generates a fine mist of saline droplets, 2 to 4 μ in diameter, which are carried down to the smallest and most distal bronchioles. This mist should be used only intermittently. Mist treatments may be administered via mask (tracheostomy mask, if tracheostomy is present) or in a mist tent. The mask is definitely preferable in the PACU to allow close direct observation of the patient.

Fluid Balance

Maintenance of Optimal Hydration

Optimal hydration of the post-thoracic surgery patient is exceptionally important to prevent increased viscosity of mucus to facilitate the removal of secretions. Oral fluids may be started as soon as the patient recovers from anesthesia and danger of nausea and vomiting has passed.

Accurate intake and output are especially important to ensure that optimal hydration is maintained without letting vascular overload develop. Removal of large segments or of the total lung significantly reduces the size of the pulmonary circulation, predisposing the patient to development of pulmonary edema if fluids are administered too rapidly or in too large a volume. Increased permeability of the capillaries that results from hypoxia increases the risk of pulmonary edema developing in this patient. Unless the surgeon specifically directs otherwise, the intravenous fluid rate should not exceed 200 ml in an hour.

Circulatory Functions

Maintenance of Adequate Circulation

Accurate assessment of the patient's cardiovascular status is important to ensure adequate circulation and thus oygen delivery to the tissues. Vital signs, including blood pressure, pulse, and respirations, are monitored frequently to detect trends that may indicate level of circulatory efficiency. The incision and the dressings should be checked frequently for drainage, and accurate intake and output records, including chest tube drainage, should be kept and evaluated.

Urine output volume is measured as an indicator of cardiac output. Level of consciousness and sensory changes are evaluated, and heart rhythm may be electrically monitored, especially if the patient is known to have underlying cardiac disease. Central venous pressure or pulmonary artery pressure is measured to assist in evaluating the patient's fluid balance.

Maintenance of Optimal Blood Volume

In addition to measuring degree of hydration, blood loss must be estimated. Blood loss during thoracic surgery is usually great because the incision is quite long and capillary oozing is significant, thoracic adhesions and tissue planes are usually extensive and quite vascular, and the thoracic arteries are large. Reexpansion of blood volume with intravenous infusions, blood, or plasma expanders is indicated if blood loss is significant and the patient shows signs of hypovolemia.

Prevention and Detection of Complications

Hypoxia and Atelectasis

These complications have already been discussed. The PACU nurse must make astute observations to identify quickly the symptoms of developing hypoxia and institute treatment to correct the cause (Fig. 22–18).

Airway obstruction leads rapidly to the development of postsurgical atelectasis, which may in turn lead to pneumonitis. The presence of decreased breath sounds and increased temperature should alert the PACU nurse to the need for greater efforts at maintaining a clear airway, since this is the essence of treatment. The stir-up regimen should be accomplished more frequently; more deep breathing, coughing, and suctioning are necessary. Bronchoscopy may be necessary to remove obstructive secretions or mucoid plugs. Respiratory therapy adjuncts, including blow bottles, mist inhalation, and IPPB, with or without the addition of detergent aerosols, may be used to increase ventilatory efforts. In addition, respiratory center stimulants such as carbon dioxide inhalation and intravenous or intramuscular caffeine or doxapram hydrochloride (Dopram) may be administered. The surgeon may elect to start the patient on antibiotic therapy to prevent the development of infection.

Infection

Fortunately, pulmonary infection following thoracic surgery is rare when preventive measures are followed. The use of sterile suctioning technique, the maintenance of sterility of the chest drainage system and of a patent airway (see above), and nose, mouth, and skin care to promote cleanliness are safeguards against the development of pulmonary infection. Definitive symptoms of infection rarely appear within the relatively short period of time the patient spends in the PACU. Nurses on the receiving unit must be alert to symptoms of hypoxia, increasing temperature, increased

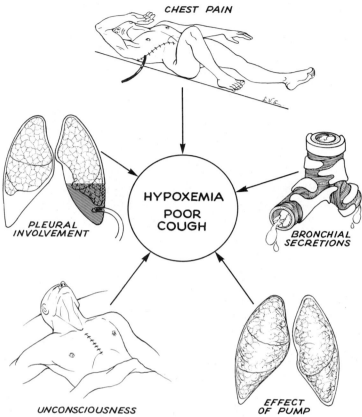

Figure 22–18. Postoperative factors leading to hypoxemia. (From Thomas, A. N. *In* Sanderson, R. G.: The Cardiac Patient. Philadelphia, W. B. Saunders Co., 1972.)

production of secretions, or a change in the color of secretions from clear or pale yellow to yellow or green. These symptoms may indicate the presence of pulmonary infection. If infection develops, culture and sensitivity studies are done to identify the causative organism and the antibiotics that will be effective.

Ventilatory Mechanical Complications

Pneumothorax, tension pneumothorax, and mediastinal shift have been discussed previously. Maintenance of the patency of chest tubes and correct positioning of the postoperative patient are preventive measures. If symptoms of these complications develop, rapid intervention to correct intrapleural pressure, including the placement of thoracotomy tubes, is necessary, since these are life-threatening conditions.

Subcutaneous emphysema, or the accumulation of air in the subcutaneous tissue

of the neck and chest, especially around the site of chest tube insertion, is common after thoracic surgery and does not usually cause serious problems. The PACU nurse should note its presence, however, and mark the boundaries of accumulation with a skin-marking pencil so that its rate of formation can be evaluated. Subcutaneous emphysema of the neck may be evaluated by measuring neck circumference. Small areas of subcutaneous emphysema are tender and may be uncomfortable for the adult but do not require specific treatment; however, compression of the vena cava or trachea by distended tissues may occur in the infant, so air must be removed. A progressive increase in subcutaneous emphysema in any patient should alert the nurse to the possibility that chest drainage tubes are not properly functioning, or that a bronchopleural fistula is present, or, in the case of the patient with pneumonectomy, that air is leaking through the bronchial stump. Treatment in these cases is aimed at correcting the underlying cause, ensuring patency of chest drains, replacing the chest tube, adding or increasing suction to the drainage system, aspirating the mediastinum, or repairing the bronchial stump to make it airtight.

Gastric dilation may occur in the postoperative period as a result of depression of gastric motility, air swallowing, or insufflation of anesthetic gases. Gastric distention is more common after surgery involving the left chest and occurs in the immediate postoperative period. Treatment involves decompression of the stomach with the use of a nasogastric tube.

Bleeding, Hypovolemia, and Shock

Blood loss or fluid depletion that results in hypovolemia is the most common cause of circulatory inadequacy in postoperative patients. Any signs and symptoms of blood loss, including increased pulse rate, decreased blood pressure, progressive oliguria, and changes in the sensorium, as well as external bleeding, should alert the nurse to possible hypovolemia, which could result in shock if the cause is not corrected. The surgeon should be notified. Preoperative and postoperative hematocrit values may assist in determining the presence of hypovolemia and the types and amounts of replacement fluids necessary to correct the problem. Vasopressors may be used to support blood pressure while waiting for fluid replacement to take effect. A return to the operating room may be necessary to correct continued bleeding.

If bleeding occurs into the intrapleural space and it cannot escape via chest tubes, a hemothorax will result. All chest tubes should be checked frequently to ensure that they are functioning correctly. If the patient becomes dyspneic, if pulse and respiratory rates increase, and if blood pressure decreases, the surgeon should be notified. Chest tubes may have to be inserted or replaced to remove blood from the intrapleural space, or surgical evacuation of the blood and direct control of bleeding may

have to be accomplished in the operating room.

Cardiac Arrhythmias

Underlying cardiac disease should be carefully evaluated and documented prior to surgery. Any patient with preexisting cardiac dysfunction should be electrically monitored on a continuous basis in the PACU, as these patients commonly develop cardiac dysrhythmias in the anesthesia recovery period. Sinus tachycardia and atrial fibrillation are the most commonly encountered dysrhythmias in the early recovery phases, but any disturbance in cardiac rate, rhythm, or electrical conduction may be cause for alarm.

Neurogenic Hypotension

Neurogenic reflexes due to pain or chest trauma may cause hypotension via vasodilatation in the postoperative period. This hypotension must be carefully evaluated to rule out other possible causes, including blood loss, volume depletion, or cardiac disease. Neurogenic hypotension may be treated by providing adequate analgesia to remove the pain stimulus. The patient must be observed carefully after administration of analgesia for depression of respiratory or cardiac function. The return of a preoperative blood pressure level should be sought.

REFERENCES

1. Allan, D.: Chest tube patient. Nurs. Times, *81*(5):24–25, 1985.
2. Bartlett, B. A.: Postoperative pulmonary prophylaxis: breathe deeply and read carefully. Chest, *81*(1):1–3, 1982.
3. Brindley, G. V.: Pulmonary resection in patients with impaired pulmonary function. Surg. Clin. North Am., *62*(2):199–214, 1982.
4. Burkhart, C.: After pneumonectomy. Am. J. Nurs., *83*(11):1562–1565, 1983.
5. Castello, R.: Chest physical therapy: Comparative efficacy of preoperative and postoperative prophylaxis in the elderly. Arch. Phys. Med. Rehabil., *66*:376–379, 1985.
6. Cimprich, B.: A program of nursing care for patients with lung cancer. Cancer Nurs., *81*:409–418, 1981.
7. Corrigan, A.: Pneumonectomy. Nursing (Oxford), *2*(12):343–345, 1983.

8. Cory, P. C.: Postoperative respiratory failure following intercostal block. Anesthesiology, *54*:418–419, 1981.
9. de la Rocha, A. G.: Pain amelioration after thoracotomy: a prospective randomized study. Ann. Thorac. Surg., *37*(3):239–242, 1984.
10. de la Rocha, A. G.: Sealing the postpneumonectomy space: use of a pectoralis major myodermal flap. Ann. Thorac. Surg., *38*(3):221–226, 1984.
11. Dumon, J. F.: Principles for safety in application of neodymium YAG laser in bronchology. Chest, *86*:163–168, 1984.
12. Duncan, C., and Erickson, R.: Pressures associated with chest tube stripping. Heart Lung, *11*(2):166–171, 1982.
13. Erickson, R.: Stripping chest tubes. Nursing, *13*(3):96–98, 1983.
14. Fry, D. E.: Systemic prophylactic antibiotics. Arch. Surg., *116*(2):466–469, 1981.
15. Lawrence, G. H.: Current management of carcinoma of the lung. J. Thorac. Cardiovasc. Surg., *88*:858–862, 1984.
16. McElvein, R. B.: Indications, results, and complications of bronchoscopic carbon dioxide laser therapy. Ann. Surg., *199*(5):522–525, 1984.
17. Mims, B.: You can manage chest tubes confidently. RN, *25*:39–42, 1985.
18. Nagasaki, F.: Complications of surgery in the treatment of carcinoma of the lung. Chest, *82*(1):25–26, 1982.
19. Nakahara, K.: A method for predicting postoperative lung function and its relation to postoperative complications in patients with lung cancer. Ann. Thorac. Surg., *39*(3):260–265, 1985.
20. Nicoll, J.: Management of underwater chest drainage. Nurs. Times, *79*(8):58–59, 1983.
21. O'Donohue, W. J.: National survey of the usage of lung expansion modalities for the prevention and treatment of postoperative atelectasis following abdominal and thoracic surgery. Chest, *87*(1):76–80, 1985.
22. Pillbeam, S. P.: Chest tubes and pleural drainage. Curr. Rev. Respir. Ther., *5*(19):151–156, 1983.
23. Saum, M.: Taking the mystery out of chest tubes. AORN J., *32*(1):86–100, 1980.
24. Stach, M.: How to work with chest tubes. Am. J. Nurs., *80*(4):685–712, 1980.
25. Warfield, C. A.: The effect of transcutaneous electrical nerve stimulation on pain after thoracotomy. Ann. Thorac. Surg., *39*(5):462–465, 1985.

Postoperative Care After Cardiac Surgery

Gayle Whitman, R.N., M.S.N., C.C.R.N.

The concept of cardiac surgery as a viable option for patients with heart disease or trauma did not develop until the late 1800s. This late birth in a profession that found its roots in the days of Hippocrates was largely due to emotional as well as technical difficulties inherent in concepts of the heart itself. The perceived seat of the soul and a vital hemodynamic structure, it was viewed as untouchable on both fronts. It can be easily appreciated, then, why trauma intervention became the first aspect of cardiac surgery to be practiced. The imminent life-and-death concerns associated with trauma supplied the practitioner with an acceptable rationale to attempt to surgically manipulate the heart. This first surgical manipulation occurred in 1896, when Rehn successfully closed a stab wound in the ventricle of an unconscious man.

As success in the treatment of cardiac trauma continued to accelerate, attention turned to concern over the low survival rates patients with valve disease were experiencing. Initial attempts at valvular repair were fraught with failures. Finally, Souttar, in 1925, performed the first suc-

cessful mitral commissurotomy by inserting his finger into the left atrial appendage and splitting the leaflets of a stenotic mitral valve. While this was a major milestone, there were still numerous myocardial structures that were technically impossible to manipulate, owing to lack of adequate access. In the 1950s, this access problem was solved by the development of the cardiopulmonary bypass machine and techniques. Now, open heart surgery became a viable option. With the development of cardiopulmonary bypass, numerous new procedures were rapidly developed and successfully performed. Today these techniques range from valve and myocardial structure repair and replacement and direct manipulation of the coronary arteries to transplantation, implantation of assist devices, and total mechanical replacement of the heart.

Many institutions currently perform cardiac surgical procedures. In most of these institutions, patients are transferred directly from surgery to a special cardiac surgery intensive care unit, where they remain for 1 to 3 days before transfer to a regular nursing floor. During this period these patients require intensive hemodynamic monitoring and rapid intervention to prevent many of their normal postoperative states (i.e., hypothermia, hypertension) from growing into postoperative complications (i.e., myocardial infarction, hemorrhage). Discharge from the hospital usually occurs within 7 to 10 days after the surgical procedure.

The length of the preoperative period can vary greatly. In some situations numerous diagnostic tests and procedures may be required to make a definitive diagnosis and to suggest an ultimate surgical procedure. In these situations, owing to the lengthy amount of time the nurse has to instruct and reinforce, both patient and family may proceed into the surgery with adequate knowledge and understanding of the procedure and its expected outcomes. In emergency situations this time period may not be available, and preoperative preparation may be minimal. The PACU nurse should be aware of the knowledge, understanding, and anxieties that both patient and family are experiencing. It is helpful, though not always practical, for the PACU nurse to perform the preoperative instruction for the patient and family or to play an introductory visit to them prior to surgery.

This chapter is designed to familiarize the beginning PACU nurse with postoperative care for the cardiac patient. Additional study is a necessity, and the reader is directed to the references at the end of this chapter for books that deal with the continuum of care needed by the patient hospitalized for cardiac surgery.

Definitions

Annuloplasty: *a surgical technique in which the annulus of the valve is manipulated to decrease the size of the valve orifice and thus limit valvular regurgitation;* this can be accomplished by suturing portions of the valve annulus. More recently, this has been done by using a plication ring, which is a cloth-covered flexible metal ring that is placed over the valve orifice, with the annulus of the valve attached to the ring (Fig. 23–1). This procedure is

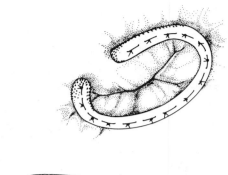

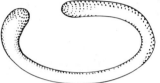

Figure 23–1. Plication ring.

most frequently performed on tricuspid and mitral valves.

Aortic regurgitation: *occurs when the aortic valve does not totally close because the cusps do not completely approximate with each other during diastole.* This can occur as a result of congenital or rheumatic heart disease, infective endocarditis, trauma, aortic dissection, or Marfan's syndrome. This lesion is also known as aortic insufficiency.

Aortic stenosis: *a narrowing of the orifice of the aortic valve itself or of the areas adjacent to the aortic valve.* These narrowings create an obstruction to left ventricular outflow and can be generally classified as three different types: valvular, subvalvular, and supravalvular. In the most common type, the valvular, there is a fusion of the commissures of the valve leaflets that leaves only a small opening. This can occur as a congenital process, as in the bicuspid valve, or owing to an acquired disease process, such as rheumatic heart disease. The second most common type is a subvalvular aortic stenosis. This is usually caused by a fibrinous diaphragm located a few millimeters below the valve leaflets. Another type of subvalvular stenosis occurs when the intraventricular septum becomes hypertrophied and creates an obstruction to left ventricular outflow. This lesion is known as idiopathic hypertrophic subaortic stenosis or hypertrophic obstructive cardiomyopathy. The most infrequently seen form of aortic stenosis is the supravalvular type in which the aorta is constricted just above the ostia of the coronary arteries. This lesion may be considered a coarctation of the ascending aorta. Figure 23–2 illustrates the different types of left ventricular outflow tract obstructions.

Aortocoronary bypass grafts: see Myocardial revascularization.

Atrial septal defect (ASD): *a hole through the atrial septum. An* **ostium secundum defect** *is a defect high in the atrial septum for which no etiologic factors are known. Some secundum defects are associated with anomalous pulmonary veins returning oxygenated blood into the superior vena cava or into the right atrium. An* **ostium primum lesion** *is a defect low in the atrial septum and may involve the tricuspid and mitral valves and the upper portion of the intraventricular*

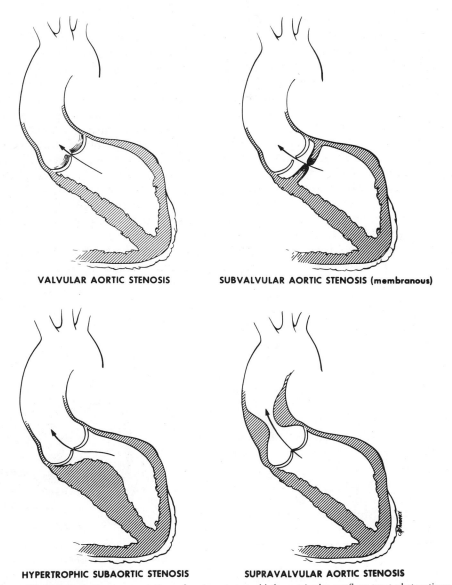

VALVULAR AORTIC STENOSIS   SUBVALVULAR AORTIC STENOSIS (membranous)

HYPERTROPHIC SUBAORTIC STENOSIS   SUPRAVALVULAR AORTIC STENOSIS

Figure 23–2. Schematic representation of various types of left ventricular outflow tract obstructions.

septum. Ostium primum defects develop following arrested embryonic development of the endocardial cushions that normally meet with the ventricular and atrial septa to form the four chambers of the heart. *Atrioventricularis communis is a severe lesion caused by extensive nondevelopment of the endocardial cushions.* In this lesion there is an ostium primum defect, portions of the mitral and tricuspid leaflets form a common valve, and a ventricular septal defect exists. Both ostium primum defects and atrioventricularis communis are also known as *endocardial cushion defects* or *atrioventricular canal defects,* owing to their similar embryonic origins. Closure of septal defects is accomplished by suturing or patching the defect with a graft of pericardium or prosthetic material. Appropriate manipulation and reconstruction of the involved valves are also performed if necessary. Anomalous pulmonary veins are diverted to the left atrium. Figure 23–3 illustrates the areas affected by these lesions.

Cardiac catheterization: *commonly referred to as a cardiac cath; a technique in which a radiopaque plastic catheter is inserted into the right or left heart via a percutaneous puncture or via a cutdown into the femoral or brachial artery or vein in order to obtain pressure, volume, and oxygen saturation determinations from the intracardiac chambers and the great blood vessels (i.e., superior and inferior vena cava, pulmonary artery, and aorta).* In addition, injection of a contrast medium can be utilized to assist in identifying intracardiac and intracoronary artery structural alterations, as well as to obtaining cardiac output and ejection fraction values and wall motion studies. Generally, a "right heart" catheterization will yield data concerning the inferior and superior vena cava, the right atrium and ventricle, and the pulmonary artery. A "left heart" catheterization yields information concerning the left atrium and ventricle, the aorta, and the coronary arteries, if a selective coronary arteriography study is performed.

Cardioplegia: *a paralysis of the heart or cardiac arrest.* While there are different methods that can be used to induce this arrest, today the term cardioplegia is most commonly used to refer to hyperkalemic solutions that produce this arrest effect. Infused into the aortic root, these solutions enter the ostia of the coronary arteries and perfuse the myocardium. In addition to potassium, these solutions can have numerous additives, such as other electrolytes, blood, or antiarrhythmic agents. The purpose of these other agents is to provide a physiologically balanced environment, to provide energy substrates, and to decrease ventricular irritability.

Cardiopulmonary bypass (CPB): *a temporary substitution for the heart and lungs by a pump-oxygenator.* With cardiopulmonary bypass, direct visualization and manipulation of a noncontracting heart is achieved. At the same time, blood is oxygenated, carbon dioxide is removed, and systemic blood flow is sustained. Venous access is achieved by placing cannulas in the venae cavae and the right atrium. Blood is then circulated through the cardiopulmonary bypass circuit where it becomes oxygenated. It is then returned to the patient via arterial cannulas that are located in the aorta or femoral or iliac arteries. Commonly used

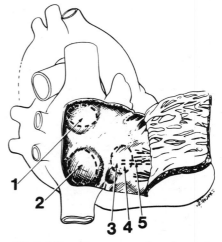

Figure 23–3. Schematic representation of areas involved with various atrial septal defects: (1) anomalous pulmonary vein, (2) ostium secundum defects, (3) ostium primum defects, (4) ventricular septal defect, (5) leaflet of mitral valve.

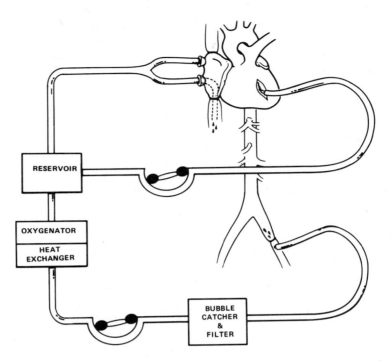

Figure 23–4. Schematic representation of a standard cardiopulmonary bypass circuit.

oxygenators are the rotating disc, the bubble, and the membrane oxygenator (Fig. 23–4).

Coarctation of the aorta: A *narrowing of the aorta that can occur anywhere between the arch to the femoral bifurcation.* There are generally two types of coarctations: preductal and postductal (Fig. 23–5). *In the* ***preductal*** *type, the pulmonary artery communicates with the distal aorta through a ductus.* In this situation, blood flow from the right ventricle and the pulmonary artery supplies the lower half of the body, while flow from the left ventricle and the aorta supplies the upper torso. With this anomaly there are usually other concurrent intracardiac defects, such as ventricular septal defects, transposition of the great arteries, and so forth. *In the* ***postductal*** *type, there is a localized constriction, usually just distal to the left subclavian artery.* This narrowing is usually followed by a poststenotic dilatation. Correction is accomplished by excising the coarctation and then performing an end-to-end anastomosis, with or without a graft, to establish continuity. In the preductal type, appropriate correction of the associated intracardiac defects is also performed.

Commissurotomy: *the opening or separation of fused valvular commissures.* Either closed or open commissurotomy may be performed. In the case of mitral stenosis, closed commissurotomy with a transventricular dilator can be performed, in which a dilator is inserted through the left atrial appendage and then through the mitral valve. The valve is then dilated to the appropriate degree. If the patient is suspected of having a left atrial thrombus that could be easily embolized, an

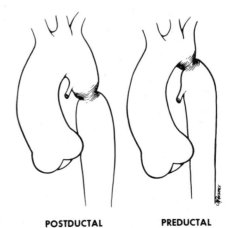

POSTDUCTAL   **PREDUCTAL**

Figure 23–5. Illustration of postductal and preductal types of coarctation of the aorta.

open procedure is performed, in which both dilator and digital pressure are utilized.

Hypothermia: *the elective cooling of the patient during cardiac surgery.* Two general methods are used: systemic and local. *Systemic cooling is accomplished by lowering the patient's temperature to 25 to 30°C with the use of the CPB circuit.* *Local cooling refers to cooling the myocardium to levels of 0 to 10°C.* This can be accomplished by placing an ice slush solution in the pericardial area as well as by administering a cold cardioplegic solution. The purpose of both the local and the systemic use of hypothermia is to diminish cellular demands and limit ischemic injury.

Mechanical assist devices: these devices can be divided into two general types: *temporary assist devices* and *permanent assist devices.* The purpose of temporary assist devices is to provide the failing heart with support over a short period of time, such as hours or days. Examples of temporary assist devices would include the intra-aortic balloon pump (IABP) and the external left and right ventricular assist devices (LVAD, RVAD).

The intra-aortic balloon is a sausage-shaped balloon mounted on a catheter which is inserted most often through the femoral artery and is then placed distal to the left subclavian artery in the descending thoracic aorta. The action of the balloon is to inflate and deflate during diastole. Inflation allows the blood to be pushed cephalad into the aortic root, which increases coronary artery blood supply. Deflation of the balloon, just prior to systolic ejection, creates a negative intra-aortic pressure and therefore decreases afterload. Afterload is simply the impedance against which the ventricle must work in order to open the aortic valve. By increasing coronary blood flow and decreasing afterload, the total work of the heart is reduced, thereby providing an environment that supports the recovery of a failing myocardium.

Another variety of temporary cardiac assist device, the external ventricular assist device, are indicated for use in patients with markedly impaired ventricular function who, following cardiac surgery, develop ventricular failure unresponsive to pharmacologic and IABP support. While these devices vary in their specific design, their technique generally consists of removing blood via cannulas from the left atrium or ventricle and reinfusing it into the aortic root. This technique bypasses the ventricle and therefore requires no ventricular contraction. Blood flow in these systems can be either pulsatile or nonpulsatile and can be propelled by roller, centrifugal, or pneumatically powered drive systems. In these temporary systems, the cannulas and pumps are most often situated outside the chest cavity.

At present, work on a permanently implantable mechanical heart assist device is advancing in two directions. The totally artificial heart, developed by Jarvik at the University of Utah, has arrived at the stage of clinical usage. This system consists of two pneumatically driven elliptical artificial ventricular chambers. Blood flows through these chambers in a manner similar to that in the natural heart, going from the right side through the lungs and then into the left chamber. At this point the blood is ejected into the systemic circulation. The pumping action in the chambers is supplied by a pusher plate system that is controlled by a console external to the patient. The chambers are attached to the console via drive lines that exit from the patient in the abdominal region. This system requires complete excision of the natural myocardium. The other thrust in the development of a permanent artificial device is toward a permanently implantable left ventricular assist device in which the natural heart would remain in place, while cannulas and a pump system would divert blood flow from the left atrium or ventricle into the aorta. Implanted in the chest cavity, this device would also require external drive lines and a drive system. The advantage to this system is that if there were a catastrophic failure of the artificial pump, the natural pump—the

Heart—could maintain the patient until arrival at a medical facility. This device currently has numerous successes in animal models. For both of these systems technology to eliminate the cumbersome drive systems is less than half a decade away.

Mitral regurgitation: *occurs when the mitral valve does not totally close because the leaflets do not completely approximate with each other during diastole.* This can occur as a result of a rheumatic process in which there is a progressive shortening of the leaflets and the chordae. The ischemia or infarction that is associated with coronary artery disease can cause a rupture or elongation of the papillary muscles or the chordae and also create a regurgitant state. In addition, connective tissue disorders, syphilis, Marfan's syndrome, and systemic lupus erythematosus can produce this state by their effect on the papillary muscles and on the chordae.

Mitral stenosis: *a narrowing of the normal aperture of the mitral valve* due to one or a combination of the following: a growth of rheumatic nodules on the valve where the leaflets meet, a thickening of the valves, a fusion of the commissures, or a shortening and thickening of the chordae tendineae. It is most frequently seen as a consequence of rheumatic heart disease.

Myocardial protection techniques: *techniques or procedures designed to expedite the surgical procedure and to limit the amount of ischemic tissue injury that can occur.* These techniques and procedures consist of the following: (1) electrical arrest of the myocardium with alternating current during diastole. This allows a quiet operative field, which will expedite surgical repair and, hence, limit ischemic time; (2) anoxic arrest, produced by crossclamping the aorta. The effect of this is similar to the above; (3) hypothermia, both local and systemic, which serves to decrease cellular metabolism and thus limits ischemic damage (see Hypothermia); and (4) chemical cardioplegia, the infusion into the aortic root of electrolyte, pharmacologic, or blood solutions that assist in chemically arresting the myocardium. This also limits the amount of cellular damage (see Cardioplegia). In addition to these techniques, care is taken to prevent ventricular fibrillation, as this will increase wall tension and increase oxygen consumption.

Myocardial revascularization: *surgical intervention in which blood flow is diverted past significant obstructions in the coronary arteries to inadequately perfused myocardium distal to the obstruction.* This allows adequate oxygenation of these ischemic sections. Most often, portions of the saphenous vein harvested from the patient's leg are used as the conduits for blood flow. One portion of the vein is anastomosed in an end-to-side fashion to the aorta, and the other end is similarly anastomosed to the coronary artery distal to the obstruction (Fig. 23–6). In addition to utilizing the saphenous vein, the right and left internal mammary arteries (RIMA and LIMA) are well suited for myocardial revascularization. Arising from the aorta, these vessels extend along the inside of the chest wall. For revascularization purposes they are distally dissected off the chest wall and are left attached proximally to the aorta. Their distal ends are then attached to vessels on their respective sides. Other conduit vessels that are attached in the same manner as the saphenous vein include portions of the cephalic vein and portions of a specially processed human umbilical vein. Bypass grafts are usually performed on the major coronary arteries, such as the right coronary artery (RCA), the two major branches of the left coronary artery (LCA), the left anterior descending artery (LAD), or the circumflex (Cx) artery. However, grafts can be attached to any vessel that has a diameter of 1 mm. Because of this, other vessels, such as the diagonal artery (Dg), or other branches of the major arteries, such as the posterior descending artery (PDA) of the RCA, also can be revascularized. Myocardial revascularization is also known as coronary artery bypass grafting (CABG) or aortocoronary grafting.

Patent ductus arteriosus (PDA): *a duct between the pulmonary artery and the aorta.*

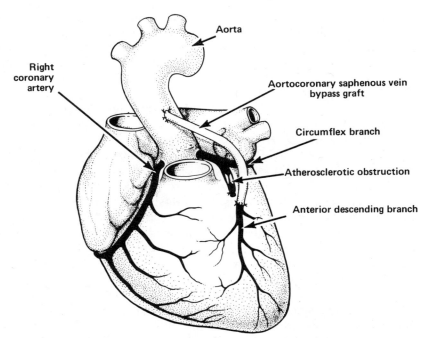

Figure 23–6. Saphenous vein bypass graft attached proximally to the aorta and distally to the anterior descending coronary artery past the atherosclerotic obstruction.

This structure, which is normally present in fetal life, usually closes within 1 to 2 weeks after birth. Failure to close can predispose the patient to the development of pulmonary hypertension or cardiac failure. Closure can be surgically achieved by ligation of the ductus or by division of the ductus followed by oversewing the ends.

Pericardiectomy: *the partial excision of an adhered, thickened, fibrotic pericardium to relieve constriction of a compressed heart and great blood vessels.* In patients with chronic cardiac effusions, the creation of a pericardial window between the pericardial sac and the pleural space can also be accomplished. The opening to the pleural space allows chronically accumulating fluid to be reabsorbed.

Pulmonary artery banding: a procedure in which the pulmonary artery is constricted with tape to reduce its diameter and to decrease the pulmonary blood flow. This is usually performed as one of several stages prior to a complete surgical correction. The goal of this technique is to prevent the development of pulmonary hypertension.

Pulmonary stenosis: *fusion of the valve cusps at the commissures,* which creates an obstruction to the right ventricular outflow tract. In infundibular stenosis, fibromuscular obstruction occurs proximal to the valve. Most frequently, repair is accomplished via an open procedure under direct visualization. The stenotic valve is opened wide and the fused commissures are sharply excised back to the annulus. Correction can also be performed by a closed procedure in which, via a right ventriculotomy, a valvulotome is inserted and the stenotic leaflets are separated when it is withdrawn.

Tetralogy of Fallot: *a congenital entity with four distinctive features* (Fig. 23–7): (1) *a high ventricular septal defect,* (2) *pulmonary stenosis,* (3) *overriding of the ventricular septal defect by the aorta,* and (4) *hypertrophy of the right ventricle.* At present, the trend is to proceed with an elective procedure for correction, generally when the patient is 3 to 5 years old. If the child is severely symptomatic prior to this age, either a corrective or a palliative procedure is performed, according to the surgeon's preference. Currently, the most frequently

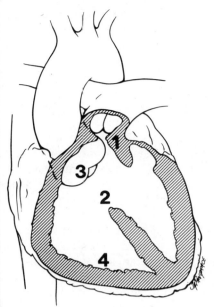

Figure 23–7. Four features of tetralogy of Fallot: (1) pulmonary stenosis, (2) ventricular septal defect, (3) overriding aorta, (4) right ventricular hypertrophy.

performed palliative procedure is the Blalock-Taussig or systemic-pulmonary anastomosed technique. In this procedure the subclavian artery is anastomosed to the pulmonary artery, thereby producing an increase in blood flow to the lungs. In a corrective procedure, a complete resection of the infundibular or pulmonary valve stenosis and closure of the ventricular septal defect are performed. If previously constructed palliative shunts are present, they are closed prior to the initiation of the corrective procedure.

Transplantation: First performed in 1967, transplantation was not an immediate success owing to problems with inadequate monitoring of rejection and infection and inadequate prophylaxis. With improvement in these therapies, cardiac transplantation 1-year survival rates are approaching 90 percent. Potential candidates are patients who are considered to be in the New York Heart Association's Functional Class IV and who have less than a 10 percent chance of surviving for 6 months. Contraindications for transplantation include significant pulmonary hypertension, presence of systemic disease, recent pulmonary infarction, or active systemic infection. Heart donors are individuals who have suffered irreversible, catastrophic brain injury, who are under the age of 30, and who are free from atherosclerotic heart disease. Removal of the donor heart is accomplished by transection of the vena cava, the pulmonary artery and veins, and the aorta. The donor heart is then transported to the recipient's institution in a ice saline bath with ischemic times of less than 4 hours. The recipient's heart is surgically removed once the donor heart has arrived in the operating room. The posterior and lateral atrial walls, the vena caval inflow tracts, the pulmonary vein orifices, and the atrial septum remain intact while the remainder of the heart is excised. The donor heart is then attached at the atria, the pulmonary artery, and the aorta. Except for the addition of infection and rejection monitoring, these patients receive the same postoperative care given other general cardiac surgery patients. If no complications ensue they are generally discharged from the hospital in 3 weeks.

Transposition of the great arteries (TGA): *a congenital anomaly in which the pulmonary artery arises from the left ventricle and carries oxygenated blood back to the lungs, and the aorta arises from the right ventricle and carries unoxygenated blood into the systemic circulation.* An uncommon anomaly, this condition is incompatible with life unless a concomitant anomalous shunt, such as a septal defect or a patent ductus arteriosus, between the systemic and pulmonary circulations is also present. These lesions allow adequate mixing of the blood between the two circulations. To maintain the patency of the atrial septal defect, a balloon atrial septostomy is usually performed. In addition, E-type prostaglandin is administered to maintain the patency of the PDA. A variety of corrective procedures can be utilized to achieve a repair, with the selection of the procedure being dictated by the patient's anatomy and the surgeon's preference. Arterial, ventricular, and intra-atrial repairs can be performed. The two intra-arterial repairs are the Senning and the Mustard procedures. In both of these, the atrial chambers are reconstructed so that pulmonary venous blood returns to the right atrium and systemic venous blood returns to the left atrium. Surgical correction for this anomaly is undertaken as early as possible.

Tricuspid regurgitation: *occurs when the tricuspid valve does not totally close because the leaflets do not completely approximate in diastole.* This lesion is more common than tricuspid stenosis and can develop because of rheumatic changes, following a right ventricular infarction, or, transiently, from annular dilatation resulting from right ventricular failure.

Tricuspid stenosis: *a narrowing of the orifice of the tricuspid valve.* Although this occurs infrequently, it can be associated with rheumatic heart disease or bacterial endocarditis.

Valve replacement: *a surgical procedure in which the natural valve is replaced with an artificial valve.* Whatever the etiology, repair consists of excising the natural valve and its attached apparatus, such as the chordae tendineae of the mitral valve, and inserting a prosthetic valve. Prosthetic valves can be classified into two groups: mechanical and biologic. Types of mechanical valves currently used are the caged-ball, the tilting disc, and the bileaflet valve (Fig. 23–8). The caged-ball valve consists of a metallic cage attached to a sewing ring. In the center of the cage is a hollow metal or plastic ball that moves forward in the cage, allowing blood to flow through the valve. When the ball rests on the sewing ring it impedes flow. An example of a caged-ball valve is the Starr-Edwards valve.

The tilting disc valve consists of a freefloating, thin, lens-shaped disc occluder made of pyrolytic carbon mounted on a semicircular sewing ring. The disc tilts or pivots upward when the valve is open, allowing blood flow, and when the valve is closed, the disc lies on the sewing ring. Examples of the tilting disc valve are the Björk-Shiley and the Lillehei-Kaster

valves. More recently, a bileaflet valve, the St. Jude Medical prosthesis, has been developed. The St. Jude valve consists of a sewing ring in which reside two semicircular leaflets that open centrally. This valve is well suited for use in children and adults with small aortic roots because of its size and design.

Mechanical valves are extremely durable and withstand wear over a long period of time. One disadvantage associated with their use is the high incidence of thromboembolic events. For this reason, patients with these valves need lifelong anticoagulation drugs. This is usually initiated 3 to 5 days after surgery, when all their intracardiac lines and chest tubes are discontinued and immediate postoperative hemorrhage is no longer a concern. Oral coumarin therapy is then started and titrated appropriately to achieve prothrombin times two and a half times normal.

Biologic valves can be classified as xenograft (from animal cadaver tissues) or homograft (from human cadaver donor tissue). Xenografts can be made from porcine aorta or bovine pericardium. The Hancock and Carpentier-Edwards valves are porcine valves. The Ionescu-Shiley valve is an example of a bovine pericardial valve. The advantage of biological valves resides largely in the decreased incidence of thromboembolic events associated with their use. Despite this, some physicians will maintain their patients on prophylactic anticoagulation drugs for 6 months after biological valve replacement, particularly if the patient has had a history of a mural thrombus, of atrial fibrillation, or of an enlarged left atrium. Disadvantages of biological valves are that they are not as durable as mechanical valves; they are prone to tissue degeneration and calcification of their leaflets and may therefore require reoperation and replacement earlier than mechanical valves.

Ventricular aneurysm (VA) repair: Ventricular aneurysms most often result from a large myocardial infarction or numerous smaller adjacent infarcts in which a por-

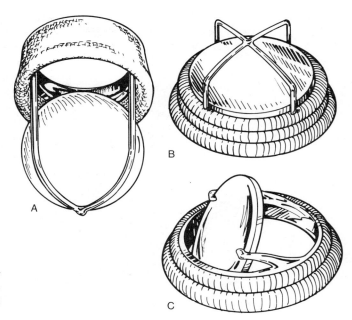

Figure 23–8. Schematic representation of various types of mechanical valves: (a) cage and ball, (b) cage and disc, (c) tilting disc.

tion of the myocardial wall becomes necrotic, thin, and weak. This portion then does not contract during systole but instead bulges outward, which decreases the patient's cardiac output. Additionally, the endothelial layers of the aneurysm become roughened, which promotes the development of large mural thrombi, leaving the patient at a high risk for an embolic event. Also, the perimeter around the necrotic area, because it consists largely of varying amounts of fibrous tissue, can alter conduction pathways and create reentrant ventricular arrhythmias. The surgical technique consists of excising the aneurysm at its perimeter, carefully removing the thrombus inside to avoid embolization. Then the edges of the ventricle are joined with suture. If the patient has been experiencing recurrent ventricular tachycardia, an endomyocardial mapping might also be performed. With this technique, the aneurysm is first removed and then a small electrode probe is attached to the surgeon's fingers and passed over the edges of the endothelial portion of the remaining ventricle, and activation potentials are observed. This procedure assists in differentiating fibrous tissue from viable tissue. The en-

dothelium is then peeled back, removing all the fibrous tissue. This eliminates tissues that are a source of reentrant rhythms. The edges of the ventricle are then closed as previously described (Fig. 23–9).

Ventricular septal defect (VSD): *a defect consisting of a hole through the ventricular septum.* Usually this defect is located in the upper portion of the septum just anterior to the membranous septum. A VSD can be congenital or acquired; those of congenital origin will sometimes close

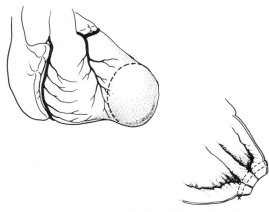

Figure 23–9. A ventricular aneurysm is illustrated in upper drawing. Repair consists of excision of the aneurysm and approximation of the edges of the left ventricle.

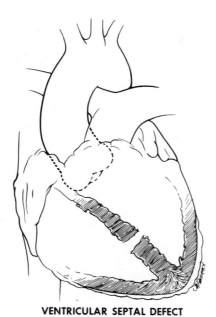

VENTRICULAR SEPTAL DEFECT

Figure 23–10. Schematic representation of a ventricular septal defect. Size and location of the defect can vary from patient to patient.

spontaneously. In an adult, these are most commonly acquired from myocardial ischemia following an infarction of the septal wall (Fig. 23–10). In both types, closure of the defect can be accomplished either with the use of a synthetic patch or by oversewing the edges, depending on the size of the defect.

INTRAOPERATIVE CONSIDERATIONS

The most commonly used approach in cardiac surgery is the median sternotomy. However, anterolateral or posterolateral thoracotomy incisions or a transverse sternotomy with a bilateral thoracotomy can also be used. The median sternotomy approach allows exposure of the anterior mediastinum without entry into the pleural cavities. With this approach, the sternum is split with a saw. At the conclusion of the procedure, the sternum is closed with stainless steel wires, and the skin is approximated subcutaneously with suture. The pericardium that was incised during the surgery is left open at the end of the procedure. Pericardial chest tubes are placed

anteriorly and posteriorly in the pericardium to facilitate drainage. They exit via stab wounds at the distal portion of the mediastinal incision. If either of the pleurae was opened during the procedure, then pleural chest tubes are also inserted.

Once the sternum is opened the patient is placed on CPB, and hypothermia and cardioplegic infusions are initiated. While CPB is an essential component of cardiac surgery, it is not without its potential problems. With prolonged use of the pump-oxygenator, usually 4 hours or longer, various coagulation, volume, respiratory, and neurologic dysfunctions may develop. Bleeding dyscrasias develop as a result of the direct trauma from the pumping to the elements of the blood. Treatment consists of replacing depleted elements with infusion of platelets, fresh frozen plasma, or fresh whole blood. With prolonged pump use, cell walls become increasingly permeable, thus allowing a capillary leak syndrome to develop. As fluid shifts from the intravascular space to the interstitial space, a relative hypovolemia develops. Administration of colloidal agents, such as albumin products, helps to reverse this situation. If this cell wall permeability extends to the lungs, a permeability pulmonary edema can develop. This is a rare occurrence. Significant atelectasis, however, can easily occur with prolonged bypass times, since the lungs are purposely kept underinflated during the surgical repair to provide the surgeon with a quiet operative field. Additionally, neurologic dysfunctions, both motor and cognitive, can occur. Air or fat emboli or inadequate cerebral perfusion during the procedure can cause various stroke-like states. Postpump psychosis with auditory and visual hallucinations has also been attributed to prolonged surgical repairs. As mentioned earlier, these complications are largely associated with CPB times of 4 hours or more. Fortunately, the majority of procedures are accomplished within a shorter period of time, and thus these complications are infrequent. However, the PACU nurse should always be aware of their potential.

Anesthesia for cardiac surgery varies

from hospital to hospital and also can vary depending on the type of cardiac repair undertaken. For example, in repair of a mitral valve when there is evidence of significant pulmonary involvement, agents that increase pulmonary vascular resistance would be avoided. Commonly employed inhalation agents include halothane, enflurane, methoxyflurane, and nitrous oxide. Barbiturates, such as thiopental and methohexital, are utilized to accomplish the rapid sequence of induction and intubation. Morphine sulfate and fentanyl are the narcotic analgesics that are most frequently used. Morphine can assist in increasing the cardiac index, since it decreases systemic vascular resistance, and since fentanyl has a negligible myocardial effect, it is also a commonly used analgesic. Antianxiety agents, such as diazepam and Ativan, in addition to narcotic analgesics, are employed in the early postoperative period.

PACU CARE

Following cardiac surgery, most patients require monitoring of their heart rate and arterial blood pressure during transport from the surgical suite to the intensive care unit. This is because these patients can develop acute circulatory instability due either to their normally recovering physiologic state or to inadvertent movement or displacement of the numerous invasive lines and tubes they require. Upon arrival at the unit, the PACU nurse should assess these parameters immediately. If either of these parameters indicates circulatory or ventilatory dysfunction, immediate resuscitative measures should be instituted.

If, at a quick glance, circulatory and ventilatory status appear adequate, then admission routines should be begun. The respiratory therapist or anesthesiologist usually attaches the patient to the ventilator and establishes the initial settings and sets the alarms. Once the patient is attached to the ventilator, the nurse auscultates both lung fields and repeats that assessment frequently until discharge. Arterial blood gases are obtained on admission and as needed thereafter. Patients remain intubated until

the effects of anesthesia subside and hemodynamic stability is achieved and maintained. Controlled ventilation is used initially. As patients begin to generate their own respirations, they are switched to intermittent mandatory ventilation (IMV) modes, in which they gradually increase their spontaneous respirations in order to maintain adequate minute ventilations. Once patients are maintaining an adequate respiratory rate they are switched to continuous positive airway pressure (CPAP) systems. With CPAP, the patient determines the respiratory rate and the ventilator provides the positive pressure to the airway that the glottis normally provides when the patient is not intubated. The use of CPAP prevents microatelectasis and increases the functional residual capacity of the lung. Once the patient maintains adequate arterial blood gases on CPAP, extubation usually follows quickly. After extubation, face masks or nasal cannulas are used to deliver supplemental oxygen.

A continuous ECG recording is established, alarm limits are set, and a strip recording is obtained. A 12-lead electrocardiogram is obtained as soon as possible and repeated daily for the first 3 days. Recorded rhythm strips are then obtained every 2 hours and documented. Lead selection varies, but MCL1, in which the LA and RA leads are in their respective places and the third lead is placed on the fourth right intercostal space, is commonly used. Electrode placement with this lead does not interfere with defibrillation procedures or with mediastinal or chest tube dressing placement. The apical pulse is auscultated and validated with the ECG recording. If the patient has a temporary external pacer in place, the nurse should check and record the type of pacing, the mode, the rate, the milliamperage (mA) and determine if the pacer is functioning adequately. If the patient is not being paced, then the nurse needs to ensure that the unused pacemaker wires are covered with gauze, placed in a plastic covering (a finger cot), and securely dressed and attached to the chest to protect the patient from electrical hazard. Usually two ventricular and two atrial pacing wires are attached to the epicardium with absorbable suture prior to closure of the chest. These wires then exit the chest via stab wounds on either side of the sternal incision. The atrial wires are usually on the right and the ventricular wires on the left. They are most often left in place for a few days after surgery and may be utilized to assist in cardiac rhythm control. Prior to discharge of the patient from the hospital, they are totally removed by gentle traction or they are clipped off at the skin level, leaving a portion of them attached to the epicardium and residing in the subcutaneous tissues.

All intravascular lines are attached to transducers or manometers. Their patency is ascertained and their values or wave tracings or both are continuously displayed and recorded. Commonly measured intravascular parameters include: mean arterial pressure (MAP), right atrial pressure (RAP), mean pulmonary artery pressure (PAM), pulmonary artery systolic pressure (PAS), pulmonary artery diastolic pressure (PAD), pulmonary capillary wedge pressure (PCWP), and left atrial pressure (LAP). In addition to providing these directly measured parameters, these values assist in calculating indirect or derived hemodynamic parameters, such as cardiac output and cardiac index (CO/CI), systemic vascular resistance (SVR), and pulmonary vascular resistance (PVR). All of these parameters assist in assessing both left and right ventricular status and are invaluable in determining pharmacologic, fluid, and mechanical therapies for the postoperative cardiac surgery patient. Once these intravascular lines are appropriately monitored, the nurse reviews and assesses with the anesthesiologist all intravascular lines and solutions in regard to type, drugs being infused, flow rates, patency, and expiration times, if applicable. Intake and output recordings are made hourly, and ongoing running totals are documented hourly. Volume administration and replacement therapies are largely determined by the individual patient's hemodynamic parameters and responses and can vary greatly from hour to hour.

The patient's neurologic status is assessed on admission and every 30 to 60 minutes thereafter until arousal from anesthesia. Once the patient has been aroused, neurologic assessments are decreased to every 2 hours. The Glasgow coma scale can be utilized for these checks.

Chest tube drainage systems are established. Water seal drainage or autotransfusion systems with 15 to 20 cm of negative suction are most frequently used. The amount and type of chest tube drainage are frequently assessed and recorded on an hourly basis. Drainage exceeding 100 ml per hour should be brought to the attention of the physician. Chest tubes are usually removed on the first or second postoperative day providing intracardiac lines have been removed, there is no evidence of fluid accumulation on the chest film, and there has been less than 200 ml of drainage in the last 6 hours. Most patients will have one to two mediastinal chest tubes that facilitate pericardial drainage after surgery. If the pleural spaces were opened during the procedure or the internal mammary arteries were dissected off the chest wall, or both, then pleural chest tubes will also be present to facilitate drainage and to prevent a pneumothorax.

An admission temperature is obtained, and rewarming therapies are instituted, if necessary. During rewarming, temperatures are recorded hourly and rewarming devices are discontinued just prior to the patient's reaching normothermia. This slightly premature discontinuation is performed to avoid a hyperthermic overshoot, which is common. In this situation, temperatures may overshoot the 37°C level and elevate to levels of 38 to 40°C. It is desirable to avoid these elevations, since hyperthermia increases myocardial oxygen consumption. Commonly employed rewarming devices include warming lights, alcohol circulating mattresses, and warmed thermal blankets.

An abdominal assessment is performed on admission and every 2 hours thereafter until bowel sounds return. A nasogastric tube is in place to relieve gastric distention ard facilitate removal of gastric contents. It is usually attached to low intermittent suction or gravity drainage and removed at the time of extubation. Analysis of pH and tests for the presence of occult blood may be performed on gastric secretions if they begin to resemble coffee grounds. Once the nasogastric tube is removed, the patient is given ice chips and resumes a clear liquid diet within the first 24 hours.

A retention catheter is in place and urinary outputs are recorded on admission and then hourly. The appearance of the urine is also monitored closely. During the first few hours after surgery, massive diuresis of 2 to 3 liters of pale, dilute urine is usually common. This is a result of use of diuretics that are generally administered during the discontinuation of cardiopulmonary bypass pumping. This is done to facilitate the removal of fluid that has sequestered during surgery in the interstitial space. Once this initial diuresis resolves, urine color and consistency return to normal. At that time it is desirable to keep urinary output at levels greater than 0.5 ml per kg per hour. Catheters are usually removed prior to patient discharge from the recovery area.

Peripheral pulses as well as skin color and temperature are assessed and recorded hourly. All incisions and intravascular and tube insertion sites are observed. The patient is placed in a semi-Fowler position with the legs supported at the knees and calves slightly elevated. This facilitates venous return from the legs and limits swelling, particularly in patients with saphenous vein incisions. Legs are wrapped from toes to hips with elastic leg wraps or with antiembolism stockings.

Following these admission routines, a written assessment is performed. The frequency of assessing and documenting the above-mentioned hemodynamic parameters and routines is dictated by the individual patient's response to and recovery from surgery. Recovery time varies from patient to patient but generally occurs within a 12-48-hour period. During that time, owing largely to the techniques of cardiopulmonary bypass, hypothermia, anesthesia, and surgical manipulation of the myocardium, numerous normal postoperative physiologic alterations occur. With correct interventions, these normal physiologic responses are short-lived and reversible. However, two problems do exist. First, while these alterations are reversible, if they are not identified early and quickly reversed they can lead to complications. Such is the case with uncontrolled hypertension that can develop into hemorrhage if fresh suture lines are disrupted. Secondly, these normal alterations frequently resemble complications and thus may be missed in their early stages. For example, the initial absence of a pedal pulse may be attributed to hypothermia and vasoconstriction only to be later traced to a vascular embolism. For these reasons it is incumbent upon the PACU nurse to be knowledgeable about the etiologies, assessment factors, and interventions for both normal physiologic alterations and complications that can occur after cardiac surgery. In the next section these alterations and potential complications will be briefly reviewed.

COMPLICATIONS

The Cardiovascular System

The major postoperative alterations and complications that develop after cardiac surgery are cardiovascular in origin and generally consist of the following: peripheral vasoconstriction, alteration in myocardial contractility, alteration in volume status, cardiac tamponade, and dysrhythmias.

Peripheral Vasoconstriction

Factors that contribute to the development of peripheral vasoconstriction include the patient's own sympathetic drive triggered by anxiety and the surgical manipulation of the heart and the great vessels with their attached pressor receptors. Additionally, CPB, systemic hypothermia, and vasoactive drugs contribute to this vasoconstriction. The patient physically presents with pale, cold extremities, temperature less than 37°C, elevated systemic vascular resistance, absent pulses, tachycardia, and vary-ing degrees of hypertension. If left unat-tended, the hypertension could disrupt new surgical anastomoses, and the elevated sys-temic vascular resistance could assist in cre-ating a state of myocardial depression due to the high afterload effect it creates. Ther-apies consist of immediate rewarming and administration of vasodilating agents. Such agents include intravenous sodium nitro-prusside, nitroglycerine, and phentola-mine. These agents have relatively imme-diate effects and can be easily reversed once their use is discontinued. The PACU nurse usually titrates the dosage of these agents to maintain mean arterial blood pressure at 60 to 120 mm Hg and to bring the systemic vascular resistance back to normal levels.

Alteration in Myocardial Contractility

Alteration in myocardial contractility with resultant low cardiac outputs and shock-like states can also develop postoperatively. Causes include a perioperative myocardial infarction or an ischemic state, faulty sur-gical repair, myocardial edema from sur-gical manipulation, metabolic disturbances, and depression from hypothermia and anesthesia. The patient will clinically dem-onstrate a decrease in cardiac output/cardiac index, hypotension, elevated SVR, elevated filling pressures, acidosis, tachycardia, and decreased urine output. If the condition is due to faulty surgical repair, the patient should immediately return to the surgical suite for correction. If other causes of de-creased contractility are suspected, then va-sopressor agents should be employed. Do-pamine and dobutamine are most often the first agents used. If they fail to produce adequate results, then isoproterenol and norepinephrine are utilized. Concurrent va-sodilator therapy may also be required to diminish the peripheral vasoconstrictive ac-tions of these inotropes. In cases of severe myocardial depression, intra-aortic balloon pump assist or left or right ventricular heart assist may be necessary. For the most part, these low-flow states are relatively short-lived. If associated with a perioperative in-farction, the shock state may be more se-

vere, depending on the size of the infarc-tion. Assessment factors used to identify the presence of a perioperative myocardial infarction include SGOT elevation greater than 140 units, development of new Q waves on the 12-lead electrocardiogram, and CPK enzyme elevations three to six times their normal values on the second postoperative day.

Inadequate Volume Status

Inadequate volume status can easily de-velop in postoperative patients. Hypovole-mia can be induced by inadequate volume management in conjunction with or follow-ing rewarming in which there is rapid va-sodilatation. Hypovolemia can also be as-sociated with diuretic and vasodilator therapies, hemorrhage from active or slow-oozing bleeders in the chest, hemorrhage from coagulopathies associated with CPB, or inadequate reversal of the effects of the heparin used during CPB. Hypervolemia develops as interstitial fluid moves back into the intravascular space or if overaggressive volume replacement occurs. Assessment of these states requires extensive hemody-namic monitoring and understanding of the numerous processes involved. Signs and symptoms specific to hypovolemia or hy-pervolemia will be sought. Interventions for hypovolemia first consist of replacement with crystalloid agents. If the patient is suspected of having a moderate capillary leak syndrome due to prolonged bypass times, of if the patient had significant pe-ripheral edema, then colloidal solutions are more appropriate. If persistent hemorrhage from coagulopathies exists, transfusion with replacement factors such as fresh fro-zen plasma, platelet concentrates, and other factors may be indicated. If hemorrhage is related to technical factors, reoperation is required and replacement solutions in the interim can be autotranfused blood, whole blood, or packed cells.

Cardiac Tamponade

A cardiac tamponade develops when there is an accumulation of blood or fluid in the pericardial cavity sufficient to compress the heart. This compression of the heart results in ineffective filling and ejection. Symptoms therefore consist of low cardiac output/cardiac index, hypotension, tachycardia, equalization of the right and left atrial pressures, development of a pulsus paradoxus, narrowed pulse pressure, muffled heart sounds, widening of the mediastinum on the chest x-ray, and alteration in neurologic status. Observation of the quality of chest tube drainage is critical in this situation. Normally, chest tube drainage in cardiac surgical patients is thin, red, and non-clotted. This is because blood resides in the chest cavity for a brief period before it exits via the chest tubes. Because of this residence time, it is exposed to the mechanical effects of the contracting heart and the motion of the lungs. This allows the blood which normally begins to clot once it leaves its vessel to defibrinoginate the clot it forms and thus become thin, nonclotted drainage by the time it exits the chest tube. If clots begin to appear in the chest tubes, this indicates that relatively fresh bleeding is occurring, since blood has no residence time in the chest cavity. In this situation, the incidence of tamponade is higher, as the chest tubes become clotted off easily. Therefore, sudden cessation of previously heavily clotted drainage is a primary indicator for the nurse at the bedside that a tamponade may be developing. Tamponade most frequently occurs in the first 6 hours after surgery. The specific cause can be either rapid, active bleeding from a suture line or a continuous, slow ooze from a coagulopathy that exceeds the ability of the chest tube to drain it. A tamponade may also develop after the removal of intracardiac lines as a result of which bleeding occurred. Treatment consists of reoperation. If the patient becomes acutely unstable, the chest will be reopened in the PACU. Opening of the chest cavity frequently relieves the compression enough that relatively stable vital signs immediately ensue. The patient can then be taken to the surgical suite for complete repair on a less emergent basis. A reoperation to relieve a tamponade does not usually delay the patient's recovery or prolong the hospital stay.

Dysrhythmias

Rhythm disturbance can occur postoperatively in as many as 30 percent of patients undergoing cardiac surgery. Caused by ischemic, pharmacologic, metabolic, or iatrogenic effects, these disturbances can range from atrial to ventricular in nature. Ischemia due to infarction, hypoxemia, or hypotension may serve as the precipitant drive for dysrhythmia. Inotropic drugs, with their contractile and chronotropic effects, or acid-base imbalances and electrolyte abnormalities may also be the causative factors. Iatrogenically, mechanical irritation from some intracardiac lines and from the patient's endogenous catecholamine release may create irregularities. Owing to this high incidence of dysrhythmia, continuous monitoring is usually performed for the first 24 to 48 hours on these patients, even if they are discharged to a regular nursing floor in that period. Aggressive treatment of electrolyte imbalances and the correction of hypoxic states are the first priorities. Owing to the massive diuresis some patients experience, hypokalemia frequently develops. This can precipitate numerous arrhythmias, and therefore potassium replacement is aggressive, and efforts are made to maintain serum potassium concentrations at levels greater than 4.0 mEq/L. If correction of these imbalances fails to eliminate the dysrhythmia, pacing may be undertaken via the temporary external pacing wires inserted during the surgical procedure. Overriding arrhythmias with the pacer is usually necessary only for a day or so. After that time, pacing can be discontinued and the pacer wires removed. If this fails to correct the bradycardias, blocks, or tachyarrhythmias, antiarrhythmic drugs will be instituted.

The Respiratory System

Moderate episodes of impaired gas exchange with concurrent moderate alterations in the arterial blood gases commonly occur after cardiac surgery, mainly owing to the effects of anesthesia, sedation, and CPB. These episodes, largely atelectatic in nature, are usually self-limiting or easily resolved with chest physiotherapy and supplemental oxygen administration. A hemothorax or a pneumothorax may develop. In these situations, more negative pressure may be added to the drainage systems, or placement of additional chest tubes may be required. A volume overload from overaggressive replacement or mobilization of fluid from the third spaces may exist that could hamper gas exchange. In this situation, diuretic therapy would be instituted. In rare instances, a noncardiac permeability pulmonary edema can develop. Since this entity is associated with a high mortality rate, mechanical ventilatory assistance, and pharmacologic and fluid therapy are quite intensive.

The Nervous System

Temporary and permanent sensory, motor, perceptual, and cognitive deficits can occur during the perioperative period. Permanent deficits can usually be attributed to a low cerebral perfusion state from inadequate cardiac output or to an embolic phenomenon from intracardiac thrombi, calcified valve fragments, plaque embolization from the aortic crossclamp, or air embolization from intracardiac lines. The magnitude of the deficit is determined by the degree of neurologic involvement. These are usually identified early in the postoperative period when the effects of anesthesia have resolved. Some of these deficits may not be identified until after extubation. Transient deficits that can last from hours to days can occur in as many as a quarter of patients undergoing cardiac surgery. These transient deficits can range from a slowness to arouse, to confusion and delirium. A second type of delirium that can develop after cardiac surgery is a postcardiotomy delirium (PCD) syndrome. Classically, PCD occurs 2 to 5 days after cardiac surgery, usually following a normal and uncomplicated arousal from anesthesia. Symptoms can range from full-blown psychosis to mild confusion. The syndrome is self-limiting, subsiding in a few days. Risk factors seem to include advanced age, duration of bypass, and severe preoperative illness.

The Renal System

Prerenal and acute renal failure states can develop after cardiac surgery. Inadequate cardiac output from myocardial depression or inadequate volume replacement can lead to prerenal oliguria. In this situation, blood urea nitrogen and serum sodium levels rise, and serum creatinine remains the same. There is a low sodium content in the urine as the body attempts to save sodium and thus increase its intravascular volume; the urine plasma osmolality ratio remains 1:1.5. If these states continue for prolonged periods, acute renal failure can ensue. Treatment centers on adequate volume replacement and on increasing cardiac output, perhaps with an inotropic agent. In addition, renal emboli from intracardiac thrombi or hemolysis from blood transfusions can also lead to the development of acute renal failure. In the event of acute renal failure, serum creatinine and urea levels elevate and remain in a 10:1 ratio, urine sodium levels rise, and the plasma urine osmolality ratio falls to a 1:1 ratio.

Transient hematuria can occur following discontinuation of CPB or after autotransfusion of shed mediastinal blood. These events are usually short-lived and clear up themselves or following infusion of an osmotic diuretic such as mannitol.

The Gastrointestinal System

Gastric complications that can develop include mesenteric or splenic ischemia or infarction from intracardiac thrombi or air emboli. Immediate surgical intervention may be necessary in these situations. Gastric distention can occur if the patient swallows air. This distention can cause cardiac problems as well as pulmonary complications. Stress ulceration can also develop; however, in recent years its incidence has decreased with the more frequent use of cimetidine.

The Peripheral Vascular System

Vascular complications can include both venous and arterial thrombus formation and embolism development. Venous thrombus can develop, owing to stasis from immobilization and inactivity in the immediate postoperative period. Arterial complications are largely associated with various intravascular devices such as intra-arterial lines, intra-aortic balloon catheters, and so forth. Assessment of pulses should be on-going, but particular attention should be given to the performance of the Allen test following radial artery line removal. The Allen test assesses for the patency of the radial and ulnar arteries. In addition, the status of lower extremity pulses, skin color and temperature, and motor activity should be monitored closely in the presence of an intra-aortic balloon catheter, particularly during insertion and removal. Passive and active range of motion exercises and early ambulation are advocated and encouraged in these patients to prevent some of the foregoing complications. In the recovery areas, the patient is instructed and assisted in performing active dorsiflexion and extension of the feet and ankles. These maneuvers facilitate venous return and decrease stasis.

CARDIAC MONITORING

The PACU nurse must have a basic understanding of cardiac monitoring and should be able to interpret the basic cardiac rhythms and dysrhythmias and correlate them with expected cardiac output and its effects on the patient's condition. This section is designed to provide an introduction to specific problems of cardiac monitoring in the PACU. A list of references is included at the end of the chapter for the reader who needs a basic review of electrocardiographic interpretation or who wishes to be informed on more advanced interpretation.

Any type of cardiac arrhythmia may be seen in the PACU. Their causes must be carefully differentiated before any treatment is instituted. Some commonly encountered problems are reviewed here, but the list is by no means complete.

All abnormal rhythms should be documented with a rhythm strip and recorded in the patient's progress record. Any questionable rhythms should be documented by a complete 12-lead electrocardiogram.

Electrical monitoring of the patient's heart is only one assessment parameter and must be interpreted in conjunction with other salient parameters before therapy is initiated. Cardiac monitors generally depict only a single lead. They will certainly not detect all rhythm disturbances and alterations and a 12-lead electrocardiogram is essential to define a conduction problem accurately.

Lead Placement. The skin where the electrode will be placed should be clean, dry, and smooth. Excessive hair should be removed; moisture or skin oils should be removed with alcohol or acetone and the

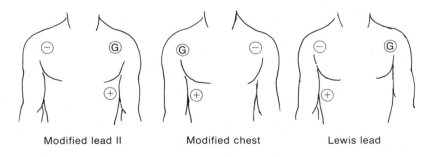

Modified lead II   Modified chest   Lewis lead

Lead I

Figure 23–11. Basic electrode placement.

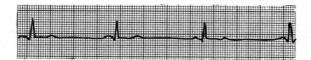

Figure 23–12. Sinus bradycardia (lead III). (From Guyton, A.C.: Textbook of Medical Physiology. 6th ed. Philadelphia, W.B. Saunders Co., 1981, p.197.)

skin mildly abraded to obtain good adherence of the electrode.

Site selection on the chest is based on a triangular arrangement of positive, negative, and ground electrodes. Avoid placing electrodes directly over the diaphragm, areas of auscultation, heavy bones, or large muscles. Allow adequate space for application of defibrillator paddles in case defibrillation should become necessary. Figure 23–11 depicts the most commonly used electrode leads. The modified lead II is the most commonly used because it is the most versatile; it is useful in assessing P waves, PR intervals, and atrial arrhythmias. The modified chest lead I (MCLI) is useful for assessing bundle branch block and differentiating between ventricular arrhythmias and aberrations. This lead is useful when the patient is known to have preexisting cardiac disease. The Lewis lead is useful when P waves are difficult to distinguish using other leads.

Sinus Bradycardia

Figure 23–12 shows a slow heart rate—less than 60 beats per minute. Its rhythm may be irregular owing to accompanying sinus arrhythmias. All other complex features are normal.

Sinus bradycardia is commonly encountered in the recovery room, owing to the depressant effects of anesthesia. Young, healthy adults, especially those who are normally physically active, often have bradycardia. Usually no treatment is necessary except to continue the stir-up regimen. Excessive parasympathetic stimulation from pain may cause bradycardia, in

which case appropriate analgesics should be administered and other pain-relieving measures initiated. If the patient shows symptoms of low cardiac output, the physician should be notified and treatment instituted using atropine to block vagal effects or isoproterenol to stimulate the cardiac pacemaker. If temporary pacing wires are available, either atrial or ventricular pacing can be attempted.

Sinus Tachycardia

Figure 23–13 shows a fast heart rate—more than 100 beats per minute. The rhythm may be slightly irregular, and all other complex features are normal.

Sinus tachycardia results from any stress and may be encountered in the PACU owing to stress of surgery, anoxia, hypovolemia, pain, anxiety, or apprehension, as well as many other causes. Treatment must be based upon removing the underlying cause. The patient should be assessed carefully for his ability to tolerate the rapid rate. Poor tolerance with a resultant fall in cardiac output occurs when the diastolic interval, and thus the ventricular filling time, is significantly impinged upon.

Sinus Arrest (Atrial Standstill)

Sinus arrest is failure of the S-A node to discharge, with resulting loss of atrial contraction. The rate remains within normal ranges. The rhythm is regular except when the S-A node fails to discharge. P waves and QRS complexes are normal when the S-A node is firing and absent when it fails to discharge.

Common causes of sinus arrest in the

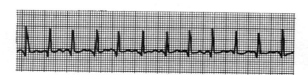

Figure 23–13. Sinus tachycardia (lead I). (From Guyton, A.C.: Textbook of Medical Physiology. 6th ed. Philadelphia, W.B. Saunders Co., 1981, p. 197.)

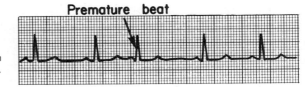

Figure 23–14. Atrial premature beat (lead I). (From Guyton, A.C.: Textbook of Medical Physiology. 6th ed. Philadelphia, W.B. Saunders Co., 1981, p. 200.)

PACU are the depressant effects of anesthesia or analgesics and electrolyte disturbances. Treatment is aimed at eliminating depressant drugs from the body and correcting electrolyte imbalances. This arrhythmia must be brought to the attention of the physician immediately, since persistent sinus arrest constitutes an emergency, and cardiopulmonary resuscitation must be initiated.

Premature Atrial Contraction (PAC)

This contraction occurs earlier than expected, resulting from an irritable focus in the atrium (Fig. 23–14). The rate and rhythm are normal except for their prematurity. The P wave configuration of the premature beat usually differs from that of the normal beat. The PAC is followed by a pause that is not fully compensatory.

This arrhythmia results from anxiety and is commonly encountered in the PACU. No treatment is necessary unless the PACs become frequent or the patient becomes symptomatic. If pharmacologic therapy becomes necessary, agents such as propranolol and verapamil can be administered.

Atrial Tachycardia

This rhythm disturbance is a rapid, regular supraventricular heart rate, resulting from an irritable focus of five or more PACs in succession (Fig. 23–15). The rate is 150 to 200 beats per minute with a regular rhythm.

This rhythm should be documented with a full 12-lead electrocardiogram. The physician should be notified to institute therapy. Maneuvers that enhance vagal tone, such as the Valsalva maneuver or carotid sinus massage, may be successful in terminating this arrhythmia. Antiarrhythmic agents such as digitalis, quinidine, or verapamil may cause the patient to revert to normal sinus rhythm. If these measures are unsuccessful, cardioversion with countershock will be necessary.

Atrial Flutter

Atrial flutter consists of rapid supraventricular contractions resulting from an ectopic focus with varying degrees of ventricular blocking (Fig. 23–16). Its etiology is the same as that of PACs and atrial tachycardia. The rhythm is usually regular; the atrial rate is 250 to 350 beats per minute. Treatment is the same as for atrial tachycardia.

Atrial Fibrillation

In atrial fibrillation, one or more irritable atrial foci discharge at an extremely rapid rate that lacks coordinated activity (Fig. 23–17).

Atrial fibrillation occurs commonly in patients with atrial enlargement from mitral valve disease or from long-standing coronary artery disease and is often preceded by atrial premature contractions, tachycardia, or flutter. Clinically, the patient will have an irregular heart beat, pulse rate, and usually, a noticeable pulse deficit. Cardiac output will decrease in varying degrees. Normally atrial filling and contraction ac-

Figure 23–15. Atrial paroxysmal tachycardia—onset in middle of record (lead I). (From Guyton, A.C.: Textbook of Medical Physiology. 6th ed. Philadelphia, W.B. Saunders Co., 1981, p. 201.)

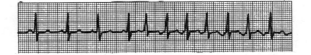

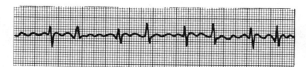

Figure 23–16. Atrial flutter—2:1 and 3:1 rhythm (lead I). (From Guyton, A.C.: Textbook of Medical Physiology. 6th ed. Philadelphia, W.B. Saunders Co., 1981, p. 202.)

count for 30 percent of ventricular filling. Without this atrial filling or "atrial kick" of volume into the ventricle, stroke volumes and thus cardiac outputs are diminished. Treatment involves digitalis, quinidine, verapamil, atrial pacing, or cardioversion.

Premature Ventricular Contractions (PVC)

This rhythm disturbance involves an earlier-than-expected ventricular contraction from an irritable focus in the ventricle (Fig. 23–18). The rhythm is regular except for the premature beat, and the rate is normal.

The P wave is absent before the premature beat. A wide, bizarre, notched QRS complex, which may be of greater-than-normal amplitude, is present. A widened T wave of greater-than-normal amplitude will be present after the premature beat and will be of opposite deflection to that of the QRS complex.

The PVC is followed by a pause that is fully compensatory; that is, the time of the PVC plus the pause time will equal the time of two normal beats.

PVCs are commonly encountered in the PACU and can occur in any patient. Occasional PVCs occur normally and need no treatment. Multiple PVCs may indicate inadequate oxygenation and the patient's respiratory status should be thoroughly assessed. Other causative factors of PVCs include electrolyte disturbances, acid-base imbalance, drug toxicity, and hypoxemia of the myocardium.

Treatment of PVCs is based upon the underlying cause and obliteration of the irritable focus. Occasional, isolated PVCs need not be treated. If PVCs occur more frequently than five per minute, if a successive run of two or more occurs, if they are multifocal or occur during the vulnerable period on the EKG complex, they must be treated, as they are the precursors of the more lethal ventricular arrhythmias.

Ventricular Tachycardia

Three or more consecutive premature ventricular beats constitute ventricular tachycardia (Fig. 23–19). The rhythm is fairly regular and P waves are not seen.

Occasionally, patients may have ventricular tachycardia and be asymptomatic, but usually they experience anxiety, palpitations, fluttering, pounding in the chest, dizziness, faintness, and precordial pain. If prolonged, cyanosis, mental confusion, convulsions, and unconsciousness develop as a result of decreased blood and oxygen supply to the brain.

The etiologic factors of ventricular tachycardia are essentially the same as those for PVCs. Most commonly, ventricular tachycardia in the PACU is due to hypoxia, drug toxicity, or underlying heart disease.

Ventricular tachycardia must be treated immediately. If the patient initially tolerates the arrhythmia, treatment should be instituted with lidocaine. If the patient has cardiac decompensation and circulatory insufficiency, cardioversion with DC electrical

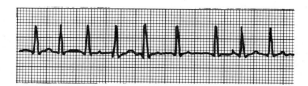

Figure 23–17. Atrial fibrillation (lead I). (From Guyton, A.C.: Textbook of Medical Physiology. 6th ed. Philadelphia, W.B. Saunders Co., 1981, p. 202.)

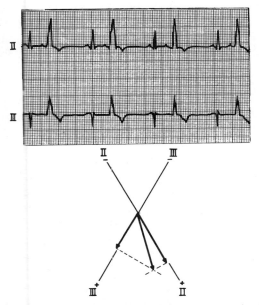

Figure 23–18. Premature ventricular contractions (leads II and III). (From Guyton, A.C.: Textbook of Medical Physiology. 6th ed. Philadelphia, W.B. Saunders Co., 1981. p. 200.)

countershock should be immediately instituted. Immediate notification of the physician is essential.

Ventricular Fibrillation

A rapid, irregular quivering of the ventricles that is uncoordinated and incapable of pumping blood characterizes ventricular fibrillation (Fig. 23–20). This is the major death-producing cardiac arrhythmia. The immediate initial treatment is external DC countershock (Fig. 23–21). Ventricular fibrillation may occur spontaneously without any forewarning, or it may be preceded by evidence of ventricular irritability. Patients likely to develop ventricular fibrillation include patients with underlying heart disease, those who evidenced ventricular irritability in the operating room during surgery, and those with symptoms of

shock. All should be monitored continuously throughout their recovery.

If ventricular fibrillation is not immediately terminated with countershock, cardiopulmonary resuscitation is instituted without delay. The anesthesiologist should be summoned immediately.

The reader is referred to the references at the end of this chapter for information on the arrhythmias and conduction disturbances originating in the atrioventricular node and the bundle branches and for detailed information on all the cardiac arrhythmias and their etiologies and treatment.

HEMODYNAMIC MONITORING

As mentioned earlier, all patients undergoing cardiac surgery require hemodynamic monitoring for variable periods postoperatively. The extent of monitoring depends upon the patient's response to surgery and the extensiveness of the procedure. Hemodynamic monitoring can be accomplished via the following invasive lines: a flow-directed pulmonary artery catheter (FDPAC), a central venous pressure catheter (CVP), a left atrial catheter (LAC) or a right atrial catheter (RAC), a pulmonary artery thermistor catheter (PATC), or a peripheral arterial catheter (A line). The parameters obtained from these various lines, the catheter insertion sites, and the placement and monitoring methods are presented in Table 23–1 and depicted in Figure 23–22. Problems associated with maintaining these lines are briefly discussed in Table 23–2.

Right Atrial Pressure (RAP). The normal right atrial pressure ranges from 0 to 7 mm Hg. Pressures exceeding that level can be due to fluid overload, right ventricular failure, tricuspid valve abnormalities, pulmo-

Figure 23–19. Ventricular paroxysmal tachycardia (lead III). (From Guyton, A.C.: Textbook of Medical Physiology. 6th ed. Philadelphia, W.B. Saunders Co., 1981, p. 202.)

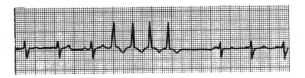

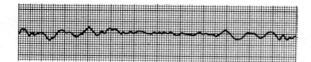

Figure 23–20. Ventricular fibrillation (lead II). (From Guyton, A.C.: Textbook of Medical Physiology. 6th ed. Philadelphia, W.B. Saunders Co., 1981, p. 203.)

nary hypertension, constrictive pericarditis or tamponade. Values in the lower range are usually indicative of hypovolemia.

Pulmonary Artery Pressures (PAP). Pulmonary artery systolic (PAS) pressures normally range from 15 to 25 mm Hg, while a normal pulmonary artery diastolic (PAD) pressure is 8 to 15 mm Hg. Hypovolemia contributes to low pressure readings. Increased volume loads that can develop with an ASD, a VSD, or left ventricular failure can create elevations. Additionally, obstructions to forward flow that can be caused by mitral stenosis or pulmonary hypertension can lead to an elevation in pulmonary artery pressures.

Pulmonary Capillary Wedge Pressure (PCWP). Normal PCWP recordings are between 6 and 15 mm Hg. Values over this range can be caused by an increased volume load, as is seen in left ventricular failure, or created by an obstruction to forward flow. Such obstructions could be caused by mitral stenosis or regurgitation, or by a pulmonary embolism. Lower values may be a result of hypovolemia or indicative of an obstruction

to left ventricular filling, which could occur with a pulmonary embolism, with pulmonary stenosis, or with right ventricular failure.

Left Atrial Pressure (LAP). Normal left atrial pressures (LAP) range from 4 to 12 mm Hg. As is seen with the PCWP, elevations in LAP are associated with volume overloads or obstructions to forward flow, the latter of which can consist of left ventricular failure states, mitral or aortic valve dysfunctions, or constrictive pericarditis. Lower recordings are generally a consequence of hypovolemia from inadequate volume or related to an obstruction to forward flow. Such an obstruction could be a pulmonary embolism, a pulmonic valve stenosis, or the result of a right ventricular failure.

Mean Arterial Pressure (MAP). Normal mean arterial pressures generally range between 80 and 120 mm Hg. In a postoperative cardiac surgical patient, pressures less than 60 mm Hg are generally avoided since coronary artery filling may be limited or impeded when parameters reach this level.

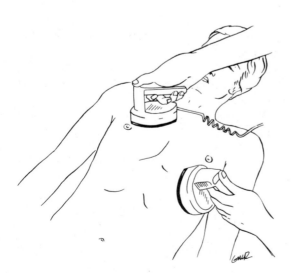

Figure 23–21. The emergency administration of external DC countershock. (From Sanderson R.C. [ed.]: The Cardiac Patient. Philadelphia, W.B. Saunders Co., 1972.)

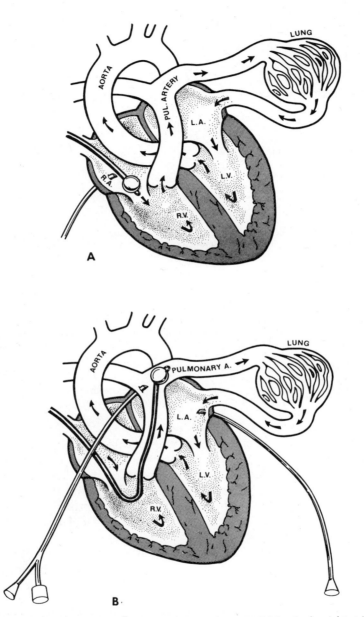

Figure 23–22. Placement of hemodynamic lines: (a) distal tip of a FDPAC lying in the right atrium as it floats toward the pulmonary artery, and the distal tip of a right atrial catheter directly inserted through the right atrial wall lying in the right atrium, (b) distal tip of a FDPAC advancing into a wedged position. This figure also illustrates the distal tip of a PATC lying in the pulmonary artery after direct insertion through the pulmonary artery wall and the distal tip of an LAC lying in the left atrium after direct insertion through the left atrial wall near or in a pulmonary vein. (From Whitman, G.R : Bedside Cardiovascular Monitoring. *In* Horvath, P.T. [ed.]: Care of the Adult Cardiac Surgery Patient. New York, John Wiley & Sons, Inc., 1984, pp. 31 and 33. Used with permission.)

TABLE 23–1. Methods for Invasive Monitoring of Hemodynamic Parameters

Parameters	Catheter Placement	Insertion Sites	Monitoring Method	Special Considerations
RAP	Proximal port of FDPAC lies in the right atrium	Brachial Jugular Subclavian	Water manometer	Intermittent readings at lowest fluctuation*
	Distal end of RAC or CVP lies in the right atrium	Direct insertion through RA wall†	Transducer‡	Intermittent or continuous readings on mean§
PAP	Distal end of FDPAC lies in right or left branch of pulmonary artery	Brachial Jugular Subclavian	Transducer	Readings on systole and diastole
	Distal end of PATC lies in main pulmonary artery	Direct insertion through PA wall†		
PCWP	Inflation of balloon on tip of FDPAC allows it to float into a wedged position in a smaller branch of the pulmonary artery	—	Transducer	Intermittent readings on mean§
LAP	Distal end of the LAC lies in left atrium	Direct insertion through LA wall†	Water manometer	Intermittent reading recorded at lowest fluctuation*
MAP	Distal end of catheter lies in a peripheral artery	Radial Brachial Femoral	Anaeroid manometer	Midpoint of needle fluctuation
			Transducer	Continuous readings on mean§

*Fluctuation indicates a patent catheter and good position in the thorax.

†Direct insertion is achieved during an open chest procedure via a median sternotomy incision. Exit site is via a stab wound at the distal portion of the median sternotomy. Catheter is attached to skin with suture. Removal is achieved by removing suture and applying gentle traction to catheter to free it from the chamber wall. Catheter is sutured to chamber wall with absorbable suture so that it releases easily. Chest tubes remain in place until such lines are removed, owing to the possibility of bleeding.

‡To convert mm Hg to cm H_2O, multiply mm Hg reading times 1.36.

§Biphasic waves are measured on mean.

Adapted from Whitman, G. R.: Bedside hemodynamic monitoring. *In* Horvath, P. T. (ed.): Care of the Adult Cardiac Surgery Patient. New York, John Wiley & Sons, Inc., 1984. Used with permission.

This could contribute to an ischemic or infarction state. Conversely, pressures higher than 120 mm Hg are avoided, as these place too much stress on newly created suture lines that could readily rupture under sustained pressures.

Cardiac Output (CO) and Cardiac Index (CI). Cardiac output is the amount of blood ejected by the ventricle in one minute. Normal cardiac output is 5 to 6 liters per minute; it is calculated by the formula:

$$SV \times HR = CO$$

where SV is stroke volume and HR is heart rate.

Cardiac index is calculated by the following formula:

$$\frac{CO}{BSA} = CI$$

where BSA is body surface area in m^2. Normal CI ranges from 2.5 to 3.5 liters per minute per m^2. Since CI takes body size into consideration, it is a better indicator of the patient's perfusion status.

Systemic Vascular Resistance (SVR). Systemic vascular resistance is the resistance the left ventricle must work against in order to eject its volume of blood. Normal SVR is 900 to 1300 dynes per second per cm -5. An elevated SVR can create enough resistance to left ventricular ejection that cardiac output and cardiac index will fall, which will lead to a state of hypoperfusion or shock. Infusion of vasodilators and afterload-reducing agents can counteract this elevation. SVR is calculated using the following formula:

$$SVR = \frac{(MAP - CVP) \times 80}{CO}$$

TABLE 23–2. Potential Problems Associated with Invasive Hemodynamic Monitoring

Potential Problems	Etiology	Precautions/Treatment
Alterations in pressure wave configurations		
Dampened tracings	**Technical**	
	Air in system	Check system for bubbles; flush bubbles out of system.
	Disconnection in system	Inspect and tighten all connections.
	Blood on transducer head	Flush until transducer dome clears of blood; change dome if necessary.
	Kinked catheter	Remove dressing to ascertain if catheter is kinked externally.
	Catheter tip against wall	Turn patient's head or reposition extremity that catheter is inserted into, watching for improvement in tracing. Gently aspirate catheter from various angles to determine at which angle the best flow is achieved; tape and redress the catheter at the angle at which the best flow is achieved. Gently flush catheter in an attempt to push tip away from vessel wall. NEVER flush a catheter in which a clot is suspected.
	Physiologic	
	Clot on catheter tip	Attempt to aspirate blood from catheter. If possible, keep aspirating until clot is retrieved or blood no longer seems thickened. Flush system until the line is cleared and a readable tracing reappears. If blood cannot be aspirated, notify the physician.
	With an FDPAC this may also indicate the catheter has advanced forward and is in a wedged position*	Make sure balloon is deflated. Recheck system and line. If no improvement, obtain a chest x-ray film and notify physician.
Abrupt exaggeration of pressure tracings	**Technical**	
	Loss of calibration of level of transducer	Recalibrate and relevel transducer.
	Physiologic	
	Slippage of catheter out of chamber or vessel	Avoid traction on intravascular lines; tape catheter to skin or secure with suture.
	FDPAC slipping from pulmonary artery to right ventricle. This is characterized by a systolic pressure that remains the same while the diastolic pressure falls into the range of the right ventricular end diastolic pressure	Inflate balloon in attempt to let catheter float back into pulmonary artery. If catheter does not migrate back into pulmonary artery, obtain a chest x-ray film and notify a physician.
	RAC, PAC or PATC has slipped out of vessel wall into thoracic cavity	Attempt to aspirate to see if catheter is still in the vessel. If blood returns, flush system and attempt to obtain readable pressure tracings. If no blood return is achieved, notify physician and remove catheter, per protocol.
Alterations in vascular integrity		
Venous and arterial spasms	Irritation to vessels during prolonged insertion attempts	Apply local anesthetic to catheter surface or administer anesthetic by IV route. Use a guide-wire to facilitate insertion. Cool catheter to make it less flexible and easier to insert.
Thrombophlebitis	Irritation to vessels from prolonged insertion attempts or from constant motion of catheter against vessel	See "venous and arterial spasm" above. Secure catheter in place with either tape or suture. Avoid prolonged infusions of chemically irritating medications. Maintain adequate dilutions. Observe for signs and symptoms of phlebitis and notify physician for possible withdrawal of catheter. Distal placement of stopcocks connecting catheters and tubing permits atraumatic blood sampling and flushing.

Table continued on following page

TABLE 23–2. Potential Problems Associated with Invasive Hemodynamic Monitoring *Continued*

Potential Problems	Etiology	Precautions/Treatment
Embolization	Clot embolization from thrombophlebitis or from clot on catheter tip	Always aspirate catheter first if clot is suspected. NEVER FLUSH.
	Pulmonary embolism with infarct from FDPAC	Observe for changes in chest x-ray film that indicate pulmonary embolization.
	Cerebral embolization from LAC catheter	Observe for neurologic changes that may indicate embolization from LAC.
	Peripheral embolization with extremity ischemia from peripheral arterial lines	Observe for ischemic changes of the extremity in which the catheter is located.
Air embolization	Loose connections	Secure and tighten all connections. Vigilantly observe LAC catheter, since even minute amounts of air in this system can lead to serious neurologic complications.
	Rupture of balloon on FDPAC due to overinflation or following normal use, since the latex layer on the balloon absorbs lipoproteins from the blood and slowly loses elasticity, thus increasing its incidence of rupture	Inflate balloon slowly and do not overinflate. Limit inflations. Allow balloon to empty air passively back into syringe. Avoid aspirating air back, as this weakens integrity of balloon. Aspirate only if air fails to return passively. If air does not return and rupture is questioned, sterile saline can be injected into balloon and attempts made to aspirate it back. Failure to aspirate fluid back indicates a leak and the physician should be notified.
Vessel erosion or hemorrhage	Inadequate hemostasis following insertion	Apply firm pressure for 15–20 min.
Bleeding from insertion site. Rupture of a branch of the pulmonary artery	Overinflation of the balloon in a normal-sized vessel	Do not attempt to inflate the balloon if tracing already appears wedged. Inject only prescribed amount of air into balloon.
	Normal inflation of balloon in a too-small vessel	Inject air slowly and stop injecting if resistance is felt. Inject only amount of air required to obtain a wedge tracing.
	Repeated normal inflations in a brittle or susceptible vessel	Limit wedge intervals in high-risk patients, such as patients with pulmonary hypertension or long-standing mitral valve disease.

TABLE 23–2. Potential Problems Associated with Invasive Hemodynamic Monitoring *Continued*

Potential Problems	Etiology	Precautions/Treatment
Dysrhythmias		
Atrial dysrhythmias	Irritation of RA from RAC or during insertion of FDPAC	Withdraw CVP catheter to level of superior vena cava and obtain readings from that area. Continue with insertion of FDPAC, as dysrhythmias are usually self-limiting and stop once catheter tip exits the right atrium.
Ventricular dysrhythmias	Irritation of RV from tip of FDPAC during insertion procedure or from catheter tip slipping out of the pulmonary artery and back into the right ventricle	Continue with insertion of FDPAC, as dysrhythmias are usually self-limiting and stop once the catheter passes into the pulmonary artery. If catheter tip falls back into the right ventricle from the pulmonary artery, inflate the balloon, as this will cushion the tip of the catheter and may alleviate the dysrhythmias. Administer lidocaine if ventricular dysrhythmias continue. Notify physician, obtain a chest film, and manipulate catheter, per hospital policy.
Infections		
Local infection	Faulty aseptic techniques during insertion or during subsequent dressing changes	Maintain sterility during insertion. Change dressings with sterile technique and tubings, per hospital policy.
Systemic infection	Faulty aseptic technique during insertion	Avoid spasms during insertion. Avoid development of thrombophlebitis along vessel. Change indwelling catheters and insertion sites every 48–72 hr. This may be impossible in patients with difficult vascular access sites. In these situations, rethreading a new catheter over a guidewire at the previous insertion site can be done every 48–72 hr. However, once the site is questionable or the patient develops symptoms of sepsis, such as elevated temperatures and WBC, a new line at a new site is required.
Endocarditis	Extension of a local insertion site. Infection along the catheter and into the circulation	Culture, per hospital policy. Observe for the development of new murmurs.

*Note: Wedging of the catheter in a postoperative patient may be a common occurrence for two reasons: (1) The catheter may have advanced forward during operative procedure when the chest was open and the lungs were not fully inflated, since there was less resistance to forward advancement; (2) as hypothermia is reversed and the patient and catheter rewarm, its increased flexibility may allow it to float forward.

From Whitman, G. R.: Bedside Hemodynamic Monitoring. In Horvath P. T.: Care of the Adult Cardiac Surgery Patient. New York, John Wiley and Sons, Inc., 1984.

Pulmonary Vascular Resistance (PVR). Pulmonary vascular resistance is the resistance the right ventricle must work against in order to eject blood into the pulmonary bed. Normal PVR is 80 to 240 dynes per second per cm −5. An elevated PVR can create enough resistance to right ventricular ejection that right-sided failure or infarction can develop. Infusion of vasodilators or pulmonary artery dilators such as aminophylline can counteract these elevations. PVR is calculated using the following formula:

$$PVR = \frac{[PAM - (PCWP \text{ or } LAP)] \times 80}{CO}$$

where PAM is the pulmonary artery mean pressure.

For a more detailed discussion of hemodynamic monitoring, the reader is referred to the references at the end of this chapter.

REFERENCES

1. Adlkofer, S. R.: The effect of endotracheal suctioning on arterial blood gases in patients after cardiac surgery. Heart Lung, 7:1011–1014, 1978.
2. Barash, P. C.: Catheter-induced pulmonary artery perforation: mechanisms, management and modifications. J. Thorac. Cardiovasc. Surg., 82:5, 1981.
3. Behrendt, D.: Patient Care in Cardiac Surgery. Boston, Little, Brown & Co., 1980.
4. Chatham, M. A.: The effect of family involvement on patient's manifestations of postcardiotomy psychosis. Heart Lung, 7:995–999, 1978.
5. Chesbro, J. H. : Effect of dipyridamole and aspirin on late vein graft patency after coronary bypass operation. N. Engl. J. Med., 310:209–224, 1984.
6. Disch, J. M.: Wound integrity in the patient undergoing cardiac surgery. Nurs. Clin. North Am. 14:743–759, 1979.
7. Fremes, S. E.: Effects of postoperative hypertension and its treatment. J. Thorac. Cardiovasc. Surg., 86:47, 1983.
8. Gershan, J. A.: Effect of positive end-expiratory pressure on pulmonary capillary wedge pressure. Heart Lung, 12:143–147, 1983.
9. Glancy, D. L.: Medical management of adults and older children undergoing cardiac operations. Heart Lung, 9:277–283, 1980.
10. Guzzetta, C. G., and Whitman, G. R.: Cardiac surgery. In Kenner, C.: Critical Care Nursing: Body, Mind and Spirit. Boston, Little, Brown & Co., 1985.
11. Horvath, P. T.: Care of the Adult Cardiac Surgery Patient. New York, John Wiley & Sons, Inc., 1984.
12. Jurkiewicz, M. J.: Infected median sternotomy. Ann. Surg., 81:738–743, 1980.
13. McCauley, K. M., and Brest, A. N.: McGoon's Cardiac Surgery: An Interprofessional Approach to Patient Care. Philadelphia, F. A. Davis Co., 1985.
14. Miller, D. C.: Discriminant analysis of the changing risks of coronary artery operation. J. Thorac. Cardiovasc. Surg., 85: 197–201, 1983.
15. Ream, A. K.: Acute Cardiovascular Management. Philadelphia, J. B. Lippincott Co., 1982.
16. Ricks, W. B., Winkle, R. A., Shumway, N. E.: Surgical management of life-threatening ventricular arrhythmias in patients with coronary artery disease. Circulation, 56:38–42, 1977.
17. Sabiston, D. C., and Spencer, F. C.: Gibbon's Surgery of the Chest. Philadelphia, W. B. Saunders Co., 1983.
18. Shellock, F. G.: Reproducibility and accuracy of using room-temperature vs. ice-temperature injectate for thermodilution cardiac output determinations. Heart Lung, 12:175–176, 1983.
19. Shinn, J. A.: Heart transplantation. In Woods, S. L.: Cardiovascular Critical Care Nursing. New York, Churchill Livingstone, Inc., 1983.
20. Stuart, E. M.: Nursing rounds: Care of the patient with a mitral commissurotomy. AJN, 80:1511–1532, 1980.
21. Sweetwood, H.: Cardiac tamponade: When dyspnea spells sudden death. RN, 35–41, 1980.
22. Underhill, S. L., Woods, S. L., Sivarajan, E. S., et al.: Cardiac Nursing. Philadelphia, J. B. Lippincott Co., 1982.
23. Whitman, G. R.: Comparison of maximal temperature elevations following reversal of hypothermia with four rewarming techniques. Circulation, 64:II–4, 1981.
24. Wulff, K. S.: Use of temporary epicardial electrodes for atrial pacing and monitoring. Cardiovasc. Nurs., 18:1–7, 1982.

Postoperative Care After Vascular Surgery

Integrity and patency of the vascular system, including the arteries, veins, and lymphatic vessels, is essential to the life of human tissues. Before 1950, the patient with impaired vascular patency was treated only medically. Loss of limb or life resulting from impaired blood flow was common, and surgery on the vascular system was only in the experimental stage. The advancement of vascular surgery from the experimental laboratory to accepted procedure in the clinical setting resulted from the successful development of diagnostic tools, such as arteriography, improved antibiotics and anticoagulants, and the perfection of vascular surgery instruments and techniques.

Definitions

Aneurysm: a localized, abnormal dilatation, distention, or sac in an artery.

Angiography (arteriography): injection of radiopaque dye into the arteries followed by rapid sequential x-rays of the vascular tree to determine abnormalities.

Bypass: rerouting of the vascular system by construction of another arterial route by use of a vein graft or a synthetic (Dacron or Teflon) artery, and reestablishment of functional integrity.

Embolectomy: the surgical removal of an embolus from a blood vessel.

Embolus: a bit of free-floating foreign matter (may be clotted blood, air, cancer, or other tissue cells, amniotic fluid, fat, or other foreign bodies) carried by the blood stream.

Endarterectomy: opening of the artery over an obstruction and removal of the obstruction, or excision of atheromatous material creating the blockage.

Ischemia: lack of adequate blood supply to meet the tissue needs.

Ligation: tying or binding of a blood vessel (Fig. 24–1).

Plication: creating of folds in the wall of a vessel or other methods of reducing intraluminal size (Fig. 24–1).

Sympathectomy: resection of selected portions of the sympathetic nervous system to denervate the vascular system, producing vasodilatation.

Thrombus: a stationary blood clot or atheromatous plaque that partially or totally occludes a blood vessel.

Thrombectomy: surgical excision of a thrombus from within a blood vessel.

GENERAL CONSIDERATIONS

Vascular surgery is now commonly practiced in most institutions and the PACU nurse must be prepared to care for these patients postoperatively and to evaluate

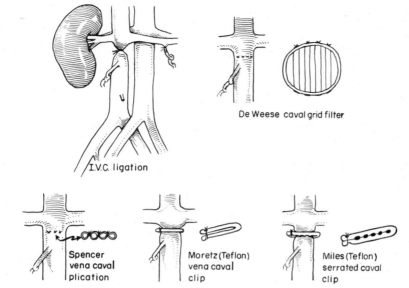

De Weese caval grid filter

I.V.C. ligation

Spencer vena caval plication

Moretz (Teflon) vena caval clip

Miles (Teflon) serrated caval clip

Figure 24–1. Drawings illustrating various surgical techniques available for preventing embolism from pelvic and lower extremity veins. (From Fairbairn, J. F., II, Juergens, J. L., and Spittel, J. A., Jr.: Peripheral Vascular Diseases. 4th ed. Philadelphia, W. B. Saunders Co., 1972).

their vascular status. Many vascular impairments are amenable to surgery, especially when localized. Vascular surgery generally involves the elimination of obstruction by excising and removing thrombi and emboli, the bypassing of atherosclerotic narrowing, and the resection of aneurysms. Occasionally, sympathectomy is performed to treat vasospastic disease, but its success is limited to patients whose vascular system are still elastic enough to dilate. Veins may be ligated or plicated to prevent emboli from passing up the vena cava into the heart and lungs. Research in vascular disease continues, and every day new techniques and surgical devices are introduced for trial. The nurse should be familiar with all of the procedures being performed in the local setting and with any specific care involved postoperatively. Only the more common procedures will be discussed here.

Vascular problems may be acute and constitute a life- or limb-threatening emergency; they may be chronic conditions for which surgery is performed only as a last resort after medical treatment has failed. In either case, the PACU nurse must be sensitive to the feelings of these patients and be prepared for the questions about limb viability that will invariably arise upon the patient's awakening.

Postoperative care following vascular surgery is determined by the surgical site, the extent of surgical revision, and the anesthesia used.

Anesthesia

Anesthesia may be local, spinal, or general, depending upon the surgical site and the patient's condition. Peripheral embolectomy may be accomplished with only local anesthesia and appropriate sedation, whereas an aortoiliac bypass graft requires prolonged general anesthesia. Anesthetic management of bypass graft patients is exceptionally important, because they are often elderly and in poor physical condition, and present with many risk factors. Patients who undergo thoracic or abdominal aortic surgery are considerably more labile than patients undergoing peripheral vascular surgery, and they are frequently transferred directly from the operating suite to the intensive care unit for monitoring and special care. The goals of treatment for vascular surgical patients are to support the vascular system, to remove the cause of the problem, and to prevent further episodes of ischemia.

DIAGNOSTIC PROCEDURES

Arteriography is commonly performed prior to any vascular surgery in order to determine the exact location of the problem.

It is usually accomplished within the x-ray department. The patient may be returned to the PACU for a brief period of observation, depending upon the policies of the hospital and the patient's PAR score. Arteriography is generally accomplished with the use of only local anesthesia at the catheter insertion site. Postarteriography care includes observation of the catheter site for bleeding. Usually, a pressure dressing is applied to the site for several hours. The injection site may become irritated or thrombosed, and, occasionally, the patient will have an allergic reaction to the radiopaque dye.

All pulses distal to the catheter site should be checked. Pedal pulses should be assessed if the femoral artery was used and brachial and radial pulses evaluated if the upper extremity is the site of catheter insertion. The cardiovascular status of the patient should be carefully monitored if pulmonary angiography was performed, because passage of the catheter may create myocardial irritability.

The patient is often apprehensive following arteriography and anxious to know the results. The nurse should be familiar with the information given to the patient by the physician and be able to reinforce or reinterpret it for the patient if necessary.

PERIPHERAL VASCULAR SURGICAL PROCEDURES

Treatment for peripheral vascular disease may be performed directly on the involved vessels or sympathectomy may be done, depending upon the nature of the problem and the age and general condition of the patient.

Peripheral procedures include embolectomy, thrombectomy, endarterectomy, and ligation and stripping of veins (Fig. 24–1). Other procedures include the femoral-popliteal bypass graft (Fig. 24–2), peripheral artery embolectomy, carotid endarterectomy or bypass, and venous ligation and stripping of the lower extremities.

Anesthesia may be local, as for embolectomy; spinal, as for surgery on the lower extremities; or general, for more extensive

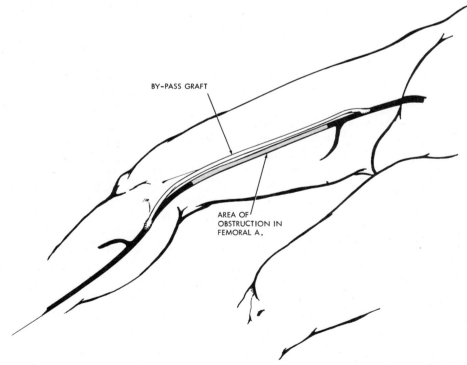

BY-PASS GRAFT

AREA OF OBSTRUCTION IN FEMORAL A.

Figure 24–2. Saphenous femoral-popliteal by-pass graft in place, going around the femoral artery obstruction. (From LeMaitre, G. D., and Finnegan, J. A.: The Patient in Surgery. 3rd ed. Philadelphia, W. B. Saunders Co., 1975, p. 276.)

procedures or when the patient cannot tolerate local or spinal anesthesia.

PACU Care

Positioning

Upon return to the PACU, the patient is placed in the supine position, with head and neck turned to the side. If the lower extremities are the site of an arterial procedure, the head of the bed is elevated on 6-inch shock blocks to aid perfusion of the legs and feet. Some controversy exists over the positioning of the patient after vein stripping. In our experience, surgeons have preferred to have the patient's legs slightly elevated (20 to 30 degrees) to aid venous return. The surgeon's preference should be followed; if preference is not specified, the nurse should ask. After surgery on the carotid arteries the patient is placed in supine position, with the head of the bed elevated 25 to 30 degrees to minimize venous oozing in the neck. Sudden changes in head position should be avoided during the immediate postoperative period. Raising the head suddenly or more than 30 degrees can precipitate hypotension, and lowering the head can precipitate hypertension, owing to a temporary inability of the great vessels to compensate for changes in head position.

Circulatory Status

Checking the circulation to the operated extremity is one of the most important nursing functions. Careful explicit recording of observations is important for determining any changes. The circulatory status of the patient and the pulses present should be reported to the nurse by the surgeon. It is helpful to PACU personnel for the surgeon to mark on the skin those places where the pulses can be evaluated best.

All pulses on the affected extremity are evaluated frequently and compared with pulses on the unaffected side (Fig. 24–3). The pulses should be checked not only for their presence but also for pulse volume and occlusion pressure. A reduction in pulse volume or occlusion pressure is more likely to be detected if the same nurse cares

for the patient during the entire stay in the PACU. If assignments need to be changed—for instance, if a shift change occurs—a direct report should be made from nurse to nurse with direct inspection, palpation, and evaluation of the pulses so that the relieving nurse has accurate baseline observations for future assessments.

The PACU should have an ultrasonic Doppler device to assist with evaluating pulses (Fig. 24–4). The Doppler can indicate the presence of adequate blood flow even when pulses are not palpable. The affected part should remain warm, dry, and normal in color. Capillary flush should be checked by the "blanch reflex": pressure applied to the skin surface over a small area with the fingers should blanch the area (produce pallor). Normal pink skin color should return quickly (the flush response) when pressure is released. Coolness, pallor, numbness, and tingling may be danger signs that vascular problems have developed. If pulses previously present become more difficult to palpate or are absent, the surgeon should be notified immediately.

After carotid endarterotomy or bypass, circulation to the head and neck is checked by assessing the patient's level of consciousness. If local anesthesia has been used, the patient's degree of orientation is a useful sign. If general anesthesia has been employed, consciousness is more difficult to evaluate; however, the pharyngeal reflexes, the lid (or "blink") reflexes, and the patient's response to pain stimuli are helpful indicators of the level of consciousness. As the patient emerges from anesthesia, specific levels of response should be noted along with the time of response, so that any relapse will be noted. Check pupillary response and motion of the extremities to further assess neurologic status.

Meticulous blood pressure monitoring must be performed for these patients, owing to the risk of hypotension or hypertension during the immediate postoperative period.

Dressings

All dressings should be checked for drainage. Dressings following bypass grafting

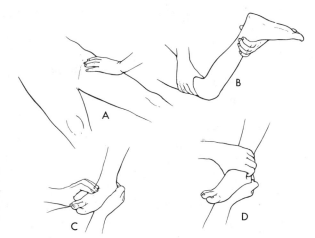

Figure 24–3. The method of palpation for pulsations in the peripheral arteries. A, Femoral artery, B, popliteal artery. C, Dorsalis pedis artery. D, Posterior tibial artery. (From Fairbairn, J. F., II, Juergens, J. L., and Spittell, J. A., Jr.: Perpheral Vascular Diseases. 4th ed. Philadelphia, W. B. Saunders Co., 1972.)

and embolectomy are usually light. They should remain dry and intact. If frank bleeding occurs, the surgeon should be notified, as this may indicate an interrupted arteriotomy or graft anastomosis site. A tourniquet or a blood pressure cuff should be kept at the bedside for immediate use if rupture on an arterial operative site should occur. If a cuff is used, it should be applied proximal to the incision site and inflated carefully and slowly until bleeding just stops.

The pressure necessary to stop bleeding will normally be just below the systemic systolic blood pressure.

After venous ligation and stripping, the legs are wrapped with Kerlex or similar elastic gauze dressings, and compression is applied with Ace wraps or antiembolic stockings from toes to groin. Some seepage of blood may occur, but the dressings should not soak through. Excessive bleeding should be reported to the surgeon.

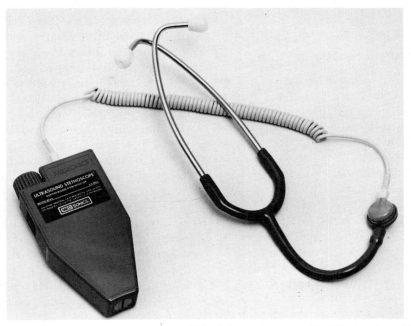

Figure 24–4. Doppler instrument for the detection of blood flow. (Courtesy of MedSonics, Inc., Mountain View, California.)

Pain Relief

Pain following any of these procedures should be mild and easily controlled with moderate doses of the narcotic analgesics. Severe unrelieved pain should be reported to the surgeon.

Intake and Output

The PACU course for these patients is usually smooth and uneventful. Fluids may be instituted orally as soon as the patient recovers the pharyngeal reflexes, and solids can then be given progressively as tolerated.

The patient may suffer urinary retention, which is especially likely to occur after spinal anesthesia. Check for abdominal distention. Some surgeons will allow male patients to stand for voiding. If measures to enhance the ability to void are not effective, a catheterization order must be obtained.

SYMPATHECTOMY

Some carefully selected cases of vasospastic disease are amenable to sympathectomy, which results in vasodilatation of the vessels in the extremity by removing the vasoconstrictive effects of the sympathetic nervous system.

Cervicodorsal Sympathectomy

Cervicodorsal sympathectomy is performed to denervate the upper extremity and improve circulation. The most common approach used is the transaxillary transpleural incision. Resection of thoracic ganglia, T_2–T_6, and half of the stellate ganglia, C_8–T_1, is accomplished.

Anesthesia is general. Upon return to the PACU, the patient is placed in the supine position until sufficiently recovered from anesthesia to be able to tolerate the head of the bed being elevated 30 to 45 degrees. A chest tube will be present since a thoracic incision has been made. This should be cared for as outlined in Chapter 22. Since the chest tube is inserted primarily for the removal of air to correct the surgically created pneumothorax, bleeding should be

negligible. Accumulation of more than 200 ml of blood in the collection receptacle in eight hours or less is excessive and should be reported to the surgeon.

Bilateral breath sounds should be evaluated. Circulation to the hand and arm must be assessed by evaluating pulses, temperature, and color. As soon as pharyngeal reflexes have returned, the patient may be started on oral fluids and diet widened as tolerated. Dressings should remain dry and intact. The patient's cardiovascular status should be assessed and any downward trends reported, as these may indicate hemorrhage from the intercostal vessels, thoracic aorta, or subclavian artery. Damage to these vessels causes excessive bleeding, and hypovolemic shock could develop quickly.

Lumbar Sympathectomy

Lumbar sympathectomy is performed to denervate the lower extremity and improve circulation. A flank incision is used to approach the lumbar ganglia (L_1–L_4) and they are resected. At present, this particular procedure is not commonly performed.

This procedure is accomplished under general anesthesia. The patient may be placed in the supine or side-lying position when returned to the PACU. The light flank dressing on the operative side should remain dry and intact. If bleeding occurs, the surgeon should be notified, as this may indicate damage to one of the lumbar veins. Drainage from the incisional site must be carefully assessed. The presence of urine in the drainage suggests that damage to the ureter may have occurred during surgery.

Postoperative pain should be minimal and easily controlled with small doses of narcotic analgesics. If the patient complains of severe flank pain not associated with the incision, the surgeon should be informed, as this may indicate inadvertent ligation of the ureter. Ligation of the ureter leads to the dilatation of the renal pelvis with urine. If unable to void normally within 8 to 10 hours, the patient will probably need catheterization.

The patient may develop an ileus and should be given nothing by mouth for the first 25 hours postoperatively. Bowel sounds should be monitored for return. Fluid intake is provided intravenously. Occasionally, a nasogastric tube is required to decompress the stomach. This should be cared for as outlined in Chapter 28. Circulation to the lower extremities should be assessed by evaluating pulse, temperature, and color.

After sympathectomy, especially lumbar sympathectomy, the patient has an increased sensitivity to changes in body position, so turning and sitting up should be accomplished slowly. This patient is also more sensitive to changes in room temperature and should be provided with warmed blankets in the PACU to conserve body heat.

OPERATIONS ON THE LARGE VESSELS

Operations on the large vessels include embolectomy and thrombectomy; bypass procedures on the aorta, iliac arteries, and renal arteries; and ligation and plication of the vena cava (Figs. 24–5 to 24–7).

Surgery on the great vessels still carries a rather high risk of mortality and morbidity. Patients are usually in a precarious physical state before surgery, owing to the cardiovascular problem. These patients are often elderly, and, in addition to the specific problem for which surgery is being performed, they often have diffuse cardiovascular and respiratory disease affecting all of the vital organs. Vascular surgery on the large vessels, especially abdominal and thoracic aortic surgery, is often prolonged and is quite shocking to the system.

As with postoperative cardiac patients, these patients should be cared for in the immediate recovery period by at least two professional nurses. All physiologic functions must be assessed accurately and continually. In some institutions, a special unit is set aside for the postoperative care of cardiac and vascular patients. If these patients are sent to the general recovery room, adequate numbers of well-trained staff must be available to manage their care. After recovery, these patients must be transferred to the surgical intensive care unit, where close monitoring and special care can be

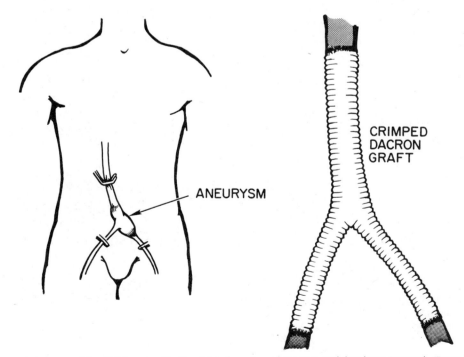

Figure 24–5. Aneurysm of the distal aorta. On the right, the crimped Dacron graft has been inserted. (From LeMaitre, G. D., and Finnegan, J. A.: The Patient in Surgery. 3rd ed. Philadelphia, W. B. Saunders Co., 1975, p. 287.)

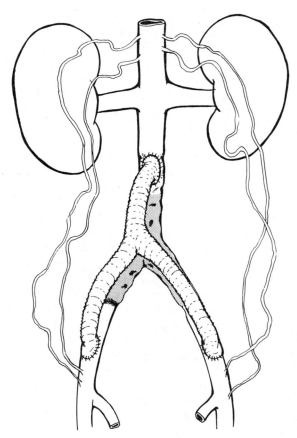

Figure 24–6. An aortoiliac Dacron bypass graft in place. (From LeMaitre, G. D., and Finnegan, J. A.: The Patient in Surgery. 3rd ed. Philadelphia, W. B. Saunders Co., 1975, p. 280.)

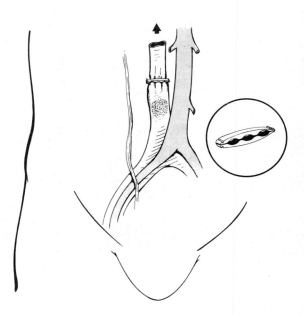

Figure 24–7. A partially occluding Teflon clip on the vena cava, preventing a caval embolism (dotted area) from reaching lungs. (From LeMaitre, G. D., and Finnegan, J. A.: The Patient in Surgery. 3rd ed. Philadelphia, W. B. Saunders Co., 1975, p. 306.)

provided until they are fully stable and until the time has passed during which the most common complications occur.

Anesthesia for these procedures is general and may be prolonged. Surgery may take as long as 10 hours in some cases. The procedure may involve extensive blood loss and the incisions used are commonly long, involving both thoracic and abdominal entrance. For a review of care of the patient and management of chest tubes following thoracic incisions, see Chapter 22.

PACU Care

Positioning and Initial Care

Upon return to the recovery room, the patient is placed in the supine position with head and neck turned to the side. As soon as the patient can tolerate it, the head of the bed is elevated 30 to 45 degrees to promote respiratory function. After vena cava plication, the patient is kept supine or may have the bed placed in the Trendelenburg position, as directed by the surgeon.

The surgeon and anesthesiologist should give the receiving nurse a detailed report on the anesthesia, the procedure accomplished, blood loss and replacement, other fluid replacement, the patient's overall condition, and any special instructions. At the same time, all necessary monitors and support systems should be hooked up, all drainage tubes and catheters cared for appropriately, and baseline measurements of all physiologic functioning determined and documented.

Cardiopulmonary Status

Most commonly, owing to systemic shock from the procedure, extent of anesthesia, and general condition of the patient, respiratory support with a volume-controlled ventilator is provided for at least 8 to 24 hours postoperatively. A 24-hour period of assisted or controlled respiration gives the patient a rest and assists in stabilizing his condition more rapidly. The reader should review Chapter 18 for information on the care of the patient with an endotracheal airway and management of the respirator.

Because of the age of the average patient undergoing this type of surgery, pulmonary care is exceptionally important. The patient should be suctioned frequently, following the guidelines in Chapter 18, and position should be changed at least every hour. Because thoracic and abdominal incisions are long and painful, adequate analgesia must be maintained to promote respiratory function as well as comfort. An order for morphine sulfate, 2 to 4 mg IV every 1 to 2 hours, gives the nurse flexibility in medicating the patient appropriately for both of these purposes while the patient is on controlled ventilation.

The patient's cardiac status should be monitored electronically. Any arrhythmias not previously present must be investigated and an explanation for their presence sought. The nurse must, of course, be prepared to treat immediately any lethal arrhythmias that develop. Frequently, the cause of premature ventricular contractions is inadequate oxygenation. Arterial samples for blood gas analysis are frequently necessary to evaluate the patient's cardiorespiratory status. It is, therefore, highly advantageous to have an arterial line present from which to draw specimens. The arterial line is also helpful in monitoring the patient's systolic blood pressure continuously. Systolic blood pressure should be recorded every 10 to 15 minutes during the first 2 postoperative hours and every 30 minutes thereafter. Since these procedures involve a moderate to extensive blood loss and are shocking to the system, a systolic blood pressure of 100 mm Hg is generally acceptable if the patient was not preoperatively hypertensive.

Hypertension control is also essential when surgery has been performed on the great vessels. Extreme elevations in blood pressure can stress the suture line, precipitating oozing and rupture of the operative site.

A pulse rate of 100 to 120 is generally acceptable. A moderate tachycardia is expected as a result of the stress of surgery. Central venous pressure on Swan-Ganz monitoring may also be instituted to assist in evaluating the patient's cardiovascular function and fluid balance.

Circulatory Status

Circulation to the extremities must be checked every hour and results recorded along with the vital signs. All peripheral pulses should be present. The surgeon should indicate the parameters within which he or she would like the patient's vital signs to remain. Trends in these measurements are more important indicators of the patient's status than the raw numbers. Any indication of hypotension or impending shock should be reported to the surgeon. Hemorrhage and shock are the most common complications of vascular surgery and may result from the primary surgery or from associated injury to the aorta, the vena cava, or the nearby vessels, including the iliac or renal arteries and veins, or the lumbar veins. Massive bleeding is particularly likely if anticoagulant therapy was instituted preoperatively.

Temperature

The temperature should be taken hourly for several hours postoperatively. An electronic axillary or rectal probe is probably the most accurate. The presence of a nasogastric tube, an endotracheal tube, and the connected respirator makes oral temperature readings impossible, and the paraphernalia present make rectal readings difficult. A temperature elevation to 101°F (38.3°C) or 102°F (38.8°C) is common after these extensive procedures and is not indicative of infection. A temperature of 103°F (39.4°C), however, is significant and may be due to respiratory problems such as pulmonary atelectasis. In this case, efforts at pulmonary toilet must be increased and the surgeon may start the patient on an antibiotic regimen if it has not already been instituted.

Intake and Output

Adequate fluid intake is provided by intravenous infusions maintained throughout the postoperative period. The quantity and content of the fluids needed are determined by the surgeon, based upon the patient's cardiovascular status and urine output. Blood replacement may be necessary. A hematocrit and a hemoglobin determination are usually performed 4 and 8 hours postoperatively. At least four units of blood, typed and crossmatched for this patient, should be kept available in the blood bank until it is released by the surgeon.

A Foley catheter should be connected to straight gravitational drainage with a calibrated measuring device. Urine output is measured and recorded hourly. At least 1 ml per kg per hour of urine output should be expected, and the surgeon is notified if any downward trend occurs. Decreased or inadequate urine output may indicate hypotension due to hypovolemia or impending shock with renal shutdown. The urine should be examined for the presence of blood or for cloudiness. Blood in the urine may indicate injury to a ureter or kidney, reaction to blood transfusion, or massive hemorrhage.

A nasogastric or long intestinal tube will be present and is cared for as described in Chapter 28. It should be connected to low intermittent suction; the drainage and all stools should be given a guaiac test for occult blood, and its presence should be reported to the surgeon immediately. The presence of blood may be indicative of impending infarction of the colon, which must be treated immediately. Occasionally, a gastrostomy must be performed in this situation; it is cared for in the routine manner.

All intake and output must, of course, be accurately measured and recorded. The intake and output record will assist in the evaluation of hypotensive states, pulmonary congestion, edema, and renal shutdown, all of which are common problems encountered after major vascular surgery.

Pain Relief

The incisions for major vascular surgery are long and painful, and, frequently, significant doses of narcotic analgesics are required to keep the patient comfortable and promote respiratory effort. All vital signs must be monitored continuously following administration of medication, as the narcotics commonly alter the patient's cardiorespiratory status. Transcutaneous electrical nerve stimulation (TENS) has been very effective in controlling incisional pain for these patients. Although not satisfactory as the sole pain relief modality, TENS in conjunction with narcotic analgesia may significantly reduce the dosage of narcotics necessary to control pain. This is advantageous, since it allows the patient to breathe and ambulate more easily.

Dressings

The abdominal incisions are not commonly drained, and all dressings should remain dry and intact. If dressings become soaked with serosanguineous drainage, the surgeon should be notified. The surgeon should change the dressing and inspect the incision.

Neurologic Status

The state of consciousness, facial function, movement, and strength of all extremities as well as pupillary size and reaction and carotid pulses must be evaluated frequently as parameters of cerebral function. Cerebrovascular accidents are not uncommon postoperatively, owing to the dislodgment of emboli during surgery.

REFERENCES

1. Allwood, A. C.: Cerebral artery bypass surgery. Am. J. Nurs., 80:1284–1287, 1980.
2. Atchison, J. S.: Post-vascular surgery: when happiness *can* be a warm foot. Nursing '78, 8:36–39, 1978.
3. Crowe, L.: Post-op care of the cineangiography patient. J. Nurs. Care, 12:21, 1979.
4. Czapinski, N., et al.: Nursing plan for abdominal aortic aneurysm. AORN J., 37(2):205–210, 1983.
5. Durbin, N.: The application of Doppler techniques in critical care. Focus Crit. Care, 10(3):44–46, 1983.
6. Fahey, V. A., and Bergan, J. J.: Venous reconstruction. AORN J., 41(2):423–434, 1985.
7. Hudson, B.: Sharpen your vascular assessment skills with the Doppler ultrasound stethoscope. Nursing '83 13(5):40–43, 1983.
8. Hurst, J. W., and Logue, R. B. P.: The Heart, Arteries, and Veins. 3rd ed. New York, McGraw-Hill, Inc., 1977.
9. Pairitz, D.: Peripheral vascular surgery: postoperative assessment. AORN J., 40(5):712–715, 1984.
10. Rutherford, R. B. (ed.): Vascular Surgery. Philadelphia, W. B. Saunders Co., 1983.
11. Slasen, R. N.: Vascular crises in the postoperative period. Curr. Rev. Recov. Room Nurses, 10(5):79–86, 1983.
12. Szaflarski, N.: Carotid endarterectomy. After surgery. AORN J., 32:48–54, 1980.
13. Webb, P. H.: Neurological deficit after carotid endarterectomy. Am. J. Nurs., 79:654–658, 1979.

Postoperative Care After Orthopedic Surgery

Pamela K. Stann, R.N., B.S.N.
and Susan B. Christoph, R.N., D.N.Sc.

Postoperative nursing care of the orthopedic patient encompasses many parameters of post anesthesia care. In addition to the general post anesthetic care, the nurse must be attentive to the particular orthopedic surgical procedure performed. The use of astute nursing observation and inspection will prove very important in ensuring a low incidence of morbidity in the postoperative orthopedic patient. Orthopedic patients often undergo a series of procedures, and the nurse must be sensitive to the anxieties of the patient who has had previous surgical experience.

Definitions
AEA: above the elbow amputation.
AKA: above the knee amputation.
Arthrodesis: surgical fixation or fusion of a joint.
Arthroplasty: surgical formation of a joint.
Arthroscopy: direct vision into a joint by means of an instrument called an arthroscope.

Arthrotomy: surgical exploration of a joint.
Articulation: the connection of bones at the joint.
BEA: below the elbow amputation.
BKA: below the knee amputation.
Cineplasty (kineplasty): surgical manipulation of muscles after amputation, so that an artificial limb can be activated.
CTS: carpal tunnel syndrome.
D/L: dislocation.
Disarticulation: amputation at a joint.
Fasciotomy: surgical separation of the fascia, a fibrous membrane that covers, supports, or separates the muscles.
Fx: fracture.
Harrington rods: used in spinal fixation for scoliosis and for some spinal fractures.
Kyphosis: an exaggeration of the posterior curve of the thoracic spine.
LE: lower extremity.
Lordosis: abnormal anterior convexity of the lower part of the back.
Luque rods: spinal fixation, applying transverse force, for scoliosis.

Meniscectomy: surgical removal of the meniscus of the knee.

Osteomyelitis: infection of the bone.

ORIF: open reduction and internal fixation.

Osteoporosis: diminished amount of calcium in the bone.

Osteotomy: surgical cutting of the bone.

Patellectomy: surgical removal of the patella.

Scoliosis: lateral curvature of the spine.

Sequestrectomy: surgical removal of necrosed bone.

Spinal fusion: a fusion of the cervical, thoracic, or lumbar region of the spine using iliac or other bone graft, primarily fusing the laminae and sometimes the joints, most often through the posterior approach.

Syme amputation: amputation of the foot at the ankle joint.

Synovectomy: surgical removal of the synovial membrane.

TKR: total knee replacement.

THR: total hip replacement.

TSR: total shoulder replacement.

UE: upper extremity.

Volkmann ischemia: swelling and edema that occur within the joint capsule or muscle coverings in the elbow and can result in paralysis of the median, radial, and ulnar nerves.

GENERAL POSTOPERATIVE CARE

Immediate postoperative nursing care of the orthopedic patient centers around proper body alignment, assessment of neurovascular status, care of the affected extremity, cast care, pulmonary care, wound care, and observation for complications.

Positioning

Proper body alignment is important for all orthopedic patients. The extremities should be supported along their entire length. The operated extremity should be elevated above the heart to increase venous return and prevent effusion. If the hand or arm was operated on, it may be suspended from an overhead frame or intravenous pole. A stockinette with a muslin bandage may be used to facilitate this position. The elbow should be supported with a pillow, and a hole should be cut in the end of the stockinette so that the neurovascular status of the fingers can be monitored.

Long leg casts usually require two or three pillows for elevation. These should be placed along the entire length of the cast to prevent muscle strain. Postoperative care of the patient with a bulky compression dressing of the leg is similar to that of the patient with a long leg cast. It must also be remembered that the leg should be kept in 15 to 20 degrees of flexion at the knee unless otherwise ordered by the physician.

The total hip replacement patient needs to be in good alignment with an abduction pillow in place between the knees at all times. It is also important to support the lateral aspect of the leg of the affected hip to prevent external rotation. This can be accomplished by using rolled towels or sheets.

The PACU nurse should also be familiar with the various types of orthopedic equipment available for use. The TKR and the knee arthrotomy patient are often placed in a constant passive motion (CPM) machine to prevent postoperative stiffening of the joint. The Circo-electric bed and the Stryker frame are used for the total hip and trauma patient. There are also various types of traction that may be used with the orthopedic patient. The PACU nurse is not usually involved in the setting up of these various types of traction but should be aware of some basic principles related to traction. The patient should be maintained in good body alignment in relation to the traction, and the weights should all be kept hanging free and not resting on the floor. One type of traction is depicted in Figure 25–1.

Cast Care

When the orthopedic patient arrives in the PACU, immediate assessment should include the type of traction and casts or splints applied. The casts should be inspected to see if the fingers or toes are visible. Has the cast been bivalved? Are

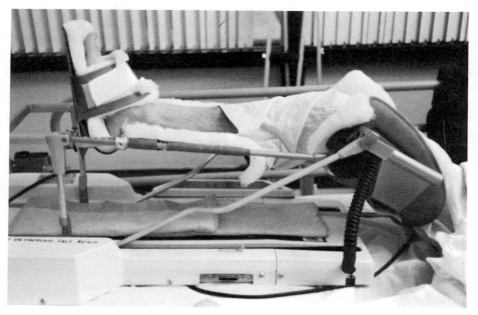

Figure 25–1. Traction.

there any bony prominences that, if not protected, could be sites for tissue breakdown? The surgical dressing should be inspected for bleeding. If the surgical incision is covered by a cast, the drainage may be circled and the time noted with a marking pen. This can provide a guide for postoperative blood and fluid loss, and can alert the nurse if the drainage appears to be excessive. Casts may not have completely dried. All casts should be handled with the palms of the hands. Handling a cast with the fingers could cause indentations that might later lead to pressure areas and consequent decubitus formation.

Assessment of the cast should include inspection of the exposed fingers or toes. The hallmarks of neurovascular changes due to constriction and circulatory embarrassment are pain, color change (cyanosis, blanching [anemia]), swelling, decreased local temperature, and diminished sensation. Comparisons should be made with the unaffected limb when possible. If any of the above-stated symptoms occur, the surgeon should be notified at once.

Complications

Postoperative complications for the orthopedic patient include fat embolism, renal shutdown, pulmonary embolism, thrombophlebitis, urinary retention, atelectasis, and compartment syndrome.

Fat Embolism. Fat embolism is a clinical state that can occur after multiple severe injuries, especially those of the long bones. It is caused by fat droplets that are released into the circulation. It usually occurs between 12 and 24 postoperative hours, and is generally less common in children and in adults past the age of 60. Because the emboli spread widely, abnormalities may develop anywhere. If the lungs are involved, symptoms such as tachypnea, tachycardia, petechiae over the chest, pallor, cyanosis, and confusion will occur. Brain involvement is evidenced by mild agitation, confusion, twitching of muscles, and coma. Immediate nursing care of this sometimes fatal complication includes administering oxygen, keeping the patient quiet, and preventing motion at the fracture site.

Renal Shutdown. Renal shutdown may occur following severe injury or shock. A 24-hour urinary output of 400 ml (18 to 20 ml per hour) or less is usually indicative of this complication. Patients with renal shutdown should be monitored closely for intake and output since intravenous therapy is usually instituted.

Pulmonary Embolism. If the patient has been inactive and movement has been restricted prior to surgery, a clot may form in the vein with little or no inflammatory reaction in the vein wall. This reaction, termed phlebothrombosis, can lead to pulmonary embolism. The patient usually displays no subjective or objective symptoms until the infarction occurs. Pulmonary embolism is usually characterized by chest pain, dyspnea, apprehension, and shock. Immediate nursing care involves administration of oxygen and relief of pain.

Thrombophlebitis. Thrombophlebitis is an acute inflammatory reaction in the wall of a vein and surrounding structures. The patient will usually complain of pain and tenderness accompanied by swelling and sometimes localized redness. A positive Homans sign may be exhibited. Venous complications can usually be prevented by exercise, but if they occur exercise should cease; anticoagulant therapy is usually instituted. Thigh-high TED hose (antiembolism stockings) should be used on all patients who will not be ambulatory, who have a hip or lower extremity injury, who are elderly, or who have a previous history of thrombophlebitis. Pneumatic hose (alternating pressure gradient stockings), along with the TED hose, are used on those patients who are at high risk for thrombus formation, including spinal surgical and total hip replacement patients with a history of thrombophlebitis.

Urinary Retention. Urinary retention may occur in adult patients on whom hip or back procedures have been performed. The retention may be due to spinal anesthesia. These patients should be monitored for bladder distention and the surgeon should be notified if distention occurs or if the patient is unable to void within 8 hours after the surgery is completed. An in-and-out catheterization is usually employed.

Atelectasis. Because it is sometimes difficult to change the patient's position postoperatively and because some orthopedic patients are of advanced age, atelectasis, which may lead to pneumonia, is a possible complication. Since anesthetic agents depress the respiratory system, it is of utmost importance to have the patient cough and breathe deeply. Sustained maximal inspirations should be encouraged, and the incentive spirometer should be used every hour postoperatively as soon as the patient is able. The position of these patients should be changed every hour when possible.

Assessment should include frequent inspection of the chest to see that it expands and contracts symmetrically and to assure that no retractions occur. Auscultation should be done after every position change or every 2 hours. Rales and rhonchi indicate increased fluid in the lungs. Decreased breath sounds, especially at the base of the lung, indicate possible atelectasis.

Compartment Syndrome. Compartment syndrome is an acute ischemic condition that can cause permanent muscle and tissue damage if a fasciotomy is not performed. This condition most often occurs in the forearm or the calf of the leg and is considered an orthopedic emergency. The symptoms of compartment syndrome are increased pain, neurologic and vascular deficits, and sharp pain upon passive flexion of the middle finger of the affected arm or the large toe of the affected leg. The physician should be notified immediately if these symptoms occur.

POSTOPERATIVE CARE AFTER HAND SURGERY

The hand surgery patient will often be admitted to the PACU with a large bulky dressing in place on the hand and forearm. An Ace wrap to apply pressure may also be in place outside of the dressing. The hand should be elevated above the level of the heart at all times to prevent edema and hemorrhage. The hand may be placed on pillows on the chest of the patient, or suspended from the bedframe or IV pole by stockinette. The elbow should be supported by a pillow. If a drain is present, it should be checked to assure that it is activated. The drain may be connected to a vacuum blood tube. This should be changed every 1 to 2 hours to maintain a proper vacuum and the output recorded on the intake and output records. The tips of the fingers should be visible, and the neurovascular status should be checked every half hour for signs of change. It should be remembered that hand surgeries are frequently done with the use of an axillary block and that sensation and movement may not fully return for several hours after surgery. Baseline neurovascular indicators should be noted in the admission nursing assessment. These can be used to establish whether or not there have been any deleterious effects from the surgery.

POSTOPERATIVE CARE AFTER SHOULDER SURGERY

Shoulder surgeries may include arthroscopies, arthrotomies, or total shoulder joint replacements. The patient will be admitted to the PACU with a bulky pressure dressing in place along with a sling-style shoulder immobilizer (Fig. 25–2). Make sure that the dressings do not interfere with chest expansion, as this would inhibit good respiratory exchange. The surgical dressing should be inspected for bleeding, as the shoulder is a vascular area and hemorrhage is very difficult to manage in this area.

Inspection should include checking to see if any skin surface is in contact with an-

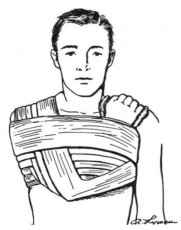

Figure 25–2. The Velpeau bandage is used temporarily to immobilize clavicle, shoulder, humerus, elbow, or forearm. Wherever skin comes in contact with skin, a protective pad should be inserted. (From Larson, C. B., and Gould, M.: Orthopedic Nursing. 9th ed. St. Louis, C. V. Mosby Co., 1978.)

other. If this is the case, a protective pad should be inserted between the two skin surfaces. The distal pulses (radial and ulnar) should be monitored because flexion of the arm in the immobilizer can reduce blood flow to the hand. Again, neurovascular observations are a very important part of the postoperative assessment of these patients. If the hand on the affected side becomes edematous, the patient should be encouraged to perform active range of motion exercises with that hand, and the immobilizer should be checked for areas that are causing pressure to the shoulder and arm.

POSTOPERATIVE CARE AFTER SURGERY OF THE ARM AND FOREARM

Postoperative care of the patient recovering from arm and forearm surgery centers around elevating the extremity, observing for excessive bleeding, and monitoring for neurovascular changes. The radial and ulnar pulses should be taken every 30 minutes and compared with those of the unaffected limb. Any decrease in intensity of the pulse or in bilateral strength of the hand, any excessive bleeding, and any changes in neurovascular status should be reported to the surgeon. Symptoms of excessive pain, weakness, or decreased sensation, especially on passive extension of the fingers, are usually indicative of Volkmann ischemia, which constitutes an orthopedic emergency.

POSTOPERATIVE CARE AFTER SURGERY OF THE HIP OR FEMUR

When the patient who has had hip or femur surgery is admitted to the PACU, nursing assessment should include pulmonary function, neurovascular function, body alignment, and the amount and type of bleeding from the surgical incision.

Respiratory function may be compromised for this patient, owing to advanced age, to preexisting respiratory disease, or to effects of the anesthetic agent itself. Cough-

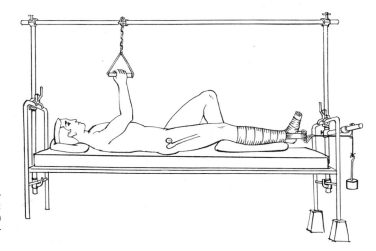

Figure 25-3. Buck's extension with overhead trapeze. (From Schmeisser, G., Jr.: A Clinical Manual of Orthopedic Traction Techniques. Philadelphia, W. B. Saunders Co., 1963.)

ing and deep breathing, SMIs, and position changes, when possible, are of utmost importance. The incentive spirometer can be used to facilitate good lung expansion. Any change in the pulmonary dynamics should be reported to the anesthetist.

Because swelling at the operative site can reduce blood flow to the feet, neurologic signs along with pulses of the affected foot should be monitored and compared with those of the unaffected foot. The dorsalis pedis pulse can be palpated on the dorsum of the foot and lateral to the extensor tendon of the great toe. The posterior tibial pulse can be palpated just behind and slightly below the medial malleolus of the ankle.

The body should be aligned as anatomically normally as possible. If the extremity is in Russell's or Buck's traction, the weight bag should hang free and not rest on the floor (Fig. 25-3 and 25-4). The skin traction may be applied with Ace wraps or straps. Make sure that the securing is not tight around the knee area, as it might compress the peroneal nerve where it crosses the fibula or the knee. Any decrease in sensation over the dorsum of the foot should be noted as indicative of injury to this nerve.

The total hip replacement patient is often placed on a Circo-electric bed immediately following surgery (Fig. 25-5). It is of utmost importance that the patient be properly secured to the bed with at least two belts. An abduction pillow should be placed between the patient's knees. The patient should not be allowed to flex at the hips at

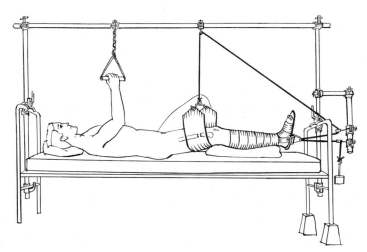

Figure 25-4. Russell's skin traction (single) with overhead frame and trapeze. (From Schmeisser, G., Jr.: A Clinical Manual of Orthopedic Traction Techniques. Philadelphia, W. B. Saunders Co., 1963.)

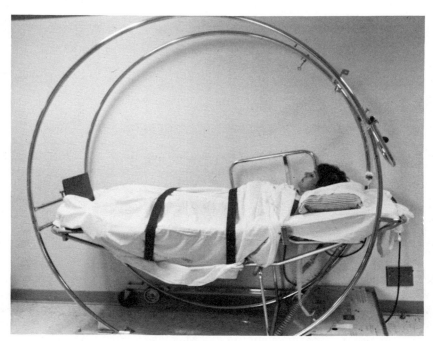

Figure 25–5. Circo-electric bed.

a greater than 30 to 40 degree angle or to adduct the leg of the affected side. This is especially important if a posterior approach to the hip was used; the muscle groups are weakened and dislocation of the joint is a potential danger with these patients.

A Hemovac drain is usually inserted at the operative site to facilitate the removal of blood; the color and amount should be inspected frequently. If the color is bright red or the drainage is more than 300 ml in an 8-hour period, the surgeon should be notified. The THR patient may experience a large blood loss. This becomes a problem if the blood loss is sustained or if it increases.

POSTOPERATIVE CARE AFTER KNEE SURGERY

Postoperative care of the patient who has had surgery of the knee involves observation for complications and proper knee positioning. The surgical procedure may involve repair of ligaments and tendons or removal of all or of a portion of the meniscal cartilage. Patients may undergo a total knee replacement when degenerative processes

have caused the knee joint to become nonfunctional.

The knee joint is formed by the articulation of rounded condyles of the femur with shallow depressions in the tibia, also called condyles. At the periphery of the articulation between the femoral and tibial condyles are the wedge-shaped meniscal cartilages that function primarily in joint lubrication and in cushioning. The medial and lateral cruciate ligaments are primarily responsible for lateral stability, and the cruciate ligaments within the intercondylar notch are primarily responsible for anteroposterior stability.

After knee surgery, the patient will arrive in the recovery room with a bulky compression dressing in place. Ice may be ordered over the surgical site, and the leg should be elevated and positioned in full extension. This can be facilitated by elevation at the ankle so that maximum extension of the leg can be accomplished. Circulation should be checked by palpation of the dorsalis pedis or of the posterior tibial artery at frequent intervals. Sensation should be assessed during the circulation check. Any decrease in sensation over the dorsum of the foot should be noted, as this can represent compression of the peroneal nerve where it crosses the fibula at the knee. The surgeon should be notified if any neurologic or circulatory change is found, as early detection and correction will prevent permanent nerve deficit or ischemic muscular injury. If the patient received a spinal or epidural anesthetic, it will be difficult to assess whether or not neurologic deficits exist. When motor function has returned to the foot of the operated extremity, neurologic tests can be initiated.

Arthroscopies of the knee are done to facilitate minor repairs and for diagnosis of more extensive damage to the knee; in general, there are fewer postoperative complications because this is a less invasive procedure. However, neurovascular assessment remains an important part of the postoperative care of these patients.

The total knee replacement patient and those patients who have undergone extensive arthrotomy knee repairs are sometimes placed in a CPM machine. This unit is used to prevent postoperative stiffening of the knee joint by providing passive flexion and extension to the knee joint. The footpiece should be adjusted to assure that the knee joint is properly aligned in the machine. The flexion and extension setting of the machine should be determined by the physician.

POSTOPERATIVE CARE AFTER SURGERY ON THE FOOT

The patient who has had a surgical procedure performed on the foot will have either a cast or a bandage over the operative site. The amount and color of bleeding should be noted. Neurovascular signs should be monitored every 30 minutes. The extremity should be elevated above the level of the heart, with pillows supporting the entire length of the leg.

POSTOPERATIVE CARE AFTER SURGERY OF THE SPINE

There are several types of spinal procedures. The important features of the post-

operative assessment relate mostly to the surgical area of the spine. Patients who have had a cervical procedure should be monitored for neurologic signs of the upper extremities. Symptoms such as weakness or radiating pain should be reported to the surgeon. Patients in halo traction should be monitored for any deficiency in the sixth cranial (abducent) nerve. Any decrease in the lateral movement of the eye is indicative of injury to the abducent nerve.

If the surgical procedure involves the third, fourth, or fifth cervical spine, respiratory movements should be monitored, as the diaphragm muscle is innervated by the spinal outflow from C_3, C_4, and C_5. The patient with this nerve deficit will exhibit lack of diaphragmatic excursion, as well as shortness of breath and the use of intercostal and accessory muscles in breathing. If these symptoms appear, oxygen should be administered and assistance in ventilation may be necessary.

Patients who have had midthoracic or lower spine surgery may develop an ileus. This complication is signaled by abdominal distention, diminished or absent bowel sounds, and tympany upon percussion of the abdomen. The usual treatment is to withhold oral food and fluids and to decompress the stomach with a nasogastric tube.

Patients who have had lumbar or sacral spinal surgery should be observed for loss of strength in the lower extremities and bladder distention. Bladder distention may be indicated by diaphoresis, hypertension, tachycardia, tachypnea, and a feeling of distress. If the patient has a catheter in place, it should be irrigated to remove any obstruction. If there is no urinary catheter and the patient cannot urinate, the surgeon should be notified.

Patients with progressive curvature of the spine (scoliosis) may undergo a Harrington or Luque rod insertion for correction or stabilization of the spine. The postoperative assessment will entail those features included in the assessment of the thoracic and the lumbar/sacral spine surgical patient.

Patients who have surgery on the spine should also be observed for bleeding from the site of the operation. The patient should be turned from side to side to help reduce stasis of fluids in the lungs. The technique for turning the spinal patient is called log-rolling. All parts of the patient's body should move in unison. To facilitate this, a pillow may be placed between the patient's knees and the knee opposite the side the patient will be turned to should be flexed. Using a draw sheet can also help to facilitate turning in one smooth motion. Pillows should be placed to support the length of the back and buttocks along with the pillow between the patient's knees. This method of turning the patient puts the least amount of pressure on the spine.

All spinal patients should have TED hose on, and ankle pumping should be encouraged to decrease the stasis of blood in the lower extremities. The patient should be encouraged to use the incentive spirometer every hour to reduce the stasis of fluids in the lungs. For additional information see Chapter 26.

POSTOPERATIVE CARE AFTER AMPUTATION OF A LIMB

Patients who have had an amputation of the leg will be admitted to the PACU with a dressing or a cast applied to the extremity. The patient with an amputation of the arm will usually have a bulky compression dressing in place. The dressing should be assessed for drainage. The extremity should be elevated and ice may be applied to reduce postoperative edema.

REFERENCES

1. Allard, J. L., and Dibble, S. L.: Scoliosis surgery: a look at Luque rods. Am. J. Nurs., 84(5):609–611, 1984.
2. Burg. M. E.: Compartment syndrome. Crit. Care Q., 6(1):27–32, 1983.
3. Drucker, M. M.: Arthroscopic surgery of the knee joint. AORN J., 36(4):585–593, 1982.
4. Farrell, J.: Orthopedic pain: What does it mean? Am. J. Nurs., 84(4):466–469, 1984.
5. Laskin, R. S., and Varrichio, D. M.: Total knee replacement. AORN J., 36(4):577–584, 1982.
6. Miller, B. K., and Gregory, M.: Carpal tunnel syndrome. AORN J., 38(3):525–537, 1983.
7. Shenkman, B., and Stechmiller, J.: Fat embolism syndrome: pathophysiology and current treatment. Focus Crit. Care, 11(6):26–35, 1984.
8. Thompson, M. B.: An overview of arthroscopy. Today's OR Nurse, 4(11):9–13, 1983.
9. Turner, P.: Caring for emotional needs of orthopedic trauma patients. AORN J., 36(4):566–570, 1982.
10. Urbanski, P. A.: The orthopedic patient: identifying neurovascular injury. AORN J., 40(5):707–711, 1984.
11. Voluz, J. M.: Surgical implants: orthopedic devices. AORN J., 37(7):1341–1352, 1983.

26

Postoperative Care Following Neurosurgery

by Marie H. Dutton, R.N., M.S.N.

Many patients seen in the post anesthesia care unit (PACU) have received insult or compromise to some aspect of the nervous system. This insult may be as dramatic and graphic as that seen in severe head trauma or as quiet and insidious as that caused by a constrictive circumferential limb cast. Individuals with neurologic trauma suffered as a result of motor vehicle accidents, gunshot wounds, or sports mishaps are seen, as well as those requiring surgical intervention for or repair of preexisting medical problems.

This chapter will be divided into two sections—cranial surgery, and spinal surgery. This division is solely for the purpose of this discussion, since there are aspects of care for each that are common to both. In addition, disease or injury of any portion of the nervous system may also affect other organs and systems of the body. In caring for the neurosurgical patient, each structure of the nervous system (see Chapter 9) must be considered as it relates to the individual as a whole.

Definitions

Baroreceptor: a sensory nerve cell aggregate present in the wall of a blood vessel, which is stimulated by changes in blood pressure.

Compliance: ability of the brain to yield when a pressure or force is applied.

Crepitus: crackling sound produced by the rubbing together of fractured bone fragments or by the presence of subcutaneous emphysema.

Decompensation: inability of the heart to maintain adequate circulation due to the impairment of brain integrity.

Diabetes insipidus: metabolic disorder caused by injury or disease of the posterior lobe of the pituitary gland (also known as the hypophysis).

Focal deficit: any sign or symptom that indicates a specific or localized area of pathology.

Gibbus: hump or convexity.

Laminectomy: excision of the posterior arch of a vertebra to allow the excision of a herniated nucleus pulposus.

365

Phrenic nucleus: group of nerve cells located in the spinal cord between the levels of C-3 and C-5. Damage to this area will abolish or alter the function of the phrenic nerve.

Pyramidal signs: symptoms of dysfunction of the pyramidal tract, including spastic paralysis, Babinski sign, and increased deep tendon reflexes.

Rhizotomy: surgical interruption of the roots of the spinal nerves within the spinal canal.

Spinal shock: state that occurs immediately after complete transection of the spinal cord. It may sometimes occur after only partial transections. All sensory, motor, and autonomic activity is lost below the level of the transection and reflexes are absent. Paralysis is of a flaccid nature and includes the urinary bladder. There is gradual resumption of autonomic activity as spinal shock subsides. Once autonomic activity has returned, bladder and bowel training programs may be begun. Flaccid paralysis may develop into varying degrees of spastic paralysis, as evidenced by spasms of flexor or extensor muscle groups. The presence of autonomic activity also allows for episodes of autonomic hyperreflexia.

Subarachnoid block: injection of a local anesthetic into the subarachnoid space around the spinal cord.

Subluxation: partial or incomplete dislocation.

Tonoclonic movements: tense muscular contractions alternating rapidly with muscular relaxation.

Valsalva maneuver: contraction of the thorax in forced expiration against the closed glottis. Results in increases in intrathroacic and intraabdominal pressures.

CRANIAL SURGERY

Diagnostic Tools

Some of the techniques used to ascertain the presence of and extent of cranial injury or disease are invasive. In many hospitals, patients on whom these procedures are performed spend a period of time in the post anesthesia care unit. A brief discussion of these and of noninvasive diagnostic procedures is included here to familiarize the PACU nurse with the techniques and the special considerations necessary in the care of these patients.

Invasive Techniques

Pneumoencephalography (PEG). General anesthesia is preferred for this procedure, as the incidence of severe headache, shock, retching, and impaired consciousness is greater when it is done under local anesthesia.

A lumbar puncture is performed and the cerebrospinal fluid (CSF) removed is replaced with air or gas. The patient is generally placed in a chair designed for easy movement and positioning while x-ray pictures are being taken. Even when performed under general anesthesia, the patient often experiences a severe headache for some time after the procedure. Therefore, it is considerate to place the patient in an area where extraneous noise and activity are at a minimum, but where frequent observations are possible.

Ventriculography. Ventriculography is usually done under local anesthetic with the patient in the same sort of chair as that used in pneumonencephalography. Ventriculogram involves puncture of the ventricle through burr holes made in the cranium. Cerebrospinal fluid is removed and replaced with gas or air. X-rays are taken, and the size, shape, and position of the ventricular, cisternal, and subarachnoid spaces are visualized, and the presence of space-occupying lesions may be noted.

As with the pneumoencephalogram patient, postventriculogram patients may experience nausea, retching, and headache, although not usually as severely. Both types of patient require frequent observation of vital signs, neurologic status, and level of consciousness. Intravenous fluids are usually continued for 24 hours or until the danger of shock reaction and vomiting have ended. This period is variable and depends on the patient's general condition and tolerance of the procedure. Headaches may persist for 2 to 4 days, and mild analgesics may be prescribed.

Arteriography. Arteriography, or angiography, is employed to visualize the pattern and patency of the cerebral vasculature. A cannula is introduced into the femoral or axillary artery and threaded to the level of the common carotid artery. Radiopaque dye is then injected and x-rays record its path through the cerebral vasculature. Arteriovenous malformations, aneurysms, thrombosis, occlusions, space-occupying lesions, and abscesses may be detected by this method (Fig. 26–1). During and after arteriography the patient may experience an allergic reaction to the dye used that may range from mild urticaria to full-blown anaphylaxis. Resuscitative equipment must be immediately available until the danger of allergic reaction has passed.

Irritation brought on by use of the dye may manifest itself by altered states of consciousness, hemiparesis, or speech difficulties, usually transient in nature. It is imperative that the site of injection be examined closely at frequent intervals for the presence of bleeding that, when present, occurs beneath the skin and defies casual detection. Often the effects of the local anesthetic used last for several hours and prevent the patient from detecting and reporting the pain caused by hemorrhage. The site is often swollen and becomes painful after the anesthetic effect has worn off. This pain and edema can be minimized by the prompt placement of an ice pack over the area when the patient arrives in the post anesthesia care unit. Intravenous fluids are maintained until the danger of untoward reaction has passed and the patient is no longer experiencing the transient nausea that occasionally occurs.

Invasive Techniques Not Usually Seen in the Post Anesthesia Care Unit

Brain Scanning. In this procedure a radioactive compound is injected intravenously and is taken up by brain tissue. The pattern of this uptake is detected by a scintillation scanner and a visual record is rendered. Uptake may be altered at the site of a disorder and may reflect the presence of cerebral neoplasms, hematomas, abscesses, and arteriovenous malformations.

CT Scanning. Computerized axial tomography (sometimes called computerized transverse axial scanning or EMI scanning) creates a cross-sectional picture that separates various densities in the brain by means of an external radiation beam. A computer-based apparatus allows the assessment of brain-emitted radiation after the intravenous injection of a radioactive isotope. The computer performs tens of thousands of

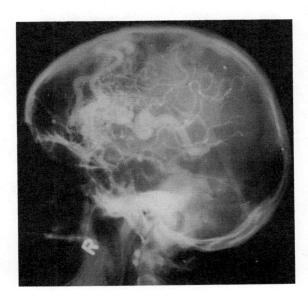

Figure 26–1. Arteriographic demonstration of an intracranial arteriovenous malformation. (From Sabiston, D. C. [ed.]: Textbook of Surgery. 11th ed. Philadelphia, W. B. Saunders Co., 1977, p. 1481.)

simultaneous equations on the radiation input and output figures stored on its tapes and delivers an accurate detailed picture of the brain and of any abnormalities (Fig. 26–2).

CT scanning has the advantages of accuracy and rapidity—both essential in emergency situations. Unfortunately, the procedure requires maximal cooperation by the patient for sustained periods of time and is therefore difficult, if not impossible, to use in an agitated, confused, or restless patient.

Nuclear Magnetic Resonance (NMR) Imaging. The NMR is a recently developed, highly promising technique for obtaining cross-sectional pictures of the human body without exposing the patient to ionizing radiation. NMR imaging yields anatomical information comparable in many ways to the information supplied by a CT scan but is, in many instances, able to discriminate more sensitively between healthy and diseased tissue.

NMR is able to visualize soft organs by differentiating the number of hydrogen molecules present in the water content of the tissues. The water content for each type of tissue, including abnormal tissue, varies and, when assessed by a skilled radiologist, serves almost as its "signature."

The patient to be scanned is placed within

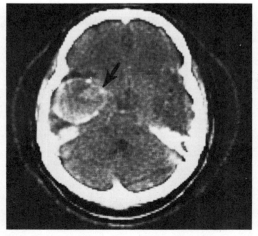

Figure 26–2. CT scan of large congenital aneurysm (arrow) of middle cerebral artery in left middle fossa. (From Sabiston, D. C. [ed.]: Textbook of Surgery. 11th ed. Philadelphia, W. B. Saunders Co., 1977, p. 1472.)

a cylindrical high-powered magnet. Body tissues are then subjected to a magnetic field, causing some of the hydrogen ions to align themselves with the magnetic field. A burst of low-energy radio waves is then applied that knocks atomic protons within the tissues out of alignment. When the radio waves are discontinued, these protons release tiny amounts of energy which are "read" by a computer. It then generates an image based on this information, yielding a detailed picture of the structural content and contours of the internal organs.

Positron Emission Tomography (PET). At present, PET scanning is used mainly in research settings and has limited, though promising, clinical application because of difficulties in interpreting its images. In this type of study, the state of the *functioning* of the tissues or organs is assessed. The patient is injected with a glucose analog that is tagged with a radionuclide. As the radionuclide decays in the tissue, the protons emitted are recorded by detectors, and a computerized picture is generated. Now used predominately in assessing brain function, PET scans have been helpful in identifying schizophrenia, Alzheimer's disease, and other brain disorders.

Noninvasive Techniques

Conventional Radiography. Skull films will show bony fragments and fractures and any shift of the calcified pineal gland from the midline. Epidural hematoma will almost always show an accompanying linear fracture across the temporal fossa. Except for nondisplaced linear skull fracture, positive skull x-rays are almost always followed up with other diagnostic tests (Fig. 26–3).

Electroencephalography. An electroencephalogram (EEG) is the tracing and recording of the electrical activity at the surface of the brain. Aberrations in the rate and amplitude signal the presence of tumors, abscesses, scars, hematomas, or infection and may aid in the localization of such lesions.

Echoencephalography (Ultrasound). This technique is used to detect shifts in the midline structures of the brain. The pineal

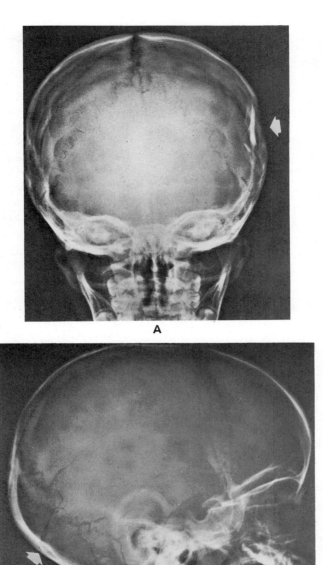

A

B

Figure 26–3. *A*, Depressed skull fracture of the left parietal bone and adjoining portion of temporal bone (arrow). *B*, Lateral view of the skull demonstrating a linear fracture of the occipital bone with no detectable depression of the fragments (arrow). (From Meschan, I.: Synopsis of Analysis of Roentgen Signs in General Radiology. Philadelphia, W. B. Saunders Co., 1976, p. 191.)

gland, septum pellucidum, and wall of the third ventricle are used as the target structures of the ultrasound waves. These waves are then echoed back to the instrument, revealing the exact location of the midline structure. When the midline structures are off center, a space-occupying lesion is assumed to have altered their position. In this manner, hematomas, massive cerebral infarcts, and neoplasms are detected. Echoencephalography has the advantages of being rapid and noninvasive, but its use is sometimes limited by imprecise or inconclusive results.

Injuries to the Brain

Types of Injuries

Following injury to the head, the most crucial concern is the extent of injury to the brain itself. Linear skull fractures in and of themselves are of little significance, but when the fracture involves depression of fragments into the brain, leakage of cerebrospinal fluid, or accumulation of hematoma, surgery is required to relieve the increased intracranial pressure that results.

Concussion, a jostling of the brain without contusion, is caused by a violent jar or shock to the skull. The patient may be dazed, "see stars," or experience a period of impaired consciousness. On regaining consciousness, these patients often experience post-traumatic amnesia, remembering nothing of the injury itself or, frequently, nothing of the events immediately preceding the injury.

More serious than concussion is *contusion*, a multiple bruising of the brain or hemorrhage on its surface. Consciousness may be lost for a considerable period of time. Death may occur within a few hours or, if less severe, stupor and confusion may persist for days or weeks. These patients characteristically resent attempts to arouse them and may be disoriented, agitated, or violent.

Contusion of the brain is usually incurred through one of two types of *blow-counterblow injury*. In a *coup-countrecoup injury* the brain is injured directly beneath the site of the striking force. As the blow thrusts the brain against bony prominences of the inner surface of the opposite side of the skull, further injury results. The vasculature of the brain may be lacerated and considerable hemorrhage may result.

The second type of blow-counterblow injury is the *acceleration-deceleration injury*. In a trauma involving abrupt impact, such as a motor vehicle accident, the internal soft tissue structures, including the brain, continue to travel for a fraction of a second longer than the external body and receive further injury as they are pressed against the rigid structures of the body. The brain is slapped *by* the surrounding skull and then is slapped *against* it. Rebound occurs and further damage is done as it strikes the unyielding bony ridges of the inside of the skull. Severe bruising or laceration may occur.

Consequences of Injury

Concussion or contusion, as well as intrinsic medical conditions, may produce different kinds of injury to the brain, including subdural hematoma, epidural hematoma, intracerebral hematoma, and supratentorial herniation, all requiring surgical intervention. The signs and symptoms of brain ischemia and increased intracranial pressure vary with the speed at which the functions of vital centers are altered. A small clot that accumulates rapidly may be fatal. On the other hand, the patient may survive a slow-developing, much larger hematoma through effective compensatory mechanisms.

An *epidural hematoma* accumulates in the epidural space (between the skull and the dura mater) and is arterial in nature. Frequently, the cause is the rupture or laceration of the middle meningeal artery, which runs between the dura and the skull in the temporal region. Bleeding along a fracture line is another possible cause. Epidural hematomas most frequently occur in the temporal area but may appear elsewhere, depending on the area of trauma or arterial rupture. Epidural hematoma requires rapid emergency surgery. Owing to its arterial nature, the hemorrhage may be massive, and neurologic deficit and death may occur imminently. Treatment consists of evacuation of the clot through burr holes made in the skull.

Subdural hematoma may result from trauma. Venous blood usually accumulates beneath the dura and spreads over the surface of the brain. A subdural hematoma may be acute, subacute, or chronic, depending on the size of the vessel involved and the amount of blood present. Acute subdural hematomas exhibit a rapid progression of signs and symptoms and the patient is critically ill.

Subacute subdural hematomas fail to show acute signs and symptoms at the outset. Brain swelling is not great, but the hematoma may become sufficiently large to produce symptoms. Progressive hemiparesis, obtundation, and aphasia often appear 3 to 10 days after injury. The degree of ultimate recovery depends on the extent of damage produced at the time of injury.

Chronic subdural hematomas are most frequently seen in infants and adults past middle age. A history of head injury may be lacking, as the causative injury is often minimal and long forgotten or deemed insignificant by the patient. The history is usually one of progressive mental or personality changes with or without focal symptoms. Papilledema may be present. As blood slowly accumulates, it compresses the brain. The blood itself becomes thicker and darker within 2 to 4 days, and within a few weeks resembles motor oil in character and color. Subdural hematoma may mimic any disease affecting the brain or its coverings, and is often incorrectly diagnosed initially as a stroke, neurosis, or psychosis. Treatment consists of evacuation of the defibrinated blood through multiple burr holes or craniotomy incision.

Intracerebral hematomas are more frequently found in the elderly, often following a fall, but are also seen as a result of spontaneous rupture of a weakened blood vessel. Hemorrhaging may be scattered or isolated. Surgical evacuation of an isolated or well-defined clot may be attempted, but the mortality rate remains high.

Supratentorial herniation is regarded as an emergency more severe than that occurring with epidural hematoma. The tentorium is an extension of the dura mater, which forms a transverse partition or shelf dividing the cerebral hemispheres from the cerebellum and brainstem. The superior portion of the brainstem passes upward through an aperture in the tentorium known as the tentorial hiatus. No space-occupying mass or lesion expanding within the cerebral hemispheres can escape upward or outward owing to the unyielding confinement of the skull. Consequently, expansion within and compression of the hemispheres causes herniation of its contents (usually a portion of the temporal lobe known as the uncus) through the tentorial hiatus.

Uncal herniation is accompanied by compression of the lateral brainstem on the same side, shutting off its blood supply and suppressing certain basic functions. The third cranial nerve (oculomotor) is in close proximity to the herniated uncus and the pupil on the injured side becomes fixed and dilated. The reticular activating system located in the brainstem that is responsible for waking and alertness becomes affected, and the patient rapidly becomes less and less responsive. Displacement of the midbrain causes compression of the pyramidal tract, resulting in contralateral hemiparesis or hemiplegia and plantar extensor responses (Babinski sign). The respiratory center in the medulla may be affected and result in changes in the respiratory pattern or cessation of respiration altogether.

In addition to these changes, the cerebellum itself may be so compressed that the cerebellar tonsil herniates inferiorly through the foramen magnum (Fig. 26–4). This usually results in immediate death, as the centers vital to life are compressed or sheared. The best treatment for supratentorial herniation is prevention through early detection and treatment of increased intracranial pressure and its causes.

If efforts to minimize edema and increased intracranial pressure fail, surgical intervention is required as a life-saving measure.

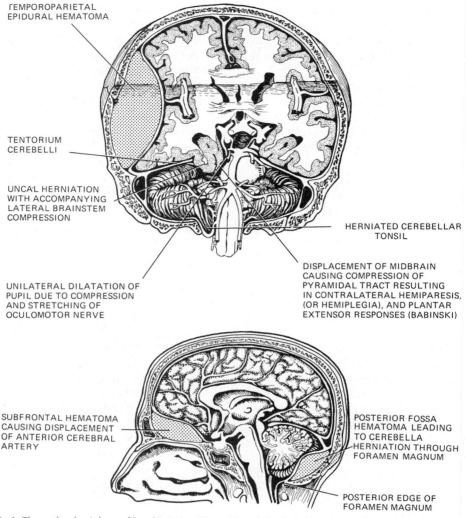

TEMPOROPARIETAL
EPIDURAL HEMATOMA

TENTORIUM
CEREBELLI

UNCAL HERNIATION
WITH ACCOMPANYING
LATERAL BRAINSTEM
COMPRESSION

HERNIATED CEREBELLAR
TONSIL

UNILATERAL DILATATION OF
PUPIL DUE TO COMPRESSION
AND STRETCHING OF
OCULOMOTOR NERVE

DISPLACEMENT OF MIDBRAIN
CAUSING COMPRESSION OF
PYRAMIDAL TRACT RESULTING
IN CONTRALATERAL HEMIPARESIS,
(OR HEMIPLEGIA), AND PLANTAR
EXTENSOR RESPONSES (BABINSKI)

SUBFRONTAL HEMATOMA
CAUSING DISPLACEMENT
OF ANTERIOR CEREBRAL
ARTERY

POSTERIOR FOSSA
HEMATOMA LEADING
TO CEREBELLA
HERNIATION THROUGH
FORAMEN MAGNUM

POSTERIOR EDGE OF
FORAMEN MAGNUM

Figure 26–4. The pathophysiology of head injuries. (From Kintzel, K. C. [ed.]: Advanced Concepts in Clinical Nursing. 2nd ed. Philadelphia, J. B. Lippincott Co., 1977, p. 679.)

Intracranial Pressure Dynamics

Intracranial pressure (ICP) is that pressure exerted against the skull by its contents: cerebrospinal fluid (CSF), blood, and brain. The volumes of these may fluctuate slightly, but despite these variations, the total volume and intracranial pressure remain nearly constant. As discussed in Chapter 9, the cerebral perfusion pressure (CPP) and resultant blood flow are normally determined by the difference between the mean systemic arterial pressure (MSAP), which is the inflow pressure, and the outflow pressure (normally the mean venous pressure). In situations where ICP is greater than venous pressure

$$CPP = MSAP - ICP$$

Consequently, any increase in ICP or reduction in MSAP will reduce CPP and resultant cerebral blood flow.

Autoregulation is capable of maintaining a constant CPP only until the finite limit of CSF compensation is reached. The spinal subarachnoid space can hold a limited amount of displaced CSF, and despite its inability to hold any more displaced fluid, autoregulation continues. In this event, autoregulation ceases to be beneficial or effective in preventing further increases in intracranial pressure; defective autoregulation aggravates pressure increase and creates critical or irreversible levels of ICP by increasing the blood volume within the cranium in an effort to maintain cerebral blood flow. Defective autoregulation generally occurs when ICP exceeds 35 to 40 mm Hg. Eventually, autoregulation ceases altogether, and blood flow fluctuates passively with changes in arterial pressure, regardless of metabolic activity or regulation.

Normal ICP ranges from 4 to 15 mm Hg. Normal CPP is 80 to 90 mm Hg. Cerebral blood flow begins to fail at a CPP of 30 to 40 mm Hg. Irreversible hypoxia occurs at a CPP of less than 30 mm Hg. When ICP = MSAP, CPP = 0 and cerebral blood flow ceases.

When intracranial pressure is increased, CPP and cerebral blood flow are reduced, rendering the tissues ischemic. Ischemic cerebral tissue releases acid metabolites that cause a relatively fixed reduction in cerebrovascular tone. Autoregulation ceases, and any increase in MSAP causes further increase in cerebral blood volume, eliciting a further rise in ICP. CPP is reduced, causing ischemic areas (such as those surrounding an expanding intracranial mass) to enlarge.

As can be seen in Figure 26–5, a pathologic cycle ensues in which ICP and MSAP eventually equilibrate, the CPP drops to zero, cerebral blood flow stops, and death occurs.

Volume may be added to any of the cerebral compartments and results in increased intracranial pressure. Brain volume can be increased by tumor, hematoma, or edema. Blood volume can be increased through dilation of the vascular bed. CSF volume can be increased through obstruction in the ventricles, resistance to reabsorption, or, in rare situations, increased production. Large brain tumors increase pressure by their mass or by blocking the rate of CSF reabsorption, or both. If the tumor is near the surface of the brain, it can cause inflamed meninges that may exude large quantities of fluid and protein into the CSF, increasing ICP. Hemorrhage or infection also causes increases in ICP. Large numbers of cells suddenly appear in the CSF and can almost totally block CSF absorption through the arachnoid villi. Regardless of the mechanism, when the volume added exceeds the volume that can be displaced, intracranial compliance is greatly reduced and ICP begins to rise.

Figure 26–6 illustrates the relationship between intracranial volume and intracranial pressure. Phase I demonstrates the success of compensatory mechanisms in main-

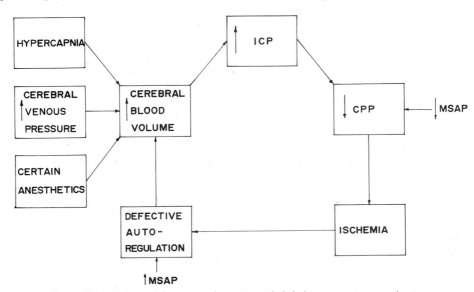

Figure 26–5. Intracranial pressure dynamics with failed compensatory mechanisms.

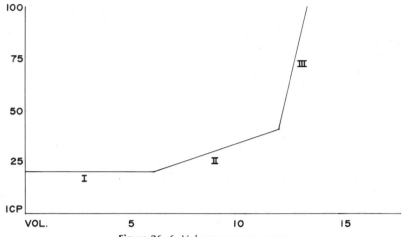

Figure 26–6. Volume-pressure curve.

taining a constant ICP despite early increases in volume. In Phase II, the limited capability of compensatory mechanisms has been exceeded, and intracranial pressure begins to rise. In Phase III, even a slight increase in volume will cause a dramatic rise in ICP, resulting in complete decompensation and death. The shape of the curve may be altered by the rate at which the volume increases. Slowly developing increases in volume will broaden the curve, whereas rapid increases will narrow it.

Anesthetic Agents and Intracranial Pressure

Anesthetic agents alter intracranial pressure by their ability to increase or decrease cerebral blood flow (CBF) and cerebral metabolic rate (CMR). In addition to their effects on ICP, some of these agents may also reduce systemic blood pressure and cause cerebral ischemia due to inadequate cerebral perfusion pressure.

Inhalation Anesthetics. The inhalation anesthetic agents, generally speaking, decrease blood pressure and may increase ICP in the cranial surgery patient. They produce a clinically significant degree of cerebrovascular vasodilatation and of metabolic depression and can modify autoregulation. In fact, high doses of volatile anesthetic agents can cause a total loss of autoregulation. The resulting increase in cerebral blood flow will ultimately lead to increased intracranial pressure. Halothane (Fluothane), in increasing doses, progressively increases cerebral blood flow (CBF) until systemic hypotension reduces cerebral perfusion pressure below the threshold of autoregulation. Enflurane (Ethrane) and isoflurane (Forane), at low doses, produce similar effects on the CBF. However, at higher doses, enflurane and isoflurane elevate CBF to a lesser extent than does halothane. In patients with decreased intracranial compliance secondary to neurologic disease, anesthetic agents that increase cerebral blood flow may produce marked changes in intracranial pressure.

Nitrous oxide, in concentrations greater than 60 percent, can cause an increase in cerebral blood flow by as much as 200 percent. However, if thiopental (Pentothal) or diazepam (Valium) are administered prior to the nitrous oxide, the rise in intracranial pressure may be blocked. Nitrous oxide should not be administered to patients with intracranial hypertension because of its cerebrovasodilatory actions.

Intravenous Anesthetics. Intravenous anesthetic agents (with the exception of ketamine) are usually the anesthetics of choice in cranial surgery. Thiopental (Pentothal), a potent cerebral vasoconstrictor, causes minimal decreases in blood pressure, significantly large reductions in ICP, and substantial increases in CPP.

Innovar (fentanyl in combination with droperidol), causes moderate decreases in blood pressure and ICP and little or no change in CPP. When used with nitrous oxide, it constitutes an acceptable alternative to the inhalational anesthetic agents. Along with this, the benzodiazepines diazepam (Valium) and lorazepam (Atavan) reduce the cerebral blood flow and ICP.

Ketamine (Ketalar, Ketaject) can rapidly increase ICP and frequently reduces CPP, despite mild increases in blood pressure. Ketamine is generally contraindicated for use in neurosurgery patients unless the fontanelles are open, CSF aspiration is instituted, or ventilatory control is maintained.

The use of controlled ventilation to produce a $PaCO_2$ in the range of 30 mm Hg and the administration of nitrous oxide and oxygen together with narcotics and/or neuroleptics and muscle relaxants is a generally accepted anesthetic technique for use in neurosurgery. Decreasing the $PaCO_2$ causes the cerebral blood vessels to constrict and helps decrease ICP. This combination avoids the problems of severely elevated ICP produced with halothane. If halothane, or any of the other inhalational anesthetics, is the agent of choice, severe elevations in ICP may be prevented if the patient is hyperventilated before and after induction and if thiopental is used as the principal induction agent.

Intracranial Pressure Monitoring

The most precise indicator of the pressure state within the cranium is the cerebrospinal fluid pressure. Measurement of this may be obtained from the lateral ventricle, lumbar subarachnoid space, cisterna magna, or epidural or subdural spaces. Values from these areas are only meaningful as indicators of ICP if pressure is freely transmitted between these compartments. Since injury and disease of the brain often create obstruction of CSF flow, the most accurate values are those obtained from the ventricle.

Lumbar puncture values reflect only a relative index of the actual intracranial pressure. These values are dependent upon the state of the spinal canal and all the factors that affect it. On the other hand, measurement of the ventricular fluid pressure gives a direct and absolute value of the intracranial pressure, regardless of the influence or condition of the spinal canal. Lumbar puncture has other limitations: Its use is limited to those patients without suspected intracranial mass or to those whose ICP is felt not to be elevated or is elevated only slightly. In patients with these conditions, there is risk of herniation of the brain tissue with the removal of CSF. Intracranial pressure monitoring does not present this risk and can be used in a variety of conditions.

Intracranial pressure monitoring requires a sensor, a transducer, and a display and recording instrument (Fig. 26–7). The sensor is usually implanted in the nondominant hemisphere in the ventricle, subarachnoid, or epidural space. The transducer itself may be implanted intracranially, or it may be placed outside the cranium. Intracranial transducers decrease the risk of infection but are often heat-sensitive and may produce false ICP readings, as they cannot be recalibrated once implanted. The greater the distance from the sensor to the transducer, the greater the incidence of artifact and imprecise wave forms. Other complications possible with any of these devices include CSF leakage, producing inaccurately low ICP readings, and contamination resulting in ventriculitis or meningitis.

The methods of continuous monitoring of the ICP include the subarachnoid screw, the subdural bolt, intraventricular catheter (IVC), and the intracranially implanted ICP transducers. The *subarachnoid screw* was developed in 1973 and requires only a twist drill hole in the skull and a nick in the dura for insertion. As the name implies, the sensor lies in the subarachnoid space. However, in the presence of moderately severe cerebral edema, a small piece of brain tissue may be driven into and occlude the proximal end of the screw, rendering it useless. The hollow *subdural bolt* is threaded into the subdural space. The bolt is then connected to an external transducer. If the seal is not water-tight, the bolt may become plugged with brain tissue which can obliterate or

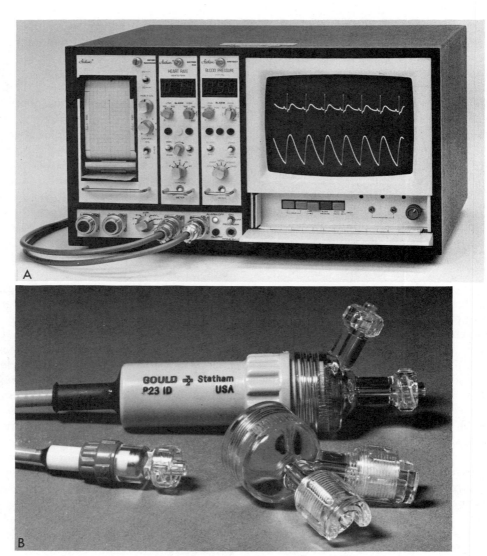

Figure 26–7. *A,* Bedside pressure display and recording monitor, showing cardiac rhythm and blood pressure wave form. It is also used to display intracranial pressure wave form. *B,* External pressure transducers capable of converting mechanical impulses transmitted from the cerebrospinal fluid into electrical impulses, which are then displayed on the bedside monitor. (Courtesy of Gould, Inc., Oxnard, California.)

dampen the recording of the ICP. The *intraventricular catheter (IVC)* is introduced into a CSF-containing ventricle via a twist-drill burr hole, and is connected to an external transducer which converts the hydrostatic pressure force into a graph and numerical readout. The advantages of the IVC are that it provides a direct ICP reading, is more easily kept patent, and CSF can be drained through the catheter to treat ICP elevations. In this way it may serve as a temporary artificial extension of the CSF-shunting compensatory mechanism. Intracranial compliance can also be tested by injecting fluid into the cranium and reading the responding pressure increase. If an abrupt and steep rise in ICP occurs, it can be assumed that compliance no longer exists and the volume-pressure curve is a steep one. When the patient's arterial pressure is being monitored simultaneously, exact cerebral perfusion pressure can be calculated at any point in time. The ventricular catheter also has the advantage of allowing instillation of contrast media or air to study the size and patency of the ventricle. The principal disadvantage of the IVC is that the technique is associated with a 5 to 10 percent incidence of central nervous system infection. The intracranially implanted *ICP transducers* are placed into the epidural space. These systems for monitoring ICP have had significant technical problems associated with calibration and stability of measurements over prolonged periods of use.

The *Ladd monitor* is useful for the noninvasive measurement of ICP in the newborn infant. The sensor of the Ladd monitor is applied to the anterior fontanelle of the newborn, and either a brief intermittent measurement or a continuous recording of the anterior fontanelle pressure can be obtained. Anterior fontanelle pressure correlates directly with ICP in the newborn. Before the sensor of the Ladd monitor is applied, the hair over the anterior fontanelle should be shaved. Also, if continuous measurements are desired, the application force on the sensor should be between 7 to 10

gm to facilitate the accurate reflection of intracranial pressure in the newborn.

Intracranial pressure monitoring is a valuable tool in assessing the efficacy of nursing interventions that are intended to decrease ICP and is essential in determining accurate assessments of the pressure state within the cranium and in treating elevations in ICP before disastrous consequences occur.

Pressure Waves in Increased ICP

Pressures waves are abnormal spontaneous variations in ICP. Three patterns have been identified. The first and most significant are *A waves*, more commonly called *plateau waves* (Fig. 26–8A). These are associated with increases in ICP between 50 and 100 mm Hg lasting for 5 to 20 minutes. They are seen only in advanced stages of increased intracranial pressure (the last phase of the volume-pressure curve) and superimpose themselves when the baseline ICP is elevated and exceeds 20 mm Hg. Early rises in MSAP do not accompany plateau waves, and autoregulation is impaired. Thus, plateau waves signal hypoxia of brain cells and a decrease in CPP. They may cause both transient and irreversible damage to the brain and may be premonitory signs of acute incidents. The cause of plateau waves is not fully understood, but they are probably a combination of transient blood volume alterations and CSF obstruction. Hypoventilation (by accumulating CO_2 and increasing intracranial blood volume) may be the cause, and the high ICP causes ischemia of the respiratory centers resulting in irregular breathing.

The second type of pressure waves are called *B waves*. These are sharp, rhythmic oscillations with a sawtooth pattern occurring every 30 seconds to 2 minutes (Fig. 26–8B). These may increase ICP up to 50 mm Hg and are more commonly seen in patients with unstable increases.

Third are *C waves* (Fig. 26–8C). These are smaller rhythmic oscillations in ICP, which occur every 4 to 8 minutes, and increase ICP as much as 20 mm Hg. They are asso-

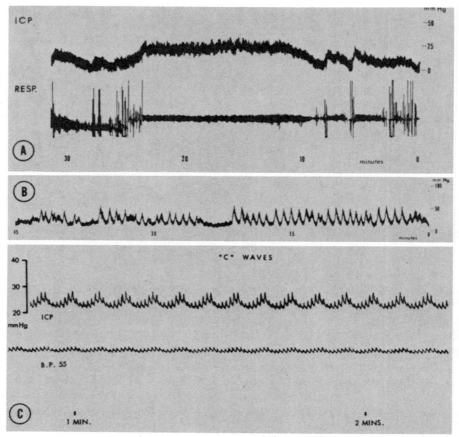

Figure 26–8. *A,* Plateau wave shown with associated respiratory changes. *B,* B waves: sharp, rhythmic oscillations with a characteristic saw-tooth pattern. *C,* C waves: smaller, rhythmic oscillations of ICP shown for comparison with the Traube-Hering-Mayer waves of blood pressure. (From Hanlon, K.: Description and uses of intracranial pressure monitoring. Heart Lung, 5:277, 1976.)

ciated with respiratory influence on the blood pressure but their significance is questionable.

Assessment

Continuous intracranial pressure monitoring is the only accurate method of assessing intracranial pressure at any given time. This method has two advantages: it provides an ongoing record of the ICP and also provides the ability to assess intracranial dynamics. In the past several years, traditional signs and symptoms have been used to indicate cerebral function and increased ICP. Research has proved the unreliability of these signs and symptoms in determining abnormal pressure situations. Their presence may or may not confirm a diagnosis of increased intracranial pressure.

The majority of these signs are manifestations of brain shift, with resultant dysfunction of the reticular activating system, brainstem, and medulla. Pressure would have to either elevate quite rapidly or be sustained at high levels to affect these structures so dramatically. Also to be considered is the fact that primary injury to these structures could elicit the same signs without appreciable increases in ICP. In this situation, they may well indicate the level of brain function and the gravity of the situation but say nothing about the pressure dynamics existing at that moment.

Just as these signs may be present without increase in ICP, it is also true that ICP may be dangerously high with few (if any) signs present. Classical brainstem signs (reflecting changes in cardiac, respiratory or vasomotor function) usually occur late, after the onset of intracranial hypertension, if at all. Several patients with benign intracranial hypertension and sustained pressures exceeding 80 mm Hg have been reported who exhibited no change in neurologic status objectively, or who complained only of headache. This was also true of a number of patients whose cerebral perfusion pressures were as low as 2 mm Hg. The most important factor in determining the degree of secondary brain damage incurred by elevated ICP is the effect of altered CPP on the circulation.

Most hospitals that have the capacity for cranial surgery also have the capacity for continuous intracranial pressure monitoring. It is not unusual, however, for a patient with multiple trauma to be treated at a smaller community hospital that lacks this capability. This patient may have received a concomitant closed head injury that does not require neurosurgery; but the patient nevertheless requires frequent nursing assessments of neurologic status.

With this in mind, the traditional signs and symptoms of increased ICP are discussed here. These are not precise or infallible as indicators of increased ICP. At the very least, they indicate that something is not right—that constant vigilance and further investigation are necessary. Even the transient appearances of these pressure signs are important. They indicate development of a highly delicate and unstable intracranial situation and that the patient may be experiencing plateau waves.

On the patient's arrival in the PACU, airway patency is verified, and electrocardiogram (EKG) monitor electrodes are attached. Vital signs, including rectal temperature, are taken and recorded. If the patient's ICP is being monitored, correct calibration of the monitor must be assured, ICP value recorded, and wave form described. The same holds true of arterial pressure recording. Reports should be taken from both the anesthesiologist and the surgeon. Of particular importance are preexistent medical problems, allergies, anesthetics used, and any problems that oc-

curred during surgery. The specific procedure performed, special positioning orders or restrictions, the presence of drains, and known CSF leaks must be noted. The dressing is described, including any visible drainage. Level of consciousness and responsiveness, motor activity, pupillary equality, size, and reactivity and the character of respirations are also documented. Continued patency of the airway is assured and the type of airway or mechanical ventilation used is noted. Urinary catheter drainage must be measured and described. Finally, the written doctors' orders must be reviewed with the physician and any questions or uncertainties clarified. Figure 26–9 is a sample form for documenting vital signs, level of consciousness, and ICP, in addition to the admitting history. The reverse side contains a standard for describing the level of consciousness (LOC) (Table 26–1) based on the Glasgow coma scale. By its inclusion on the form, this serves as a ready reference and satisfies medical-legal requirements.

TABLE 26–1. Standards for Describing the Levels of Consciousness

1. The patient does not respond to painful stimuli, not even by a change in pulse or respirations. Corneal, pupillary, pharyngeal, cough, and swallowing reflexes absent.
2. The patient responds to strong painful stimuli by increased pulse or respiratory rate.
3. The patient responds to painful stimuli by decerebrate posturing of the extremities.
4. The patient responds to painful stimuli by decorticate posturing of the extremities.
5. The patient responds to painful stimuli by movements not decorticate or decerebrate, yet not purposeful.
6. The patient responds to painful stimuli with purposeful movements aimed at defending himself.
7. The patient responds to voice, but the response is inadequate or inarticulate.
8. The patient responds to verbal command but is unable to respond to more than one command at a time (orders are extremely simple, e.g., open your eyes, stick out your tongue, blink your eyes, squeeze my hand).
9. The patient is able to follow more than one command at a time but does not express himself spontaneously and requires prodding.
10. The patient is sleepy but, when stimulated, answers questions adequately and can follow more complicated orders.
11. The patient is fully oriented, cooperative, and considered normal.

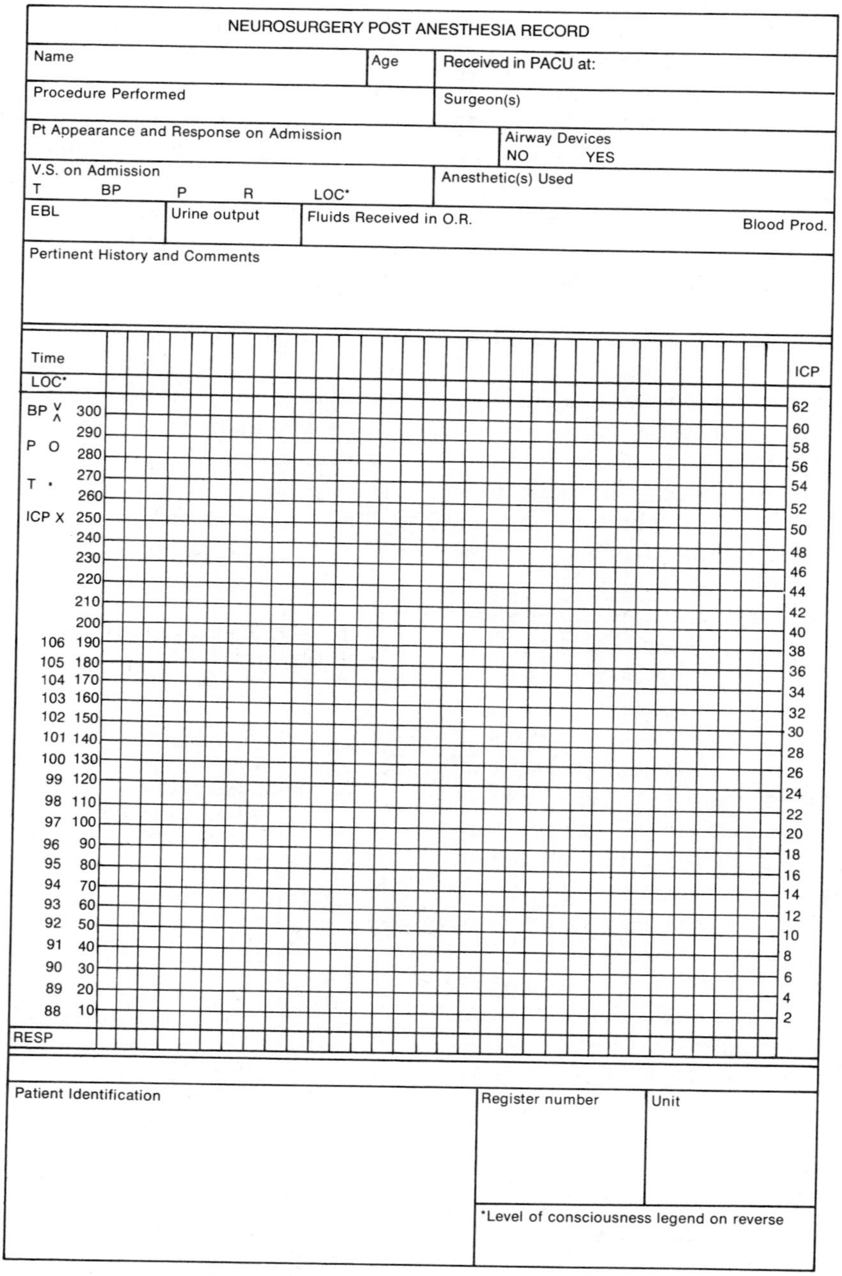

NEUROSURGERY POST ANESTHESIA RECORD			

Name | **Age** | **Received in PACU at:**

Procedure Performed | **Surgeon(s)**

Pt Appearance and Response on Admission | **Airway Devices**
NO   YES

V.S. on Admission
T   BP   P   R   LOC* | **Anesthetic(s) Used**

EBL | **Urine output** | **Fluids Received in O.R.** | **Blood Prod.**

Pertinent History and Comments

Time

LOC*

		ICP
BP ᵛ 300		62
Λ 290		60
P O 280		58
270		56
T • 260		54
ICP X 250		52
240		50
230		48
220		46
210		44
200		42
106 190		40
105 180		38
104 170		36
103 160		34
102 150		32
101 140		30
100 130		28
99 120		26
98 110		24
97 100		22
96 90		20
95 80		18
94 70		16
93 60		14
92 50		12
91 40		10
90 30		8
89 20		6
88 10		4
		2

RESP

Patient Identification | **Register number** | **Unit**

*Level of consciousness legend on reverse

Figure 26–9. Sample neurosurgery post anesthesia record.

Four major areas of assessment are required in PACU care of the cranial surgery patient: vital signs, level of consciousness, motor and sensory functioning, and pupillary signs. These should be routinely assessed at least every 15 minutes for the first 2 hours postoperatively. Then, if they are within normal limits or unchanged since surgery, every half hour. Of course, if the patient's condition is unstable or deteriorating, or if the surgeon specifies, assessments should be made more frequently.

Vital Signs. Assessment of vital signs includes blood pressure, pulse, respirations, and ICP (if monitored). Changes in vital signs may be indicative of increasing ICP, shock, hemorrhage, electrolyte imbalance, or other disturbances. Keep in mind that the injured patient may have other pathophysiologic processes occurring unrelated to his head injury. Comparisons should be made with the preoperative and intraoperative values. The character of the pulse as well as the rate and rhythm should be noted. Blood pressure and ICP readings may be used to calculate the cerebral perfusion pressure. Temperature is always taken rectally, and an elevation usually represents an infectious process, most often in the respiratory or urinary tract. Infrequently, elevations are attributable to direct damage to the temperature regulating center in the hypothalamus. Temperature elevation also increases the metabolic rate of the brain, adding further insult.

Airway patency is assured and the rate, depth, and rhythm are noted. Do not be deceived by apparent excursions of the thorax. Movement of the chest may occur without the exchange of air. The patient may exhibit substernal retractions; in this event chances are that the airway is obstructed. Place your hand in front of the mouth and nose or airway to ascertain movement of air. If the rhythm is irregular, try to determine its pattern. If no irregularity is evident, so state. If the patient is on a ventilator, check the machine for proper functioning and settings.

Research has identified four stages of vital sign changes that correlate with progressively increasing intracranial pressure. In the first two stages compensatory mechanisms are intact, and vital signs show only mild to moderate changes, while the ICP increases gradually. The third and fourth stages show sharp elevations in blood pressure and widening pulse pressure. At this point, ICP generally exceeds 50 mm Hg. At the end of Stage 3 (preterminal stage) respirations become markedly slowed and sometimes irregular. Bradycardia as low as 40 bpm accompanied by a rising MSAP and cardiac arrhythmias may occur. The fourth stage terminates in death following supratentorial decompensation.

The clinical sequence of events is thought to begin with respiratory slowing followed much later by pupillary dilation, bradycardia, and increased MSAP. Of course, mechanical ventilation will mask changes in the respiratory pattern.

Pressure signs are often transient in nature, occurring most often at the peak of plateau waves. Vital sign changes do not correlate consistently with these episodes. Indeed, there may not even be a change in behavior or neurologic status evident in the patient. The symptoms seen during plateau waves are probably triggered by transient cerebral hypoxia.

Level of Consciousness. The single most important indicator of brain function is the level of consciousness (LOC), but it is not necessarily indicative of altered ICP. A decreased level of consciousness in the PACU may be caused by the lingering effects of the anesthesia or by neuromuscular blocking agents sometimes used with individuals on mandatory controlled ventilation. Words such as "stupor," "coma," or "unconscious" have no place in the PACU or any unit caring for neurosurgical patients. Instead, a standard list of descriptions (as in Table 26–1) for detailing the level of consciousness should be available. An added advantage of this assessment tool is that it functions much the same as an Apgar score in indicating the gravity of the situation. A score of one through five indicates a poor prognosis, whereas the higher numbers indicate a more favorable one.

Motor and Sensory Functioning. Assessment of these areas can provide clues to extending hemorrhage, or expanding edema. Focal changes, such as decreased hand strength unilaterally or inability to move one side of the body, often accompany these events. Sensations may be decreased owing to brain involvement, not just to cord injury. Observe whether the patient can move all four extremities. Check both hand grasps simultaneously. Are they weak or strong, equal or unequal? Foot strength can be tested by having the patient push or pull against your hands. (Be sure he uses only the foot and ankle, not the entire leg.) If the patient does not respond to simple commands, test to see if a painful stimulus such as a pin prick or pinch will induce movement. (Test both sides to determine sensory impairment.) If he does not respond to pain, test for motor function by raising both arms or both legs and let them fall together. A paralyzed limb will fall to the bed more quickly than an unaffected one. To further check leg motor ability, flex both of the patient's knees with the feet flat on the bed; release them at the same time. The normal leg will maintain its position momentarily and then resume the original position. The affected limb will abduct while falling and will maintain knee flexion.

Facial muscle movement should also be tested. If possible, ask the patient to wrinkle his forehead, shut his eyes tightly, smile, and show you his teeth. Any asymmetry should be noted. If the patient is not responsive to verbal commands, pressure on both supraorbital ridges may elicit a grimace or other facial movement. The presence of a Babinski reflex is pathologic and indicative of pyramidal tract dysfunction in any individual over the age of 18 months. Starting at the heel and using a moderately sharp object such as the rounded tip of a bandage scissor or the tip of a retracted pen, stroke the lateral sole and proceed to the ball of the foot. Firm pressure is necessary to elicit an accurate response. The Babinski reflex is present when the great toe dorsiflexes (bends towards the head) and the remaining toes "fan out". The Babinski reflex is not present when the stimulus elicits a plantar or downward flexion of the big toe.

Motor response to a painful stimulus may be one of decerebrate or decorticate rigidity, or these postures may exist in the absence of any stimulation. Decerebrate posturing is characterized by rigidity and contraction of all the extensor muscles. The legs are stiffly extended with the feet plantar flexed. The arms are extended and hyperpronated. Decerebrate rigidity is usually the result of upper brainstem damage; this means the cerebral hemispheres are functionally cut off. Decorticate posturing indicates that function has been cut off at a lower level, that the entire cortex is cut off physiologically. In this instance, legs are extended and internally rotated and the feet are plantar flexed. The arms are flexed at all joints and the hands are frequently held beneath the chin.

Pupillary Activity. Pupillary reactions are controlled by the oculomotor or third cranial nerve. When assessing the pupils, examine both simultaneously for shape, size, and equality. Normal pupils are round and at a midpoint diameter within the range of 1 to 9 mm. Rather than use terms like "constricted" or "dilated," it is more precise to measure their diameters directly with a pocket millimeter ruler. Test the direct light reflex of each pupil with a small, bright flashlight. Normally, the pupil will constrict briskly. If it reacts sluggishly or not at all, it is abnormal. To test the consensual light reflex, hold both eyelids open, shine the light in one eye, and observe the other pupil. The opposite pupil should constrict simultaneously with the lighted one, though perhaps not to the same degree.

Normal pupillary size and reactivity can be altered by some medical situations and by certain drugs. Previous surgery or direct injury to the eye may alter or abolish reactivity. Blindness will abolish reactivity to light because the sensory part of the reflex pathway is absent.

Unusual eye movements should be noted. Normal gaze in an awake and alert individual is straight ahead, with no involuntary movements. This is generally true of the unresponsive patient, although his eyes may rove slowly and in random fashion. (When detecting this movement do not be misled into thinking that the patient is actually following you or your movements.) His eyes should move together in the same direction (conjugate gaze). If they are dysconjugate, gaze deviates from the midline, or they move in a jerky, oscillative fashion (nystagmus). These ocular movements are abnormal and should be detailed in the nursing notes.

Nursing Care

The PACU nurse has three primary responsibilities in the care of the neurosurgical patient: to institute measures of care to sustain optimal physiologic function in the helpless patient; to recognize and prevent, as much as possible, conditions that increase intracranial pressure beyond normal limits; to detect and communicate signs and symptoms of the patient's condition to the physician.

Ideally, the nurse:patient ratio in the PACU should be 3:2. The minimal ratio is 2:3 A patient's condition can change dramatically in as little as 15 minutes. His protective reflexes are impaired and he may be unable to perceive or communicate problems such as an obstructed airway or a distended bladder. Vigilant surveillance and high quality care by the nurse may determine the eventual outcome for the patient.

When caring for the cranial surgery patient, look for drainage from the suture line, from the nose, or from the ears. CSF may leak from any of these locations and, despite its benign appearance, may threaten the patient's life. The patient must be prevented from blowing or picking his nose, and suctioning through the nose is absolutely contraindicated, because CSF may leak through a fracture in the cribriform plate and drain from the nose. This is particularly applicable in patients whose surgery was performed transnasally. If drainage is present, it may be wiped from the nares, or a moustache type dressing applied. If drainage is from the ear, cover it with sterile 4 × 4 gauze. Do not pack the ear or the nose. When doubt exists as to the origin of rhinorrhea, the drainage may be tested with a dextrose stick. If positive for sugar, the drainage is probably cerebrospinal fluid, as mucus does not contain sugar, whereas CSF does. Examine dressings and linen for the "halo sign," a central blood-tinged spot surrounded by a ring of a lighter color (reminiscent of serous fluid). Save any such material for the physician's examination. This patient should be kept at absolute bed rest, and as quiet as possible, with the head of the bed raised 30 degrees. This position is most conducive to the spontaneous healing of the leak source.

Respiratory Status. Meticulous pulmonary care is essential in all patients. Morbidity and mortality in the neurosurgical patient are most frequently attributed to pulmonary complications and urinary tract infections. Airway patency is of primary importance. If there is no artificial airway, the patient may obstruct his airway as his tongue falls into the posterior pharynx. This is less likely to occur if he is prevented from assuming a supine position. Unless contraindicated by the physician, the patient should be placed on his side or in the swimmer's position, with his head slightly elevated. This promotes drainage of saliva and vomitus out of the mouth rather than into the airway. Endotracheal tubes must be kept free of secretions. Mucus plugs occur as readily in a plastic tube as they do in the trachea, and the patient will be unable to cough or expel them.

Suctioning may be necessary, but it has been proven to increase intracranial pressure. Therefore, it should be done as needed rather than according to a fixed schedule. To minimize pressure increases, hypercapnia and Valsalva effects must also be minimized. This is best accomplished by manual inflation with 100 percent oxygen for one minute prior to suctioning and limiting suctioning to 15 seconds. Hyperinflation is then repeated with 100 percent oxygen.

Cranial surgery patients are frequently maintained on mandatory ventilation into the first postoperative day, or longer, to prevent hypoventilation and to assure low Pa_{CO_2} levels (to aid in keeping ICP within acceptable limits). All settings on the ventilator must be checked for accuracy at least every hour. The cascade must also be checked for proper functioning and an adequate water level. In addition, serial arterial blood gases should be taken in order to detect and correct respiratory acidosis and to verify low Pa_{CO_2} levels.

Fluid and Electrolyte Balance. Prevention of fluid and electrolyte abnormalities is very important. Oral or nasogastric feedings are prohibited during the acute phase, owing to the danger of regurgitation and aspiration. Intravenous fluids are severely restricted but are maintained at a rate sufficient to ensure an adequate urinary output of 30 ml per hour. A delicate balance exists between overhydration and dehydration in these patients. Overhydration produces or accentuates cerebral edema and causes hyponatremia. It may also decrease the level of responsiveness. Dehydration may follow profuse diaphoresis or inadequate intravenous fluid therapy. If allowed to persist, electrolyte disturbances and renal failure will result. Serial blood urea nitrogen (BUN), electrolyte, and pH determinations of the blood, and hourly measurement of urine output are the most valuable indices in determining fluid and electrolyte imbalances.

Diabetes insipidus exists in some patients following trauma, surgery, or anoxia of the brain, most particularly to the posterior lobe of the pituitary gland. Antidiuretic hormone (vasopressin) production is markedly reduced and urinary output increases, reaching as much as 2 liters per hour. In diabetes insipidus, restricting fluid intake does nothing to alleviate urinary losses; it simply worsens dehydration. Diabetes insipidus is usually transient in nature and subsides when cerebral edema does. However, if anoxia is severe and generalized, diabetes insipidus may occur irreversibly. Treatment consists of preventing dehydration and electrolyte disturbances. Vasopressin (Pitressin) may be administered intramuscularly in an effort to correct and stabilize water metabolism.

The cranial surgery patient will have an indwelling urinary catheter during the acute phase of care. Its main advantage lies in the accurate determination of hourly urine output. Rarely are three-way tidal drainage sytems used in the PACU. In fact, catheters are removed as soon as possible to prevent urinary tract infections. The integrity of the closed drainage system must not be broken. In addition, local application of a bacteriocidal ointment at the urethral meatus also helps prevent urinary tract infection.

Temperature. Significant temperature elevations are rarely seen in the cranial surgery recovery patient, as they are most frequently caused by respiratory or urinary tract infections, which usually appear after the second or third postoperative day. When temperature elevations do occur in the acute phase, they may indicate damage to the hypothalamus and may exceed measurable values. If aggressive attempts at lowering the temperature fail, the increased metabolic demands of the body will overburden brain circulation and the patient's condition will deteriorate, causing death. Because this hyperthermia is due to central derangement rather than to an infectious process, conventional measures, such as antibiotic and aspirin therapy, fail to reduce temperature. The most effective means of lowering this patient's temperature is through the use of hypothermia blankets, and removal of the primary disorder, if possible.

When hypothermia blankets are used, they should be set no cooler than 1 degree below the patient's current body temperature; this prevents shivering or thermal crisis. A constant rectal temperature probe is essential. Many sets are available in which the temperature probe relays its information to, and automatically adjusts, the blanket temperature regulator. Do not allow the patient to shiver. Cold burns may be prevented by placing a bath blanket between the patient and the hypothermia blanket. The use of mineral oil instead of water or alcohol in the blanket system renders more even temperature conduction and less abrupt temperature changes, but its use may be contraindicated by the manufacturer.

Positioning. The patient must never be placed flat on his back. Other positioning restrictions may be communicated by the surgeon, depending on the nature and location of the surgery. Be sure these are clearly understood before the surgeon leaves the PACU. Frequently, positioning is somewhat limited by the monitoring devices in use. Whether or not the patient is being ventilated or has other injuries also enters into positioning considerations.

Generally, the surgeon specifies that the head of the bed be elevated to 30 degrees, which helps keep intracranial pressure within normal limits. If hemorrhagic shock occurs, the foot of the bed may be elevated and the arms raised above the patient's head to return blood to the heart without increasing intracranial pressure. Positioning should always allow proper drainage of secretions from the mouth and airway. Patients who have had suboccipital craniectomy are sometimes dressed with a cervical collar and adhesive stripping to restrict movement of the head and neck. When turning this patient, it is important to support the head and turn it in unison with the body. This prevents any strain on the wound or suture line. To gain proper access to the head, remove the headboard from the bed and stand behind the patient.

A patient who is unresponsive or paralyzed will be unable to move his or her limbs from uncomfortable or dangerous positions. Muscle tone will be insufficient to prevent dislocation of the shoulder should the arm fall from the side of the bed. If the patient is able to move spontaneously and respond to uncomfortable stimuli, advantage may be found in placing him or her in a safe but slightly uncomfortable position. This encourages active movement and exercise of the limbs and joints. Of course, this is contraindicated if the patient is agitated or if the physician objects.

Skin Care. Though the patient may be in the PACU less than 24 hours, it is necessary to initiate joint and skin care measures as soon as possible. It takes only 48 to 72 hours for a joint to begin to ankylose, and it is not unusual for decubiti to begin forming on the operating table. Skin over bony prominences may already be broken by the time the patient comes into the PACU. This is particularly true of elderly, very young, and dehydrated patients. Cover any broken areas with a sterile dressing and try to prevent further irritation. No salve, ointment, or individually devised remedy has proved completely successful in treating decubiti. Prevention is the best treatment. This requires turning the patient at least every 2 hours and protection of susceptible areas through frequent massage and the use of air mattresses and sheepskin pads. Footdrop and external hip rotation may be prevented by using a footboard and trochanter rolls respectively. Hand deformities may be avoided through the use of hand rolls or contoured splints placed so that the hands appear to be grasping them.

If the corneal or blink reflex is absent, the eyes must be irrigated with sterile saline and lubricated with mineral oil. In no case should the eyes be taped shut, as a lid may open under the tape and the cornea suffer abrasion. The patient may have significant periocular edema and ecchymosis following cranial surgery or trauma. Cold compresses may be used if care is taken to avoid contact with the cornea.

The lips and mucosa of the mouth must be kept moist and free of encrustations. Hyperplastic, sensitive gum tissue may be found in any individual who has been on phenytoin (Dilantin) for significant periods of time. Normal saline or lemon and glycerine swabs may be used to keep the mouth moist. Petrolatum should be applied to the lips. The patient should never be given water by mouth until it has been established that his cough and swallow reflexes are intact and until the surgeon permits oral fluids.

Neurologic Status. Electrical disturbances in the brain may manifest themselves as seizures in the PACU. These disturbances may be due to the operative lesion, trauma, anoxia, or hematoma. The seizure itself may be focal, grand mal, Jacksonian, petit mal, psychomotor, or autonomic.

The patient must be observed constantly during a seizure. The nurse's responsibility is twofold: the patient must be prevented from injuring himself, and the seizure activity must be described in detail from beginning to end. At no time should the patient be left alone. Siderails should be padded in order to protect the limbs. No attempt should be made physically to restrict motion. This will serve only to injure the patient further. Instead, try to protect the head and limbs from sharp or unyielding objects. Try to protect arterial, intravenous, and intracranial lines from being pulled out. Do not attempt to insert any sort of airway or tongue blades into the mouth after the seizure has begun. If the patient is being ventilated, remove him from the ventilator and try to protect the endotracheal tube. Begin manual inflation of the lungs as soon as the seizure subsides sufficiently to allow this. Use 100 percent oxygen to overcome the anoxia and hypercapnia induced by the seizure.

In describing the seizure, state if the patient reported an aura beforehand. If responsive and capable, he may have said only, "My hand is tingling," "I smell bacon," or something similar. His statement may have seemed totally insignificant at the time but may aid the physician in localizing the causative lesion. Also describe the actual seizure. Did it begin in one area of the body and "march" to another? Was it simply a persistent twitch in a facial muscle? Was the patient incontinent of stool or urine? How long did tonoclonic movements persist? Describe the postictal state and monitor the patient closely after a seizure. A grand mal seizure may be the precipitating factor of a sudden deterioration in the patient with cerebral anoxia or increased ICP.

Frequently, patients are placed on prophylactic anti-convulsants postoperatively. These may be combined with a barbiturate such as phenobarbital. Some surgeons order their patients to be given intravenous diazepam (Valium) if a seizure occurs. While this will control muscle activity, the causative electrical disturbance in the brain will persist nonetheless.

Some degree of hyperactivity or agitation is seen in 50 percent of all cranial surgery patients. Investigate all possible causes. The patient may have an obstructed airway, distended bladder, or overlooked bleeding or fracture. He may be too cold or too warm; he may be disoriented or fearful; or he may be experiencing slowly developing hypoxia.

If no cause for his agitation can be identified, meningeal irritation must be considered. Personality and behavior can be markedly affected by organic lesions of the brain—temporal lobe problems commonly cause resentment of interference and hostility or aggressiveness. Repetition of words or phrases (perseveration) indicates damage to the speech area, as do aphasia and dysarthria. Always remember that the patient's behavior and reactions are beyond his control.

Every attempt should be made to calm and reassure the patient. Hyperactivity increases metabolic rate and the release of metabolic wastes within the body, which cause increases in intracranial pressure. Try to avoid restraining the patient, as this is usually met with rebellion and worsened agitation, which may lead to self-injury and dangerous increases in intracranial pressure. However, it will be necessary to protect monitoring lines and endotracheal tubes.

If danger of the patient's falling out of bed is great, remove him and his mattress from the bed and place them on the floor, if possible. Mild sedation may be prescribed by the surgeon. The most effective agents are small doses of chloral hydrate, paraldehyde, or the ataraxic drugs. Narcotics are never given because of their respiratory depressant action and their effect on pupillary responses.

Intracranial Pressure. Prevention of increased intracranial pressure requires identification of its causative factors. Increased ICP may be detected most accurately through objective ICP monitoring systems. Relationships between various internal and external stimuli and intracranial pressure variations have been delineated by this method. Several factors are now known to precipitate sustained pressure increases as evidenced by plateau waves. These are inhalation anesthetics, hypercapnia (Pa_{CO_2} greater than 40 mm Hg), hypoxia (P_aO_2 less than 50 mm Hg), and Valsalva maneuvers. Factors that sometimes precipitate sustained pressure elevations include turning, painful stimulation or manipulation, arousal from sleep, agitation, neck flexion or hyperextension, extreme hip flexion, and the supine position.

Hypoxia may or may not accompany hypercapnia. They are each capable of increasing intracranial pressure. Hypercapnia may occur during normal sleep as a result of hypoventilation. It may also occur as a compensatory mechanism in response to metabolic alkalosis, or it may be the prevailing condition in the patient with severe pulmonary emphysema. In addition, it may be due to sedation or an improperly set ventilator.

Hypoxia sufficient to cause sustained pressure peaks has been reported during intubation, inadequate ventilation, or improper suctioning. Suctioning should be done only when indicated by chest sounds or arterial blood gases, not on a fixed schedule.

The Valsalva maneuver increases intracranial pressure by increasing intrathoracic pressure. The increased pressure within the thorax impedes venous return and increases cerebral blood volume and ICP. The patient may perform this maneuver during turning or painful manipulation, or if agitated. If the patient is responsive and cooperative, Valsalva effects can be minimized by instructing him to exhale during turning and not to hold his breath during painful manipulation. Neck flexion and hyperextension and hip flexion increase intracranial pressure by obstructing venous return to the heart. Extreme hip flexion impedes venous return from the leg to the heart. As a result, arterial blood volume and pressure increase within the thorax and they increase intracranial pressure much as the Valsalva maneuver does.

If intracranial pressure is measured continuously, identification and treatment of increasing ICP are made easier. Treatment can be instituted before the signs of transtentorial herniation appear.

The attending nurse can correlate and document particular activities that prompt pressure increases in the patient. The effectiveness of nursing measures designed to decrease ICP can also be evaluated and documented.

If the baseline pressure is rising gradually but persistently, the surgeon should be notified. He may order hyperventilation, controlled drainage of cerebrospinal fluid, or administration of osmotic diuretics or corticosteroids to decrease pressure.

"Negative" intracranial pressure readings have been reported in certain cranial surgery patients. Some pediatric patients have been seen to have monitor readings below zero as they sat up in bed and cried. This is believed to be due, at least in part, to the upright position assumed and to the hyperventilation that accompanies crying. Whether or not the true pressure was below zero is open to question.

Calling the Physician. The physician should be called whenever the patient's condition appears to be deteriorating. The earliest indicators of unstable pressure are often benign in appearance but must be recognized immediately. Any patient who exhibits a slight change in alertness, an increased restlessness, or a slight asymmetry in motor function must be watched closely for other signs of deterioration. Other events that should be brought to the attention of the physician include decreased responsiveness, elevated baseline pressures or sustained peak pressures on the ICP monitor, CSF leaks, copious drainage on dressings, initial seizure activity, new focal deficit, restlessness or agitation or asymmetrical motor function unknown to the surgeon, projectile vomiting, pupillary changes in one or both eyes, severe headache (note onset and location), and changes in vital signs, i.e., temperature greater than 38.5°C rectally, systolic pressure increase of 30 mm Hg or more, pulse decrease of 20 bpm or more, respiratory rate of 12 or less, or irregular respirations. The progression of any signs or symptoms should also be noted, as this is frequently important diagnostically. If the nurse has any doubt about the circumstances in which the physician is to be notified, it is better to consult him than to let an incident pass.

SPINAL SURGERY

Surgery is performed on the spine to treat injuries or remove tumors and to correct developmental abnormalities.

Diagnostic Tools

Several methods are used in diagnosing injury or disease involving the spine or spinal canal.

Conventional x-ray and *fluoroscopy* identify fractures and fracture-dislocations (Fig. 26–10). Narrowing of an intervertebral space is sometimes evident as a result of a herniated nucleus pulposus (HNP) or "slipped disc."

Fluoroscopy is used to demonstrate instability of the injured part on manipulation.

Splintered or displaced bone fragments and radiopaque foreign bodies (such as bullets or other metal fragments) are also seen on x-ray.

X-ray also demonstrates abnormalities such as scoliosis and osteoporotic and arthritic changes. Tumors may be evidenced by erosion, calcium deposits within the mass, increased interpedicular distance, enlargement of an intervertebral foramen, or collapse of a vertebra.

Computerized Tomography (CT scanning) is used to delineate mass lesions existing in the same plane as the spine and spinal cord. Large blood clots may also be localized with this method.

Nuclear Magnetic Resonance (NMR) Imaging is being used increasingly to accurately detect and assess space-occupying lesions of the spine, such as HNPs and tumors.

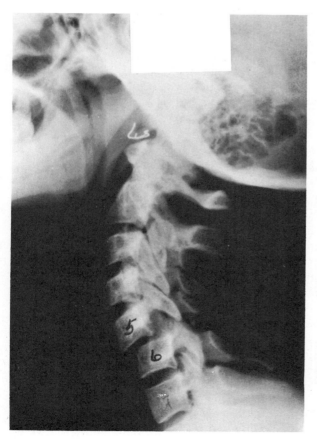

Figure 26–10. A dislocation of the cervical spine. This injury may or may not produce cord or nerve root damage. Reduction is usually achieved by relaxation and skull traction with tongs. Surgery is sometimes necessary to achieve reduction and stabilization. (From Sabiston, D. C. [ed.]: Textbook of Surgery. 11th ed. Philadelphia, W. B. Saunders Co., 1977, p. 1528.)

Electromyography is employed in evaluating muscle function as a means of detecting the nature and location of motor unit lesions. Tumors and HNPs compressing the cord or motor nerve roots will effect the function of the muscle groups they innervate.

Myelography is one of the most valuable tools available in diagnosing compression of the spinal cord due to tumor, fracture-dislocation, or HNP. A lumbar puncture is performed, at which time a Queckenstedt test may also be done. The veins of the neck are compressed on one or both sides. In a healthy individual, the cerebrospinal fluid pressure rises rapidly and then quickly returns to normal when the pressure is taken off the neck. In a patient whose cord is obstructed, little or no increase in pressure is found. This test is diagnostically accurate for most cord compressions. However, false negatives may be obtained if the lesion is located high in the cervical spine area. Needless to say, the Queckenstedt test is not performed in patients with known or suspected increased intracranial pressure. The myelogram itself consists of the injection of a radiopaque dye into the cerebrospinal fluid canal and the fluoroscopic observation of its flow over the suspected area. Cord compression is evidenced by an interruption in the contour of the cord (Fig. 26–11). Disruption of the contours of the spinal nerve roots may also be found.

Injuries of the Spine

The spine protects the spinal cord and the terminal nerve roots. Injuries to the spine and spinal cord exist as a result of acceleration-deceleration accidents, torsion injuries, penetrating wounds, or blunt trauma. Frequently, head injuries accompany injuries to the spine, and vice versa. The cervical spine is extremely mobile and therefore particularly susceptible to accel-

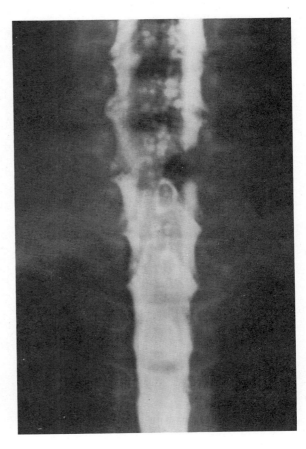

Figure 26–11. Pantopaque cervical myelogram with filling defect due to a unilateral ruptured intervertebral disc between sixth and seventh cervical vertebrae on the right. (From Sabiston, D. C. [ed.]: Textbook of Surgery. 11th ed. Philadelphia, W. B. Saunders Co., 1977, p. 1495.)

eration-deceleration and torsion injuries that hyperflex or hyperextend the neck. Propulsion may occur anteroposteriorly or laterally. The cord is relatively large in this area and sustains damage after injury to the spine fairly easily. The area is unique, in that the superior portion of the second cervical vertebra lacks a vertebral body. Rather, it has a dens, or projection, called the odontoid. Many injuries to the odontoid extend into the first cervical vertebrae or atlas, which has no vertebral body at all.

The thoracic spine is fixed by the ribs, but the lumbar spine is not, so there is an increased incidence of fracture dislocations of the twelfth thoracic and the first and second lumbar vertebrae. These fracture-dislocations are found particularly in patients involved in motor vehicle accidents who wore lap seatbelts but not shoulder restraints.

Consequences of injury to the spine are many and varied. The seriousness of the injury depends on the extent and level of involvement of the cord or spinal nerves rather than on the degree of bony destruction alone.

Injury to the bones of the spine include subluxation, dislocation, compression fractures, and fracture-dislocations (comminuted fracture-dislocations).

Subluxation is the complete or partial dislocation of a vertebrae from its normal alignment. It is caused by a fracture of the articulating facets.

Compression fractures are fractures of the vertebral body without subluxation. The articulating facets are intact unless the fracture is comminuted.

Fracture-dislocations are displaced fractures of the vertebral bodies. Any of the other vertebral elements may also be fractured.

The cord may suffer *concussion* much as the brain does. This results in transient paralysis and loss of sensation without anatomically demonstrable changes. Function and sensation generally return within an hour, unless the cord has suffered more serious injury. Blunt trauma is usually the cause, such as when a football player is struck in the midspine by the helmet of another player.

Contusion of the cord is a bruise associated with some swelling and hemorrhage that results in some degree of permanent injury. More serious is a contusion that results in *spinal shock*. This may result in a partial or complete physiologic transection of the cord. Contusion usually occurs at the site of a fracture-dislocation or penetrating wound.

Lacerations are usually the result of fracture-dislocations and are irreparable, as no method of restoring axonal continuity has been devised.

Hematomyelia, or blood within the cord, is not common but, when seen, usually accompanies blunt trauma to the cervical spine.

Cord injuries may manifest themselves as a result of an HNP, a tumor, or trauma. Several forms of HNP are illustrated in Figure 26–12. Pathologic conditions affecting the cord manifest themselves according to the portion of the cord involved. Neurologic loss in trauma to the spine may be partial or complete, permanent or transient.

Anterior cord injury can be the result of acute flexion injury, HNP, or tumor. Motor function is lost, but sensation remains. Pain and temperature sensations are diminished below the level of the injury.

Central cord injury follows acute hyperextension injury to the neck. Ligaments posterior to the cord impinge on it. Motor function is lost in the upper extremities; lower extremities may also be involved, but to a lesser extent. Sensory function is compromised similarly. Pain and temperature sensation remain in the lower extremities, but are lost in the upper extremities. The disproportionate loss of function and sensation in the upper and lower extremities is explained by the fact that the fibers to the nerve roots of the upper extremities are more centrally located within the cord.

Posterior cord injuries result in loss of sensory function, with motor function remaining intact.

Lateral cord transection (Brown-Séquard syndrome) results in loss of motor function on the injured side, and lost sensory function on the opposite side, including pain and temperature sensation. This is com-

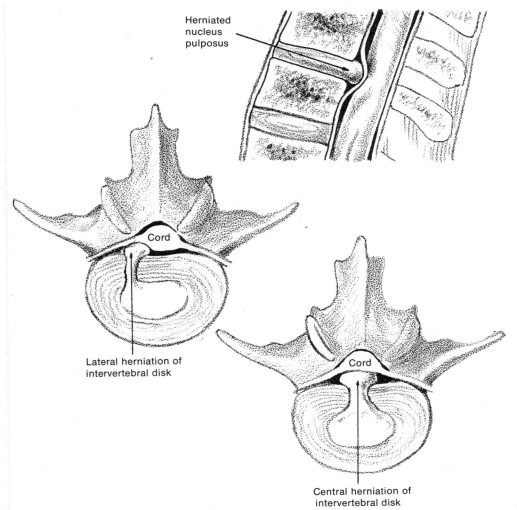

Figure 26–12. Forms of vertebral herniation. (From Luckmann, J., and Sorenson, K. C.: Medical-Surgical Nursing. Philadelphia, W. B. Saunders Co., 1973, p. 523.)

monly the result of injury sustained in motor vehicle accidents, or is the result of an acute HNP.

Complete transection results in loss of all sensation with complete paralysis at and below the level of the lesion. This occurs after anatomic severance of the cord or as a physiologic result of cord edema.

All cord injury signs and symptoms are found at and below the level of the lesion. Motor and sensory function are unimpaired above the level of the lesion.

Clinical findings during the acute phase after total cord transection include:

1 Immediate loss of all sensory, motor, autonomic, and reflex function below the level of the injury owing to spinal shock. Spinal shock may persist for days or weeks, depending on the injury and the patient's general state of health. It usually lasts from 4 to 8 weeks.

2. Urinary retention due to bladder sphincter paralysis.

3. Paralytic ileus with progressive abdominal distention.

4. Respiratory insult or cessation. Injury to the lower cervical spine or upper thoracic spine results in cessation of intercostal function. In this event respiration is under the sole stimulus of the phrenic nerve and breathing is diaphragmatic. Injury to the cord at the levels of the third, fourth, or

fifth cervical vertebrae injure the phrenic nucleus, paralyzing the diaphragm and causing respiratory failure.

5. Loss of sweating below the level of the lesion.

6. Point tenderness over the injured part. Gibbus or crepitus may or may not be present.

Initial therapeutic efforts are directed at preserving life and residual function (which may develop more fully with later rehabilitation). Mechanical stability, protection of nervous tissue, and freedom from pain are long-term therapeutic goals.

Surgery is indicated immediately after injury in these instances:

1. When the signs and symptoms of an incomplete transection of the spinal cord are observed to worsen. Myelography usually precedes surgery.

2. When a fracture-dislocation cannot be completely reduced by skeletal traction alone. If the injury is to the thoracic or lumbar spine, surgery is indicated if the reduction is inadequate after immobilization on the Stryker or Foster frame and the administration of muscle relaxants.

3. When myelography indicates complete obstruction of the cord due to bony compression, hematoma, or protruded disc.

4. When a fragment of bone or foreign body lies in a position where it could cause further cord injury or will later cause chronic myelopathy or radiculopathy.

5. When surgical fusion will prevent a marked kyphotic deformity, which may follow skeletal traction and natural fusion. This kyphotic deformity might later produce chronic myelopathy or radiculopathy.

6. When there are open penetrating injuries requiring surgical débridement.

7. When there is an acutely herniated nucleus pulposus.

Neurosurgeons differ in their opinions as to whether or not emergency surgery is indicated in those patients with immediate and complete transection injuries. Although there is at present no hope of restoring function, some surgeons believe exploratory surgery is justified to assure themselves, the patient, and the family that everything possible is being done to fully assess and correct the injury.

General contraindications to surgery are the existence of associated life-threatening injuries, and depressed respiratory function owing to high cervical injuries. Cord edema, which worsens during the first 48 to 72 hours, may extend the degree of respiratory difficulty. Such a patient is usually intubated and placed on assisted ventilation prophylactically. In these situations, immediate treatment of the cord injury consists of stabilizing the fracture by immobilizing the neck with skeletal traction. Surgery is postponed until edema has subsided and ventilatory status can be controlled.

Exploration, débridement, or laminectomy may be performed through a posterior incision. Fusion is accomplished by the placement of a bone graft fashioned from tibial or iliac bone into the involved interspace, or by placement of a fixation device.

The anterior operative approach to the cervical spine allows direct visualization of and access to the lesion responsible for cord compression. This is its major advantage. Anterior fusion generally provides greater stability than posterior, and skeletal traction and Stryker frame immobilization are sometimes unnecessary postoperatively.

Nursing Care and Considerations in the Patient with Spinal Cord Injury

In the United States alone, over 10,000 individuals per year become quadriplegic or paraplegic. Of these, 56 percent sustain injuries to their spinal cords in motor vehicle accidents, and 85 percent are male. With increased use of motorcycle helmets, many individuals survive what would otherwise have been fatal head injuries, only to be left to deal with cervical cord injuries. Permanent injuries of this nature are devastating to the patient and the family. The nursing responsibilities are great during the acute phase, the rehabilitative phase, and the chronic phase. Spinal cord–injured patients may be sent to the PACU in any of these phases, and their care requires special consideration and knowledge of pathophysiology.

Neurogenic Shock

In neurogenic shock the vascular tone is decreased, resulting in generalized vasodilation. Blood pools in the capillaries of the voluntary muscles and the gastrointestinal system prohibiting adequate circulating volume to the vital centers. The large voluntary muscles lose their tone and no longer assist the heart in pumping blood throughout the body.

Clinically, the blood pressure falls, the pulse increases, and the respirations become deep with frequent sighs. The skin becomes cool and moist, pallor and cyanosis are evident, and the patient may complain of extreme fatigue. Conditions for thrombus formation are optimal. This is not hemorrhagic shock; therefore, the patient must not be overloaded with intravenous fluids in a misguided attempt to overcome it.

Treatment consists of combating hemostasis; oxygen is given to combat hypoxia. Emergency aid may require the use of a shock suit (applied only after the fracture has been stabilized). Once stabilization of the shock has been achieved, antiembolism stockings and passive range of motion exercises are used to combat hemostasis and thrombus formation.

Intramuscular medications should never be administered below the level of the lesion, as they will only cause local inflammation and tissue breakdown, and absorption will be negligible or nil.

Edema of the Spinal Cord

Cord edema is most pronounced within the first 48 to 72 hours after injury or trauma. Profound danger lies in its ability to advance to the brain, to physiologically extend injury, or to anatomically promote the possibility of shearing the cord upon bone fragments or fracture edges. If edema extends to the level of the phrenic nucleus, respiration is threatened. Astute observation of the respiratory pattern may reveal shallow and rapid respirations or flaring of the nares before complete respiratory failure ensues.

Vital capacity should be measured with a Wright respirometer every 2 hours during the acute phase. A downward trend in the values obtained indicates development of respiratory distress and should be reported to the physician immediately. Articles necessary for emergency intubation or tracheostomy and mechanical ventilation must be readily available. Some physicians place the patient on mechanical ventilation prophylactically, when the danger of the development of respiratory distress is high.

Concomitant Head Injury

Every patient with acute injury to the spine must be observed for signs and symptoms indicative of head injury. Evaluation of cranial status should be done at the same intervals as the vital sign measurements. An abnormal "cranial check" should be reported to the physician immediately, as it may indicate injury to the brain or increased intracranial pressure resulting from the upward expansion of cord edema.

Skeletal Tong Traction

Skeletal tong traction is used in the treatment of subluxations or fracture-dislocations of the cervical spine. It is also used after some posterior fusions of the cervical vertebra. The tongs grasp the skull firmly on both sides and traction is applied by weighting the tongs so that a pulling force is exerted in the superior direction. The weight of the body serves as the countertraction. Extreme care must be taken that the traction weight be continuous and even. Ropes must be free from snags and without frays. Knots must be tied securely, and the ropes themselves must lie in the proper grooves of the pulley system. The patient's body must be aligned with the long axis of the cervical spine. Any defect in the traction system may result in the sudden release of traction. Injury to the spine or cord so incurred may prove disastrous.

Several varieties of tongs are currently in use. Crutchfield tongs are frequently used (Fig. 26–13). Vinke tongs are not used as

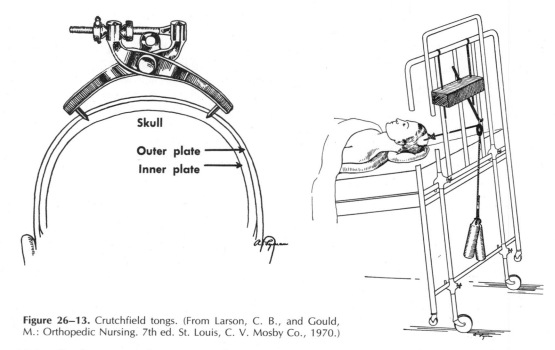

Figure 26–13. Crutchfield tongs. (From Larson, C. B., and Gould, M.: Orthopedic Nursing. 7th ed. St. Louis, C. V. Mosby Co., 1970.)

widely. Gardner tongs have grown in popularity because they have a safety bolt that prevents them from slipping out of the skull or penetrating the brain.

In some instances skeletal immobility is obtained by the use of a halo cast (Fig. 26–14). A metal band is anchored by the use of skeletal pins to the head at a level just above the eyebrows. Rigid metal rods attach to the halo and are anchored to a plaster cast, or plastic and metal jacket, which encases the shoulders and chest. This alone is sufficient immobilization after some anterior cervical spine fusions and has the advantage of dispensing with the necessity of Foster or Stryker frame immobilization and allows early ambulation.

The area surrounding skeletal pins is generally shaved to prevent contamination. Some surgeons prefer to shave the entire head. "Pin care" should be given immediately after tong insertion and at 6- to 8-hour intervals thereafter. The area surrounding the pins is cleansed of any dried blood or encrustations using sterile saline or equal parts sterile saline and hydrogen peroxide. Then a bacteriocidal ointment is applied to the sites and they are covered with sterile 2 × 2 sponges. Sterile technique is always used when administering pin care.

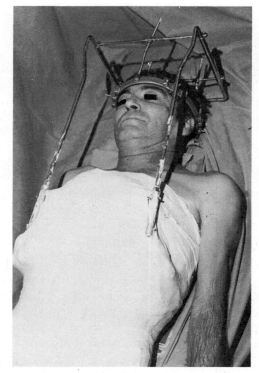

Figure 26–14. Halo cast. The halo, which has four screws inserted in the outer table of the skull, provides for rigid fixation of the cervical spine. The halo may be used for cervical traction in the recumbent position or attached to a cast. The patient may be ambulatory in the halo cast. (From Sabiston, D. C. [ed]: Textbook of Surgery. 11th ed. Philadelphia, W. B. Saunders Co., 1977, p. 1526.)

Stryker and Foster Frame Precautions

The patient with acute spinal cord injury will arrive in the PACU on a Stryker or Foster frame (Fig. 26–15). Circo-electric beds are never used, as the axis in which they turn prevents the maintenance of skeletal traction and puts the stress of the body weight on the spinal column.

While in the upright position the frame should be situated so that adequate space for turning is assured at both ends and both sides. Certain safety measures are required when using these frames: First, the patient must be strapped securely to the frame with web-type belts at all times. This is especially important when turning the patient. While the patient is sandwiched tightly between the frame halves, some have been known to shift or slip out between them as they are being turned. Therefore, belts should be placed around the upper and lower frame halves and secured as tightly as possible before any attempt is made to turn the patient.

The patient's arms must be placed securely beside the body and must not be allowed to drop from the side of the frame or shoulder dislocation will result.

Turning of the frame requires coordination between the individuals at the head and foot of the bed. It is most comfortable and least dangerous for the patient if the actual turning is done in one swift, smooth movement. Check that the frames are locked securely, that belts are fastened tightly, and that the patient's arms are secured. Anticipate the direction in which the frame will turn, and move intravenous tubing and urinary catheter collection bags to the opposite side of the bed in that direction. When you are ready to turn the frame, do so "at the count of three." Turn rapidly and smoothly and continue to hold your end of the frame until the lock holding the frame in place has been tested on both ends. Remove the upper frame half and again secure the patient with belts.

Always have the turning technique

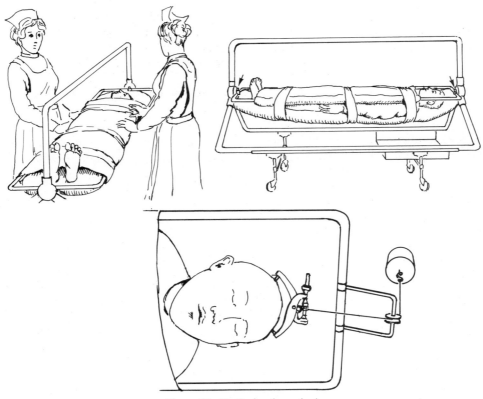

Figure 26–15. Stryker frame bed.

worked out before approaching the patient. The patient's anxiety is greatly increased by the sound of two people out of his or her line of vision arguing about the safest way to turn the frame, or voicing uncertainties about how it is done. Never attempt to turn a frame alone. If you have never turned a frame before, ask someone who is experienced to guide you until you are certain of the procedure. In all situations in which the patient is aware of his or her surroundings, he or she should be informed of every step of the turning motion. Express that the patient is safe and that no pain will be felt on turning. Every honest reassurance is warranted and necessary for the patient in this situation.

Contractures

Contractures result from disuse atrophy and improper positioning of the limbs. They may be minimized through the use of regular passive range of motion exercises, footboards, trochanter rolls, and hand rolls or specially fabricated splints.

Demineralization of Bone

Long-term immobility causes demineralization of bone tissue. Calcium is freed into the circulation and osteoporosis, "silent fractures," and renal calculi result.

Sensory Loss

The patient with a spinal cord transection experiences an abrupt cessation of all tactile and proprioceptive stimulation below the level of his lesion. Particularly in the patient with a cervical cord injury, visual stimuli are limited to those received from the small patch of floor below or the area of ceiling within his or her limited view. Hearing is intact, but much of the auditory stimuli that is perceived by the patient is foreign and unmeaningful. The patient experiences a true isolation from his or her environment and a psychologic loss of body image. This is often compounded by feelings of guilt and fear and creates an environment which fosters emotional withdrawal, reality distortion, and the development of stress ulcers.

When you approach the patient always situate yourself so that you are in his or her visual field. Speak to the patient, even one who is unable to answer because of endotracheal intubation or tracheostomy. The patient will answer with his or her eyes or will form silent words with the lips. Orient to time and place, and give tactile stimulation to those areas above the level of injury. These measures may help allay some fears and help prevent or alleviate the devastating isolation that can result from sensory deprivation.

Respiratory Complications

The incidence of respiratory complications is high, owing to immobility, incomplete postural drainage, and the patient's inability to cough up secretions effectively. A lack of muscular control creates insufficient negative pressure within the chest to cough well. Any secretions the patient cannot expectorate must be suctioned from the airway. The lungs should be auscultated every 2 hours for the presence of ronchi or rales. Ultrasonic mist is helpful in loosening secretions and in preventing tenacious mucus plugs. Gentle frappage of the chest may be permitted by the physician but is inadvisable when the jarring it creates would cause further damage to an unstable or acute fracture site.

Gastrointestinal Complications

Generalized atony and loss of motility render the stomach and intestines distended and highly susceptible to fecal impactions and obstructions. Distention is relieved by intermittent nasogastric suction. Programs of bowel training are initiated on the parent ward.

There is a high incidence of stress ulcers, especially in quadriplegic patients. Here, parasympathetic vagal action is unopposed because of sympathetic block from the ascending and descending visceral nerve paths, and gastric acid secretion by the parietal cells of the stomach is increased. This stressful situation is further compounded by the administration of corticosteroids used to reduce cord edema, which are singularly capable of inducing hyperacidity of gastric juices. Antacids or cimetidine (Tagamet), or both, are given but are generally withheld until all the effects of general anesthesia have worn off. Statistically, the incidence of acutely bleeding stress ulcers is highest between the sixth and fourteenth days postinjury. Serial hematocrit determinations establish a baseline and may be the first indicator of a "silent" gastrointestinal hemorrhage.

Urologic Complications

After transection of the spinal cord the bladder sphincter becomes paralyzed and urinary stasis develops. Indwelling urinary catheterization is necessary to prevent bladder distention during the acute phase. Catheters made of inert material are preferred over those made of rubber, which are irritating to the bladder and urethra. The catheter balloon should not be inflated with more than 5 ml of fluid. Inflation in excess of this amount aggravates bladder spasticity. A three-way tidal drainage system may be instituted as a means of irrigating the bladder with an antibiotic solution. Care should be taken that the amount of irrigant solution instilled does not overdistend the bladder and create bladder spasms.

Long-term catheterization, osteoporosis, decreased muscle tone, fluid and electrolyte abnormalities, alterations in cardiovascular dynamics, anemia, and catabolism contribute to urologic complications. Stasis, calculi and fistula formation, and chronic urinary tract complications leading to septicemia make urologic complications the leading cause of death in the paraplegic and quadriplegic population.

Temperature Elevations

Temperature elevations after spinal cord injury may be due to any infectious process, the most common being urinary tract and respiratory infections. If this is the case, treatment consists of the administration of antipyretics and the eradication of infection through the administration of appropriate antibiotics.

Unique to the paraplegic and the quadriplegic is the loss of sweating below the level of the lesion. Lacking this important body cooling mechanism, alarmingly high temperature elevations may occur. Treatment

in this situation consists of tepid water spongings, administration of antipyretics, and removal of blankets and as much clothing as possible. These methods are usually quite effective in reducing fever, but occasionally a cooling blanket is also required.

Autonomic Hyperreflexia

Autonomic hyperreflexia is a condition believed to be due to the release of norepinephrine at the ganglia of the sympathetic nervous system, which is no longer under spinal control in the paraplegic or quadriplegic. Autonomic hyperreflexia is not generally seen until the period of spinal shock has elapsed.

The stimulus that triggers autonomic hyperreflexia usually arises from mucosa or muscle tissue and is relayed via the pelvic and presacral nerves to the spinal cord superior to the transection. These impulses stimulate the inferior cord stump where they initiate the sympathetic reflexes of arterial spasm and constriction of the skin and viscera. If the lesion is above the level of the splanchnic outflow (at the seventh thoracic vertebra) the brain cannot compensate by causing vasodilation.

Clinical signs and symptoms of autonomic hyperreflexia are progressive, though somewhat variable. The patient complains of headache: blotching of the skin and "goosebumps" appear. Diaphoresis of the face occurs, and the patient may complain of nasal congestion or obstruction. Severe blood pressure elevations are found, and may exceed 300 mm Hg. The patient is bradycardic and restless; headache becomes severe. Seizure, loss of consciousness, stroke, and death may evolve.

Autonomic hyperreflexia may be triggered by a variety of stimuli. The most common offenders are bladder distention (due to a plugged catheter or excessive irrigant solution), fecal impaction, or decubiti. However, reflexive overresponse may also be triggered by conditions as seemingly innocuous as an ingrown toenail, a jarred bed, or even a draft.

Nursing care centers around the routine prevention of known precipitants of autonomic hyperreflexia. For example, the bladder must not be allowed to become distended, and decubiti must be prevented. If signs and symptoms appear, the stimulus must be sought and removed as rapidly as possible. If the symptoms cannot be alleviated, notify the physician, elevate the head of the bed (if not contraindicated), and monitor the blood pressure every five minutes. Severe cases can require treatment by spinal anesthesia and the administration of ganglionic blocking agents. For chronic problems, subarachnoid blocks or rhizotomy may be necessary.

Anesthetic Considerations

The most influential factors in the anesthetic management of paraplegic and quadriplegic patients are the fluid and electrolyte abnormalities seen (particularly in the first 3 months after injury), the frequent occurrence of heart block, and the dangers of autonomic hyperreflexia.

Patients injured less than 3 months prior to surgery frequently have elevated serum potassium levels. The elevated potassium level causes an abnormal response to depolarizing blocking agents, further elevating the potassium level. Values as high as 11 mEq/L have been reported and may lead to ventricular fibrillation. Because of this, only nondepolarizing muscle relaxants are recommended for use in these patients.

The frequent incidence of heart block during anesthesia requires that every spinal cord–injured patient be monitored by continuous EKG in the PACU. Heart block is probably induced as a baroreceptor response to vasoconstriction above the level of the lesion. Spinal anesthesia may eliminate heart block, but because of technical difficulties, such as distorted skeletal structure and vascular instability, it is frequently considered too hazardous to risk.

Herniated Nucleus Pulposus (HNP)

A herniated nucleus pulposus (Fig. 26–12) may occur in any of the intervertebral discs but is most commonly found in one of the last two lumbar interspaces. Pain and some degree of compromise of sensory or motor function along the distribution of the involved nerve are common findings pre-

operatively. Before operative intervention is undertaken, diagnostic confirmation is sought and the suspected HNP is differentiated from tumor, subluxation of the facets, or rheumatoid spondylitis.

Surgery consists of partial hemilaminectomy and removal of the diseased disc. If fusion is necessary to prevent recurrence of pain or deformity, a bone graft is removed from the iliac crest or tibia and placed as a bridge over the defective space. Spinal fusion lengthens the operative procedure and requires a second operative wound site. Therefore, postoperative complications have a greater potential for occurring and the recuperative phase may be lengthened. The threat of shock is also greater, owing to increased blood loss and pain.

Movement restrictions in the PACU are determined by the surgeon and depend on the extent of the surgery and whether or not a fusion was done. If fusion was not done, the patient is often allowed to stand at the beside and ambulation is allowed as soon as the effects of the anesthetic have subsided. If the spine is fused, mobility restrictions are more severe. Usually, turning is allowed if done in the "log rolling" fashion.

As in all spinal procedures, sensory function and motor strength of the extremities should be assessed with the vital signs in the PACU. Evidence of cerebrospinal fluid leaks must be sought on dressings and bed linens.

Intraspinal Neoplasms

Intraspinal neoplasms may occur at any level of the cord from the foramen magnum to the sacral canal. The largest number of tumors are found in the thoracic region, as this is the longest subdivision of the spine. Cord compression and neurologic deficit produce symptoms that are similar to those produced by displaced fracture of the spine, but they usually develop and progress at a slower pace. The exact location of the lesion is determined by neurologic examination, myelography, and sometimes tomography.

Intraspinal tumors may arise from the cord or its coverings, from fibrous tissue, or as a result of metastatic disease. For

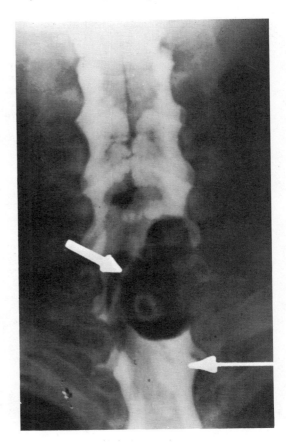

Figure 26–16. Myelogram showing an intradural-extramedullary meningioma at the seventh cervical segment. The thin arrow shows a broad dye column on that side of the spinal canal with the halftone shadow of the cord displaced toward the opposite side. The broad (upper) arrow shows the medial border of the tumor mass itself. (From Sabiston, D. C. [ed.]: Textbook of Surgery. 11th ed. Philadelphia, W. B. Saunders Co., 1977, p. 1490.)

descriptive purposes they are placed in the following subdivisions:

Intramedullary Tumors. Those arising solely from the substance of the cord.

Intraspinal Extramedullary Tumors. Those arising from within the spinal canal but not invading the dura or the cord.

Intradural Extramedullary Tumors. Those arising within the dura but not invading the cord (Fig. 26–16).

Dumbbell Tumors. Those arising within the spinal canal and extending extraspinally (or vice versa) through a vertebral foramen.

Early diagnosis and treatment are essential to prevent irreversible damage to the spinal cord. Sixty to 70 percent of intraspinal neoplasms are benign in nature. The remainder are either primarily malignant or secondary to metastasis. The decision to intervene surgically is made after considering the patient's general condition and life expectancy. Also considered are other metastases and the type and location of the primary tumor.

Treatment consists of laminectomy, surgical exploration, and excision of the mass. Most benign tumors can be excised completely. Prognosis depends on the location of the tumor, severity and duration of the preoperative neurologic deficit, and whether or not the tumor is completely removable. Intramedullary tumors carry a more guarded prognosis, because they can rarely be excised without increasing neurologic deficit.

REFERENCES

1. Brown, S.: Practical points in the postanesthetic assessment and care of the patient with increased intracranial pressure. J. Post Anesth. Nurs., 1(1):37–40, 1986.
2. Brunner, L., et al.: Textbook of Medical Surgical Nursing. 2nd ed. Philadelphia, J. B. Lippincott Co., 1970.
3. Eliasson, S., et al. (eds.): Neurological Pathophysiology. New York, Oxford University Press, 1974.
4. Fell, T., and Cheny, F.: Prevention of hy-

poxia during endotracheal suction. Ann. Surg., *174*:24, 1971.

5. Hanlon, K.: Description and use of intracranial pressure monitoring. Heart Lung, 5:277–282, 1976.
6. Hekmatpanah, J.: Sequence of alteration of vital signs during acute experimental increased intracranial pressure. J. Neurosurg., *32*:16, 1970.
7. Johnston, I., et al.: Intracranial pressure changes following head injury. Lancet, 2:433, 1970.
8. Katz, J., Benumof, J., and Kadis, L.: Anesthesia and Uncommon Diseases: Pathophysiologic and Clinical Correlations. 2nd ed. Philadelphia, W. B. Saunders Co., 1981.
9. Kintzel, K. (ed.): Advanced Concepts in Clinical Nursing. Philadelphia, J. B. Lippincott Co., 1971.
10. Mauss, N., and Mitchell, P.: Increased intracranial pressure: an update. Heart Lung, 5:919, 1976.
11. Miller, R.: Anesthesia. 2nd ed. New York, Churchill-Livingstone, Inc., 1986.
12. Mirr, M., Jankowski, K., and Taylon, M.: Nursing management for barbiturate therapy in acute head injuries. Heart Lung, *12*:(1):52–60, 1983.
13. Norrell, H., and Wilson, C.: Early anterior fusion for injuries of the cervical portion of the spine. JAMA, *214*:525, 1970.
14. Paltsev, E., and Sirovsky, E.: Intracranial physiology and biomechanics. J. Neurosurg., *57*:500, 1982.
16. Plum, F., and Posner, J.: The Diagnosis of Stupor and Coma. 2nd ed. Philadelphia, F. A. Davis Co., 1972.
16. Pykett, I.: NMR imaging in medicine. Sci. Am., *246*:(5):78, 1982.
17. Raju, T., and Vidyasagar, D.: Intracranial

and cerebral perfusion pressure: methodology and clinical considerations. Med. Instrum., *16*(3):154, 1982.
18. Saul, T., and Ducker, T.: Intracranial pressure monitoring in patients with severe head injury. Am. Surg., *48*(9):477, 1982.
19. Shapiro, H., et al.: Acute intraoperative hypertension in neurosurgical patients. Anesthesiology, *37*:399, 1972.
20. Sorensen, K., and Luckmann, J.: Basic Nursing: A Psychophysiologic Approach. 2nd ed. Philadelphia, W. B. Saunders Co., 1986.
21. Stephens, G., and Parsons, M.: A delicate balance managing chronic airway obstruction in a neurosurgical patient. Am. J. Nurs., *75*:1492, 1975.
22. Sutton, A.: Bedside Nursing Techniques in Medicine and Surgery. 2nd ed. Philadelphia, W. B. Saunders Co., 1976.
23. Swift, N.: Head injury: essentials of excellent care. Nursing, *4*:26, 1974.
24. Tate, G.: Assessment and direction of nursing care for patients with acute central nervous system insult. Nurs. Clin. North Am., *6*:165, 1971.
25. Trubuhovich, R. (ed.): Management of acute intracranial disasters. Int. Anesthesiol. Clin., *17*(2,3), 1979.
26. Varkey, G. (ed.): Anesthetic considerations in the surgery of atherosclerotic cerebrovascular disease. Int. Anesthesiol. Clin., *22*(3), 1984.
27. Wilson, J. (ed.): Handbook of Surgery. 5th ed. Palo Alto, Lange Medical Publications, 1973.
28. Youmans, J. (ed.): Neurological Surgery: A Comprehensive Reference Guide to the Diagnosis and Management of Neurosurgical Problems. 2nd ed. Philadelphia, W. B. Saunders Co., 1982.

Postoperative Care After Thyroid and Parathyroid Surgery

Surgery of the thyroid gland has been performed since the early 1800s and perfected to the degree that postoperative complications are rare. Preoperative preparation of the patient for thyroid or parathyroid surgery is extremely important and includes ensuring that the patient is euthyroid, well rested, at optimum weight, and in good health.

Definitions

Euthyroid: having normal thyroid secretion and function.

Parathyroidectomy: excision of one or more diseased, hypertrophied parathyroid glands.

Thyroidectomy: total excision of the thyroid gland. Total thyroidectomy is normally performed only in cases of thyroid malignancy.

Thyroglossal duct cystectomy: complete excision of all portions of the pretracheal cystic pouch sac and a portion of the hyoid bone to avoid recurrent cystic formation and to prevent infections.

Thyroid lobectomy: *partial thyroidectomy* is removal of a lobe of the thyroid gland. The objective in the patient with hyper-

thyroidism is to resect enough of the gland (*subtotal thyroidectomy*) to reduce the level of circulating hormones to normal, yet leave sufficient amount of the gland to secrete a supply of the hormone.

ANESTHESIA

Surgery on the thyroid and parathyroid glands is most commonly performed under general endotracheal anesthesia. Therefore, all postoperative care indicated for a general anesthesia patient is instituted. A transverse neck incision is utilized during the surgical process.

NURSING CARE

Positioning

Upon return from the operative suite, the patient should be placed in the side-lying position if unconscious. He or she should be placed in a semi-Fowler position to promote venous return as soon as condition permits. The patient should be moved carefully, with support to the head so that no tension is placed on the suture line. Firm

401

support of the head should be continued and can usually be accomplished by placing a firm pillow under the shoulders and head. The patient should be taught to support the head when moving by placing the hands at the back of the neck.

Cardiorespiratory Assessment and Care

Immediate postoperative observations should include close attention to respiratory function, which may be compromised by hemorrhage, venous oozing, laryngeal edema, and cord paralysis. Discourage the patient's talking to excess. A tracheostomy set should be immediately available at the bedside of any patient undergoing thyroid or parathyroid surgery.

Signs and symptoms of respiratory obstruction such as stridor, air hunger, laryngeal spasm, or inability to speak should be reported immediately to the anesthesiologist or the surgeon and appropriate measures instituted. A cool mist humidifier at the bedside is routinely ordered postoperatively to ease the sore throat expected after endotracheal intubation and to promote general respiratory well-being.

The patient should also be checked for the development of subcutaneous emphysema, which may indicate a pneumothorax or rupture of the trachea.

Pain

Pain should be minimal following thyroidectomy and parathyroidectomy, but small doses of narcotic such as meperidine or morphine may be required during the first 24 hours. Severe pain should be reported.

Dressings

Postoperative dressings are no longer bulky, and drains are generally not required. A simple "thyroid collar" including a gauze square over the incision secured with a sterile surgical towel crossed over the gauze is usually used. Drainage should be minimal and should not visibly soak through the dressing. The usual signs and symptoms of hemorrhage should be assessed, and the nurse should watch for swelling of the neck and feel the back of the neck for drainage. Any excess bleeding should be reported immediately.

Intake and Output

Intake and output should be carefully assessed. The postoperative patient can be expected to retain some fluid, and this will be manifested as a low urinary output. Caution must be exerted, therefore, to avoid overhydration. Oral fluid can usually be tolerated as soon as the patient regains consciousness and nausea has subsided. Ice chips may be offered to soothe the throat. Warm saline gargles may be comforting.

Complications

Complications are infrequent, but may include obstruction of the airway, postoperative bleeding, pneumomediastinum, and pneumothorax. Although rare with today's advanced surgical techniques, damage to the recurrent laryngeal nerve may occur. Hoarseness or "whispery voice" may indicate unilateral damage that is usually temporary. Hoarseness and bilateral flaccid paralysis may indicate bilateral nerve injury and should be reported immediately, since serious airway obstruction could develop rapidly. Following assessment of the voice, the patient should be discouraged from excessive talking, since this will aggravate the hoarseness.

Tetany. Although tetany due to hypoparathyroidism is rare, the patient should be evaluated for signs and symptoms that may indicate its development. The signs and symptoms of tetany include tingling of the toes, fingers, and around the mouth; apprehension; positive *Chvostek's sign* (tapping the cheek over the facial nerve causes a twitch of the lip or facial muscle); and positive *Trousseau's sign* (carpopedal spasm induced by occluding circulation in the arm with a blood pressure cuff or tourniquet). Calcium lactate or calcium gluconate should be readily available for use if signs of tetany develop. Calcium is administered slowly intravenously, and the patient's electrocardiogram should be monitored continuously before, during, and after the infusion.

Thyroid Storm. In thyroid crisis, or storm, a very rare complication, all the symptoms of hyperthyroidism are exaggerated. An increase in pulse, blood pressure, pulse pressure, and temperature, plus air hunger and restlessness, may indicate its development. Treatment includes the intravenous administration of sodium iodide, corticosteroids, and reserpine, as well as supplementary oxygen and cooling with a hypothermia unit. Lithium is the drug of choice for patients who are sensitive to iodine.

REFERENCES

1. Ashkar, F. S.: A better outlook in thyroid cancer. Consultant, 12:148, 1972.
2. Evangelisti, J. T., and Thorpe, C. J.: Thyroid storm—a nursing crisis. Heart Lung, 12(2):184–193, 1983.
3. Foster, R. J.: Morbidity and mortality after thyroidectomy. Surg. Gynecol. Obstet., 146:423, 1978.
4. Katz, A. D., and Bronson, D.: Total thyroidectomy. Am. J. Surg., 136:450, 1978.
5. Mannix, J., Pyrtek, L. J., and Crobie, H. D.: Hyperparathyroidism in the elderly. Am. J. Surg., 139:581–585, 1980.
6. Marchetta, F. C., and Sako, K.: The diagnosis of thyroid carcinoma during the postoperative period after less than total thyroidectomy. Am. J. Surg., 136:455, 1978.
7. Perry, H. A.: The postoperative care of patients after thyroid, parathyroid, and adrenal operations. Curr. Rev. Recov. Room Nurses, 4(8):59–63, 1982.

Postoperative Care After Gastrointestinal, Abdominal, and Anorectal Surgery*

Care of the patient following abdominal surgery or surgery on the gastrointestinal tract is an extremely broad subject. In this chapter we will discuss the care involved after surgery on the gastrointestinal tract, including the esophagus and the anus, even though they are not contained within the abdominal cavity, as well as the liver, gallbladder, pancreas, and spleen (Fig. 28–1). Surgery on the female reproductive organs, which are also contained within the abdominal cavity, is discussed in Chapter 30. The care common to all patients undergoing abdominal surgery will be discussed here, and only the most important variations related to specific procedures will be included.

Surgical intervention within the abdominal cavity is generally directed toward restoring normal function and therefore

involves repair of abnormalities, reconstruction of deformities, removal of obstructions to restore patency of the gastrointestinal tract and the biliary tract, and maintenance of the integrity of related organs, such as the liver, pancreas, and spleen.

Definitions

Antrectomy: removal of lower part of the stomach.

Appendectomy: removal of the vermiform appendix.

Cecostomy: creation of an opening for insertion of a tube into the cecum to decompress the bowel by removing air and accumulations of digestive juices.

Cholecystectomy: removal of the gallbladder.

Cholecystostomy: establishment of an opening into the gallbladder to permit drainage of the organ and the removal of stones. This is not performed very frequently except to provide relief in an extremely debilitated patient.

Colostomy: opening of the colon onto the abdomen; may be permanent or temporary.

---

*The authors gratefully acknowledge the expert review of this chapter by Dorothy M. Williams, R.N., Head PACU Nurse, and Denise A. Lowe, R.N., C.C.R.N., M.A., Clinical Instructor, Critical Care & PACU, Memorial Sloan Kettering Cancer Center, New York.

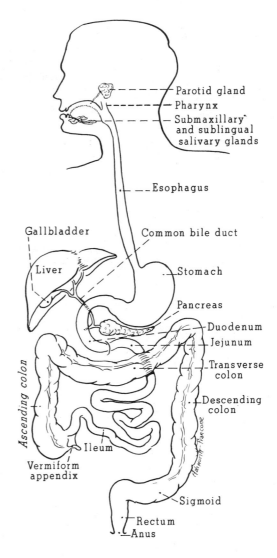

Figure 28–1. The digestive system and its associated structures. (From Jacob, S. W., Francone, C. A., and Lossow, W. J.: Structure and Function in Man. 4th ed. Philadelphia, W. B. Saunders Co., 1978, p. 453.)

Diverticulum: a pouch opening from a hollow viscus, most commonly in the sigmoid colon.

Endoscopy: visualization of a body cavity with a lighted tube or scope.

Esophagoscopy: direct visualization of the esophagus and cardia of the stomach by means of a lighted instrument (esophagoscope). Esophagoscopy may be used to obtain a tissue biopsy or secretions for study to aid in diagnosis.

Gastrectomy: removal of the stomach. Usually a subtotal gastrectomy is done, in which part of the stomach is removed, expressed as a percentage (usually 60 to

80 percent); also called gastric resection (Fig. 28–2).

Gastroenterostomy: creation of an anastomosis between the posterior wall of the stomach near the antrum and the jejunum, used to treat pyloric obstruction (Fig. 28–3).

Gastroscopy: direct inspection of the stomach and removal of a tissue specimen, if necessary, by means of a lighted instrument (gastroscope) (Fig. 28–4).

Hemorrhoidectomy: surgical excision of dilated veins of the rectum.

Hernia: the displacement of any viscus (usually bowel) or tissue through a con-

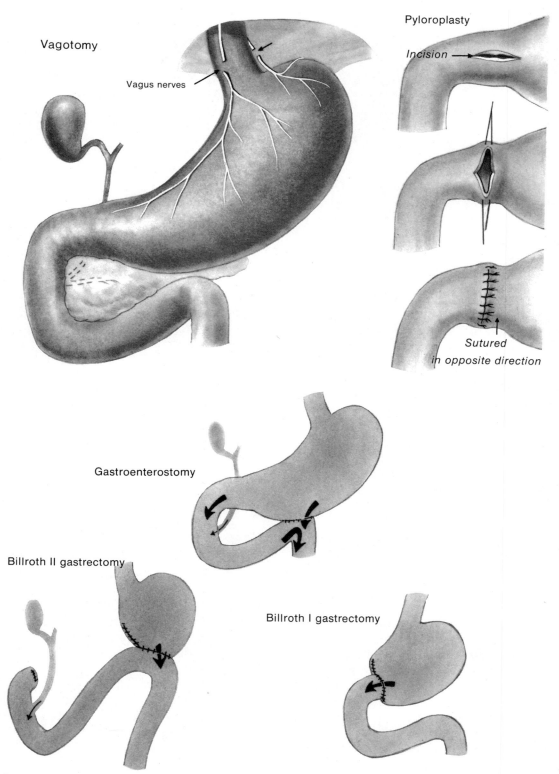

Figure 28–2. Gastric surgical procedures. (From Luckmann, J., and Sorenson, K. C.: Medical-Surgical Nursing. Philadelphia, W. B. Saunders Co., 1974, p. 1091.)

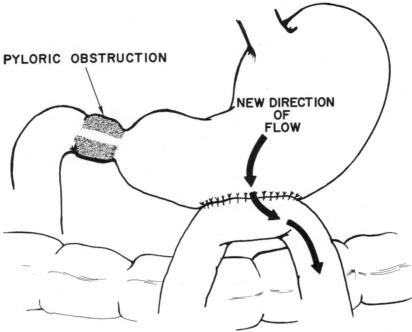

PYLORIC OBSTRUCTION

NEW DIRECTION OF FLOW

Figure 28–3. Gastroenterostomy for pyloric obstruction. (From Le Maitre, G. D., and Finnegan, J. A.: The Patient in Surgery. 3rd ed. Philadelphia, W. B. Saunders Co., 1975, p. 210.)

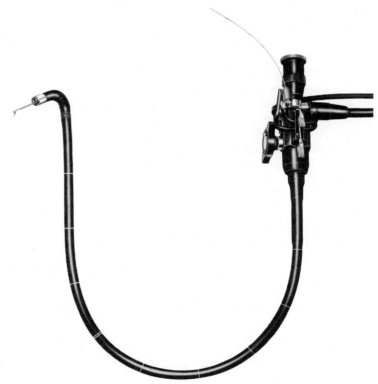

Figure 28–4. Fiberscope for gastric examination. (From Luckmann, J., and Sorensen, K. C.: Medical-Surgical Nursing. Philadelphia, W. B. Saunders Co., 1974, p. 1058.)

genital or acquired opening or defect in the wall of its natural cavity. Usually this term is applied to protrusion of abdominal viscera; however, it is actually the defect itself through which abdominal contents have protruded.

Herniorrhaphy: correction of a hernia, also termed hernioplasty. Hernias and herniorrhaphies are classified according to their anatomic sites and the condition of the viscus that has protruded. *Reducible hernias* are those in which the bowel or contents of the hernial sac can be replaced into their normal cavity. An *irreducible* or *incarcerated hernia* is one in which the contents cannot be replaced. A *strangulated hernia* is one in which the blood supply to the protruding segment of bowel is obstructed. When a segment of bowel becomes strangulated, it rapidly becomes necrotic. A strangulated hernia constitutes a surgical emergency.

Herniorrhaphy, diaphragmatic: replacement of abdominal contents that have entered the thorax through a defect in the diaphragm, and repair of the diaphragmatic defect.

Herniorrhaphy, epigastric and hypogastric: ligation of the peritoneal fat or hernial sac, with repair and closure of the abdominal wall.

Herniorrhaphy, femoral: removal and replacement of peritoneum that has protruded through the femoral ring, which is located just below Poupart's (the inguinal) ligament and medial to the femoral vein, and repair of the defect in the transverse fascia at the exit of the femoral vessels. Femoral hernias are seldom found in children and occur most frequently in women.

Herniorrhaphy, hiatal: repair of herniation of a portion of the stomach through the esophageal hiatus of the diaphragm. Repair involves reduction through an abdominal or thoracic incision.

Herniorrhaphy, incisional: reunion in layers of the abdominal wall.

Herniorrhaphy, inguinal: direct or indirect reconstruction of a weakened area in the abdominal wall, after reduction or repair of the opening through which tissue was protruding.

Herniorrhaphy, sliding: the freeing and reducing of sliding viscus, and repair of abdominal tissues surrounding and overlying the inguinal canal.

Herniorrhaphy, umbilical: closure of the peritoneal opening and reconstruction of the abdominal wall surrounding the umbilicus (umbilical ring); usually occurs in pediatric patients and is most common in black female babies.

Ileojejunal shunt: an anastomosis of the jejunum approximately 14 inches from the beginning to the terminal ileum about 4 inches above the ileocecal valve. This is used as a treatment for exogenous obesity, and patients selected for this procedure usually weigh in excess of 300 pounds.

Ileostomy: opening of the ileum to the surface of the abdomen. Used to treat inflammatory conditions of the bowel, ulcerative colitis, regional enteritis, and cancer; usually a permanent surgical construction.

Intussusception: telescoping of the bowel into itself.

Laparoscopy (peritoneoscopy): direct visualization of the peritoneal cavity by means of a lighted instrument inserted through the abdominal wall via a stab wound.

Laparotomy: an opening made through the abdominal wall into the peritoneal cavity, usually for exploratory purposes. If repairs are done, the operation is usually named according to the procedure or procedures carried out.

Pancreatoduodenectomy (Whipple's procedure): removal of the head of the pancreas, the entire duodenum, a portion of the jejunum, the distal third of the stomach, the lower half of the common bile duct, and a portion of the pancreatic duct, with reestablishment of continuity of the biliary, pancreatic, and gastrointestinal systems. The procedure is used primarily for treatment of malignancy of the pancreas and carries with it a high risk of mortality. Although this procedure was named for Whipple who first described it, surgeons modify the operation as needed and rarely perform it in the original manner. The surgeon should explain to the PACU nursing staff exactly what procedures were performed.

Pyloromyotomy (Fredet-Ramstedt's operation): enlarging the lumen of the pylorus by longitudinally splitting the hypertrophied circular muscle; used as treatment for pyloric stenosis. Pyloric stenosis is most common in first-born male babies.

Pyloroplasty: longitudinal incision made in the pylorus, and closed transversely to permit the muscle to relax and to establish an enlarged outlet.

Splenectomy: removal of the spleen.

Transduodenal sphincterotomy: partial division of the sphincter of Oddi and exploration of the common duct to treat recurrent attacks of acute pancreatitis due to formation of calculi in the pancreatic duct or blockage of the sphincter of Oddi.

Vagotomy: removal of branches of the vagus nerve that innervate the stomach, to reduce secretions and movements.

Volvulus: twisting of the bowel.

GENERAL CARE FOLLOWING ABDOMINAL SURGERY

Abdominal or gastrointestinal surgery may be performed with local, spinal, or general anesthesia. Usually, only the simpler procedures are performed under local or spinal anesthesia. Diagnostic procedures such as endoscopy, biopsies, and gastrostomy are frequently performed under local anesthesia with appropriate sedation. Appendectomy and inguinal or femoral herniorrhaphies are often performed with spinal anesthesia and sedation. Most other abdominal surgery is performed under general anesthesia.

A number of abdominopelvic incisions have been developed and are commonly used (Fig. 28–5). An ideal incision ensures

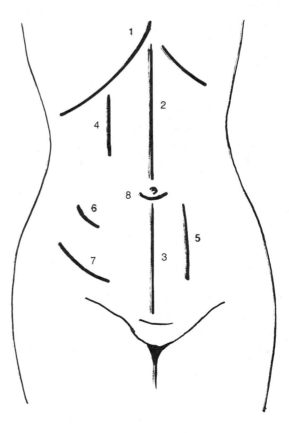

Figure 28–5. Commonly used abdominal incisions: (1), Kocher's incision: right side, gallbladder and biliary tract surgery; left side, splenectomy, (2) upper abdominal midline incision: rapid entry to control bleeding ulcer, (3) lower abdominal midline incision: female reproductive system, (4) upper paramedian incision: right side, biliary tract surgery, cholecystectomy; left side, splenectomy, gastrectomy, vagectomy, hiatal hernia repair, (5) lower paramedian incision: right side, appendectomy, small bowel resection; left side, sigmoid colon resection, (6) McBurney's incision: appendectomy, (7) inguinal incision: inguinal herniorrhaphy, (8) infraumbilical: umbilical herniorrhaphy.

ease of entrance, maximum exposure of the operative site, and minimal trauma. It should also provide good primary wound healing with maximum wound strength.

The reader should review Chapters 17 through 19 for general care following surgery.

PACU Care

As with any procedure, the surgeon and anesthetist should give the receiving nurse a full report on the anesthesia used and the procedure performed. With complicated abdominal procedures, especially those that involve extensive resection or rerouting of the gastrointestinal tract, or both, we have found it very useful to have the surgeon draw a diagram of the procedure performed, along with the incisions and drainage tubes present. This assists those caring for the patient in assessment of wounds, dressings, and expected drainage. The surgeon can draw this diagram right on the nursing care plan, which should be started upon the patient's admission to the PACU so that continuity of information is assured.

Positioning

Following abdominal surgery, patients are often positioned on the side until laryngeal reflexes have started to return. They are then placed in a semi-Fowler position to ease the tension on suture lines and to promote respiratory effort. Following surgery on the esophagus, however, the patient should be kept flat to avoid tension on the suture line. Following hemorrhoidectomy, the patient may assume any position of comfort, which will most likely be on the side.

Dressings and Drains

All dressings should be checked. It is important for the nurse to know what kind of incision was used and whether or not any drains are in place. If drains are in place, considerably more drainage can be expected than if there are none. These are discussed in more detail under the specific procedures. Drainage should be assessed

for character, volume, and odor. Some surgeons reinforce the abdominal incision and dressing with a binder. They feel that this gives the incision valuable support. However, others feel that binders restrict respiratory effort, and that this disadvantage outweighs the limited advantage of incisional support.

Since drainage is often copious after gastrointestinal surgery, frequent reinforcement of dressings may be necessary. If drainage becomes excessive, more than expected from the particular procedure, the surgeon should be notified and the incision directly inspected.

All tubes should be connected to straight gravity drainage or suction drainage, as the surgeon specifies. Maintenance of the patency of these tubes is one of the most important nursing functions following gastrointestinal surgery.

Respiratory Function

The promotion of good respiratory function is a nursing priority for the patient who has had abdominal surgery. Painful abdominal incisions cause the patient to restrict chest expansion voluntarily. This is especially true with high abdominal incisions. The patient must be coached frequently in doing sustained maximal inspirations, coughing, and changing position to prevent respiratory complications. Assisting the patient by the splinting of the incision and the judicious use of pain medications aid in deep breathing and coughing and prevent development of atelectasis. Frequent assessment of breath sounds during the postoperative period can alert the nurse to impending respiratory problems. Owing to the possibility of an accidental nick into the diaphragm during abdominal surgery, breath sounds must be monitored closely in order to check for a pneumothorax.

Fluid and Electrolyte Balance

Fluid and electrolyte losses are substantial during gastrointestinal surgery. Losses continue postoperatively through gastrointestinal tubes or other drains. For this reason, accurate intake and output records are mandatory. All drainage from incisions should be included in the assessment of electrolyte balance. Frequent serum electrolyte determinations may be necessary if losses are great. Intravenous fluids are used for replacement for at least the first 24 hours postoperatively and until the nasogastric tubes are removed. The reader is referred to Chapter 17 to review the specific problems in electrolyte loss from the gastrointestinal tract.

Urinary retention may become a problem following abdominal surgery, owing to incisional pain and physiologic splinting. Urine output should be checked frequently and accurate records kept. The nurse should also check for bladder distention. Especially with spinal anesthesia, the patient may not recognize the need to void. The patient should void within 10 to 12 hours postoperatively. If the patient has not voided by the time he or she leaves the PACU, the receiving ward should be notified so that they will check specifically for urinary retention. If permissible, it may help the male patient to stand to void. If urinary retention causes pain, distends the abdomen, or becomes prolonged, urinary catheterization may become necessary. Patients who have had extensive surgery will often return to the PACU with a urinary catheter in place. Accurate output records should be maintained.

Care of the Patient with Nasogastrointestinal Tubes

Anesthesia and manipulation of the viscera during surgery cause peristalsis to diminish or to disappear completely for 24 to 48 hours afterwards. Nasogastrointestinal or nasogastric tubes are commonly used postoperatively to prevent the sequelae of this hypomotility. Edema at the operative site can result in obstruction, too. Decompression of the stomach, with removal of accumulated fluid and air, not only prevents vomiting and eases tension on the abdominal suture line but also increases the area's vascularity and so improves its nutrition and hastens healing.

Both short and long tubes are used, depending on the operative site. Short tubes used include the Levin, the Rehfuss, and the plastic Salem sump, which is a double-lumen nasogastric tube. The double lumen prevents excessive negative pressure from developing when the tube is connected to suction. Long tubes that may be used to decompress the intestine include the Harris, Cantor, Miller-Abbott, and Abbott-Rawson.

When the patient returns from the operating suite with a nasogastric tube in place, the nurse must ascertain why the tube was placed, where it was placed, and whether it should be connected to suction or to straight gravity drainage. Frequently, the physician will order the tube to be connected to low intermittent suction (20 to 40 mm Hg). Usually, only low-pressure, intermittent suction is used because excessive negative pressure in either the stomach or the bowel pulls the mucosa into the lumen of the tube and can cause traumatic ulcers. For double-lumen nasogastric tubes, continuous suction at 20 mm Hg is usually ordered.

Tube Patency

Patency of the tube must be ensured. The nurse should observe for drainage from the tube. All characteristics of the drainage must be noted: consistency, color, odor, quantity, and any deviations from the expected drainage. After gastrointestinal surgery, drainage will be bright red at first, but it should become dark after 24 hours. Bloody drainage should not be expected from a nasogastric tube placed only for decompression of the stomach after biliary tract, liver, or splenic surgery. If no drainage is present, if the patient's abdomen becomes distended, or if the patient vomits around the nasogastric tube or complains of nausea, the tube may be clogged or the suction machine may be malfunctioning—check both. To maintain the patency of the nasogastric tube, irrigation with 30 ml of normal saline may be done every hour or more frequently if necessary. Plain water should never be used. Frequent irrigations increase the loss of electrolytes from the gastrointestinal system. Some surgeons advocate the use of air to irrigate the nasogastric tube to maintain patency.

Irrigation

The amount of irrigating solution instilled should be recorded as such, unless its equivalent is aspirated by syringe. All gastrointestinal drainage should be accurately measured and recorded. The long gastrointestinal tubes can be irrigated in the same way as nasogastric tubes; however, since the tube is so much longer, the irrigating fluid rarely fully returns, so it should always be noted on the intake and output sheet how much irrigating fluid was instilled. If irrigations do not increase drainage, the tubing should be checked for clogs by milking it toward the machine in order to dislodge any obstruction. The suction machine is checked by disconnecting the nasogastric tube at the junction of the nasogastric tube and the drainage tube leading to the bottle. With the machine turned on, the end of the drainage tube is placed in a glass of water; if the water is sucked up, the machine is functioning. If these measures fail, gastric mucosa may be occluding the lumen of the tube. In this case, the patient or the tube may need to be repositioned. If the patient has had gastric or esophageal surgery, the tube should not be manipulated; the physician should be notified of its malfunctioning.

Patient Comfort

The presence of a nasogastric or long gastrointestinal tube is a most uncomfortable experience for the patient. However, appropriate nursing care can relieve sore throat, dry mouth, hoarseness, earache, sore nose, and dry lips. Ensure that the tube is taped securely in a position to prevent pressure on the naris. The tube may be secured to the upper lip or nose in the position it naturally assumes. The tube should not be taped to the patient's nose and then to the forehead. This causes pressure on the underside of the nostril and can cause tissue necrosis. To lessen the pressure and pull on the patient's nose, either tape or pin the tube to his or her gown. Hypoallergenic tape is best used.

Apply petrolatum ointment to the tube where it enters the nose and around the naris. The tube is kept free on the outside from mucus or other drainage. This prevents encrustations from forming and reduces irritation of the nostril. Petrolatum ointment, cream, or Chap Stick is applied to the lips to keep them soft and prevent cracking. Good, frequent mouth care is essential for the comfort of the patient and to prevent parotitis. Lemon glycerine swabs, mouthwash, or even a toothbrush may be used to provide mouth care to the patient. Simply ensure that he or she understands not to swallow any of the material used. This, of course, would not be fatal, but could be detrimental to fluid and electrolyte balance.

Gargles with warm tap water or warm saline, or with viscous lidocaine (Xylocaine), or applications of a local anesthetic spray will relieve the patient's sore throat. A physician's order should be provided for these measures. Some surgeons will allow their patients to suck on isotonic ice chips or hard candy or to chew gum. Anesthetic throat lozenges, if allowed, provide a great deal of comfort to the patient. All patients with a gastrointestinal tube in place are given essentially nothing by mouth until the tube is removed.

DIAGNOSTIC STUDIES

Invasive diagnostic surgical procedures are occasionally done at the patient's bedside on the general ward, but they are more frequently done in a special procedures room, often located within the surgical suite. They require local anesthesia and appropriate sedation or sometimes general anesthesia. Patients are sent to the PACU for a short observational period. Care after endoscopy includes all of the general care afforded a post anesthesia patient. After esophagoscopy and gastroscopy, the nurse should be alert for the return of the gag reflex. When pharyngeal reflexes have returned, unless contraindicated by the diagnosis or in anticipation of further surgery, the patient may be started on liquids and may progress to a regular diet as tolerated. Rest is the most important treatment for this patient. There may be bleeding, swelling, or dysfunction of the involved area, indicating complications from the procedure.

The patient who has had peritoneoscopy will have only a small bandage dressing over the stab wound used for entry of the peritoneoscope. This should remain clean and dry. This patient will probably be apprehensive about what was discovered about his or her condition during the diagnostic procedure and should be given accurate information following the procedure by the surgeon. The nurse should be familiar with what the patient is told, in order to be able to interpret or repeat the information for the patient.

PATIENT CARE FOLLOWING SURGERY ON THE GASTROINTESTINAL TRACT

Esophagus

Surgery on the esophagus includes repair of hiatal hernia, repair of various forms of tracheoesophageal fistulas, excision of esophageal diverticula, treatment of stenosis of the lower end of the esophagus, esophagomyotomy, and cardiomyotomy.

Postoperative care depends upon the kind of incision used to expose the operative site—abdominal or thoracic. Surgery on the esophagus frequently involves a thoracic incision. Care for the patient following a thoracic incision is discussed in Chapter 22.

Procedures on the esophagus are performed under general anesthesia. Frequently, a tracheostomy is performed (see Chapter 20 for care of the patient following tracheostomy). Upon return to the PACU, the patient should be placed in a semi-Fowler position. This aids in the drainage of blood from the pleural space and prevents tension from impinging on the suture lines. The incision is generally long (from the tip of the scapula to the seventh or

eighth rib area) and painful. Analgesics must be given in adequate doses to promote rest and adequate respiratory effort. TENS often provides considerable relief of pain from long incisions.

A nasogastric tube will be in place and should be cared for as previously discussed. It should not be manipulated by the nurse. A large sterile dressing should be in place, and it should be checked frequently for drainage and reinforced as necessary. Excessive bloody drainage should be reported to the surgeon.

Stomach

Surgery on the stomach involves procedures to treat ulcers (antrectomy and vagotomy, gastric resection, gastrectomy); removal of portions of the stomach, because of cancer; and rerouting of the gastrointestinal system at this point to treat pyloric stenosis. All postoperative care of the patient is generally the same. Anesthesia will be general. The patient should be placed in a semi-Fowler position postoperatively to relieve tension on the suture line and to promote drainage. The abdominal incisions are fairly high, long, and painful, and particular attention must be paid to pulmonary toilet. This patient must be encouraged more frequently than any other to expand the lung and to cough and must generally have assistance to change position. Assistance in splinting the wound with the hands or with a firm pillow will be most appreciated by the patient. These procedures generally produce considerable postoperative pain, and analgesics should be used generously but judiciously. A nasogastric tube will be in place and should be cared for as previously discussed. Bright, bloody drainage from the nasogastric tube can be expected for the first 2 to 3 hours, since it is not uncommon to have bleeding at the anastomosis site in these procedures. However, bright bleeding that does not decrease after this period or bleeding that becomes excessive (more than 75 ml per hour) should be reported immediately to the surgeon. Since blood easily clots and clogs the nasogastric tube, an irrigation order should have been left and instructions should be followed. As blood loss may be highly significant in this patient, cardiovascular status must receive careful scrutiny. Vital signs are checked frequently, and a certain amount of hypotension and tachycardia is to be expected. If hypotension and tachycardia persist or maintain a downward trend, the surgeon should be notified.

Blood replacement may have to be instituted. Hemoglobin and hematocrit levels should be determined 4 to 6 hours postoperatively and the surgeon notified if they are significantly lower than previous determinations. Little or no drainage should be expected from the incision unless drains are in place. If drainage does appear, the dressing should be reinforced, and the surgeon notified. The initial dressing should not be replaced by the nurse in the PACU unless so directed by the surgeon.

Urinary retention is commonly a problem, and many surgeons prefer to insert a Foley catheter while the patient is in the surgical suite. Accurate measurements of output should be ascertained. If a urinary catheter is not in place, the patient should be checked frequently for abdominal distention, which may indicate an overfull bladder. If the patient is unable to void, a catheterization order should be obtained.

Perforated Ulcer. Perforation of an ulcer is usually a surgical emergency, and neither the patient nor the family members will be adequately prepared, either physically or emotionally, for the surgery. This is of concern to the PACU nurse since complications, especially hypovolemia and shock, may more readily occur in this patient.

Pyloric Stenosis. Specific care for the infant following surgery for pyloric stenosis is detailed in pediatric texts. However, the PACU nurse should be aware of their general care. Position is important. The infant should be kept either on the right side or on the abdomen until the danger of vomiting and aspiration has subsided, then should be placed in an upright position. Plastic infant seats are perfect for this purpose, and no PACU should be without one of these devices. Careful placement of the

diaper is important to avoid contamination of the wound. Sometimes the surgeon will waterproof the incision with a collodion dressing. It may also be helpful to apply a pediatric urine collector not only to prevent contamination of the wound with urine but also to determine accurate output. Feedings are usually begun for these infants 4 to 6 hours postoperatively, but the surgeon's instructions should be explicitly followed.

Small Bowel

Operations on the small bowel include resection for obstruction or perforation, ileostomy for regional ileitis, and ileojejunal shunt for obesity. Care following these procedures is essentially the same as that already mentioned. The patient may have a long gastrointestinal tube in place that should be cared for as noted earlier. No excessive drainage from incisions should be noted, unless drains have been placed. Fluid and electrolyte balance must be monitored carefully. Remember that the loss of sodium and bicarbonate ions will be great, resulting in imbalance, and that fluid losses during surgery may be significant, but fluid overload must be avoided.

The patient with an ileostomy will enter the PACU with a bag in place over the stoma, and returns may be expected almost at once; these should be recorded. Particular attention must be paid to this wound, and no leakage onto the skin should be allowed, as this causes significant injury to the skin. Karaya gum or paste should be applied to the skin surrounding the stoma to protect the skin. In some hospitals, a silver anhydrous ointment has been used instead of karaya gum with considerable success.

Large Bowel

Surgery on the large bowel includes appendectomy, colostomy (for obstruction), sigmoid colon resection, herniorrhaphy, removal of tumors or correction of deformities, and abdominoperineal resection (Fig. 28–6).

Appendectomy and herniorrhaphy are frequently done under spinal anesthesia with appropriate sedation. All other surgery is usually performed under general anesthesia. Upon return to the PACU, the patient is kept flat and on one side until reflexes have returned; he or she may then assume a position of comfort unless otherwise specified by the surgeon. Postoperative care is essentially the same as for small bowel surgery.

If the patient returns from surgery with a colostomy, some special care is required. It is unusual for the colostomy to start functioning; however, spillage must be prevented from contaminating the incision or excoriating the skin. Often, a catheter will have been inserted into the colon and may extend from the colostomy. The colon catheter should be connected to low, intermittent suction and should be gently irrigated with small amounts of warmed saline to prevent it from becoming blocked by fecal particles. The skin around the stoma should be protected with karaya gum and glycerine. A mixture is made by adding small amounts of glycerine to the karaya powder until a peanut butter consistency is obtained. This is then applied around the stoma.

Fluid and electrolyte balance must be monitored carefully. If diverticula were resected, the nurse must watch carefully for blood in the urine. Some blood-tinged urine may be expected after colectomy, since retractors used in surgery may have caused contusions of the bladder; however, gross blood may indicate that the bladder was more severely injured. Dressings should remain dry, unless drains were placed in the wound. If drains were placed, some bloody drainage may be expected, and dressings should be reinforced as necessary. If dressings soak through, the drainage should be considered excessive and be reported to the surgeon.

Abdominoperineal Resection. Abdominoperineal resection for cancer of the rectum is a most traumatic procedure. Vital signs must be monitored very carefully and any adverse trend reported. Shock is one of the frequent complications encountered following this procedure. Blood loss may exceed 2000 ml, and transfusion during surgery is often inadequate, owing to inaccurate loss estimates. Perineal drains will be in place, and this fact should be noted on the patient's chart and nursing care plan. The perineal dressings frequently become saturated with bloody drainage and must be reinforced. If drainage remains bright and obviously new bleeding is occurring, and if frequent dressing changes are required, the surgeon should be notified. If sump catheters are used to drain the perineal wound, they should be attached to a Hemovac apparatus or low continuous suction; when attached to suction, an accurate measurement of drainage may be obtained.

The abdominoperineal surgery patient will have a colostomy. Check the blood

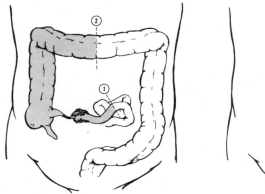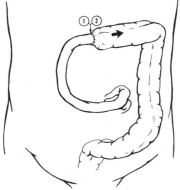

Figure 28–6. *A*, Resection of diseased ileum and right colon for obstructing regional ileitis. *B*, End-to-end ileotransverse colostomy. (From LeMaitre, G. D., and Finnegan, J. A.: The Patient in Surgery. 3rd ed. Philadelphia, W. B. Saunders Co., 1975, p. 226.)

supply to the stoma frequently, as impaired blood supply is an early and serious complication. Pain may be severe and should be relieved with adequate doses of narcotic analgesics to ensure comfort of the patient and promote respiratory sufficiency.

Appendectomy and Herniorrhaphy. Patients who have undergone surgery for appendectomy or herniorrhaphy usually return to the PACU almost fully awake and without serious postoperative complications. No nasogastric tube, Foley catheter, or drain will be in place, and recovery is generally uneventful. The patient may assume a position of comfort as soon as pharyngeal reflexes have returned and may start on a progressive diet as tolerated. All postoperative care outlined in Chapters 17 and 18 applies. Dressings should remain dry and intact, and any postoperative incisional bleeding or drainage should be reported to the surgeon. The most important postoperative complication is bleeding. The nurse should watch for urinary retention. If necessary, the male patient may stand to void if he has not had spinal anesthesia. If the patient has undergone inguinal hernia repair, the nurse should watch for development of scrotal edema or hematoma, which may indicate slow bleeding from the operative site.

Lower Rectum and Anus

Surgery on the lower rectum and anus includes excision of pilonidal cysts, rectal fissures, rectal abscesses, tumors, and hemorrhoids. Recovery room care is the same as for any patient undergoing anesthesia, which may be spinal or general, and, in some cases, local. Dressings should be checked frequently for undue drainage and bleeding. Urinary retention may be a problem, since the proximity of the bladder and operative site may make urination difficult. Pain is exquisite, but patients are often embarrassed by the location of the operative site and may not ask for analgesia. The nurse should be alert to signs and symptoms of pain and discomfort and administer analgesia as necessary for relief.

SURGERY ON RELATED ORGANS WITHIN THE ABDOMINAL CAVITY

Liver

Surgery on the liver includes biopsy, small wedge biopsy, excision of tumors, major resection, repair of traumatic lacerations (Fig. 28–7), and, although not common, hepatic transplant.

Liver biopsy is a common procedure, usually performed at the bedside; however, occasionally a patient may be taken to the operating suite and may return to the PACU for a short period of observation. Postoperative care depends on the type of anesthesia used; it is usually local but may involve other types if the patient cannot or will not cooperate. The patient should remain positioned on the right side for 2 to 3 hours. Vital signs should be determined frequently: every 10 to 15 minutes for the first hour and every 30 minutes for the second hour. Complications include hemorrhage due to penetration of a blood vessel and peritonitis due to accidental puncture of the bile duct. If the patient's vital signs take a downward trend or if he or she complains of severe abdominal pain, the surgeon should be notified immediately.

Open surgery on the liver for the excision of tumors or the repair of lacerations is

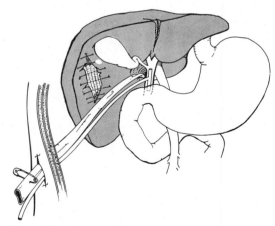

Figure 28–7. Repair of lacerated liver. (From LeMaitre, G. D., and Finnegan, J. A.: The Patient in Surgery. 3rd ed. Philadelphia, W. B. Saunders Co., 1975, p. 201.)

done under general anesthesia and involves a fairly long upper abdominal vertical incision. All care previously discussed for patients following general anesthesia and upper abdominal incisions applies. Respiratory care is of paramount importance. The liver is an extremely vascular and friable organ. It is difficult to suture, and gross bleeding is common and frequently involves large blood losses, especially when surgery is necessitated by traumatic injury. Large drains of the Penrose type are placed in the region of the laceration or excision of the tumor and are brought through the incision to the skin surface. Because of the drains, postoperative dressings will commonly be soaked with blood and bile. These should be reinforced as necessary to keep the surrounding skin dry. If bleeding becomes excessive, the surgeon should be notified to change the primary dressing and assess the patient's status.

Coagulation studies must be performed frequently and monitored closely, as many patients develop coagulation abnormalities during and after liver surgery. Specific coagulation factors may be administered, according to the results of the coagulation tests.

Vital signs must be determined frequently and any downward trend reported to the surgeon at once. Blood replacement or hemostasis may be inadequate. Frequently, this patient will also have a T tube in place in the common bile duct. This tube should be attached to straight gravity drainage, and accurate measurements of the output should be made. A nasogastric tube will be in place and should be cared for as discussed previously. Pain is usually severe, and narcotic analgesics are necessary to promote rest and respiratory effort.

Spleen

Surgery on the spleen involves general anesthesia and removal of the organ. The spleen is removed owing to rupture from trauma, to accidental trauma from associated surgery, to diseases that cause damage, such as mononucleosis and malaria, and to hypersplenism. A left upper abdominal vertical or subcostal incision is used. Postoperative care for the postsplenectomy patient is the same as that for the patient following repair of a lacerated liver. Dressings should remain dry and intact, unless a drain is placed in the subdiaphragmatic space, which may be done to prevent the collection of blood under the diaphragm and to detect unrecognized injury that may have occurred to the pancreas.

The PACU nurse should be well aware of the circumstances leading to the patient's splenectomy. If it was necessitated by trauma, the nurse must be particularly alert for signs indicating that unrecognized complications from the accident may have developed. Vital signs should be determined frequently and trends watched, especially those indicating progressive bleeding. Neurologic signs should be checked, and the patient should be assessed carefully for any signs of injury to the extremities. Any arrhythmia should be reported, as this may indicate cardiac injury.

Observe the patient carefully for abdominal distention and pain. The intestines and stomach may expand to fill the space left by removal of an enlarged spleen and cause considerable discomfort. This can be prevented by the application of an abdominal binder (bandage) and by the administration of neostigmine. The use of a binder, however, may be disadvantageous, in that it restricts respiratory effort.

Pancreas

Surgery on the pancreas is precarious. It involves general anesthesia, and care for these patients is the same as for other postoperative patients. If surgery done is to remove malignant tumors, the mortality risk is high, owing to extensive resection and poor general condition of the patient.

Postoperative care of the patient following a pancreatoduodenectomy (Whipple or modified Whipple procedure) is one of the greatest nursing challenges. All postoperative care for the abdominal surgery patient applies. Particular attention must be paid to drains and catheters. The surgeon should augment his or her report to the nurse by explaining exactly what procedure was performed, where drains or wound catheters were placed, and how to care for them. He or she should brief the nurse on expected drainage and what should be considered excessive. As with all abdominal surgery patients, intravenous lines and intravenous therapy will have already been initiated. Because of the generally low nutritional status of these patients, hyperalimentation may be started almost immediately postoperatively.

All respiratory, cardiac, and renal functioning must be monitored carefully and the surgeon notified of any untoward signs. Frequently, assisted ventilation is required for at least 24 hours following this procedure (this type of care is discussed in Chapter 18). Blood gas analysis should be performed frequently for this patient, and an arterial line should be in place for this purpose. Blood gas analysis will yield valuable information about the patient's respiratory acid/base status, which may be precarious. Urine output should be deter-

mined hourly, and at least 1 ml per kg per hour should be expected.

Frequent assays of blood glucose levels should be ordered on all patients following pancreatic surgery. Most of these patients will need to receive intravenous insulin during the postoperative period. Insulin doses are titrated to maintain the blood glucose levels between 200 and 300 mg per dl. This aids in the prevention of hypo- and hyperglycemia.

Large fluctuations in serum glucose levels or acid/base balance can precipitate electrolyte abnormalities in these patients. Potassium and calcium levels, in particular, should be monitored closely.

Biliary Tract

Surgery on the biliary tract includes exploration for removal of stones from the gallbladder and the ducts and removal of the gallbladder. Anesthesia is general, regional, or a combination of both. The incision is either a right subcostal or a right upper paramedian incision. Upon return to the PACU, the patient is placed in a semi-Fowler position. All tubes must be appropriately cared for. A nasogastric tube will

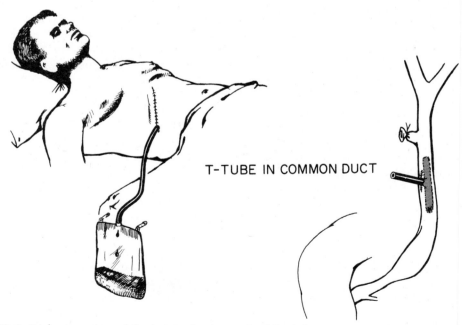

T-TUBE IN COMMON DUCT

Figure 28–8. T-tube in common bile duct, and postoperative bile drainage system. (From LeMaitre, G. D., and Finnegan, J. A.: The Patient in Surgery. 3rd ed. Philadelphia, W. B. Saunders Co., 1975, p. 188.)

be in place and should be connected to low intermittent suction and cared for as previously described. A T tube will have been placed in the common bile duct with the arms toward the hepatic duct and the duodenum (Fig. 28–8). This tube is usually connected to straight gravitational drainage. Usually, this can be accomplished conveniently by attaching a small plastic T-tube bag to the end of the tube. Careful attention must be paid to maintaining patency of this tube.

Bile drainage should be carefully measured and accurately reported. Between 200 and 500 ml of bile drainage can be expected within a 24-hour period. If more than 25 ml of bile per hour is drained, the surgeon should be notified, since this may indicate severance of the common bile duct, obstruction, or biliary fistula. Dressings should remain dry and intact, unless Penrose drains have been placed. If drains are placed, a blood bile drainage may be expected, and dressings should be reinforced as necessary to keep surrounding skin dry.

As with all upper abdominal incisions, pain is a problem, and analgesics, TENS, and relaxation exercises should be utilized to promote rest and respiratory effort. Morphine sulfate should not be used for analgesia, since it may cause biliary spasm. Any downward trend in vital signs, excessive bleeding from the incision, or bleeding noted in the bile drainage from the T tube should be reported to the surgeon. Bleeding from the cystic artery is a serious complication and can lead to rapid deterioration of the patient's status.

REFERENCES

1. Amato, E. J.: A nursing reference: gastrointestinal tubes and drains. Crit. Care Nurse, 2(6):50–57, 1982.
2. Amato, E. J.: A nursing reference: Gastrointestinal tubes and drains, Part II. Crit. Care Nurse, 3(1):46–48, 1983.
3. Given, B., and Simmons, S.: Gastroenterology in Clinical Nursing. 4th ed. St. Louis, C. V. Mosby Co. 1984.
4. McClelland, D. C.: Kock pouch: a new type of ileostomy. AORN J., 32:191–201, 1980.
5. Moss, G.: Mini-trauma cholecystectomy. Am. J. Surg., 25:66–74, 1983.
6. Patras, A. Z., and Brozenec, S. A.: Gastrointestinal assessment. AORN J., 40:726–731, 1984.
7. Salmond, S. W.: How to assess the nutritional status of acutely ill patients. Am. J. Nurs., 80:922–924, 1980.
8. Schumann, D.: How to help wound-healing in your abdominal surgery patient. Nursing '80, 10:34–40, 1980.
9. Shea, M., and McCreary, M.: Early postop feeding. Am. J. Nurs., 84(10):1230–1231, 1984.
10. Sleisenger, M. H., and Fordtran, J. S.: Gastrointestinal Disease. 2nd ed. Philadelphia, W. B. Saunders Co., 1978.
11. Smith, C. E.: Abdominal assessment: a blending of science and art. Nursing '81, 11(2):42–49, 1981.

Postoperative Care After Genitourinary Surgery

Genitourinary surgery involves procedures performed on the kidney, ureters, bladder, urethra, and male genital organs. Problems may be congenital or acquired. Adrenalectomy is included in this chapter for convenience and because of proximity of the adrenals to the kidneys.

Definitions

Cystoscopy: direct visualization of the urethra, prostatic urethra, and bladder, by means of a tubular lighted telescopic lens.

Operations on the Kidneys and Ureters

Heminephrectomy: partial excision of the kidney.

Kidney transplant: removal of a donor kidney by means of a nephrectomy and ureterectomy, followed by transplant of the donor kidney in the recipient's iliac fossa.

Nephrectomy: removal of a kidney; used to treat some congenital unilateral abnormalities causing renal obstruction or hydronephrosis; sometimes necessitated by the presence of tumors and following severe injuries.

Nephrostomy: an opening into the kidney to maintain temporary or permanent drainage.

Nephrotomy: an incision into the kidney.

Nephroureterectomy: removal of a kidney and the entire ureter that drains it.

Pyeloplasty: revision or reconstruction of the renal pelvis.

Pyelostomy: an incision into the renal pelvis to establish drainage or to permit irrigation of the renal pelvis.

Pyelotomy: incision into the renal pelvis.

Ureterectomy: complete removal of one or both of the ureters.

Ureterolithotomy: incision into the ureter and removal of stones.

Ureteroneocystostomy (ureterovesical anastomosis): division of the ureter from the urinary bladder and reimplantation of the ureter into the bladder at another site.

Ureteroplasty: reconstruction of the ureter.

Ureterostomy (cutaneous) (anastomosis of transplant; Bricker operation, ureteroileostomy): diversion of the urinary stream by anastomosing the ureters into an isolated loop of ileum which is brought out through the abdominal wall as an ileostomy (Fig. 29–1).

Operations on the Bladder

Bladder neck operation (Y-V plasty): a plastic repair of the bladder neck done to correct stricture.

Cystectomy: excision of the bladder and adjacent structures; may be partial, to

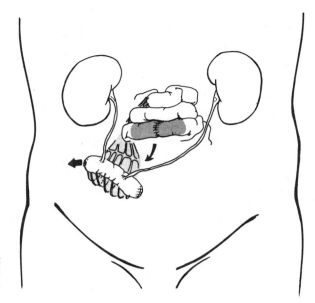

Figure 29–1. Ileal conduit, showing ileal segment with anastomosed ureters. (From LeMaitre, G. D., and Finnegan, J. A.: The Patient in Surgery. 3rd ed. Philadelphia, W. B. Saunders Co., 1975, p. 355.)

excise a lesion, or total, for excision of malignant tumors. This operation usually involves the additional procedure of ureterostomy.

Cystolithotomy: the bladder is opened to remove stones.

Cystotomy: incision into the bladder.

Vesical-urethral suspension (Marshall-Marchetti operation): suspension of the bladder neck to the posterior surface of the pubis in the female patient to treat stress incontinence.

Operations on the Prostate

Prostatectomy: enucleation of prostatic adenomas or hypertrophied masses.

Operations on the Scrotum

Epididymectomy: excision of the epididymis from the testis. This procedure is rarely done but may occasionally be indicated to treat persistent infection.

Hydrocelectomy: excision of the tunica vaginalis of the testis to remove a hydrocele (a fluid-filled sac).

Orchiectomy: removal of the testis or testes. This procedure renders the patient sterile.

Orchiopexy: suspension of the testis within the scrotum. This procedure is used to treat an undescended or cryptorchid testis to bring it into the normal intrascrotal position.

Spermatocelectomy: the removal of a spermatocele, which usually appears as a cystic mass within the scrotum, attached to the upper pole of the epididymis. A spermatocele is usually caused by an obstruction of the tubular system that conveys the sperm.

Varicocelectomy: ligation and partial excision of dilated veins in the scrotum.

Vasectomy: excision of a section of the vas deferens. This procedure is carried out electively for birth control or prior to prostatectomy to prevent the spread of infection from the urethra to the epididymis.

Disorders of and Operations on the Penis and Urethra

Chordee: downward bowing of the penis, owing to congenital malformation or to hypospadias with fibrous bands.

Circumcision: excision of the foreskin (prepuce) of the glans penis.

Epispadias: urethral meatus situated in an abnormal position on the upper side of the penis. Surgical procedure involves plastic repair.

Hypospadias: a deformity of the penis and malformation of the urethral wall in which the urinary meatus is located on the underside of the penis, either short of its normal position at the tip of the glans, or on the perineum or scrotum. This condition is often associated with chordee. Surgery involves plastic repair. Penile straightening and urethral reconstruction (urethroplasty) are usually done in two or more stages.

Phimosis: tightness of the foreskin, so that it cannot be drawn back from over the glans; also, the analogous condition in the clitoris.

Transurethral surgery: piecemeal resection of the prostate gland and of tumors of the bladder and bladder neck, and fulguration of bleeding vessels and of tumors, by means of a resectoscope passed into the bladder via the urethra.

Urethral meatotomy: incisional enlargement of the external urethral meatus done to relieve stenosis or stricture.

Operations on the Adrenal Glands

Adrenalectomy: partial or total excision of one or both adrenal glands.

GENERAL POSTOPERATIVE CARE

Assessment of the patient following genitourinary surgery involves particular attention to fluid and electrolyte balance. Intake and output records are especially important and must be accurately maintained. Postoperative care is directed primarily at maintenance of an adequate "waterway," which is second in importance only to cardiorespiratory function. Maintenance of patency of the waterway is often dependent upon the use of catheters which come in a variety of shapes and sizes (Fig. 29–2).

Urethral catheters are used to drain urine from the bladder to keep it decompressed and to measure urine output accurately. A retention catheter is used postoperatively and left in place until the patient's status is stable and the surgeon orders its removal. The catheter is attached to a sterile, closed gravitational drainage collection system. The urine collection reservoir may be a large

(usually 2000 ml) container, or a small calibrated chamber that can be emptied into a large reservoir after timed urine output volumes have been determined and recorded (Fig. 29–3).

The catheter itself should be anchored securely to the thigh with adhesive tape and the tubing brought over the leg. Loop the catheter over once before taping to prevent undue tension on the urinary meatus. Loop a rubber band around the connecting tubing, and then attach it to the bed linens with a safety pin. No proximal loops of tubing should lie below distal tubing; this is a straight gravity drainage system. Check frequently for kinks; the tubing should never be under the patient, as compression of the tubing would obstruct the flow of urine. The urine receptacle should always be kept below the bladder level to prevent urine reflux up the tubing. Particular attention must be paid to this principle when transferring patients, since attendants typically pick up the receptacle to transfer it to the new setting.

Mucus or blood, or both, can clog the tubing and prevent urine flow. Irrigations should be carried out only according to the physician's orders. All irrigations are sterile procedures. A large sterile Toomey syringe and sterile irrigating solution (usually normal saline or normal saline with a selected antibiotic) are used. Care must be taken to keep all parts of the drainage system sterile. This may be accomplished by placing a small sterile plastic cover on the drainage tubing while performing the irrigation. Irrigations should never be given under pressure, and when irrigating the bladder, no more than 30 ml should be instilled at one time, unless ordered otherwise by the physician.

To obtain a urine specimen from the closed system, use a sterile syringe and needle. Some catheters have a small, specially constructed spot from which to draw specimens. On those that do not, use the distal part of the catheter, close to the drainage tubing. Cleanse the area with alcohol or povidone-iodine preparation (Betadine), insert the needle, and withdraw a specimen.

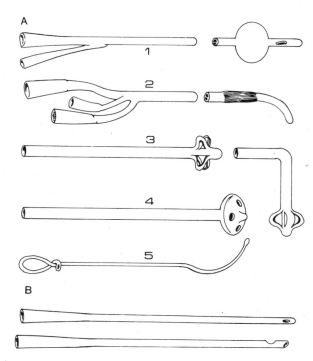

Figure 29–2. *A*, Self-retaining catheters: (1) the Foley catheter, (2) three-way Foley catheter, (3) Malecot catheter, (4) Pezzer catheter. The self-retaining protuberance at the tip of the Malecot and Pezzer must be elongated with a stylet (5), which is passive through the lumen before insertion. After insertion, the stylet is removed and the protuberance secures the catheter in place. *B*, Straight catheters. The straight catheter may have a single eye or many eyes; it may hve a round tip or a whistle tip. These catheters are not self-retaining and must be secured with adhesive tape when being used as indwelling tubes. (From Whitehead, S.: Nursing care of the Adult Urology Patient. New York, Appleton-Century-Crofts, 1970.)

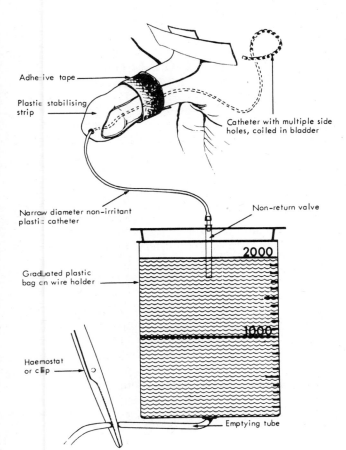

Figure 29–3. Closed drainage of the bladder. (From Douglas, A.P., and Kerr, D. S.: A Short Textbook of Kidney Disease, London, Pitman Medical Publishing Co., Ltd., 1968.)

Ureteral Catheters

Ureteral catheters are used to drain urine or to splint the ureters while they heal. They may be placed through the urethra or through abdominal or flank incisions. Care of these catheters is essentially the same as that for urethral catheters. Attention to patency must be especially scrupulous, since the renal pelvis can hold only 5 ml without becoming overly distended and causing damage to the kidneys.

Sterile irrigations are undertaken only under physicians' orders. Only 5 ml of fluid should be used for the irrigation via gravitational flow. Irrigations should never be given under pressure, such as with a syringe and plunger. The nurse must be sure that situations that could cause dislodgment or displacement of these catheters are avoided, as this could be disastrous to the outcome of the surgery. Special care must be taken when transferring the patient to ensure that these catheters stay in place. It is wise to assign this particular duty to one person while the patient is being transferred. If the catheters should become dislodged in spite of all the precautions taken, the surgeon must be notified immediately.

Intake

Optimal fluid intake is exceptionally important for this patient postoperatively; increased fluids are the general rule. If the patient can tolerate oral fluids, they should be given by this preferred route, and intake should be increased to total 3000 ml in a 24-hour period. Parenteral fluid therapy is indicated for a short time until the effects of anesthesia have passed, and it is continued only if the oral route of intake is inadequate.

Dressings

Care of dressings will vary according to the procedure. Dressings following urinary tract surgery often become soaked with blood and urine. They should be reinforced as necessary, and surrounding skin should be kept clean and dry to prevent unnecessary excoriation and breakdown. (If excessive staining is unexpected for a particular procedure and indicates a complication, it will be so indicated in the discussion of the specific procedure.) Excessive bleeding and hemorrhage are ever-present dangers of this surgery, since the kidneys and prostatic bed are extremely vascular. Vital signs must be monitored closely, and all avenues of output, especially the incisions and drainage tubes, should be evaluated frequently for bleeding.

Abdominal Distention

All patients should be assessed for abdominal distention following surgery involving abdominal and flank incisions. The reader might wish to refer to Chapter 28 for care of the patient following an abdominal incision, as the same care applies following genitourinary surgery. Frequently, these patients return with a nasogastric tube, which is cared for as discussed in Chapter 28. In addition, the patient should be assessed for distention due to overfilling of the bladder because of inability to void or malfunction of catheters.

NURSING CARE AFTER DIAGNOSTIC TESTS

Several invasive diagnostic procedures are used for patients with genitourinary disease. If general anesthesia is required, they are commonly received in the PACU for a short period of observation.

Renal Angiography

For a renal angiogram, a small catheter is threaded through the femoral artery into the aorta or renal artery; radiopaque dye is instilled, and x-rays are taken. Local anesthesia is usually all that is needed; however, general anesthesia may be used for children or patients who cannot cooperate during the procedure. When the patient returns to the PACU, check the groin area for bleeding. A pressure type of dressing will usually be present and may be replaced by a simple bandage after a few hours. Pedal pulses should be checked to ensure that no interruption of blood supply to the extremities has occurred. If possible, the leg should be kept straight.

Renal Biopsy

Renal biopsy is usually performed at the bedside with only local anesthesia, although general anesthesia may be used for children. The patient should be kept at bedrest in a prone position for at least one hour afterwards and the site of biopsy checked for bleeding. Fluids should be increased to 3000 ml daily, and the urine should be observed for occult blood.

Cystoscopy

Cystoscopy may be performed in a special procedures room with only local anesthesia and appropriate sedation. Children and patients who cannot or will not cooperate during the procedure may need general anesthesia. This procedure may also be performed under spinal anesthesia. It may be performed simply for diagnosis, or it may be used for treatment, such as resection of tumors, removal of stones and foreign bodies, or dilation of the ureters.

Upon return to the PACU the patient is placed in a side-lying position if general anesthesia was used or flat on his back if a spinal anesthesia was used. After the effects of anesthesia have been eliminated, the patient may assume a position of comfort. The patient may complain of back pain, a feeling of bladder fullness, and bladder spasms. These symptoms may become severe enough to require analgesia, in which case the agent of choice is codeine.

Fluids should be increased and started as soon as the effects of anesthesia are gone. Urine output should be checked carefully. The patient can expect frequency of urination and a burning sensation due to trauma to the mucous membranes from the procedure, which may inadvertently cause voluntary retention. The urine may be pink-tinged for several voidings; this is to be expected. Bright blood or clots in the urine, however, should be reported to the surgeon. If the patient complains of severe abdominal pain, this should be reported, as it may indicate accidental perforation of the ureters or internal hemorrhage.

NURSING CARE AFTER SPECIFIC PROCEDURES

Operations on the Kidneys and Ureters

Procedures on the kidneys and ureters involve excision of tumors and obstructions to urine flow (such as stones), reconstruction of urine outflow tracts, repair of lacerations, correction of deformities, excision of a kidney, and total organ transplant.

Anesthesia is almost always general for surgery on the kidneys and ureters. The kidneys are usually approached posteriorly through an incision that requires resection of the eleventh or twelfth rib. The surgical approach to the ureters is usually made through muscle-splitting flank incisions (Fig. 29–4). The recovery room course for these patients is usually smooth and involves general care for the post anesthesia patient and maintenance of the waterway. The patient should be placed in a position that avoids tension on suture lines or as indicated by the surgeon.

Exceptionally accurate intake and output records must be maintained. Low urine output should be reported to the surgeon.

Dressings should remain dry and intact unless drains are used, in which case dressings should be weighed when they are removed to determine output via this route. When determining output from the dressings, weigh the dressings before applying and then when removing, and subtract the difference. One gm equals 1 ml of output. Patients with drains or stomas may require the use of a small plastic bag over the area for collection of drainage that will consist primarily of urine. Drainage bags should be emptied frequently; if allowed to fill to capacity, the continual flow of urine will be interrupted.

Skin care for these patients is very important. Urine should not be allowed to remain on the skin. Plain water should be

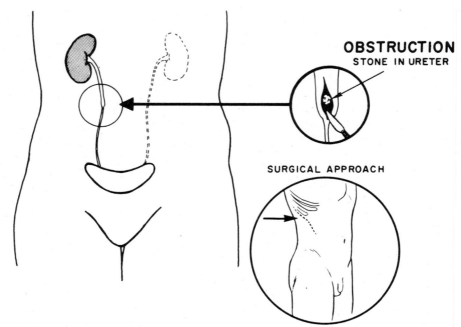

Figure 29–4. Right hydroureter due to obstructing calculus. Inset shows incision in ureter for removal of stone. (From LeMaitre, G. D., and Finnegan, J. A.: The Patient in Surgery. 3rd ed. Philadelphia, W. B. Saunders Co., 1975, p. 341.)

used to cleanse the skin, and it should be carefully dried. No powders, lotions, or harsh skin preparations should be applied to the skin. If a ureteroileostomy has been performed, the stoma must be inspected frequently to ensure adequate vascularization. If it turns a bluish hue, the surgeon should be notified immediately.

A Foley catheter is generally in place and is cared for as previously discussed. Fluid intake is increased both orally and parenterally to keep blood clots from forming in the ureters or bladder. Intestinal decompression may be necessary and is accomplished by nasogastric tube (see Chapter 28). This is essential when an ileal conduit procedure (ureterostomy) is performed to allow healing of the intestinal anastomosis. Any evidence of abdominal distention should be reported to the surgeon at once.

Kidney Transplantation

The kidney is the most frequently transplanted organ and the only one that can be preserved in a viable state for some time (Fig. 29–5). The kidney is relatively easy to remove and implant. Most people have two functioning kidneys and need only one to sustain life; therefore, kidney transplant is done only for patients who need the organ to replace a diseased or nonfunctioning solitary kidney. Tranplantation can be accomplished two, three, or even more times in the same patient with the use of hemodialysis when a functioning kidney is not in place.

Many kidney grafts come from cadaver donors. Some, however, come from live donors, usually a blood relative of the recipient. The closer the recipient and donor in blood line, the better the chances for survival of the kidney graft. Postoperatively, the donor is usually the forgotton member. His care is essentially the same as for the patient who has had a single kidney removed. All care considered previously for the urologic patient applies, as does care for the patient following abdominal incision. Because postoperative care is routine, this patient often feels a lack of self-esteem. Before surgery he was the hero and got a generous helping of attention and glory, whereas postoperatively, attention is directed primarily to the organ recipient. The donor patient feels this, even in the PACU. For this reason, it is extremely important that the PACU nurse be aware of the needs of the postoperative donor and demonstrate concerned care for his or her physical and psychologic well-being. It is wise to assign the care of these patients to separate teams. In addition to normal self-concern, the donor will be concerned about the recipient and should receive factual information.

General anesthesia is used for both the donor and the recipient in kidney transplantation. If possible, these patients should be placed in a reverse or protective isolation room with all protective isolation measures instituted. Many PACUs do not have protective isolation capabilities, and therefore these patients are returned directly from the operating suite to the surgical intensive care unit where protective isolation can be instituted.

Protective isolation is necessary because these patients are placed on immunosuppressive therapy, which reduces the white blood count. The commonly used immunosuppressive agents, including azathioprine (Imuran), cyclophosphamide (Cytoxan), and cyclosporine (Sandimmune), are nonspecific and suppress the entire immune system. It is therefore imperative that meticulous aseptic technique be used when handling these patients to prevent the introduction of infection.

Upon return to the PACU, the recipient should be kept in a flat position for 12 hours to allow the kidney to "set." The head of the bed may be elevated 30 degrees for comfort and respiratory care. After 12 hours the patient may turn to the side of the transplant. Turning to the opposite side may dislodge the graft.

All vital signs are monitored continuously. A Foley catheter is in place and all urine should be carefully monitored for volume and specific gravity. The kidney from

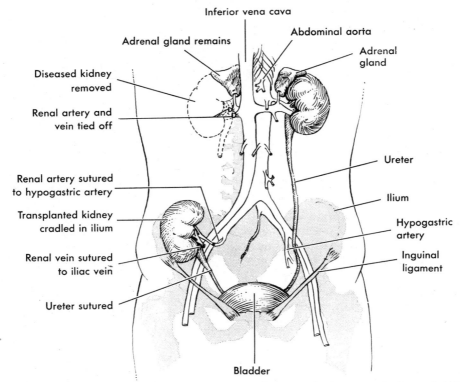

Figure 29–5. Transplanted kidney in place. (From Samartino and Preston: In Bergerson, B. S., et al. (eds): Current Concepts in Clinical Nursing. St. Louis, C. V. Mosby Co., 1967.)

a living donor may start to function almost immediately after tranplant, and diuresis will occur. The volume of urine output may be great enough to warrant measurement every 15 minutes. The cadaver kidney, on the other hand, will react more slowly, depending upon the cold ischemic time spent during transportation.

Urine samples are generally sent hourly to ascertain electrolyte content, creatinine level, and osmolarity. Once daily, the total 24-hour urine collection (minus the small samples sent hourly) is sent for creatinine clearance test and culture. Urine output less than 1 ml per kg per hour should be reported to the surgeon, since any decrease in urine output may be a sign of early rejection. A baseline weight postoperatively should be ascertained as soon as feasible.

A nasogastric tube will provide intestinal decompression and is cared for as previously discussed.

A central venous pressure (CVP) line will be present to further assess the patient's cardiovascular status.

Dressings cover the flank incision. Small plastic bags may be used to collect urine from the ureterostomy and cystostomy. Because all output must be carefully measured, all dressings that are removed are weighed to determine output.

Intravenous fluids provide the majority of intake for these patients until the nasogastric tube can be removed. Intravenous replacement fluid composition is determined by serum and urine electrolyte content, hematocrit, and the clinical course of the patient. Volume is determined from necessary fluid requirements of the patient in normal status plus replacement on a volume-to-volume basis from drainage from the Foley catheter, nasogastric tube, ureterostomy, and cystostomy. For the first 72 hours after operation, the major source of output will be from the ureterostomy. Meticulous handling of the closed urinary drainage system is mandatory to prevent the introduction of infection.

Vigorous pulmonary toilet should be instituted immediately to prevent atelectasis. The patient may be turned to the side of the kidney graft and back every half hour to provide for change of position. The painful flank incision can be splinted either with the nurse's hands or with a firm pillow or a rolled blanket to assist the patient with efforts to cough.

The threat of graft rejection is ever-present and it must be observed for closely. Hyperacute allograft rejection can occur within minutes of the completion of the vascular anastomosis or in the first few hours postoperatively. Signs and symptoms of hyperacute rejection are noted in Table 29–1. It is of utmost importance to treat a threatened rejection as soon as it appears, in order to prevent irreversible damage to the kidney.

The postoperative kidney transplant patient is usually transferred to the surgical intensive care unit for several days following surgery for close observation and intensive care.

Operations on the Bladder

The bladder is a smooth-muscle storage tank that holds urine until a reflex, normally under voluntary control, releases the urine to pass through the urethra to be eliminated. Surgery on the bladder includes removal of stones, foreign bodies, and tumors; repair of strictures at the bladder neck; repair of injuries, such as lacerations; and removal of the bladder.

Anesthesia for these procedures may be either spinal or general. Upon return to the

TABLE 29–1. Signs and Symptoms of Allograft Rejection

Irritability on the part of the patient
Anxiousness
Restlessness
Lethargy
Swollen, tender kidney
Decreased urine output
Fever; may be low grade
Increased blood pressure
Weight gain
Anorexia
Increased BUN and serum creatinine
Decreased creatinine clearance
Increased urine protein and lysosyme activity
Lymphocytes in the urine

PACU, the patient is placed in a supine position. The head of the bed may be raised 30 degrees as soon as feasible. The removal of stones or foreign bodies and the resection of selected tumors may be accomplished via cystoscopy, which has already been discussed. After the repair of lacerations or after cystotomy to remove stones, the patient will return to the PACU with a Foley catheter in place, and a urinary diversion such as a suprapubic cystostomy will usually be in place. Urine from these drainage systems will be pink-tinged but should not become grossly bloody. Dressings should remain dry and intact, fluids should be increased, and oral fluids should be started as soon as the effects of anesthesia have passed.

Lacerations or ruptures of the bladder are often the result of accidental trauma; they require emergency surgery, and the postoperative patient should be assessed carefully for any unrecognized associated injuries. Pain should be minimal for these patients and easily controlled with mild analgesics. If severe pain is present, it may represent a complication, such as internal hemorrhage or damage to a ureter, and should be reported to the surgeon.

Cystectomy requires the construction of an ileal conduit. Care for an ileal conduit was discussed in the section on surgery on the ureters.

Operations on the Prostate

The prostate is a small, walnut-sized male reproductive organ. Its sole function is to manufacture a secretion that becomes part of the semen; it is a nonessential organ. Surgery on the prostate gland includes excision of tumors, resection of the gland, or total removal of the gland.

Anesthesia may be general or spinal. Several different approaches are common in surgery on the prostate. Most frequently, the *transurethral approach* is used, especially if only minor obstructive lesions or small portions of the gland are to be removed. A resectoscope is introduced through the urethra, and the surgeon excises the tissue with a moveable tungsten wire, which operates on high frequency current controlled with a foot pedal.

When the patient returns to the PACU after transurethral resection of the prostate (TUR or TURP), a three-way Foley catheter will be in place (Fig. 29-2A). One lumen allows filling of the retention balloon, one lumen allows outflow of the urine and irrigation fluid from the bladder, and one lumen is attached to the irrigation fluid system. Irrigation fluid, which is usually room temperature normal saline, comes in 2000 ml plastic bags, and it may be regulated like intravenous solutions. The three-lumen catheter is advantageous in that blood clots do not regularly form and block the system when the flow is continuous. The irrigation rate should be regulated so that drainage remains a light pink, watermelon color. If drainage becomes bright bloody, speed up the irrigation; if returns are clear, slow the irrigation down. Some institutions utilize a Y-connecting system with one arm of the Y connected to the irrigating fluid and the other to straight gravitational drainage from the bladder. In either case, a fair amount of bleeding can be expected following TURP, since the prostatic bed is so highly vascular.

If the catheter becomes clogged, it may be necessary to irrigate it with a piston syringe using the same normal saline irrigating solution. If patency of the catheter cannot be reestablished, the surgeon must be notified.

The patient's vital signs should be monitored closely. Observe for signs and symptoms of hyponatremia or fluid overload that may occur as a result of venous absorption of the irrigation fluid through the vascular bed of the prostate gland. Serum sodium and potassium levels should be checked during the postoperative period, as changes in fluid balance may affect these electrolytes. Oral fluids should be started and increased as tolerated as soon as possible. Diet may be progressed as tolerated.

Pain should be minimal and easily controlled with mild analgesics. Analgesics or tranquilizers may be administered to control the discomfort of bladder spasms and the

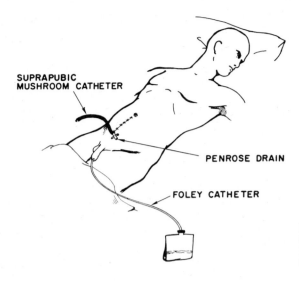

SUPRAPUBIC
MUSHROOM CATHETER

PENROSE DRAIN

FOLEY CATHETER

Figure 29–6. Postoperative positions of drainage tubes following suprapubic prostatectomy. (From LeMaitre, G. D., and Finnegan, J. A.: The Patient in Surgery. 3rd ed. Philadephia, W. B. Saunders Co., 1975, p. 347.)

presence of the catheter, which makes the patient feel an urgency to void even though the bladder is being emptied. Complaints of abdominal pain, abdominal rigidity, a rise in pulse rate, and other signs of shock should alert the nurse to the possibility that the bladder wall or the capsule of the prostate was accidentally perforated during surgery; these symptoms should be reported to the surgeon at once.

Other approaches to prostatic surgery include the retrograde or suprapubic incision, perineal incision, and retropubic incision. When the *suprapubic approach* is used, a midline vertical incision is made in the lowest part of the abdomen, then the bladder is incised, and the tumors are removed. This is the procedure of choice when 60 gm or more of tissue are to be removed. The patient will return to the PACU with a Foley catheter in place that may or may not be attached to an irrigation system. If not connected to an irrigation system, the catheter will have to be irrigated frequently with a syringe to prevent clots from clogging the drainage system. The patient will also have a suprapubic catheter in place that should be connected to straight gravitational drainage, and output should be measured carefully (Fig. 29–6). In addition, a small Penrose drain is inserted in the suprapubic space and brought out through the incision. A dressing of several layers of 4 × 4 gauze

should cover the incision and the drain. A moderate amount of serosanguineous drainage can be expected owing to the presence of the drain. This dressing should be reinforced as necessary to keep the skin clean and dry. If excessive bright red bleeding occurs, the surgeon must be notified.

The surgeon may apply traction to the Foley catheter by taping the catheter to the inner thigh. This puts tension against the vesicle outlet and promotes hemostasis. This traction may produce painful bladder spasms that may be relieved by the use of codeine. After traction is removed, a small increase in bleeding may be expected for a short time.

The *perineal approach*, used for removal of large amounts of tissue, is the approach of choice for prostatic cancer. A V-shaped incision is made above the rectum in this approach. The patient will return to the PACU with a Foley catheter and a perineal drain in place. Because of the perineal drain, a moderate amount of serosanguineous drainage can be expected, and the dressing should be reinforced as necessary.

When a *retropubic approach* is used, a small incision is made above the pubis, and a capsular incision is made into the upper surface of the prostate. A Foley catheter will be in place, and a small drain will have been inserted in the incision.

As with all urologic patients, accurate

intake and output records must be maintained following prostatic surgery. The nurse must be sure to indicate whether or not irrigation solution is included in the output.

Most prostatic surgery is performed on adult males over the age of 50, since prostatic hypertrophy is most common after 40 years of age. Therefore, assessment of cardiorespiratory status should be frequent. Astute observation of vital signs is imperative to monitor cardiovascular function, because it may be impaired by postoperative bleeding. Watch carefully for decreasing blood pressure and rising pulse, which may indicate impending shock.

Operations on the Scrotum

The scrotum is a sac separated into two pouches, externally by the median raphe and internally by the dartos tunic. Each pouch contains a testis, epididymis, and spermatic cord. The vas deferens, which is continuous with the epididymis at the lower end of the testis, together with the arteries, veins, nerves, and lymphatic vessels held together by spermatic fascia, forms the spermatic cord. Operations on the scrotum include excision of masses and tumors, correction of deformities, and excision of diseased or abnormal structures that interfere with normal function.

Anesthesia for surgery on the scrotum may be general or spinal. Spinal anesthesia is commonly used for adult patients, while general anesthesia is usually preferred for children under 12 years. Occasionally, only local anesthesia is required, as for vasectomy and epididymectomy.

The PACU course following surgery on the scrotal structures is usually smooth and uneventful. Care is dictated primarily by the agent of anesthesia and its method of administration. Postoperatively, the patient may assume a position of comfort. Any dressings present should remain dry and intact. Oral food and fluids may be reinstituted as soon as tolerated by the patient. Commonly, a Bellevue bridge is applied to provide scrotal support and elevation (Fig.

29–7). This device is suspended from thigh to thigh with a tight sling across the expanse, upon which the scrotum is supported. A T binder may also be used (Fig. 29–8).

The application of a *light* crushed-ice bag helps to relieve scrotal edema, enhances hemostasis, and promotes comfort. Pain should be minimal following these procedures and easily controlled by mild analgesics. Complaints of severe pain not controlled with mild analgesia should be reported to the surgeon.

As with any genital surgery, the patient's body image concerns and particularly questions of fertility may be of paramount importance. These concerns are not usually addressed in the PACU, but the nurse must be sensitive to them and prepared to assist the patient with factual information and reassurance should they arise. Often, these patients feel an urgency to inspect the operative site and should be assisted, if necessary, to do so.

The patient may be embarrassed by this type of surgery and reluctant to ask the nurse for assistance or to complain of pain, and he may hesitate to allow the nurse to inspect the incision area. A matter-of-fact attitude on the part of the nurse and efficient care promote a sense of well-being for

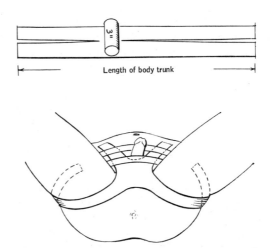

Figure 29–7. Bellevue bridge for scrotal support. (From Sutton, A. L.: Bedside Nursing Techniques in Medicine and Surgery. 2nd ed. Philadelphia, W. B. Saunders Co., 1969, p. 278.)

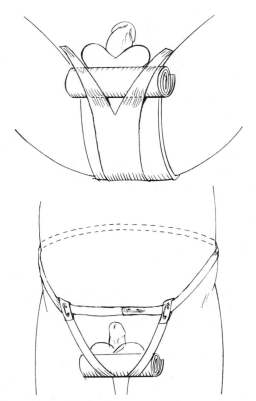

Figure 29–8. T-binder for scrotal support. (From Sutton, A. L.: Bedside Nursing Techniques in Medicine and Surgery. 2nd ed. Philadelphia, W. B. Saunders Co., 1969, p. 277.)

the patient and may help alleviate these feelings. The nurse should keep in mind that boys in the preteen and teenage group are especially sensitive about the genital area. If at all possible, a male nurse should be assigned to these patients to alleviate their anxiety.

Operations on the Penis and Urethra

Operations on the penis and urethra involve removal of tumors or obstructons to urinary flow, plastic repair of deformities, and circumsicion or excison of the foreskin. Rarely, partial or total amputation of the penis is necessary for malignancy, which is essentially skin cancer.

Anesthesia for these procedures is general or spinal. The PACU course is usually smooth, and care is determined primarily by the type of anesthesia used. Physical care for the patient who has had a plastic repair of hypospadias or epispadias will be dictated by the surgeon. Care for the patient following cystoscopy was discussed at the beginning of this chapter; the same care applies for patients undergoing cystoscopy for the resection of tumors.

Following circumcision, which may be performed for correction of phimosis or for elective reasons, the nurse should check for bleeding. Usually, only a small band of vaseline-impregnated gauze is applied as a dressing around the glans. This should be changed as directed. Bleeding that soaks this dressing is excessive and should be reported.

Patients who have undergone surgery on the penis should avoid erection during the PACU phase and at least a week postoperatively. Pain may be significant but should not be severe. Scrotal and penile support with a Bellevue bridge and the application of a light ice pack will provide some relief; however, analgesia with small doses of narcotics may be necessary. Food and fluids may be restarted as soon as tolerated by the patient. Urine output should be checked and recorded. Check for low abdominal distention, which may be due to voluntary retention. This is not uncommon, owing to fear that micturition will create pain.

Adrenalectomy

Adrenalectomy involves the removal of one or both of the adrenal glands, which are situated on top of the kidneys. Adrenalectomy, which is an extensive and shock-producing procedure, may be performed for several reasons, including metastasized cancer from the reproductive organs, hyperfunction due to hyperplasia of the organ, or hyperfunction caused by adrenal tumors. Two adrenal tumors are of major consequence; pheochromocytoma, a usually benign tumor that causes hyperfunction resulting in severe symptoms, and neuroblastoma, a malignant tumor that is a major cause of childhood death.

General anesthesia is used for adrenalectomy and may include the use of cortisone titrated to maintain catecholamine levels and blood pressure. Cortisone is usually necessary only when bilateral adrenalectomies are performed or when the uninvolved adrenal gland has poor function. The administration of cortisone, which is continued in the recovery room, is an extremely important nursing procedure. Specific instructions should be given by the anesthesiologist and surgeon as to titration of the solution. Failure to maintain postoperative levels of cortisone leads to hypovolemic and hyponatremic shock. Postoperative care of these patients is a real nursing challenge—observations must be especially astute.

The surgical approach for adrenalectomy may be either anterior or posterior. In either case, drains are placed through the bilateral incisions upon closure. Upon return to the PACU, the patient is placed in the side-lying position until reactive from anesthesia, at which time he or she is placed in a semi-Fowler's position. Assessment is aimed primarily at the cardiovascular status of this patient, since hemorrhage and shock are the two most common and most disastrous complications. Profound shock may develop, owing to the reduction of circulating catecholamines precipitated by removal of the glands as well as to the effects of the drugs used preoperatively for the control of hypertension. The effects of these drugs usually last for a few hours after surgery. Because most of these drugs produce vasodilation, they are usually a factor in postoperative hypotension. Therefore, a fluid challenge will usually be given in an attempt to treat hypotension. If fluid is not successful in increasing the blood pressure, then vasoactive drugs will be utilized. Norepinephrine in an intravenous solution may be titrated to maintain blood pressure, according to the surgeon's instructions.

Shock may also result from hemorrhage.

The adrenal glands are extremely vascular. Intravenous fluids, including hypertonic saline solutions, blood, plasma, dextran, and glucose in water, may be used to maintain blood volume and prevent shock. Dressings over the bilateral incisions should remain relatively dry even though drains are placed. If these dressings become soaked, the surgeon should be notified, since this represents excessive bleeding. If the patient complains of abdominal pain, abdominal distention, nausea, or vomiting, development of abdominal hematoma may be indicated; these signs should be reported to the surgeon.

Other parameters of the patient's status that may give clues to the development of shock should also be assessed. Dehydration (increased urine specific gravity) and restlessness may indicate developing shock. Central venous pressure should be checked. A Foley catheter will be in place, and urine output should be monitored hourly. The development of oliguria or output of less than 1 ml per kg per hour may indicate shock and subsequent renal shutdown. Serum and urine electrolyte levels, especially sodium, should be determined hourly.

All care outlined for the patient following high abdominal incisions in Chapter 28 is applicable to this patient. Good pulmonary toilet should be instituted immediately in the PACU. A nasogastric tube is frequently required until normal intestinal peristalsis returns. Incisional pain may require the use of narcotic analgesics. Since many narcotics have a hypotensive effect, they should be used judiciously, and blood pressure must be monitored continuously for at least 30 minutes after their administration.

The patient is frequently placed in protective isolation to avoid the introduction of infection. Meticulous sterile technique must be used when changing or reinforcing dressings. Because of their extreme lability, which lasts for approximately 48 hours, these patients should be transferred to the surgical intensive care unit for continued monitoring.

REFERENCES

1. Camunas, C.: Pheochromocytoma. Am. J. Nurs., *83*(6):887–891, 1983.
2. Gradus, D. and Ettenger, R. B.: Renal transplantation in children. Pediatr. Clin. North Am., *29*(4):1013–1038, 1982.
3. Hemstreet, G., Bailey, M., and Pegram, S.: Postoperative care of the urologic patient. Curr. Rev. Recov. Room Nurses, *17*(1):131–135, 1980.
4. McConnell, E. A., and Zimmerman, M. F.: Care of Patients with Urologic Problems. Philadelphia, J. B. Lippincott Co., 1982.
5. Rees, P. L.: Nursing assessment in follow-up care of the renal transplant recipient. Nephrol. Nurse, 2:47–50, 1980.
6. Stewart, B. H.: Operative Urology: Lower Urinary Tract, Pelvic Structures and Male Reproductive System. Baltimore, Williams & Wilkins, 1982.
7. Stillman, M. J.: Pre- and post-op care of a kidney donor: What you need to know. RN, 42:59–76, 1979.

CHAPTER

30

Postoperative Care After Obstetric and Gynecologic Surgery

Surgery on organs of reproduction most commonly involves an adult patient. The PACU nurse, however, may encounter pediatric or adolescent female patients undergoing gynecologic surgery for repair or correction of congenital or traumatic deformities. Surgery on the female genital organs may be conveniently divided into three major categories: (1) obstetric surgery, (2) lower genital operations and vaginal surgery, and (3) upper genital and abdominal surgery.

Definitions

Obstetric Surgery

Cesarean hysterectomy: incision of the abdomen and the uterus, extraction of the baby and the placenta, and performance of a hysterectomy.

Cesarean section (C-section): delivery of an infant through an incision made in the abdominal and the uterine walls.

C-section, classic: a midline inision between the umbilicus and symphysis pubis and an anterior incision through the uterine walls.

C-section, low segment: an incision in the lower part of the uterus made after the abdominal incision.

Ectopic pregnancy: implantation of the fertilized ovum in any site other than the upper half of the uterus (Fig. 30–1).

McDonald (Shirodkar) operation: the placement of a pursestring suture or collar-type ligature on the cervix at the level of the internal os to maintain closure.

Uterine aspiration (suction curettage): the dilatation of the cervix and the vacuum removal of the uterine contents.

Lower Genital and Vaginal Surgery

Bartholin duct cyst: a cyst that results from chronic inflammation of one of the major vestibular glands at the vaginal introitus (Fig. 30–2).

Bartholinectomy: removal of a Bartholin cyst.

Colporrhaphy: repair of the vaginal wall. May be anterior, as for cystocele repair, or posterior, as for rectocele repair.

Culdoscopy: an operative diagnostic procedure in which an incision is made into the posterior vaginal cul-de-sac, through which a tubular instrument similar to a cystoscope is inserted for the purpose of visualizing the pelvic structures, including the uterus, fallopian tubes, broad lig-

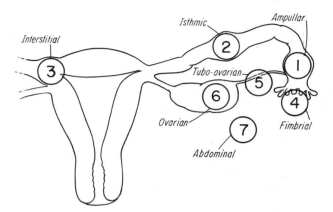

Figure 30–1. Ectopic pregnancy. Diagram shows the various implantation sites, numbered in order of decreasing frequency of occurrence. (From Sabiston, D. C. [ed.]: Textbook of Surgery. 11th ed. Philadelphia, W. B. Saunders Co., 1977, p. 1715.)

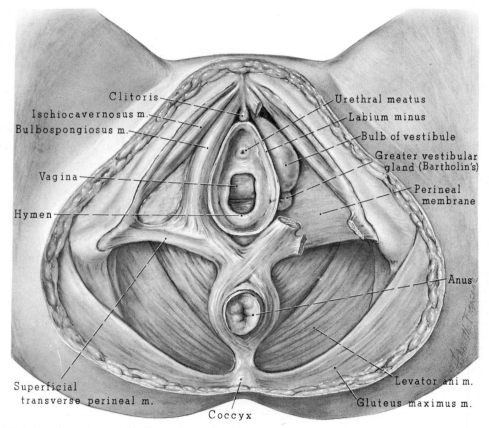

Figure 30–2. Female perineum with skin and superficial fascia removed. (From Jacob, S. W., Francone, C. A., and Lossow, W. J.: Structure and Function in Man. 4th ed. Philadelphia, W. B. Saunders Co., 1978, p. 548.)

ments, uterosacral ligaments, rectal wall, sigmoid colon, and, sometimes, the small intestines.

Cystocele: prolapse of the bladder into the anterior vaginal wall.

Dilatation of the cervix and curretage of the uterus (D&C): introduction of instruments (dilators) through the vagina into the cervical canal, and scraping of the uterus to remove substances including blood. This procedure is used for diagnostic purposes, as well as for treating conditions such as incomplete abortion, abnormal uterine bleeding, or primary dysmenorrhea.

Enterocele: prolapse of intestine into the pouch of Douglas.

Hysterectomy: removal of the uterus.

Procidentia: herniation of the uterus beyond the introitus.

Prolapse of the uterus: downward displacement of the uterus. Vaginal hysterectomy is often recommended for a prolapsed uterus when childbearing is no longer desired or when marked prolapse is present.

Rectocele: prolapse of the rectum into the posterior vaginal wall.

Trachelorrhaphy: removal of torn surfaces of the anterior and posterior cervical lips and reconstruction of the cervical canal.

Urethrocele: prolapse of the urethra into the anterior vaginal wall.

Vaginal plastic operation (anterior and posterior [A&P] repair): reconstruction of the vaginal walls (colporrhaphy), the pelvic floor, and the muscles and fascia of the rectum, urethra, bladder, and perineum. Used to correct cystocele or rectocele, restore the bladder to its normal position, and strengthen the vagina and the pelvic floor.

Abdominal Gynecologic Surgery

Abdominal myomectomy: removal of fibromyomas.

Laparoscopy (peritoneoscopy, celioscopy): endoscopic visualization of the peritoneal cavity through a small incision of the anterior abdominal wall after the establishment of a pneumoperitoneum.

Oophorectomy: removal of an ovary.

Oophorocystectomy: removal of a cyst on the ovary.

Salpingo-oophorectomy: removal of fallopian tube and all or part of the associated ovary.

Salpingostomy (tubal plasty): removal of the obstructed portion of the fallopian tube, and suspension of the remaining portion from the side of the pelvic wall or placement of it into the uterine cavity.

Total abdominal hysterectomy (panhysterectomy): removal of the uterus, including the corpus and the cervix, with or without the adnexa, through an abdominal incision.

Tubal ligation: interruption of fallopian tube continuity resulting in sterilization. The most commonly used technique is the *Pomeroy procedure*, which is done through a laparoscope. A segment of the fallopian tube is ligated and excised. Reversal procedures are now being performed with microsurgery.

OBSTETRIC SURGERY

Obstetric surgery involves procedures in pregnant women to promote full-term pregnancy, to provide an alternative means of delivery when normal vaginal delivery is not feasible for reasons of either fetal or maternal well-being, and to interrupt pregnancy.

Care After Specific Procedures

Cesarean Section

The incidence of cesarean sections performed both on an emergency and on an elective basis has nearly tripled in the United States.* These patients have very special physical and psychologic needs. An extensive reference list is included at the end of this chapter to assist the reader who cares for families experiencing cesarean birth.

---

*National Institutes of Health Consensus Development Conference Summary. Caesarean childbirth. DHEW 3(6), 1980.

Cesarean sections are indicated for dystocia (usually due to cephalopelvic disproportion); antepartum bleeding; some cases of toxemia; certain medical complications, especially diabetes mellitus; and previous cesarean section. The low segment C-section is usually the procedure of choice. Anesthesia may be general inhalational, spinal, or local infiltration of the operative field.

Postoperative care following cesarean section includes all care rendered to a patient undergoing abdominal surgery as well as post-partum care.

Upon return to the PACU, the patient should be placed in the side-lying position. As soon as her condition permits, she can assume any position of comfort.

Parenteral fluids are usually administered during the first 24 hours postoperatively, but oral fluids can usually be resumed as soon as the patient desires. Intravenous fluids often contain pitocin and should be administered very carefully. A progressive diet is advised, pending the return of bowel sounds.

The patient will have an abdominal dressing as well as a perineal pad; both should be inspected for drainage. The abdominal dressing should remain dry and intact. A moderate amount of lochia rubra is normal. Saturation of two or more perineal pads with blood during the first hour should be considered excessive. The area underneath the buttocks should be checked for pooling of blood.

The fundus should be checked frequently to ensure that it is firmly contracted. This is an uncomfortable procedure for the patient, and therefore its importance should be carefully explained before proceeding. The patient should be encouraged to relax her abdominal muscles as much as possible. Instructing her to take slow, deep breaths with her mouth open will facilitate relaxation of those muscles. If the uterus is firmly contracted, it need not be massaged, and in fact should not be, since this may cause uterine muscle fatigue and subsequent relaxation and bleeding. If the uterus is soft and "boggy," it should be gently but firmly massaged through the abdominal wall to stimulate contraction. The patient may be instructed to do this herself under supervision, which may allay anxiety and be less uncomfortable for her. Frequently, oxytocic drugs are administered intravenously and titrated to maintain the uterus in a state of contraction. If oxytocics are employed, the uterus should be checked for firmness, but it usually does not need to be massaged.

An indwelling urethral catheter is commonly left in place for the first 12 hours postoperatively. Urine should be monitored for volume and color.

Warmed blankets should be available as a comfort measure to the new mother, because tremors that resemble shivering are common following delivery.

Many hospitals have separate PACUs for post-partum patients, so the special considerations for the cesarean patient pose no significant problems. The nurse caring for the cesarean patient within the general post anesthesia care unit must be judicious and often be very innovative in order to meet the needs of not only the mother, but also the new family. Mother, baby, and father should be together as soon as possible to allow for the bonding experience. This may be accomplished by using a quiet corner of the unit (if such a thing ever exists) or by drawing curtains around the family. Mother and father will be anxious to review the details of the birth together, and the PACU nurse should be prepared to answer their questions. Consistent communication between OR nurse and PACU personnel makes answering these questions much easier.

Ectopic Pregnancy

Faulty implantation of the ovum may take place in the fallopian tube (this occurs in approximately 98 percent of all ectopic pregnancies), in the ovary, in any part of the abdominal cavity, or in the uterine cervix.

The treatment of choice for ectopic pregnancy is laparotomy, with removal of the involved fallopian tube (see Abdominal Gynecologic Surgery). Preferably, the ovary is not resected or removed, but this may be necessary if the ovary is involved. If implantation occurs in the cervix, a hysterectomy is usually indicated to control hemorrhage. If abdominal implantation has occurred, the fetus is removed, and often the placenta is left within the cavity to be reabsorbed.

Laparotomy for ectopic pregnancy is performed under general anesthesia, and postoperative care is the same as that for the patient undergoing abdominal surgery. The PACU nurse should be especially observant for signs of intra-abdominal hemorrhage and shock, as these are not uncommon complications of ectopic pregnancy, especially one that has ruptured preoperatively. All patients with ectopic pregnancy should have complete typing and crossmatching done for whole blood, which should be kept available in the laboratory for 24 hours. Rh-negative women should receive RhoGAM to prevent sensitization.

McDonald Operation

The McDonald, or Shirodkar, procedure is used to treat an incompetent cervix and is fairly successful in maintaining pregnancy. The suture is usually placed between the fourteenth and eighteenth week of gestation. This procedure is most commonly performed under general anesthesia.

Upon return to the PACU, the patient is placed in the side-lying position. Food and fluids may be resumed as soon as the patient is conscious and the laryngeal reflexes have returned. A perineal pad should be kept in place. Only a minimal amount of bloody spotting should be considered normal. Pain should be minimal and easily controlled with a simple analgesic such as aspirin or acetaminophen. Any gross vaginal bleeding or abdominal cramping should be reported to the surgeon, since this procedure may induce labor and expulsion of the uterine contents. If labor begins, the suture must be removed immediately.

Uterine Aspiration

Uterine aspiration is used to terminate early pregnancy (i.e., first trimester) or to treat incomplete spontaneous abortion. It is a type of D & C. A general anesthetic may be used, but the trend has been toward the use of a paracervical block and sedation only. Nursing care in the PACU is essentially the same as after dilatation and curettage by conventional means. The patient should have complete blood typing done prior to surgery and the Rh-negative woman should receive RhoGam to prevent sensitization. Complications of this procedure include incomplete evacuation and hemorrhage, which may be treated with oxytocics, and uterine perforation, which must be treated surgically.

GYNECOLOGIC SURGERY

Certain problems are inherent in gynecologic disease processes and the operations devised to deal with them. The patient is frequently more chronically anemic than even the peripheral blood indices may show, because of prolonged or heavy menstrual periods. In addition, large amounts of blood may have accumulated within the pelvic organs at the time of operation and may not be reflected in the external blood loss. Consequently, shock out of proportion to the estimated or measured blood loss may ensue. Many gynecologic operations, although elective procedures, are associated with significant hemorrhage owing to their location, to the large vascular pedicles with their increased blood supply because of the menstrual cycles, and to the large capillary bleeding that complicates hemostasis.

Because of the proximity of the female genital organs to the urinary tract, great care must be taken during surgery and in the observation period afterward to ensure the integrity of this system. Therefore, in addition to overall assessment and general care of these patients, the PACU nurse should direct specific attention toward the patient's cardiovascular status, renal function, and fluid balance.

Laparoscopy

Laparoscopy is commonly being performed as outpatient surgery to diagnose and treat gynecologic problems. A small single incision (approximately 1 cm) is made in order to insert the laparoscopic needle. After a pneumoperitoneum is established, the surgeon can visualize all the organs within the peritoneum. In this case, the surgeon can examine the ovaries, tubes, and uterus; differentially diagnose PID; and perform simple procedures, such as aspiration of cysts, adhesiolysis, tissue biopsies, or tubal ligation. Closure of the skin wound involves only a couple of sutures or staples, and the dressing is a Band-Aid. There should be no drainage or bleeding. Pain should be minimal and easily controlled with ASA or mild narcotics. Severe pain may indicate inadvertent perforation of an intestine and, if such pain is present, the surgeon should be notified. Postoperative care instructions should be discussed with the patient and a significant other both preoperatively and postoperatively. Instructions should be written so that they may be reviewed as necessary after discharge. Special care of the patient undergoing day surgery is outlined in Chapter 34.

LOWER GENITAL AND VAGINAL SURGERY

The conditions that require this type of surgery occur most commonly in parous and older women. Primarily, they are due to an exaggeration of the normal relaxation of the pelvic ligaments and support, which occurs during childbirth and after menopause. A number of specific procedures, named after their developers, may be encountered, including the following:

Baldy-Webster procedure: shortening the round ligaments and changing the direction of their pull by attaching them to the back of the uterus.

Fothergill-Hunter procedure: complete repair of the vaginal walls, from above downward toward the vulva, to correct faulty supportive structures of the pelvic floor.

Gilliam procedure: shortening the round ligaments by attaching them to the abdominal wall.

Le Fort operation (colpocleisis): closure of the vagina by approximation of the anterior and posterior vaginal walls, with or without attendant vaginal hysterectomy.

Radical vulvectomy: abdominal and perineal dissection of the superficial and deep inguinal nodes and portions of the saphenous veins, reconstruction of the vaginal walls and pelvic floor, and closure of the abdominal wounds.

Vulvectomy: removal of the labia major, labia minor, and possibly the clitoris and perianal area, with a Z-plasty closure. Used to treat leukoplakia vulvae, carcinoma in situ of the vulva, and Paget's disease of the vulva.

Other vaginal operations include fistula repairs, operations for urinary stress incontinence, excision of fibromas and tumors, and vaginal reconstruction to repair congenital or acquired defects.

GENERAL POSTOPERATIVE CARE

Anesthesia for lower genital and vaginal surgery may be local, general, or regional, but it is most often general, owing to the extent of pelvic relaxation necessary to perform these procedures. Upon return to the PACU the patient should be placed in the side-lying position until the laryngopharyngeal reflexes have returned. She may then assume a position of comfort. After making a general assessment of the patient's condition, check all dressings carefully. Frequently, a vaginal packing will be in place with a perineal pad as the only dressing. Saturation of the vaginal packing may be expected after any vaginal surgery; however, saturation of the perineal pad when vaginal packing is in place should be considered excessive bleeding and should be reported. Vaginal and groin wounds frequently have drains, and care must be exercised to avoid dislodging them. If drains are in place, a moderate amount of drainage may be expected.

Food and fluids may be safely resumed after the minor procedures, such as D&C

or bartholinectomy, once the pharyngeal reflexes have returned. After more extensive procedures, the patient is usually not given anything by mouth until peristalsis is reestablished; intake is supplied by intravenous fluids. Urine output should be monitored carefully for amount and for the presence of blood. If a Foley catheter is in place, care must be taken to ensure its patency.

Pain must be carefully evaluated and may be alleviated by appropriate analgesics. Abdominal cramping is common after gynecologic surgery. For these patients, relaxation exercises are often helpful if they have been learned preoperatively. Because the patient is often sleepy owing to the anesthesia, she will need coaching, especially during the first hour. If cramping is not relieved by relaxation exercises, analgesics ordered, or other comfort measures, the surgeon should be notified, since this may indicate a perforated uterus. After removal of tumors or cysts from the vaginal area, ice may be applied to reduce edema and provide comfort.

ABDOMINAL GYNECOLOGIC SURGERY

Abdominal gynecologic surgery may be performed alone or in conjunction with vaginal surgery.

General Postoperative Care

Postoperative care after abdominal gynecologic surgery involves all the care and considerations rendered to the patient undergoing any abdominal surgery. Anesthesia is most often general.

Overall assessment of the patient, with special emphasis on the cardiovascular status, should be undertaken as soon as possible.

As mentioned previously, the most common and dangerous complications of any obstetric or gynecologic surgery are excessive hemorrhage and shock. Therefore, the PACU nurse should direct assessment to full evaluation of the patient's circulatory

status at frequent intervals. All dressings should be checked for drainage. Pain should be evaluated, and appropriate comfort measures and analgesics should be administered.

Following hysterectomy and other major abdominal procedures, the patient is usually not given anything orally until peristalsis has returned and nausea has subsided. Intake is supplied by intravenous fluids. Occasionally, the patient returns to the PACU with a nasogastric tube in place to prevent abdominal distention. If abdominal distention develops, nasogastric and rectal tubes may be used to relieve it.

Frequently, a Foley catheter is in place, and its patency must be ensured. The PACU nurse should accurately document the amount of urinary output as well as the presence of blood. A not uncommon complication of hysterectomy is accidental perforation or ligation of a ureter. Inadvertent injury to the bladder wall or the bowel may also occur.

To help prevent vascular disorders, especially in the lower extremities, the patient's position should be changed frequently, high Fowler's position should be avoided, and passive range-of-motion exercises of the lower extremities should be instituted in the PACU as soon as possible.

REFERENCES

1. Affonso, D.: Impact of Caesarean Childbirth. Philadelphia, F. A. Davis Co., 1981.
2. Cranley, M. S., Hedahl, K. J., and Pegg, S. H.: Women's perceptions of vaginal and cesarean deliveries. Nurs. Res., 31:10–15, 1983.
3. deTornyay, R.: Nursing decisions. Helping your patient through elective hysterectomy. RN, 42:75–80, 1979.
4. Hallmark, G., and Findlay, M.: Cesarean birth in the operating room. AORN, J., 36:978–984, 1982.
5. James, F. M., and Wheeler, A. S.: Obstetric Anesthesia: The Complicated Patient. Philadelphia, F. A. Davis Co., 1982.
6. Kehoe, C. F.: The Cesarean Experience: Theoretical and Clinical Perspectives for Nurses. New York, Appleton-Century-Crofts, 1981.

7. Loughlin, Sr. N.: Cesarean childbirth: current perspectives. Today's OR Nurse, 4:8–13, 46, 49, 1982.

8. Marut, J. S.: The special needs of the cesarean mother. MCN, 3:202–206, 1978.

9. McClellan, M. S., and Cabianca, W. A.: Effects of early mother-infant contact following cesarean birth. Obstet. Gynecol. 56:52–55, 1980.

10. Rogers, S. F., and Moore, J.: Variations in vaginal surgery: severe uterine prolapse and vaginal wall defects. Today's OR Nurse, 21(1):8–10, 1984.

11. Schlosser, S.: The emergency C-section patient. Why she needs your help . . . what you can do. RN, 41:52–57, 1978.

12. Shipley, Susan, B.: Patient teaching and day care anesthesia. FOCUS AACN, 9(4):14–16, 1982.

13. Stanto, S. L., and Cardozo, L. D.: Surgical treatment of incontinence in elderly women. Surg. Gynecol. Obstet., 150:555–557, 1980.

14. Tilden, V. P., and Lipson, J. G.: Caesarean childbirth: Variables affecting psychological impact. West. J. Nurs. Res., 3:127–149, 1981.

31

Postoperative Care After Breast Surgery*

Breast surgery is very common today. It is performed when disease or other physical or psychologic determinants are present. Surgery on the breast is most common in adult women but may occasionally be performed on adult males and on children.

The psychologic ramifications of breast surgery in both male and female patients are numerous. These patients need a great deal of quiet acceptance and reassurance. The reaction of PACU personnel to breast surgery is often an important determinant in the patient's entire course of rehabilitation.

Definitions

Augmentation mammoplasty: enlargement of the breasts for cosmetic reasons; usually a soft bag of medical-grade silicone rubber is placed beneath the breast tissue and the pectoral fascia.

Breast biopsy: partial or total removal of an unidentified lump within the breast. This is usually followed immediately by a frozen section to determine etiology.

Mammoplasty: reconstruction of the breast.

*The authors would like to gratefully acknowledge the contribution of illustrations and the review of this chapter by Colonel Alan Seyfer, M.C., Chief, Division of Plastic and Reconstructive Surgery, Walter Reed Army Medical Center, Washington, D.C.

Mastopexy: uplifting the sagging breasts by surgically tightening the skin (Figs. 31–1 and 31–2).

Modified radical mastectomy: removal of the breast and axillary lymph nodes; the pectoralis major muscle is left intact.

Radical mastectomy: removal of all breast tissue, axillary lymph nodes, portions of the greater and smaller pectoral muscles, and the rectus sheath (Fig. 31–3).

Reduction mammoplasty: removal of large

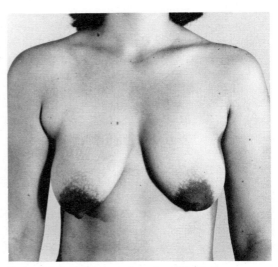

Figure 31–1. Mastopexy (breast uplift). Before surgery, this patient complained of sagging (ptosis) of the breasts.

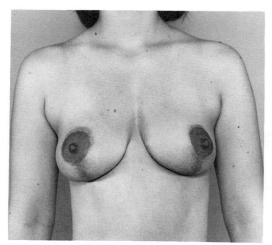

Figure 31–2. Mastopexy—same patient, several weeks postoperatively. The scars are beginning to fade.

portions of the breast because of extreme enlargement, heaviness, or other associated problems.

POSTOPERATIVE CARE AFTER SPECIFIC PROCEDURES

Breast Biopsy

Lumps are a prime symptom of breast disorder and are generally biopsied for definitive diagnosis. Fibrocystic disease accounts for approximately 45 percent of all biopsied female breast lesions, and benign lesions are generally excised. Fibrocystic disease describes a variety of benign and localized tumors or swellings within the breast tissues. It is thought to be due to sensitivity to normal hormones and is usually not considered to be related to the development of breast cancer.

The breast biopsy patient is usually advised of all the risks before surgery, and her main concern when awakening in the PACU will be whether she had a lump or an entire breast removed. Breast biopsies are generally performed under general anesthesia, not because of the nature of the surgery, which is minor, but because the patient's tension and anxiety are almost always high, and because of the possible necessity of performing a radical mastectomy if the frozen section should prove positive for malignancy. If only a biopsy has been performed, the patient recovers from anesthesia rapidly, and has very little pain and a very small incision.

The incision should be inspected for excessive drainage, but this is very rare. Upon return to the PACU, the patient may assume a position of comfort and can resume fluid and food intake as soon as the cough and gag reflexes have fully returned.

Mastectomy

Breast cancer is common and affects thousands of women each year. Mastectomy, sometimes in association with radiation, is the treatment of choice. Controversy continues over whether or not a simple mastectomy is sufficient in selected cases. Nursing care after either modified radical or radical mastectomy is essentially the same, except that, of course, the radical mastectomy involves more gross excision of tissue and demands more detailed observation of viability of remaining tissue.

Following mastectomy the patient should be placed on her back with the head turned to the side. As soon as she begins to respond, her head may be elevated in order to assist respiration, unless another position is advised by the surgeon.

Dressings are usually bulky and should be checked frequently for excessive serosanguineous drainage and for constriction. Dressings are necessarily snug but should not impair respiration or circulation to the upper extremity. The arm on the operative side should be supported and elevated on a pillow; it must be checked frequently for cyanosis or pallor, and the pulse palpated for intensity. If signs of respiratory distress or impaired circulation arise, the surgeon should be notified in order to rearrange the dressing. Unless a true emergency arises, the post anesthesia nurse should not attempt to loosen the dressing, since skin grafts may inadvertently be disrupted.

When a radical mastectomy is performed, there is extensive excision, and skin grafting is usually required (see Chapter 32). Donor sites (usually the thigh) should be checked

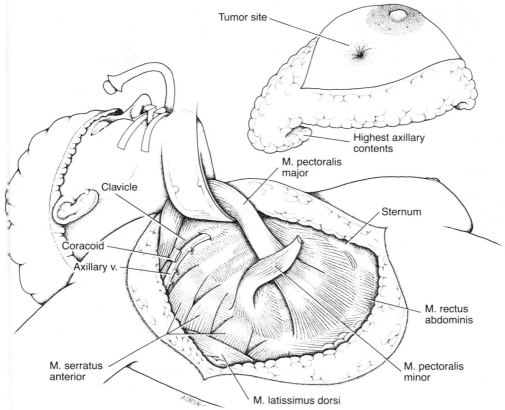

Figure 31–3. Mastectomy.

for drainage and treated according to hospital policy.

Drains are usually placed under the skin flaps to remove excess blood and serum that would ordinarily collect under the wound site, causing edema, infection, and sloughing of the skin graft. The drains may be connected to Hemovac suctions. Generally, additional vacuum is needed the first 8 hours postoperatively, and the Hemovac is connected to vacuum pressure of 20 to 30 mm Hg.

The patient should be advised to avoid excessive motion in the immediate postoperative period. She should not strain the pectoral girdle by levering herself on the bed with her arms to change position. These patients usually need intravenous fluid augmentation for the first 24 hours postoperatively. There is no reason to refrain from oral feeding after cough and gag reflexes have returned and if there is no nausea.

Small sips of fluids may be offered and taken as desired and diet resumed as tolerated. Postoperative pain is moderate to severe and can usually be controlled with narcotics such as meperidine (Demerol) or morphine.

The most important postoperative complication is hematoma occurring below the skin flaps. Attention to the drains and the maintenance of free drainage within the vacuum system prevent this. Bleeding may be a problem, owing to inadequate hemostasis. If gross bleeding occurs, the surgeon must be notified in order to assess the need for operative control.

Mastopexy

Postoperative care following mastopexy is generally not demanding. General anesthesia is most commonly used, and only

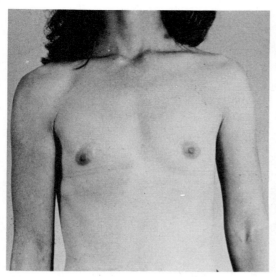

Figure 31–4. Appearance of patient before breast augmentation.

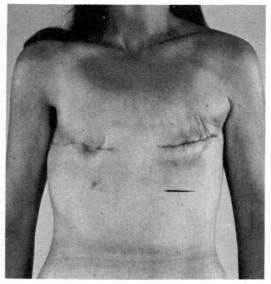

Figure 31–6. Appearance of patient after healing from bilateral mastectomies for cancer.

minor adjustments in breast tissue are made.

Postoperatively, the patient is positioned on her back and may assume a semi-Fowler to high Fowler position for comfort as soon as she awakens. The motion of the arms is restricted to below shoulder level.

Postoperative dressings are minimal, and drains are rarely required, since the entire procedure, with the exception of nipple release, is at the level of the dermis. Drain-

age should be minimal, and if frank bleeding occurs, the surgeon should be notified. Pain is usually not a problem and discomfort can be controlled with the mild analgesics. Food and fluids may be resumed as tolerated after nausea has disappeared.

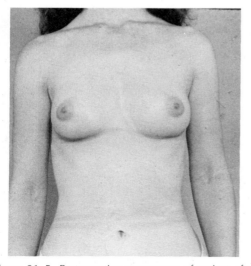

Figure 31–5. Postoperative appearance of patient after breast augmentation with silicone bag prostheses.

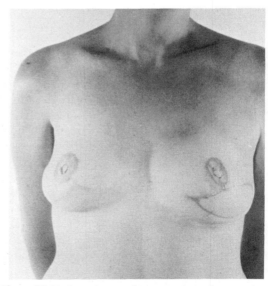

Figure 31–7. Appearance of same patient after muscle-skin flap (latissimus) reconstruction and nipple reconstruction. The patient has gained much weight and later delivered a healthy baby. She is free of disease at six years post mastectomy.

Mammoplasty

Nursing care for reduction and augmentation mammoplasty is essentially the same.

Anesthesia may be local, in combination with appropriate sedation, or general for breast augmentation. Breast reduction is usually carried out under general anesthesia and may require more extensive manipulation of tissue. Regional anesthesia with intercostal block may be used for either procedure if the patient is not fearful of being conscious during the operation.

Upon return to the PACU, the patient is positioned on her back, and as soon as her condition warrants, placed in a low Fowler position. Dressings may be of any variety, but most commonly wide strips of Elastoplast, which readily conform to the patient's new skin contours, is used. A Velpeau bandage should be in place to restrain the patient from raising her arms, and she should be advised of this. Drains are rarely required and drainage should be minimal. If drains are present, they should be connected to a vacuum source such as the Hemovac. As after mastectomy, the patient should be advised to do nothing that puts strain on the pectoral girdle.

Pain after augmentation is generally minimal and can be relieved with mild analgesics. Light ice packs may be used to relieve discomfort and to minimize tissue swelling. Pain after reduction may be more significant and usually requires the use of narcotic analgesia for the first 24 hours.

Breast Reconstruction

One of the advances in breast surgery during recent years is the availability of effective means for reconstructing the breast after removal for cancer. This can be done by a variety of methods in which the plastic surgeon tailors the operation to the patient's deformity.

For reconstructive augmentation mammoplasty, a pocket is made under the remaining tissues into which a soft silicone bag is made to simulate the natural contour (Figs. 31–4 and 31–5). The pocket can be

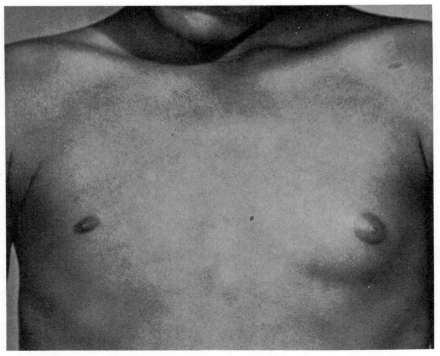

Figure 31–8. Gynecomastia (idiopathic hypertrophy of the breast) in a boy aged eight years. (From Haagensen, C. D.: Diseases of the Breast. 2nd ed. Philadelphia, W. B. Saunders Co., 1971, p. 81.)

made at the time of surgery or before the surgery by means of an inflatable "tissue expander." The expander method requires several injections of gradually increasing volumes of saline over a period of weeks. Then the expander is replaced surgically with a soft silicone bag prosthesis.

Muscle flap/skin flap reconstruction (Figs. 31–6 and 31–7) involves moving nearby muscle and skin into the area of the mastectomy in order to replace the lost volume. Commonly used muscle and skin flaps include the latissimus dorsi and rectus abdominis muscles with attached skin. Nipple/areola reconstruction may be accomplished by using small portions of the labia and grafting to the selected location.

Postoperative care is generally the same as for the patient experiencing other types of breast surgery, with attention to graft and flap donor sites.

These operations have served to provide a measure of comfort to patients whose body image was significantly disrupted by mastectomy. They report a return of their sense of femininity and confidence. Many women do not choose to undergo additional surgery after mastectomy, but knowing that the operation is available is reassuring to them.

Surgery in Gynecomastia

Gynecomastia, or hypertrophy of one or both breasts in the male, is relatively common (Fig. 31–8).

In extreme instances, or when it causes problems in psychologic adjustment, this excess tissue can be excised. The surgical procedure is similar to that of breast reduction in the female patient. A periareolar incision is made and tissue removed. Suction drainage of the incision site is usually necessary and may be conveniently accomplished by use of a Hemovac.

Postoperative care is essentially the same as that for the female patient undergoing breast surgery.

REFERENCES

1. Georgiade, N. G.: Reconstructive surgery of the breast. *In* Sabiston, D. C. (ed.): Textbook of Surgery. 13th ed. Philadelphia, W. B. Saunders Co., 1986.
2. Koch, S. J.: Augmentation mammoplasty. Am. J. Nurs., *80*:1480–1484, 1980.
3. Lierman, L. M.: Support for mastectomy. AORN J., *39*(7):1150–1157, 1984.
4. Miller, S. H., Graham, W. P., Tepsich, J., et al.: Breast reconstruction following mastectomy. AORN J., *25*(5):945–960, 1977.
5. Rubin, L. R.: Reconstruction of the breast after mastectomy. Clin. Plast. Surg., *6*:13–17, 1979.
6. Walsh, M. H., and Stefanski, D. M.: Breast prosthesis. AORN J., *37*(7):1381–1392, 1983.
7. Wilson, R. E.: The breast. *In* Sabiston, D. C. (ed.): Textbook of Surgery. 13th ed. Philadelphia, W.B. Saunders Co., 1986.

32

Postoperative Care After Plastic Surgery

LTC. Susan B. Christoph, R.N., D.N.Sc., C.C.R.N., and COL. Alan Seyfer, M.C.

Plastic surgery has achieved the status of a major surgical specialty after many years without such recognition. The techniques of plastic surgery are most often applied to the skin and soft tissues. Correction of congenital anomalies in infants and children composes the majority of modern plastic surgery procedures performed, in addition to repair of many acquired deformities. Plastic surgery techniques deal with the body in its entirety, striving to restore normal appearance as well as normal function.

There are few absolutes in plastic surgical techniques and in preoperative or postoperative care. Therefore, only the very basics of postoperative care for the plastic surgery patient will be presented here. Some elements of care related to specific body parts are discussed in related chapters, and the reader is referred to them.

The most basic techniques of plastic surgery relate to excision of skin lesions, to closure of skin wounds, and to placement of skin grafts and skin flaps. Minor plastic surgery is often performed under local anesthesia. Postoperative nursing care is minimal, primarily involving observation of the surgical site for untoward symptoms. When the patient must undergo general anesthesia, postoperative care includes all the considerations discussed under general care of the postoperative patient, in addition to attention to the surgical site. Postoperative vital signs, including accurate temperatures, are especially important in the case of the postoperative plastic surgery patient, since these signs provide baselines from which to judge the possible later complications of an immunologic reaction.

SKIN GRAFTS

Most superficial layers of the skin may be removed as sheets and transposed to fill in an area of skin shortage. These grafts will "take" on the recipient locale, but will require several days of immobilization so that the microscopic blood vessels can bridge across from the recipient bed to the newly grafted skin. Tieover dressings are often employed, and these require little, if any, care. However, if the graft is left open, then

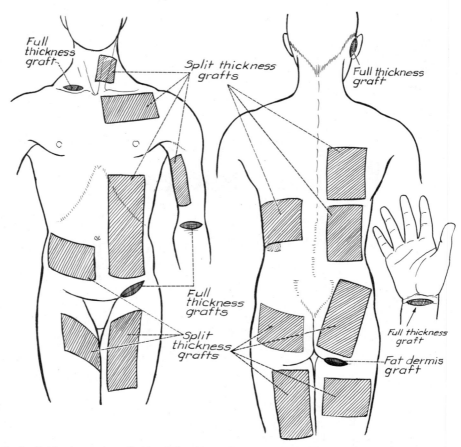

Figure 32–1. Available donor sites of skin grafts. (From Converse, J. M.: Reconstructive Plastic Surgery. 2nd ed. Philadelphia, W. B. Saunders Co., 1977, p. 176.)

one must frequently check the sheet of skin for the presence of blood or serum under the graft. This is especially important in the PACU and on the ward during the first 24 hours postoperatively. If blood or fluid lifts the graft off its bed, the graft will die owing to lack of circulation. Therefore, any accumulation of fluid under the graft must be removed, either by gently rolling a cotton-tipped applicator over the graft to express the fluid from under the graft, or by "pie crusting" (incising) the graft with a needle over the collection of fluid. The fluid is then gently expressed from the small opening. The donor site (from which the skin was harvested for use) is akin to a partial-thickness burn and, if kept clean, will heal with a new layer of skin. (See Chapter 33 for additional discussion of care for grafts and donor sites.)

Composite grafts may be performed, consisting of either skin and fat, or skin, fat, and cartilage. These are dressed and cared for in the same manner as that for skin grafts.

Postoperatively, the grafted area should be elevated, if possible, and protected from both pressure and motion. The patient should be positioned to prevent pressure on, or other trauma to, either the graft or the donor site. The physician may order cold packs to reduce the metabolic requirements of the graft and enhance its survival. These can be made by partially filling a rubber glove with cracked ice and cool water or saline, which makes a light, moldable cold pack. Dressings over grafts should be observed closely for drainage, and any excess should be reported to the physician.

Donor sites should be treated according

to hospital policy. The split-thickness donor site may be left open or covered with a single layer of fine-mesh gauze. Several new products are currently on the market for use as donor site dressings, but these have yet to demonstrate any outstanding advantages over the traditional dressings that could account for their increased cost.

Full-thickness donor sites may be sutured closed and treated as a surgical wound if the donor site is small. If a large area is used for full-thickness grafting, it may be necessary to graft the donor site with split-thickness grafts (Fig. 32–1).

FLAPS

Local flaps are large areas of skin or muscle, or both, that are partially attached to the body and rotated to a nearby position in order to cover an open area (Fig. 32–2). If the flap is nourished by a single artery, the artery is carefully preserved and left undisturbed so that it will serve as a lifeline to the newly positioned skin and muscle. Another type of flap is a *free flap*. It is usually a piece of skin and muscle that is taken off one area of the body (along with the artery and vein that supply it), and placed on another area that needs coverage. After it has been placed in its new location, its tiny artery and vein are sutured to a new artery and vein found in the new location—this procedure is done with the aid of the operating microscope. Whichever type of flap is utilized, the newly positioned flap is kept under constant observation by PACU personnel. Sometimes, an electronic flow meter or temperature probe is placed on the graft to assess its viability by checking tempera-

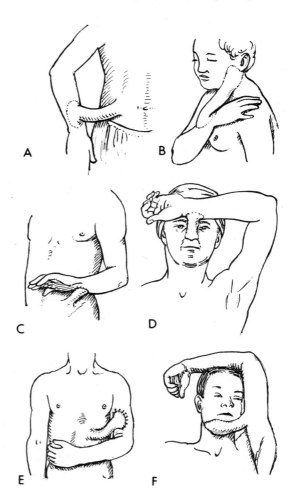

Figure 32–2. Various methods of transfer of tubed pedicle flaps: *A* and *B*, transfer via the wrist; *C* and *D*, the "salute" position of Kilner; *E* and *F*, transfer via the arm (Schuchardt). (From Converse, J. M.: Reconstructive Plastic Surgery. 2nd ed. Philadelphia, W. B. Saunders Co., 1977, p. 211.)

ture and capillary blood flow. However, many times just observing the flap and gently feeling it with the back of the hand to assess its warmth will suffice. The flap must be handled with extreme caution, and no pressure must be allowed directly on or near it; such pressure would cause the circulation to be interrupted, and the flap would then die.

Pain at the sites of skin grafting or flaps is usually minimal; donor sites ordinarily generate the more painful stimuli, which should be managed with the mild analgesics and attention to comfort measures.

BONE GRAFTS

When bone grafts have been performed, the graft site must be immobilized and excessive movement of the patient avoided. The patient may experience considerable pain at the donor site and must be moved very carefully. Pain can be managed with narcotic analgesics after assessment of the patient's overall condition is made. If split-rib grafts are used, the patient should be placed in a low Fowler's position, respiratory status should be checked frequently, and signs of possible pneumothorax, such as tachycardia and tachypnea, should be reported to the surgeon immediately.

COSMETIC SURGERY

Cosmetic surgery is becoming more and more commonplace. In America this may be due, in part, to the national preoccupation with youth and the desire to remain forever youthful in appearance.

Whatever the reasons, one must recognize that such surgery does take place, and that, since it is a surgical procedure, it cannot be taken lightly. These patients have been screened by their surgeon and found to be acceptable in terms of risk, psychologic testing, and anatomic "deformity." The patients place an enormous importance (and often expense) on their surgery and should not be looked down upon or made the object of insensitive remarks about their vanity. Those associated with postoperative care of the cosmetic surgery patient should give the same professional care as that provided any other patient. If the nurse has significant biases against these procedures, reassignment should be considered.

Dermabrasion

Dermabrasion is the surgical planing of the skin, with removal of the epidermis and portions of the superficial dermis, in order to remove high spots or other irregularities in an uneven skin surface. Enough of the dermal and epidermal elements are preserved to allow reepithelialization, and the result is smooth healing and blending of the scarred areas with the surrounding skin surface.

Usually the dermabraded areas are treated by the open method, and postoperative care includes protection of these areas from abrasion caused by rubbing on pillows or bed clothing. Facial edema, especially of the eyelids, may be expected, and the patient must be reassured that this will subside rapidly. The dermabraded area should be observed closely for the development of moisture. If moisture develops, it should be dried with heat lamp or a warm hair dryer. This procedure may produce an uncomfortable burning sensation for the patient that may be minimized by holding the lamp or dryer a considerable distance from the area to be dried. Analgesics should be administered as necessary to manage burning-type pain sensations.

Facelift

The facelift operation is usually done under local anesthesia with supplementary sedation. Although some "lift" is accomplished around the cheek areas, the most important and long-lasting change is in the loose skin of the neck. The facial/neck skin is freed from the underlying tissues and pulled upward and backward toward the postauricular scalp. Excess skin is trimmed off, and meticulous suturing is performed. The procedure takes from 2 to 4 hours, and the patient comes to the PACU with a large, fluffy bandage about the neck and cheeks. Surprisingly, such extensive surgery is not usually associated with significant pain. Pain, especially on one side, is *unusual* and may be the first sign of a complication. It may mean that the skin is being tightened by active bleeding—the most common serious complication of facelift. The surgeon should be notified at once, and he may decide to open the dressing to assess the situation. It should be noted that bleeding is more common in patients with high blood pressure. Sedation, a quiet atmosphere, and continued elevatiuon of the head of the bed will go a long way in helping these patients avoid problems.

Liposuction

Liposuction is a relatively new technique for removing subcutaneous fat in order to improve facial or body contours. It may be used in conjunction with other techniques. Anesthesia may be local or general.

Pain should be minimal. However, if large areas are treated, analgesia with meperidine may be required. Drugs containing aspirin should be avoided so as not to increase bleeding time. If large areas are suctioned, the patient will need intravenous fluid replacement. The patient can usually start oral fluids and a progressive diet as soon as pharyngeal reflexes have returned.

Relatively few complications of this procedure have been reported; however, postoperative bleeding and infection are possible.

SURGICAL REPAIR OF INJURIES TO THE FACIAL BONES

Repair of injuries to the facial bones often requires general anesthesia. If damage is extensive and airway obstruction or concomitant cranial or intrathoracic injury is present, a tracheostomy must be performed. All patients who have facial, jaw, or neck surgery should have a tracheostomy set kept at the bedside in the PACU, in case an airway emergency should occur. If a tracheostomy is not performed, the endotracheal tube or nasotracheal tube should be left in place until the laryngopharyngeal reflexes have fully returned. Since the apparatus may be most uncomfortable, the nurse must explain the need for it to the patient and enlist his or her cooperation. The reader is referred to Chapters 17 and 18 for the essential procedures.

Upon return to the PACU, the patient who has undergone repair of the facial bones is placed in a low Fowler position as soon as his condition warrants. This aids in minimizing the development of head and neck edema. Careful monitoring of the airway is mandatory.

If interdental wire fixation was performed, a pair of wire clippers should be affixed to the head of the bed (where clearly visible to all personnel) in case rapid opening of the jaws is needed. Opening of the jaws may become necessary if an airway emergency develops.

Good oral hygiene is a priority for these patients and may be accomplished with lemon-glycerin swabs and a weak solution of hydrogen peroxide. Petrolatum ointment should be applied to the lips to prevent drying and cracking. Frequent suctioning of secretions may be necessary during the first postoperative hours. Once nausea has subsided and the gag reflex has fully returned, the patient may be allowed small sips of fluids.

CLEFT LIP AND PALATE

Repair of the cleft lip (Figs. 32–3 and 32–4) is usually accomplished when the child is about 3 months old. He or she should

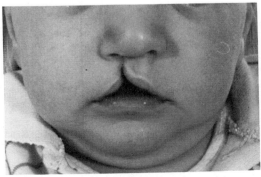

Figure 32–3. Preoperative appearance of a unilateral cleft lip.

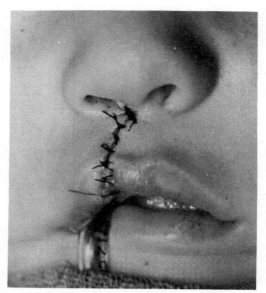

Figure 32–4. Post-operative appearance of unilateral cleft lip. The incision is covered with an antibiotic ointment to prevent crusting.

weigh at least 10 pounds and have a hemoglobin level of at least 10 gm per dl. Repair is accomplished under general anesthesia. Upon return to the PACU, the child is placed in a semiprone position. The baby's arms should be restrained to avoid disruption of the newly repaired lip, and he or she should not be allowed to cry, because crying puts excessive tension on the newly repaired lip. If possible, the mother or father should be allowed in the PACU to hold the child, since this often prevents crying. A rocking chair may prove invaluable in comforting the child, who may be sedated, if necessary.

The most important nursing activity, in addition to preventing trauma to the lip, is airway management. A mist humidifier at the bedside (or rocking-chair side) should be used at least 12 hours postoperatively to aid in clearing of secretions and general respiratory well-being. Hemorrhage may occur as a complication but is, fortunately, rare. It should be remembered, however, that the loss of even a few milliliters of blood in an infant may be important, and any bleeding requires definitive control. Once the child has fully awakened from

anesthesia, small sips of clear fluids may be given.

Pain is usually minimal. Iced normal saline–soaked gauze may be applied to the suture areas to reduce swelling and promote comfort. Analgesia may be provided with the milder oral analgesics.

Repair of a cleft palate is usually completed when the child is 12 to 18 months of age, preferably before the beginning of speech. It is advantageous, again, to have a parent accompany the child in the PACU if possible. Upon return to the PACU, the child is placed in the semiprone or "tonsil" position, and careful attention is given to airway maintenance. As in cleft lip repair, the child's arms should be restrained and crying avoided. The head should not be flexed, since this will tend to occlude the airway.

Suctioning of secretions may be necessary and may be accomplished with a metal tonsil sucker. It must be performed very gently and only if the nurse's view is unobstructed. The sucker should be passed over the dorsum of the tongue and only minimal vacuum pressure used. A mist tent or cold-mist humidifier should be used for at least 12 hours postoperatively to aid in the elimination of tenacious secretions.

Hemorrhage may occur as a complication and requires control. Any bleeding should be recorded and reported to the surgeon. Pain may be managed with mild analgesics such as Tempra drops. Rarely, a stronger analgesic is needed.

MICROSURGERY

Microsurgery is performed with the aid of the dissecting microscope, which greatly improves visualization and detail of small structures. It greatest value in plastic surgery has been in the area of repair of small blood vessels and nerves. Postoperative care for the patient who has undergone microsurgery is the same as that for the principal procedure, with emphasis on notation of color changes in the skin at the operative site. *White* indicates that no blood is entering the area, owing to probable arterial blockage. *Pink* is normal. Check for branch reflex. Momentary pressure on the skin should produce white blanching, which should return to normal pink color within seconds after release of pressure. *Blue* indicates the presence of blood that is low in oxygen and suggests trouble. *Dark blue to black with swelling* indicates impending death of tissue caused by venous obstruction. Any color change from the normal pink should be reported to the surgeon immediately.

REFERENCES

1. Arnet, G. F., and Basehore, L. M.: Dentofacial reconstruction. Am. J. Nurs., *84*(12):1488–1490, 1984.
2. Baj, P. A.: Lipo-suction: "new wave" plastic surgery. Am. J. Nurs., 84(7):892–893, 1984.
3. Chang, W. H. J. (ed): Fundamentals of Plastic and Reconstructive Surgery. Baltimore, Williams & Wilkins, 1980.
4. Fraulini, K. E.: Nursing care of the plastic/reconstructive surgery patient. Curr. Rev. Recov. Room Nurses, 2(6): 11–15, 1984.
5. Grazer, F. M., and Klingbeil, J. R.: Body Image: A Surgical Perspective. St. Louis, C.V. Mosby Co., 1980.
6. Levy, D. M.: Cosmetic surgery patients: They need nursing care, too! J. Pract. Nurs., *30*:13–27, 1980.
7. Rees, T. D.: Aesthetic Plastic Surgery. Vol. 1. Philadelphia, W.B. Saunders Co., 1980.

33

Postoperative Care of the Burn Patient*

Burns are the third leading cause of accidental death in the United States and the leading cause of death in children from birth to 5 years. Care of the postoperative burn patient can be most challenging to the post anesthesia nurse. A burn, no matter how small, represents a total body assault. Burn patients present a very complex array of problems, from deranged fluid and electrolyte balance, respiratory complications, and disrupted temperature regulation, to psychologic disturbances. It is important that the post anesthesia nurse understand integumentary anatomy, physiology, the pathophysiology created with burn injuries, and the systemic ramifications of such injuries.

Types of Burn Injuries

Burn injuries may result from heat, cold, electrical, or chemical sources. A *cold* injury is trauma caused by exposure to cold. Conditions such as immersion foot, trench foot, childblain, and frostbite are the result. *Im-*

mersion foot and *trench foot* occurs when the skin of the foot is exposed to cold (50° F) in damp surroundings with prolonged immobility. *Chilblains (acute and chronic pernio)* involve focal injuries to epidermal and dermal structures which result from exposure to above-freezing cold temperatures associated with high humidity. Because these injuries are focal and superficial, they tend to heal without incident. Therefore, these conditions are rarely seen in the post anesthesia care unit. *Frostbite* results from the crystallization of intracellular fluids and regional ischemia. In particularly severe cases of frostbite, in which necrosis of epidermis, dermis, or deeper structures has occurred, débridement or amputation of the part may be necessary.

Chemical burns are caused by caustic agents, either acid or alkali. Chemical burns cause necrosis of the tissue protein by coagulation and degradation through various chemical reactions. Chemical burns may be devastating because, without appropriate emergency treatment, causatic agents continue to cause destruction of fascia, fat, muscle, and bone. The severity and depth of the injury are directly related to both the concentration of the agent and the duration of contact.

Electrical burns result from contact with a

---

*The authors would like to acknowledge the assistance of CPT. Bryan S. Jordan, A.N.C., and MAJ. Steven Schmidt, M.C., of the United States Army Institute of Surgical Research, Fort Sam Houston, San Antonio, Texas, for assistance in review and revision of this chapter.

source of electricity. The effects of electricity are dependent upon the type (direct or alternating), voltage, frequency, and pathway of the current; duration of contact; and environmental conditions. Although the only visible wounds may be those of entrance and exit sites, massive deep damage is often sustained because of the resistance afforded by bone, muscle, and nerve tissues. Heat created by this resistance to the electrical current is the chief cause of tissue damage. Heated tissue cools unevenly, the superficial portions cooling more rapidly than the deeper portions. Therefore, the deeper tissues are more liable to severe injury. Concomitant thermal injury may occur with electrical burns from the heat of arcing and from clothing ignition.

The most common type of burn injury is the *thermal* burn. It is caused by contact with hot liquids and flames or conduction from a heat source. Thermal energy causes cell injury and cell death by coagulation necrosis. The severity of injury, duration of functional impairment, and completeness of recovery are directly related to the intensity and duration of the thermal insult.

Indices of Severity and Depth of Burn Injury

The severity of any burn injury depends on the extent and depth of the injury. The extent of the burn is calculated as a percentage of the total body surface area (TBSA). The two methods that may be used are the "rule of nines" and the Lund and Browder method. The rule of nines provides a rapid but not precise estimate of body surface burned. It does not take into consideration the influencing factor of age (Fig. 33–1). The Lund and Browder method of estimating the area of body surface involvement is more accurate and should be used whenever possible (Fig. 33–2). This method defines each body part or location, specifically taking into account the changes in surface area that occur with age.

The depth of a burn depends upon the depth of penetration by heat and the resultant extent of damage through the layers of the skin. There is a preferred nomenclature for describing such depth of injury:

A *partial-thickness burn* is a wound that extends through some, but not all, of the epidermal or dermal elements. A partial-thickness burn injury has the ability to heal without grafting. Because only a portion of the integument has been damaged or destroyed, the epithelial cells remaining below the level of damage will provide new epidermis.

Partial-thickness burns can be divided into three categories: (1) *superficial burns*, in which there is partial skin loss but not dermal death and therefore no slough formation; (2) *partial-thickness* burns, characterized typically by healing from the level of the hair follicles; and (3) *deep dermal* burns, which heal typically from the level of the sweat ducts. A deep dermal burn can heal without grafting; however, infection, poor wound management, inadequate nutrition, advanced age of the patient, or additional mechanical trauma may convert a deep dermal burn to a full-thickness burn requiring

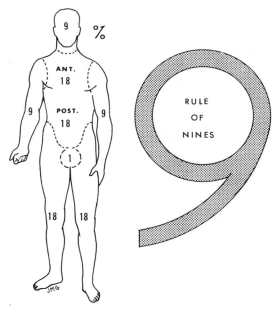

Figure 33–1. Schematic outline of the Rule of Nines. Use of the rule provides a rapid method for determining percentage of body surface burned, but it is of limited accuracy. (From Sabiston, D. C. [ed.]: Davis-Christopher Textbook of Surgery. 11th ed. Philadelphia, W. B. Saunders Co., 1977, p. 298.)

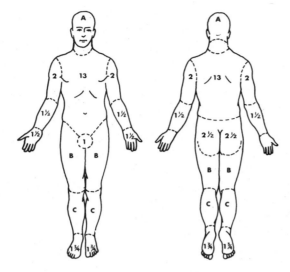

Relative Percentages of Areas Affected by Growth
(AGE IN YEARS)

	0	1	5	10	15	ADULT
A: 1/2 of head	9 1/2	8 1/2	6 1/2	5 1/2	4 1/2	3 1/2
B: 1/2 of thigh	2 3/4	3 1/4	4	4 1/4	4 1/2	4 3/4
C: 1/2 of leg	2 1/2	2 1/2	2 3/4	3	3 1/4	3 1/2

Total Per Cent Burned _____ 2° + _____ 3° = _____

Figure 33–2. Classic Lund and Browder chart. The best method for determining percentage of body surface burn is to mark the areas of injury on a chart and then compute total percentage according to the patient's age. Every emergency room should have such a chart for plotting the burned area soon after the patient is admitted. (From Sabiston, D. C. [ed.]: Davis-Christopher Textbook of Surgery. 11th ed. Philadelphia, W. B. Saunders Co., 1977, p. 298.)

grafting, or grafting may be required to improve either function or cosmetic results.

A *full-thickness burn* results in total destruction of all epithelial elements, and there may be destruction of the subcutaneous tissue, muscles, and bones. This type of wound must be grafted, as the skin will not regenerate.

PATHOPHYSIOLOGY

A burn is a systemic injury because, irrespective of the size of the burn, there are systemic ramifications. In the first 24 to 48 hours post burn, these include loss of vascular integrity, hemoconcentration, and decreased cardiac and urine output. The vasculature exposed to the heat source demonstrates a temporary loss in vessel integrity, which results in a massive shift of plasma, plasma proteins, and electrolytes into the third space. This produces the characteristic edema so often associated with initial burn wound appearance. Hemoconcentration is the result of decreased intravascular volume caused by the shift of plasma into the third space. As a result of hemoconcentration, the cardiac output decreases, and, accordingly, urine output decreases.

After the initial 24 to 48 hours, a reverse process begins. The damaged vessel regains its integrity and the third space fluid volume pours back into the vascular tree. The result is hemodilution, increased cardiac and urine output, and a loss of body edema. The initially depressed metabolic rate now increases in relation to burn size. The increased metabolic rate is expressed by an increased heart and respiratory rate, an increased oxygen consumption and carbon dioxide production, and an enormous increase in caloric consumption.

Various configurations of fluid and electrolyte imbalances and cardiovascular, pulmonary, renal, and hepatic dysfunction may occur singly or in combination and may remain present throughout the patient's hospitalization. The ever-present threat of infection cannot be overemphasized. Burn wound sepsis remains a leading cause of mortality following burn injuries. Protection from pathogens in the environment must be a priority for nursing intervention throughout the patient's hospitalization.

The initial postburn stage is extremely stressful for the patient, particularly in cases with extensive TBSA involvement. Preexisting or concomitant pathologic conditions, extremes in age, general debilitation, and diminished coping mechanisms must be considered in the overall patient assessment. The complexities inherent in the medical management of the burn-injured patient, including the considerations for comprehensive nursing care, are staggering

SURGERY

Burn patients rarely go to surgery during the first 72 hours because of cardiovascular instability. The first 18 to 24 hours post burn are the most critical. Cardiovascular instability is usually associated with problems in capillary permeability or with lesions in the cardiovascular system that begin to stabilize after 24 hours. Exceptions to this general 72-hour rule occur when the burn patient has associated injuries that require immediate surgery to control hemorrhage, fix fractures, or complete partial amputations.

The most common surgical procedures performed on burn patients are escharotomies, fasciotomies, excisions, and grafting. The decision to intervene surgically in the management of the burn wound is based upon many factors, including the extent and severity of the burn wound, the age of the patient, the patient's nutritional status, the incidence of infectious processes, the general condition of the patient, postburn functioning, and cosmetic considerations.

Anesthesia

General anesthesia is usually administered to the burn patient, although regional anesthesia may sometimes be utilized. Regional anesthesia may be used for local débridement. When grafting is to be accomplished, regional anesthesia is not usually satisfactory, since the donor site is frequently remote from the excision site. In some instances, ketamine may be administered to the burn patient. For the pediatric patient, emergence from ketamine anesthesia is usually smooth. Premedication of the adult burn patient with a benzodiazepine reduces the incidence of hallucinations or emergent reactions. The advantages of using ketamine in the burn patient include the intense analgesia produced, with maintenance of normal pharyngeal and laryngeal reflexes, and cardiac stimulation. For additional information on ketamine anesthesia see Section III.

Excision and Grafting

Excision and grafting may be accomplished independently but are usually performed together through sequential or tangential removal of each successive layer of nonviable tissue, working downward toward viable tissue and then applying a graft. This type of débridement and grafting may be utilized for either partial- or full-thickness wounds. When the depth of injury includes significant subcutaneous necrosis or damage, deep excision is employed. The excised wound may then be grafted with either the patient's own skin— an *autograft*—or with a temporary graft, with autografting delayed until a later time.

Autografts, both split- and full-thickness, are harvested from nonburned tissue from areas known as donor sites. There are two forms of autograft. The first form, a *sheet graft*, is removed in a predetermined thickness from the dermis, leaving epithelial remnants for donor site regeneration. The second form, a *mesh graft*, is removed in the same way but is subsequently placed in a device that cuts small slits in the graft in a crosshatched manner. Meshing the skin allows expansion of the graft for covering a larger surface. These grafts can be expanded up to nine times the original surface area, but expansions of one and one-half and three times the original surface area are most commonly used. The grafts may be held in place by staples, sutures, or immobilizing dressings.

POSTANESTHESIA CARE
Room Preparation

Often, burn patients are cared for in special burn units. When a burn patient will be cared for in the general post anesthesia care unit, a certain amount of preparation will be necessary. The room should be checked for and stocked with supplies and special equipment, such as ventilators, cradles, warming lights, and medications. Ambient air temperature should be maintained at approximately 85°F. If the temperature of the room cannot be separately controlled, the nurse should attempt to maintain a warm temperature. Drafts should be avoided by closing or blocking air vents and by closing the doors.

Infection Control

Infection is the most common and the most dreaded complication following a burn injury; therefore, asepsis is most important. Upon arrival in the PACU, the patient should be placed in strict protective isolation, and the nurse should wear a cap, mask, and gown. No more than two persons should be responsible for the patient care there, and the movement of personnel into and out of the room should be limited. Handwashing is a *must*, and its necessity can never be overemphasized. Sterile surgical gloves should be used when touching any exposed area or dressing on the burn patient. The gloves should be changed frequently. Gloves must always be changed when moving from one burn area on the patient to another.

Assessment

As with any patient recovering from anesthesia, vital signs must be assessed every 5 to 15 minutes. Attention must be directed

toward maintenance of a patent airway and adequate respiration. Respiratory rate and pattern as well as blood gases should be monitored closely.

Care necessary to prevent pulmonary complications should include deep breathing and sustained maximal inspiration (SMI) exercises. The patient should be encouraged and stimulated, if necessary, to cough.

In the burn patient, the acute respiratory distress syndrome, which is sometimes referred to as "shock lung," can develop as a result of interstitial edema soon after injury or at any time during the recovery from a severe burn. An alveolar-capillary block results when sequestration occurs in the interalveolar spaces of the lungs. This creates a fluid interface where carbon dioxide and oxygen interchange in the lungs. The carbon dioxide is readily diffusible, the oxygen is much less diffusible, and the end result is hypoxemia and hyperventilation. Signs of oxygen hunger including tachypnea, dyspnea, tachycardia, stridor, chest pain, and anxiety or restlessness may indicate development of this complication. The surgeon should be notified, and, meanwhile, oxygen should be provided to the patient by mask or nasal catheter.

The burn patient may already have some compromised pulmonary function from such causes as burns of the upper torso, smoke inhalation, or overloading of fluids during the initial phase of burn treatment. Hypoxemia may be present owing to the increased metabolic rate and oxygen consumption or edema due to increased pulmonary capillary permeability. These patients will often require mechanical ventilation (see Chapter 18). In some instances the burn patient will have a tracheostomy tube in place (see Chapter 20 for tracheostomy care). Because of the high incidence of infection in the burn patient, aseptic technique should be meticulously adhered to when administering tracheostomy care.

Circulatory dynamics may change frequently during the postoperative period. The blood loss during burn procedures is often significant. Fluid and electrolyte balances shift quickly.

Many burns occur on the extremities, and it may be impossible to utilize a pneumatic blood pressure cuff. It is generally felt that extra invasive lines will lead to extra sources of sepsis, and they are usually avoided in the burn patient whenever possible. However, the advantages may outweigh this disadvantage; if the physician deems it necessary because of the patient's condition, an arterial pressure line may be inserted to determine blood pressure measurements and to obtain frequent blood gas samples. A central venous pressure line or a flow-directed catheter might also be used.

In the burn patient, hypovolemia, hemolysis, muscle injury, and sepsis may contribute to kidney failure. Kidney function should be monitored via urine output.

In patients whose burns cover 20 percent or more of the total body area or in those in whom the perineum was burned, an indwelling urinary catheter is usually inserted. Urine should be assessed for quantity, color, specific gravity, acetone level, and the presence of occult blood. Urinary output of 0.5 to 1 ml per kg per hour for the adult patient is a reasonably safe indication that the kidneys are functioning normally. *Anuria*, a complete absence of urinary output, and *oliguria*, which is less than 400 ml of urine in 24 hours for the adult, are indicators of renal failure and if encountered should be reported to the surgeon. *Polyuria*, increased urinary output greater than 2000 ml in 24 hours, can also be a complication and should be reported to the surgeon.

Disrupted temperature regulation is a problem in burn patients. In addition, these patients tend to lose heat through radiation because a large amount of the body surface is exposed to the air. The burn patient must be kept warm with body core temperature maintained at 99.6° F to 100.0° F. The patient's temperature should be taken every 30 to 60 minutes. Heat shields and heat lamps may be used to ensure the patient's warmth.

Wound Care

Wound care in the PACU is dependent upon the type of surgical procedure performed and the surgeon's preference. Generally, graft sites must be immobilized and the joints are usually splinted. Care must be taken to ensure that patient movement does not dislodge fresh grafts. The burn patient should not be repositioned, turned, or moved, unless these changes are cleared by a physician. The patient who becomes restless during emergence, owing to anxiety or pain, may require a tranquilizer.

Grafts should be observed to ensure their adherence and survivability. Dressings should be intact and free of any discoloration. Autografts should be cared for as described in Chapter 32. Hematoma or seroma accumulation under a graft will separate it from the recipient bed and requires evacuation in order to achieve adherence and prevent loss of the graft. Sheet grafts are generally not dressed in order to provide for direct visualization. Hematoma or seroma accumulation is either rolled with a cotton-tipped applicator to express the fluid or aspirated with a very small-gauge needle.

Areas where burned tissue has been excised will be covered with dressings. Dressings will vary depending upon surgeon preference and individual patient requirements. The dressing may consist of dry or moist gauze, synthetic skin substitutes (Biobrane), or biologic coverings, including pigskin (a *xenograft*) or cadaver skin (an *allograft*). Even though hemostasis has been achieved intraoperatively, postoperative increases in blood pressure and movement of the affected part may cause bleeding in the excised area. If bleeding occurs, the surgeon should be notified.

Donor sites may present a special problem. The resultant raw surface may be likened to a giant rug burn. The wound is very painful and may be dressed with a single layer of gauze. Donor areas should receive heat and aeration to promote drying and healing. These sites must be guarded against infection. For the severely burned patient, care of the donor sites becomes a top priority, since these sites may very well be reharvested to provide grafts for subsequent procedures.

Pain Management

Postoperatively, the patient may experience pain or discomfort, typically at donor sites. The pain may be very intense, as evidenced by tachycardia, hypertension, increased anxiety, and restlessness. Restlessness from pain must be differentiated carefully from restlessness due to other causes, such as hypoxemia and gastric or bladder distention, prior to the administration of analgesia.

Pain may best be managed with intravenous administration of narcotic analgesia (morphine is the drug of choice) in incremental doses.

Positioning of the Patient

Care must be taken to ensure that patient movement of any type does not dislodge the fresh graft. Immobility of the grafted area is critical for the graft to be able to "take". The position of the patient as when presenting in the PACU is dependent upon the type and location of the surgical procedure. Splints or traction, if required, are generally applied in the operating room but may require some readjustment in the PACU. The extremities may require repositioning to decrease edema, protect grafted areas, and reduce the potential for contractures. The patient may return to the PACU in a prone position if posterior débridement and grafting were performed. In this case, the patient may be placed in a Circo-electric bed. If the patient returns to the PACU in a prone position, ventilation may be compromised. The nurse must make even more frequent assessments of respiratory status to assure adequacy of ventilation.

Psychosocial Considerations

Burn patients often experience a succession of operative procedures requiring multiple trips to the operating room. Coordination of the burn victim's care requires particularly close collaboration between nursing staff and other team members who will care for these patients.

The PACU nurse must be familiar with the history of the burn, the patient's hospital course, and his or her response to injury and hospitalization. Of particular importance is the patient's present stage of psychologic response to the injury. Each burn patient will view the steps of his or her rehabilitation in a different light, and each surgical procedure will have a different meaning for each patient. The PACU nurse will get the assessment and care information from the burn nurse who usually cares for the patient.

Family members will naturally be anxious to receive word of how the burn victim has fared through surgery, and the nurse should ensure that the surgeon or another responsible team member has spoken to the family following surgery.

REFERENCES

1. Artz, C. P., Moncrief, J. A., and Pruitt, B. A.: Burns: A Team Approach. Philadelphia, W. B. Saunders Co., 1979.
2. Bessey, P. Q.: The patient with major burns in the recovery room: the first five days. Curr. Rev. Recov. Room Nurses, 2(17):131–135, 1980.
3. Engeman, S. A.: The burned patient: perioperative nursing care. AORN J., 40(1):36–41, 1984.
4. Kothary, S. P., and Zsigmond, E. K.: Prevention of ketamine-induced psychological sequelae by diazepam. Clinical Pharmacology and Therapeutics, 17(2):238, 1975.
5. Park, R. P.: Anesthesia for the burned patient. AORN J., 40(1):42–47, 1984.
6. Pruitt, B. A.: Electrical injury. In Wyngaarden, J. B., and Smith, L. H. (ed.): Textbook of Medicine. Philadelphia, W. B. Saunders Co., 1982.
7. Pruitt, B. A.: The Burn Patient: 1. Initial Care. In Ravitch, M. M. (ed.): Current Problems in Surgery. Chicago, Year Book Medical Publishers, Inc., 1979.
8. Robertson, K. E., Cross, J. P., and Terry, J. C.: The crucial first days. Am. J. Nurs., 81(1):30–50, 1985.

Postoperative Care of the Ambulatory Surgical Patient

The concept of outpatient or ambulatory surgery was introduced by J. H. Nicoll in 1909 and by Ralph Waters in 1918; however, by the 1930s, most surgical procedures were performed in the inpatient hospital setting. In the 1960s, because of the advent of Medicare and Medicaid, a movement was begun to enlarge the medical services. In 1968, Dornette initiated the free-standing ambulatory surgical centers (FASCs). The significance of the FASCs is that they are not physically or administratively associated with a particular hospital. In 1971, the American Medical Association passed Resolution 33, which endorsed the concept of surgery being performed on an outpatient basis under select circumstances as a part of good medical practice. Ambulatory surgical care has become one of the fastest-growing areas in the health care delivery system. With the added attractions of reduced costs and the emphasis on a safe environment and efficient care, ambulatory surgery has met with enthusiasm among the general public. Since post anesthesia care is an integral part of ambulatory surgery, it is important for the PACU nurse to understand the major concepts presented in this chapter.

PREOPERATIVE PERIOD

Patient Selection for Ambulatory Surgery

Most ambulatory surgical facilities will treat patients who are in good health. Specifically, candidates for outpatient surgery must be in stable health and, according to the Physical Status criteria of the American Society of Anesthesiologists (ASA), must be of either ASA class I or II. Occasionally, an ASA class III patient with no acute life-threatening condition (i.e., diabetes or moderate pulmonary insufficiency) can qualify as a candidate for outpatient surgery.

The types of operations performed in an ambulatory surgical setting are summarized in Table 34–1. The criteria for surgical procedures appropriate to ambulatory surgery are summarized in Table 34–2. The preoperative evaluation of the ambulatory surgical patient usually includes the medical history, physical examination, laboratory studies, and, if required, a radiologic and electrocardiographic examination. The history and physical examination are usually conducted within 48 hours of surgery to determine if there are any intercurrent problems, such as fever or upper respiratory

TABLE 34–1. Types of Surgical Procedures That Are Performed in the Ambulatory Surgical Setting

Dental	**Otolaryngology**
Extraction of teeth, restorations	Septoplasty
General	Myringotomy—drainage tube insertion/removal
Pediatric herniorrhaphy, orchiopexy	Otoplasty
Incision and drainage of abscess	Removal of foreign bodies
Suture of lacerations	Reduction of nasal fracture
Breast and node biopsy	Laryngoscopy
Nerve and muscle biopsy	T and A
Hemorrhoidectomy	**Plastic**
Fissure and fistula procedures	Excision of skin lesions
Gynecology	Augmentation mammoplasty
D and C, excision of cervical polyp	Scar revisions
Bartholin cyst excision	Rhinoplasty
Laparoscopy	Cosmetic procedures
Abortion	**Thoracic**
Ophthalmology	Esophagoscopy
Eye muscle procedures	Bronchoscopy
Tear duct probing	Esophageal dilation
Eyelid ptosis procedures	**Urology**
Iridectomy	Cystoscopy
Orthopedic	Meatotomy
Cast change, manipulations	Orchiopexy
Fracture reduction	Circumcision
Carpal tunnel procedures	Vasectomy
Removal of hardware	
Removal of plantar neuroma	
Trigger finger and de Quervain's disease repair	
Ganglion excision	
Arthroscopy	

From Dripps, R., Eckenhoff, J., and Vandam, L.: Introduction to Anesthesia: The Principles of Safe Practice. 6th ed. Philadelphia, W.B. Saunders Co., 1982.

infection (URI). Laboratory data generally include a determination of the patient's hemoglobin and hematocrit and a urinalysis. If the patient is more than 35 years old, a preoperative chest x-ray and ECG are performed. Some institutions require performance of an ECG and chest x-ray for all patients; however, in other institutions, in the case of ASA class I patients, this decision is left to the physician. Overall, the decision for the performance of laboratory and radiologic tests is made by the physi-

TABLE 34–2. Criteria for Surgical Procedures Appropriate to the Ambulatory Surgical Setting

1. There should be no major intervention into the abdomen, thorax, or cranium.

2. The procedure should be associated with a reliably low incidence of postoperative complications and physiological derangement.

3. Minimal blood loss is anticipated.

4. The procedure should last less than 90 minutes, except for some plastic and dental cases.

From Allen, B.: Anesthesia and ambulatory surgery. AANA J., 52(3):303–308, 1984.

cian responsible for the surgery or anesthetic, the main consideration being that outpatient care should meet the same standards that apply to inpatients.

Outpatient Fasting (NPO) Period

Adult patients are usually requested to fast for at least 10 hours before surgery. Children present problems in this area because they become dehydrated faster than adults and do not completely understand the importance of the fasting period. The usual fasting procedure for ambulatory surgery calls for the infant less than 5 months old to have milk up to 4 hours before surgery and clear fluids up to 3 hours before surgery and then be completely NPO. Infants 6 months to 2 years of age can have clear fluids up to 4 hours before surgery and then be NPO. Children scheduled for surgery in the early morning should be fed at midnight, then NPO thereafter. However, if the child is scheduled for afternoon surgery, clear liquids should be given until 8:00 A.M. on the day of surgery and then NPO.

One of the more serious implications of PACU nursing care for the ambulatory surgical patient concerns patient compliance during the fasting period. Adults, and more often infants and children, may sneak off at home and eat or drink something. This happens because the patient does not understand what behavior is expected or does not realize the importance of the fasting period. Therefore, in the post anesthesia care unit every ambulatory surgical patient, especially the pediatric patient, should be monitored for vomiting and aspiration. If active vomiting occurs, the patient should be placed in a head-down position, and the vomitus should be mechanically cleared from the upper airway. Then 100 percent oxygen should be given and the anesthesiologist notified immediately.

Preoperative Medication

Philosophies differ on the administration of the premedication; they range from no premedication to premedication of some patients to premedication of all ambulatory surgical patients. In many cases, however, the decision on giving premedication is based on the patient's degree of anxiety, and whether the patient is expected to experience postoperative pain. If the physician determines that a preoperative medication is needed, it may be administered intramuscularly 1 hour prior to surgery or be given intravenously just before the beginning of the anesthetic. The drugs used in most premedications for ambulatory surgical patients are opioids, such as fentanyl; tranquilizers, such as diazepam (Valium) or lorazepam (Ativan); or barbiturates given alone or in combination. Many physicians avoid a premedication that contains an opioid because the incidence of postoperative vomiting is about 40 percent in ambulatory surgical patients given an opioid premedication, as compared with only 4 percent in patients who are not given

opioids. Therefore, patients who are given an opioid premedication should be monitored continuously for signs of vomiting. If vomiting occurs, the nursing interventions should consist of placing the person in head-down position, clearing the airway, administering 100 percent oxygen, and summoning the anesthesiologist.

INTRAOPERATIVE PERIOD

Patients who were not premedicated can walk to the operating room with their anesthesiologist or nurse anesthetist. This gives the ambulatory surgical patient a sense of self-control, which is extremely important psychologically for facilitating a rapid recovery from anesthesia and surgery. General inhalational and regional anesthetics with or without intravenous sedation are used in the ambulatory surgical setting.

For the pediatric patient under the age of 6 years, a gas induction will be done without the use of needles. Nitrous oxide with either halothane or enflurane is generally used for induction and maintenance of anesthesia. An intravenous solution is usually started after the pediatric patient reaches surgical anesthesia. Skeletal muscle relaxants are rarely used and, if indicated, oral endotracheal intubation will be performed. Pediatric patients usually emerge from anesthesia rather rapidly and can take fluids within 30 minutes after most surgical procedures.

For the adult ambulatory surgical patient receiving a general inhalational anesthetic, the induction of anesthesia is ordinarily done by intravenous injection of an ultra-short-acting barbiturate, such as methohexital (Brevital) or sodium thiopental. After induction, the patient is given nitrous oxide with oxygen. In addition, narcotics, muscle relaxants, anticholinergic drugs, or 100 percent potent inhalational anesthetics may be administered. Narcotics, such as fentanyl or meperidine, may be used in small doses to supplement the inhalation anesthesia. Small doses of d-tubocurarine, pancuronium bromide (Pavulon), or metocurine iodide (Metubine) may be given to facilitate the inhalational anesthesia and to make assisted or controlled ventilation easier. The nondepolarizing muscle relaxants are favored because they have direct antagonists. The depolarizing skeletal muscle relaxant succinylcholine is not pharmacologically reversible (see Chapter 14). If endotracheal intubation is deemed necessary, a one-time dose of succinylcholine preceded by a small dose of d-tubocurarine is usually given. This nondepolarizing skeletal muscle relaxant will block the fasciculations produced by succinylcholine that cause muscle pain and soreness. The anticholinergic agents such as atropine or glycopyrrolate (Robinul) may be administered to reduce upper airway secretions, especially in patients having surgery of the mouth or pharynx and to treat intraoperative bradycardia. Unless indicated, anticholinergics are frequently avoided in the ambulatory surgical setting because of the side effects of dryness of the mouth and general discomfort that can be experienced in the postoperative phase as a result of their use.

The 100 percent potent inhalational anesthetic agents act rapidly and are well suited for the patient in the ambulatory surgical setting. They offer a low blood-gas partition coefficient and thus are eliminated rapidly, leading to a rapid emergence from anesthesia. Some clinicians prefer enflurane (Ethrane) and isoflurane (Forane) because of their low lipid solubility (see Chapter 12), which allows for rapid emergence. Halothane (Fluothane) has a higher lipid solubility and so may have the disadvantage of a slightly longer emergence time. However, halothane does have the advantage during gas inductions without the use of IV agent of being a little more easily tolerated by the patient at high concentrations.

Regional anesthesia is used often in the ambulatory surgical setting. It offers the advantage of a selective local action since only the actual area or extremity involved in the surgery is anesthetized. In additon, the patient who receives a regional anesthetic will not experience the "hangover" or nausea associated with general inhalational anesthesia. Another distinct advantage of regional anesthesia is that it provides postoperative pain relief, reducing the need for analgesics in the immediate postoperative period.

The intermediate-acting amide local anesthetics, such as lidocaine (Xylocaine) and mepivacaine (Carbocaine), are drugs of choice in the ambulatory surgery setting. They are relatively safe, and if epinephrine is not used to prolong the duration of the block, the recovery time is not unduly long. Procaine (Novocain) and 2-chloroprocaine (Nesacaine) have the briefest action but, because of their ester linkage, are associated with allergic reactions. Long-acting local anesthetic agents, such as bupivacaine (Marcaine), tetracane (Pontocaine or Amethocaine), and etidocaine (Duranest), are generally not used in ambulatory surgery because of their lengthy duration of action.

The regional anesthetic techniques used in the ambulatory surgical setting are local infiltration, intravenous regional (Bier) block, brachial plexus (axillary) block, intercostal nerve blocks, femoral-sciatic nerve block, and spinal and epidural blocks. Opinions vary in regard to the use of spinal and epidural blocks because they require a significant amount of time to administer and to produce an appropriate level of anesthesia. Other problems with their use include a significant failure rate and complications such as postspinal headache and puncture of the dura by an epidural needle. The focus of the argument for the use of spinal and epidural blocks centers around the fact that if they are administered by anesthesia personnel who are experienced in these regional block techniques, the incidence of failure and complications is reduced.

POSTOPERATIVE PERIOD

Recovery of the ambulatory surgical patient generally occurs in two stages, with the first stage commencing when the patient arrives in a fully equipped and fully staffed post anesthesia care unit (PACU). The second stage begins when the fully dressed patient leaves the PACU, goes to the lounge-chair recovery area, is reunited with a family member, and is offered light refreshment.

Stage One—The PACU

When the ambulatory surgical patient arrives in the post anesthesia care unit, the nurse should start the patient on oxygen, assess the patient's current physiologic status, and then be given a report by the anesthetist. The report on the patient should include (1) name, age, and weight; (2) surgical procedure, including the length of time the patient was under anesthesia; (3) preoperative information, including diagnosis, premedication, ASA class, baseline vital signs, allergy and drug history, and any unusual problems, such as blindness; (4) intraoperative information, including anesthetic agents used, narcotic and skeletal muscle relaxant reversal, changes in vital signs, dysrhythmias, estimated blood loss, and fluid therapy; and (5) suggestions on specific PACU care, such as a more vigorous stir-up regimen, narcotic reversal, or use of peripheral nerve stimulator to assess the status of the reversal of the skeletal muscle relaxant.

After the nurse has received the report on anesthesia and surgery, the stir-up regimen of turn-cascade-cough and sustained maximal inspiration (SMI; see Chapter 18) should be instituted and repeated every 5 to 10 minutes. The PACU nurse should monitor the patient specifically for complications associated with the ambulatory surgical experience in the immediate postoperative period (Table 34–3). The two most common complications related to ambulatory surgery are nausea and vomiting and postoperative bleeding. More specifically, if a patient has received drugs that could increase the incidence of postoperative nausea and vomiting, such as meperidine (Demerol) or morphine, close monitoring for such untoward sequelae is necessary. Halothane anesthesia is associated with vomiting more frequently than is enflurane. Adequate hydration is usually accom-

TABLE 34–3. Complications Associated with the Ambulatory Surgical Experience

Persistent nausea and vomiting
Bleeding or hemorrhage (T and A, laparoscopy, mammoplasty)
Perforated uterus (D and C)
Delirium
Infection
Bowel burn, distention, pain (laparoscopy)
Airway edema (intubation)
Chemical phlebitis
Delayed recovery from anesthesia

Adapted from Dripps, R., Eckenhoff, J., and Vandam, L.: Introduction to Anesthesia: The Principles of Safe Practice. 6th ed. Philadelphia, W. B. Saunders Co., 1982.

plished by the IV route, so that there is no urgency to force fluids, which can lead to nausea and vomiting. If the patient complains of nausea or is still NPO, ice chips should not be given since they are fluid and could initiate severe nausea and vomiting. Once the laryngopharyngeal reflexes have returned, the resumption of oral fluid should be very slow with intermittent periods of NPO to make sure the patient can tolerate the intake of fluid. Postoperative bleeding should be assessed routinely and any abnormal bleeding should be reported to the surgeon. This is especially true for the patient who has undergone a dilatation and curettage (D & C), since a perforated uterus is a major complication of this procedure. Specific signs and symptoms of a perforated uterus include vaginal bleeding, abdominal pain and rigidity, hypotension, and tachycardia.

In the pediatric population the most frequent problems in the immediate postoperative period are croup, nausea and vomiting, and fever of unknown etiology. These problems, which are also the most frequent reasons for admission to the hospital among pediatric patients, should be specifically monitored in the PACU, and the anesthesiologist or attending surgeon should be notified if any of these problems arise.

Another complication that can occur in the PACU is caused by the delirious patient who creates a disturbance and poses potential harm to himself by thrashing about. If this happens, the anesthesiologist should be notified and the patient restrained and protected from injury. Physostigmine (Antilirium) in a dosage of 1 to 2 mg given either intramuscularly or intravenously will usually reverse the delirium, and the patient will become cooperative and pleasant.

For some patients, anesthesia and surgery can be devastating to the body, even though the surgical procedure is considered minor. In these patients, the central nervous system and other organ systems may take considerable time to return to homeostasis. As a result, they may experience a delayed recovery from anesthesia (up to 24 to 48 hours). Ordinarily, they will be admitted to the hospital for extended postoperative care.

If the patient complains of postoperative pain, injectable analgesics, such as meperidine (Demerol) or morphine, should be avoided because they significantly prolong the recovery time in the PACU. Most ambulatory surgical patients undergo short surgical procedures that do not involve the upper gastrointestinal tract. Consequently, in the postoperative phase, these patients can generally tolerate the administration of oral analgesics such as aspirin, acetaminophen, codeine, and meperidine. Given orally, the opiate drugs do not have the same additive effect as when given intravenously. After the administration of one of these drugs, the patient may continue to experience some pain. However, the patient usually rests and breathes quietly, responds to the spoken word or to a gentle stimulus, and can be discharged after a substantially shorter stay in the PACU than would be the case with injectable analgesics.

Stage Two—The Lounge-Chair Recovery Area

When the patient arrives in the lounge-chair recovery area, his vital signs and dressings should be evaluated. After that, the patient can visit quietly with family members and take light refreshments. The usual time in the second stage is about one to two hours after the administration of the anesthetic.

Certain criteria are used to determine if the patient can be discharged from the ambulatory surgical unit. The patient's ability to ambulate successfully and stand with his eyes closed without unsteadiness are crude but effective methods to determine the patient's recovery from sedation. Other discharge criteria are listed in Table 34–4. If any criteria are not met by the patient, the physician responsible for the patient's care must either justify or delay the discharge.

If regional anesthesic technique on an extremity was used intraoperatively, residual anesthesia may be present. If the extremity is a leg, the anesthesia should have dissipated enough so that the patient can ambulate without assistance. If the extremity is an arm, the residual anesthesia works to the patient's advantage in delaying postoperative pain. The PACU nurse must instruct this patient to be careful to avoid injury and must provide the patient with a sling and some protection for the numb extremity. If the patient has received an epidural or spinal anesthetic, full motor function must have retruned before he can be discharged from the PACU. This is required because otherwise sympathetic blockade and orthostatic hypotension will be a problem if ambulation is attempted.

At the time of discharge, the patient should be given oral instructions reinforced by printed material cautioning against driv-

TABLE 34–4. Criteria for Discharge from the Ambulatory Surgical Unit

1. Vital signs are stable and blood pressure is within 20 percent of preoperative supine value.
2. Nausea and vomiting are under control, and the patient is able to take fluids orally.
3. The patient has voided—especially after cystoscopy and spinal or epidural anesthesia.
4. The patient is steady when upright and can ambulate without fear.
5. Mental status approaches preoperative status.
6. The operative site is dry, and circulation is not impaired by casts or dressings.
7. Pain is reasonably controlled.
8. Full motor function has returned after regional anesthesia.

From Allen, B.: Anesthesia and ambulatory surgery. AANA J., *52*(3):303–308, 1984.

ing a car or operating heavy machinery, ingesting alcohol or other depressants, or making any important decisions in the ensuing 24 hours. The patient should be told how and at what intervals body temperature should be taken. Also, the patient should be given the telephone number of the ambulatory surgical unit to call if questions or problems, such as temperature elevation, arise. Valuables and any other clothing should be returned to the patient, and, upon discharge, the patient should be driven home by a responsible adult.

Discharge criteria for the pediatric patient should be adapted to the age and abilities of the particular child. The pediatric patient should be discharged into the care of two adults, one to drive the car and one to remain with the child.

REFERENCES

1. Allen, B.: Anesthesia and Ambulatory Surgery. AANA J., 52(2):303–308, 1984.
2. Detmer, D., and Buchanan-Davidson, D.: Ambulatory Surgery. Surg. Clin. North Am., 62(4):685–704, 1982.
3. Dornette, W.: Planning Tomorrow's Hospital Today. Paper presented at ASA Meeting, Washington, D.C., 1968.
4. Dripps, R., Eckenhoff, J., and Vandam, L.: Introduction to Anesthesia: The Principles of Safe Practice. 6th ed. Philadelphia, W. B. Saunders Co., 1982.
5. Miller, R. (ed.): Anesthesia. 2nd ed. New York, Churchill-Livingstone, Inc., 1986.
6. Wetcher, B.: Anesthesia for Ambulatory Surgery. Philadelphia, J. B. Lippincott Co., 1985.
7. Woo, S. (ed.): Ambulatory Anesthesia Care. Int. Anesthesiol. Clin. Boston, Little, Brown & Co., Inc., 20(1):1–162, 1983.

Special Considerations

CHAPTER

35

Postoperative Care of the Substance Abuser

THE DRUG ADDICT

The great increase in the number of persons using narcotics, amphetamines, cocaine, hallucinogens, and barbiturates has created new problems in postoperative nursing care.

Drug abuse is the nonmedical use of a drug and consists of the self-administration of any drug in a manner that deviates from the approved medical or social practices within a given culture. *Physical dependence* is an altered physiologic state caused by repeated administration of a drug, which necessitates the continued administration of the drug in order to prevent the appearance of the withdrawal or abstinence syndrome characteristic for that drug. *Psychologic dependence* is a habituation-compulsive drug use. In this case, a drug is used to alter mood and feeling, and eventually, dependent individuals come to believe that the effects of the drug are necessary to maintain an optimal state of well-being. Another term that should be defined when discussing substance abuse is tolerance. *Drug tolerance* is a state in which, after repeated administration of a drug, a given dose produces a decreased effect or, on the other hand, increasingly larger doses are needed to obtain the same effect as that of the original dose.

The pharmacologic agents that are most commonly abused can be grouped as follows: (1) the *opioid analgesics;* (2) *general CNS depressants,* such as alcohol and the barbiturates; (3) *CNS sympathomimetics,* such as amphetamines and cocaine; (4) the *cannabinoids,* such as marihuana; and (5) the *psychedelics,* of which LSD and phencyclidine are the prototype drugs.

Opioid Analgesics

Opioid analgesics (narcotics) will cause very strong psychologic dependence. Physical dependence is manifested by the withdrawal syndrome of autonomic storm and central nervous system irritability. Also, there is a strong tolerance for these drugs as well as a cross-tolerance with other drugs of the same classification of opioid analgesics. Interestingly, studies indicate that in persons who are chronically addicted to opioid analgesics such as morphine, the minimum alveolar concentration (MAC) of halothane (Fluothane) is increased, indicating that a cross-tolerance with general inhalational anesthetics may exist.

Heroin, an opioid analgesic that is derived from morphine, is degraded in the body to morphine about 30 minutes after injection. The most common problem associated with the use of heroin and other opioid analgesics is pulmonary edema; other dysfunctions include superficial bacterial infections, adrenal insufficiency, bacterial endocarditis, liver disease, urinary abnormalities (proteinuria and glycosuria), and false-positive serology. In addition, about 30 percent of the opiate abusers have positive results on VDRL test for syphilis, but only about 25 percent of these are true-positive when checked by the treponema immobilization test.

PACU care of an opiate abuser, such as the heroin addict, centers around monitoring the patient for complications. Probably foremost is monitoring for the withdrawal (abstinence) syndrome. The abstinence syndrome after opiate abuse occurs in two phases. The acute phase occurs during the first few days. The protracted phase, which is not readily treatable, can persist for up to 2 to 6 months. The acute opiate abstinence phase is not dangerous to life because it is usually not associated with convulsions and delirium. Instead, the symptoms are anxiety, nervousness, jittery behavior, anorexia, rhinorrhea, hypotension, muscle twitching, insomnia, sweating, pupillary dilation, gooseflesh, and nausea and vomiting. Symptoms during the protracted phase include those of the acute phase, along with convulsions and delirium. Treatment for the acute opiate abstinence phase is accomplished with any narcotic analgesic; recent reports indicate that clonidine has proven to be most effective in attenuating the symptoms. Treatment for the protracted phase centers around protection of the patient and abating the symptoms demonstrated by the patient. If a patient is a suspected opiate abuser, narcotic antagonists such as naloxone (Narcan) should not be administered, as the withdrawal syndrome can be precipitated. No attempt should be made at withdrawal of the active abuser during the PACU period. Liberal use of morphine or methadone in the post anesthesia care unit appears to be satisfactory. The former abuser should not receive narcotics; analgesics, such as pentazocine (Talwin) or butorphanol (Stadol), should be utilized in their place.

General CNS Depressants

The *barbiturate addict* may only present as nervous and anxious before surgery. However, the patient should be monitored postoperatively for anxiety, tremors, and hallucinations. These symptoms usually develop on the second or third postoperative day and can be treated with a barbiturate until acute illness has passed. These patients also appear to have an increased tolerance to anesthesia and therefore have an increased chance of anesthetic toxicity.

Alcoholism has long been widespread, yet it is very difficult to define. An *alcoholic*, for purposes of this discussion, is an individual who is excessively dependent on alcohol and who has developed a noticeable degree of mental, physical, psychologic, or pathologic disorders. It is interesting to note that alcohol was the first anesthetic; it can produce anesthesia, respiratory depression, and hypotension.

Alcohol affects many of the body's major systems. It is well known that in the later stages of alcoholism, cirrhosis of the liver is quite common. This is of importance to the PACU nurse because the liver detoxifies many drugs administered during the perioperative period (see Chapter 7). Hepatic cirrhosis may produce significant alterations in pulmonary and cardiovascular functions. Hyperventilation and arterial oxygen desaturation are very common findings caused by an increase in shunting of blood away from areas in the lung where diffusion of oxygen takes place. Concomitant with this is an increase in blood volume that may lead to cardiac hypertrophy and, eventually, to congestive heart failure. Fluid balance is affected by the presence of alcohol, since alcohol exhibits antidiuretic effects by inhibiting the release of antidiuretic hormone (ADH). Alcoholic cirrhosis (Laennec's cirrhosis) is also associated with portal vein hypertension, renal failure, hypoglycemia, duodenal ulcer, esophageal varices, and hepatic encephalopathy.

The alcoholic, when compared with the nonalcoholic, will usually require a larger amount of sodium thiopental for induction and a higher concentration of anesthetic agents during surgery. It is difficult to predict the time or the character of emergence from anesthetic in the alcoholic patient. This patient may be anxious and might possibly have a stormy emergence and postoperative phase.

During the PACU phase, the alcoholic patient should be monitored for withdrawal symptoms. The *minor alcohol withdrawal syndrome* is characterized by symptoms such as tremulousness, insomnia, and irritability. Because of autonomic nervous system imbalance, signs such as tachycardia, hypertension, and cardiac dysrhythmias are often observed. The minor alcohol withdrawal syndrome can occur within 6 to 8 hours after abstinence by the alcoholic patient. The signs and symptoms of this syndrome will usually disappear within 48 hours without treatment.

In about 5 percent of the alcoholic population, when the ingestion of alcohol is abruptly ceased, the *severe alcohol withdrawal syndrome,* or *delirium tremens,* will occur. The mortality rate from this syndrome is about 15 percent, and it is considered a medical emergency. The time of onset of delirium tremens is about 48 to 72 hours after the abrupt discontinuation of alcohol ingestion.

The patient will be difficult to manage if withdrawal symptoms are allowed to develop. The severe withdrawal syndrome should be suspected if symptoms occur, such as restlessness, disorientation, tremulousness, and hallucinations. Along with this, because of activation of the sympathetic nervous system, symptoms such as diaphoresis, hyperpyrexia, tachycardia, and hypertension will be seen. When any of these symptoms is observed, hypoxia should first be ruled out, as the symptoms of withdrawal can be confused with those of hypoxia. The treatment used to control the withdrawal symptoms is sedation with diazepam (Valium), along with intravenous fluids and electrolytes, vitamin replacement (i.e., thiamine), and glucose. If deemed necessary by the attending physician, propranolol may be given to suppress the clinical manifestations of the increased sympathetic nervous system activity. Along with this, should cardiac dysrhythmias occur,

lidocaine may be administered intravenously.

CNS Sympathomimetics

Cocaine has a two-pronged effect: (1) vasoconstriction, and (2) mood alteration, because it inhibits the reuptake of catecholamines. The mood-altering effect is similar to the psychologic effect produced by amphetamines. Cocaine is steadily becoming one of the most popular drugs among substance abusers. Patients who are known abusers of cocaine should be closely monitored in the post anesthesia care unit for hypertension and cardiac arrhythmias. Also, these patients are very prone to frequent nosebleeds. Hence, care should be taken when administering nursing care near or to the nose and nasal cavity.

Central nervous system stimulants, which include amphetamines, tend to be long-acting vasopressors. The patient will have dilated pupils, tachycardia, palpitations, cardiac arrhythmias, changes in temperature regulation, and will appear to be very anxious. If the stimulant is wearing off, the patient will be lethargic and very depressed. Continuous electrocardiographic monitoring for cardiac arrhythmias is necessary coupled with frequent blood pressure and pulse measurements. The mental sensorium should also be monitored throughout the patient's stay in the PACU.

The Cannabinoids

The hemp plants, of which cannabis is the generic name, contain about 30 active substances that are called cannabinoids. Of these, tetrahydrocannabinol (THC) is the most active. Marihuana is the generic term applied to the hemp plants. The marihuana cigarette contains rolled up or crushed dried leaves from the hemp plant. Each marihuana cigarette contains about 0.005 gm of THC. The cannabinoids are three times more potent when inhaled than when ingested orally. Psychologic changes occur minutes after inhalation of marihuana and the effects peak in an hour, with a duration of up to three hours.

The peripheral effects of THC on the autonomic nervous system include vagal blockade and beta-adrenergic stimulation. Hence, the abuser of marihuana will experience tachycardia, peripheral vascular dilation, bronchodilatation, conjunctival congestion, and a dry mouth. The actual effects of THC on the central nervous system are not known.

Because of the rapid effects of the drug, along with the short duration of action and the absence of physiologic dysfunction or changes, abusers of marihuana do not seem to present any added problems in the post anesthesia care unit. However, because of the chronic irritation produced by the inhalation of smoke from the marihuana cigarette, chronic abusers should be monitored for chronic bronchitis.

Psychedelics

Phencyclidine is the hallucinogen most commonly used today. This drug is a very popular veterinary anesthetic agent (Sernylan) and is related pharmacologically to the drug ketamine. It can be ingested, taken parenterally, or inhaled. The sensory effects have a rapid onset and last approximately 1 to 2 hours, and the CNS effects can last for 1 or more days. The CNS activation usually produces sympathetic nervous system activation.

It is not very likely that the PACU nurse will have much contact with a patient under the influence of this drug. However, if a patient who abuses this drug should require PACU care, the nurse must monitor this patient for sympathetic activation, and symptoms such as dilated pupils, increased pulse, and elevated blood pressure should be reported immediately to the attending physician.

Lysergic acid diethylamide (LSD) is a hallucinogen that seemed to reach its peak of use in the late 1960s. Since then, the use of LSD has generally declined. This drug is ingested orally, and its major effects occur in a dose-related manner. Moderate dosage of the drug will cause euphoria, marked sensory distortion, which includes heightened awareness of sensory stimuli, and occasional visual hallucinations. Large doses of LSD usually lead to frightening hallucinations and a distorted body image—what is commonly referred to as a "bad trip." This drug also will produce some hypertension, dilated pupils, and increased temperature, by virtue of its stimulation of the central hypothalamic area of the brain. The onset of the psychologic effects of LSD is after about 40 minutes, and the duration is about 2 hours. Some of the milder effects of LSD have been reported to last up to 8 hours postingestion.

The primary focus of PACU nursing care for the patient who is in the hallucinogenic state is to prevent self-injury and sedation. The "bad trip" effects can be managed with chlorpromazine (Thorazine) or diazepam (Valium). Other considerations in regard to the patient who has ingested LSD are that the analgesic effects of narcotics are potentiated by LSD, and that the plasma cholinesterases are somewhat inhibited by LSD. Hence, narcotic dosage may need to be reduced in these patients, and if succinylcholine is to be administered to the patient, a possibility of prolonged apnea does exist.

REFERENCES

1. Brangman, G.: Drug addiction and anesthesia. AANA J., 39(1):43, 1971.
2. Heerdt, M.: Drug Addiction and Anesthesia. AANA Annual Meeting Summary, 1981.
3. Katz, J., Benumof, J., and Kadis, L.: Anesthesia and Uncommon Diseases. 2nd ed. Philadelphia, W. B. Saunders Co., 1981.
4. Miller, R.: Anesthesia. 2nd ed. New York, Churchill-Livingstone, Inc., 1986.
5. Stoelting, R., and Dierdorf, S.: Anesthesia and Co-Existing Disease. New York, Churchill-Livingstone, 1983.
6. Weiss, S.: Anesthesia for the alcoholic and addict. AANA J., 47(3):309–312, 1979.

36

Postoperative Care of the Patient with Chronic Disorders

CHRONIC OBSTRUCTIVE PULMONARY DISEASE

Chronic obstructive pulmonary disease (COPD) is a term that describes respiratory diseases of the bronchial obstructive type. It is characterized by dyspnea, with or without cough and sputum. The two major clinical manifestations of COPD are airway obstruction and airway destruction. The magnitude of the various disease entities that come under the term COPD is great. Therefore, it is difficult to elaborate individually on the diseases, as each deserves separate attention. Rather, we will describe briefly the overall characteristics of COPD and general care required in the post anesthesia care unit (PACU). It must be remembered that variations exist among patients diagnosed as having COPD. It is important for the PACU nurse to consult with the physician about the specific nursing care to be administered to the patient with COPD. For discussion of specific COPD diseases, see the references listed at the end of the chapter.

Description of COPD

Three major diseases are part of COPD: asthma, emphysema, and chronic bronchitis. All are characterized by airway obstruction. These diseases may have medically reversible components, such as bronchospasm, or they may have irreversible components, such as alveolar septal destruction. Some of the reversible components of *asthma*, such as retained secretions, bronchospasms, and infections, can be corrected by the interaction of the physician, nurse, physical therapist, and respiratory therapist. The treatment of asthma may include oxygen therapy, bronchial dilators, chest physiotherapy, and proper hydration.

Chronic *bronchitis* is associated with chronic cigarette smoking. The nurse can contribute greatly to the patient's future health by strongly influencing him or her to refrain from smoking. Other therapy for the reversible components may include the use of bronchial dilators, chest physiotherapy, and oxygen.

The patient with *emphysema* usually has

airway destruction that is irreversible. As the alveolar septa are destroyed, insufficient alveolar ventilation ensues and eventually leads to hypercarbia. As the disease progresses, carbon dioxide cannot be expelled from the lungs and is retained there. The patient usually increases his minute ventilation to try to compensate for the hypercarbia. Respiratory acidosis develops slowly as the various acid-base buffer systems try to neutralize the accumulated acid. In this compensated state, the patient will usually have a near-normal pH, a high plasma bicarbonate, low chloride concentrations, and a high total carbon dioxide. The Pa_{CO_2} will usually be low, as some inspired oxygen is unable to cross into the blood from the lungs, owing to the decrease in respiratory diffusion membrane surface area in the lungs. Pulmonary hypertension usually appears as the disease progresses. Cor pulmonale may develop and, because of the pulmonary venous engorgement, the right heart may begin to fail. The patient with emphysema who has irreversible destruction may be treated with chest physiotherapy, bronchial dilators, and steroids.

Surgical Considerations

The incidence of pulmonary complications in patients who have undergone abdominal or thoracic surgery is high. Changes occur in the pulmonary status of the patient who undergoes anesthesia and surgery. In the postoperative phase, these changes are characterized by gradual or abrupt alveolar collapse. The patient with COPD, when subjected to surgery, then represents an even higher risk for postoperative complications. It is very important that these patients be given meticulous preoperative care so that they may be in the best possible health when they enter surgery. This preoperative medical treatment usually includes hydration, nutrition, chest physiotherapy, bronchial dilators, and prophylactic antibiotics if an infection is present. Serial pulmonary function tests and arterial blood gases are used to monitor the progression of the preoperative treatment.

When the patient's pulmonary function reaches a peak preoperatively, that is, when the pulmonary function tests and arterial blood gas test results no longer show continued improvement, then surgery is considered, because the patient has reached his optimal pulmonary status.

PACU Care

PACU care of the COPD patient centers around prevention of complications. The post anesthesia care unit stir-up regimen should include frequent cascade coughing, sustained maximal inspirations (SMIs), and repositioning of the patient (see Chapters 4 and 18). An appropriately implemented stir-up regimen is of great importance, especially in patients recovering from upper abdominal or thoracic operations. Surgery at these sites can cause decreased ventilatory effort and a complete absence of sighs by the patient. Given that the patient already suffers from compromised respiratory function, the possibility of retained secretions and atelectasis is certainly magnified. Hence, these patients represent a significant challenge to the PACU nurse.

When the patient is completely reactive, the use of the incentive spirometer may be helpful in reducing the incidence of atelectasis. Consequently, the PACU nurse who is responsible for supportive measures should assist and encourage the patient in using the SMI with or without the incentive spirometer. Based on subjective research findings, it is believed that if the PACU nurse explains the rationale of the SMI maneuver and properly instructs the patient in the use of the technique *preoperatively*, the patient is more likely to correctly utilize the SMI maneuver postoperatively with or without coaching. The performance of the SMI maneuver, with or without mechanical devices, should be monitored by the nurse to ensure proper production of a sustained inspiration with a three-second inspiratory hold. The PACU nurse should also encourage and monitor the patient's performance of the cascade cough to facilitate early secretion clearance.

The cardiac status should be monitored meticulously because of the frequent involvement of the heart in the pathologic disorders of these patients. Kidney function should also be monitored because it may be altered, especially in patients who exhibit fluid retention and edema of the extremities

The patient with severe COPD who has marked hypercarbia can present difficulties in the PACU. Patients who have severe emphysema usually fall into this category. Their ventilatory effort is stimulated by the hypoxic drive, in which lack of oxygen serves as the stimulus to ventilation. Hypoxia indirectly stimulates the respiratory center by means of chemoreceptors in the carotid bodies located at the bifurcation of the carotid artery. When oxygen tensions rise in the inspired gas, owing to the patient's being given 100 percent oxygen to breathe in the PACU, the carotid and aortic chemoreceptors will cease to function and the patient will quickly become apneic. The patient's respiratory status should be assessed carefully and the physician consulted before 100 percent oxygen is administered. Mist therapy postoperatively will aid in liquifying the secretions and help in the all-important maintenance of a patent tracheobronchial tree. If excessive bronchial drainage is not removed, it will provide a convenient avenue for bacteria and it may also obstruct the airways, leading to insufficient alveolar ventilation and hypoxia.

The COPD patient should be under constant surveillance for signs of cardiopulmonary decompensation, including shallow, rapid, gasping respiration, severe dyspnea, substernal retraction, and disorientation. Blood pressure may be elevated or low, but the patient will usually have tachycardia, fever, and muscle rigidity. Cyanosis may or may not be present.

It should also be noted that respiratory depressant drugs, such as narcotics, should be given in low doses, or, if the COPD is severe, they should be completely avoided. Repositioning of the patient and splinting of the incision site, along with reducing the anxiety usually seen in these patients, will reduce the need for narcotic drugs.

MYASTHENIA GRAVIS

The patient with myasthenia gravis (MG) deserves special consideration in the PACU because of the respiratory dysfunction and possible pharmacologic ramifications of the disease. It is a chronic disease characterized by progressive muscle weakness and easy fatigability. The majority of the patients with MG have developed antibodies to muscle acetylcholine receptors. Interestingly, the antibody does not bind exactly on the site that binds the acetylcholine, but very close to it. The acetylcholine receptors are steadily destroyed, with a resulting reduction in the binding of acetylcholine at the postsynaptic myoneural junction. The myasthenic patient will sometimes have a lesion in the myocardium that is a spotty, focal necrosis accompanied by an inflammatory reaction. An alteration in the S-T segment and T wave is sometimes seen in these patients.

The incidence of myasthenia gravis has been estimated to be between 1 in 15,000 and 1 in 40,000. It occurs twice as frequently in females as in males and at an earlier age. The main symptom is weakness involving one or more of the muscle groups, with ptosis of the eye the most frequent sign of the disease.

Ptosis is usually accompanied by diplopia, blurred vision, or nystagmus. Ocular signs and symptoms are frequently worsened by bright light. The patient may also have "myasthenic facies," which is caused by weakness of the facial muscles. This can progress to dysphagia and difficulties in speech.

Respiration is often affected in the myasthenic patient. Dyspnea can be either inspiratory, if the diaphragm is involved, or expiratory, if the intercostal and abdominal muscles are affected. The patient may also have emotional disturbances caused by anxiety and depression.

Diagnosis of MG is made on the clinical symptoms and the characteristic electromyogram (EMG). The clinical symptoms can be assessed by the neostigmine test or by the edrophonium test, both of which involve anticholinesterases that produce an increase in the strength of the myasthenic muscle. Muscle relaxants, such as d-tubo-curarine chloride (curare) or gallamine trie-thiodide (Flaxedil), given in very small doses will cause an exaggeration of MG symptoms and can be used in the diagnostic work-up of the patient.

Treatment for this disease consists of various pharmacologic interventions designed to enhance neuromuscular transmission and slow the progression of the disease. Anticholinesterase drugs, which slow down the enzymatic destruction of acetylcholine at the neuromuscular junction, are commonly utilized. Oral pyridostigmine and the shorter-acting neostigmine are the anticholinesterases of choice. MG patients seem to favor pyridostigmine over neostigmine because of its length of action and its less unpleasant side effects. Steroids and other immunosuppressive agents may be used in some cases to reduce antibody production responsible for the disease.

The thymectomy seems to be an appropriate therapeutic mode, as the thymus gland appears to be intimately involved in the disease process. About 67 percent of the MG patients who do not have thymoma will experience improvement after a thymectomy. On the hand, about 25 percent of the MG patients with thymoma will have improvement in the disease process after thymectomy.

Since the thymectomy has been utilized as a therapeutic intervention in the treatment of MG, the PACU nurse will probably render nursing care to many MG patients. Because of the location of the incision, the MG patient does not usually receive any intraoperative skeletal muscle relaxants. These MG patients can experience an exacerbation of symptoms in the post anesthesia care unit. Hence, critical monitoring of the patient's ventilatory status should be the primary focus of the PACU nursing care. It should also be stated that MG patients who are recovering from any type of surgical procedure and who have been administered any form of anesthesia (general, inhalational, or regional) can develop an exacerbation of symptoms, as well as myasthenic

crisis, in the PACU. Consequently, respiratory support should always be available for these patients.

PACU Care

The patient with myasthenia gravis can present various difficulties because of an impaired respiratory system, possible poor nutrition, susceptibility to infection, altered psychiatric status, and possible altered response to drugs used during anesthesia. The patient should be placed in a quiet area, where no direct light will shine in his eyes. The patient's respiratory effort and exchange should be monitored continuously. Oxygen should be administered with humidification, and secretions should be removed by frequent suctioning and postural drainage. Any change in respiratory status should be reported to the physician immediately.

Cardiac monitoring should be instituted for every myasthenic patient in the PACU, because cardiac mechanisms may be responsible for some sudden deaths encountered in myasthenic patients. It is also important to monitor the fluids administered to these patients. Hypovolemia and hypervolemia must be avoided because of their deleterious effects on the already compromised heart and lungs.

The patient should be kept as pain-free as possible to facilitate good respiratory exchange. Morphine and other narcotics are often potentiated by anticholinesterases. Therefore, the initial narcotic dose should be reduced to half the normal dose and then increased if required. If the patient is receiving continuous mechanical ventilation, the normal amount of medication can be given without compromising the patient's respiratory status.

The emotional status of the myasthenic patient is of considerable importance. As few individuals as possible should be responsible for the myasthenic throughout his recovery phase because he is likely to be distrustful of anyone he does not know. Communication is very important, and the patient should be informed about any nursing procedure to be performed. If the myasthenic has a tracheostomy, paper and pencil should be utilized to facilitate communication between nurse and patient.

DIABETES MELLITUS

Diabetes mellitus is a chronic metabolic disease associated with insulin deficiency or insensitivity, hyperglycemia, and glycosuria. It occurs in about 2 to 3 percent of the general population. One important aspect of this disease is an associated degeneration of the small blood vessels (microangiopathy) that is most marked in the retina, kidneys, and nervous system.

The focus of the physiologic activity of insulin is to "open the door" of the cell to let glucose enter. In the diabetic state, the patient will have an elevated blood glucose because of a defect in the cellular response to insulin and the "door" remains closed. Sources of the excess glucose are dietary carbohydrate, liver glycogen, and glucose formed by the fatty acids metabolized to acetone, or β-hydroxybutyric acid. These three products are known as ketone bodies. The degree of insulin deficiency is reflected by hyperglycemia, glycosuria, and ketoacidosis exhibited by the patient.

Anesthesia and Diabetes

The goals of anesthetic management of the diabetic patient are prevention of diabetic acidosis, hypoglycemia, and severe fluid loss. Clinicians differ regarding the specific method to be utilized to achieve these goals. One method is to withhold the usual dose of long-acting or intermediate-acting insulin. Two liters of 5 percent dextrose, with 10 to 15 units of crystalline regular insulin added to each liter, are given to the patient during surgery. In another method, the patient is administered 5 percent dextrose in Ringer's lactate at 125 ml per hour. Regular insulin, in 5-unit increments, is administered as needed to keep the patient's blood sugar at or above 200 mg/dl. A more widely used method consists of giving half the daily dose of insulin on the morning of surgery or a third of the

daily dose if the surgery is scheduled later in the day. The patient is given 500 to 1000 ml of 5 percent dextrose and water prior to surgery and at least 1000 ml of 5 percent dextrose and water during surgery. This method avoids hypoglycemia during surgery but increases the need for careful nursing attention in the post anesthesia care unit.

These methods are used in the patient who is undergoing elective surgery. Emergency surgery for the uncontrolled diabetic patient is an entirely different situation. Before the patient undergoes anesthesia and surgery, treament of the diabetes should be instituted, if possible. Frequent blood glucose levels are usually taken along with a blood urea nitrogen to indicate the proper amount of regular insulin to be administered intraoperatively on a sliding scale. Intravenous solutions are given to treat dehydration.

PACU Care

The patient should be monitored for fluid and electrolyte balance, and degree of glycosuria. Most authors agree that mild glycosuria is more desirable than glucose-free urine. Hypoglycemia should be avoided. Patients who have had a stressful problem relieved—for example, the removal of an intra-abdominal abscess—may have a reduced insulin requirement postoperatively. This may be as much as a 50 percent reduction in the first 24 hours. However, because of the stress of surgery, insulin requirements postoperatively are usually increased.

Urine glucose can be monitored by the Clinitest method. This method does not monitor the blood glucose directly, but does provide a rough indicator of insulin requirements. Blood glucose can be monitored closely in the PACU by using a Dextrostix with blood from a finger stick. Blood glucose laboratory determinations should be done at least twice daily for 2 to 3 days postoperatively. A sliding scale that is usually utilized for the Clinitest method is seen in Table 36–1.

TABLE 36–1. Sliding Scale of Insulin Determinations

Urine Glucose (Trace %)	Regular Insulin Dose (Units)
0.25	5
0.50	8
1	10
2	15

Respiratory acidosis should be prevented by aiding the patient to cough and breathe deeply to promote adequate pulmonary ventilation and carbon dioxide elimination. Metabolic acidosis must be prevented by administration of fluid and electrolytes. Therefore, very strict monitoring of intake and output should be instituted on every diabetic patient admitted to the post anesthesia care unit.

There is a strong possibility that the diabetic patient will receive an insulin preparation in the recovery phase. The types of insulin, along with times of onset, peak effects, and duration of action, are summarized in Table 36–2.

Observation of the diabetic patient for possible diabetic coma (hyperglycemia) or insulin reaction ensures his proper recovery. The symptoms of each complication are summarized in Table 36–3. It is sometimes difficult to detect hyperglycemia or hypoglycemia by symptoms when a patient is recovering from an anesthetic. Therefore, frequent tests of blood and urine glucose are most helpful in determining the patient's state. It is also important to keep in mind that any patient who arrives in the PACU, especially in the older age groups, may have undiagnosed diabetes.

RHEUMATOID ARTHRITIS

Rheumatoid arthritis is a relatively common disease that affects the connective tissue of the body. The clinical course varies, but it tends to be progressive, leading to characteristic deformities. A large proportion of the patients become incapacitated over time. The disease affects more women than men, and its incidence in temperate climates is about 3 percent. The etiology is not completely understood, but it is thought to be an autoimmune phenomenon. The outstanding clinical feature of this disease is proliferative inflammation. The patient often appears chronically ill, undernourished, and anemic.

These patients often undergo surgery to correct restrictive deformities caused by the disease process (see Table 36–4). Upon arrival in the post anesthesia care unit, they require comprehensive nursing management. Some of the hazards to be aware of in patients with rheumatoid arthritis are listed in Table 36–5.

PACU Care

Airway. Extubation is often deferred in these patients until they are unquestionably able to maintain their own airways. This is of prime importance, as these patients are often extremely difficult to intubate and are very prone to airway obstruction.

Lungs. The patient with rheumatoid arthritis usually has such pulmonary dysfunction as diffuse interstitial fibrosis, granulomatous lesions, or large silicotic nodules. These pulmonary dysfunctions lead to what is termed stiff lungs, and these patients are prone to atelectasis, hypoxemia, and hypercarbia in the PACU (see Chapter 4). Postoperative blood gas analysis and good, pulmonary support are therefore important. Respiratory depressant narcotics should be given with caution, if at all. Deaths in rheumatoid arthritic patients have resulted from

TABLE 36–2. Time of Action of Various Insulin Preparations

Types of Insulin	Time of Onset (Minutes)	Peak Effects (Minutes)	Duration of Action (Hours)
Insulin injection, U.S.P. (regular)	0.50	2–4	6
Crystalline zinc insulin	1	2–4	8
Globin zinc insulin	2–4	8	18–24
Isophane insulin injection (N.P.N.)	2	8–20	20–30
Protamine zinc injection (P.Z.I.)	6–8	12–24	24–36
Lente insulin (insulin zinc suspension)	2–4	8–20	20–28

TABLE 36–3. Symptoms of Complications of Diabetes

	Diabetic Coma	Insulin Reaction
Onset	Slow	Sudden
Skin	Flushed, dry, hot	Pale, moist
Behavior	Drowsy	Excited
Breath	Acetone (sweet)	Normal
Respirations	Kussmaul's (air hunger)	Normal–rapid, shallow
Pulse	Rapid, weak	Normal–slow, full bounding
Blood pressure	Low	Normal
Vomiting	Present	Absent
Hunger	Absent	Present
Thirst	Present	Absent
Urine glucose	Large amount	Absent

drug-induced respiratory failure during this period.

Heart. Disease of the pericardium, myocardium, endocardium, and coronary vessels is usually associated with rheumatoid arthritis. Therefore, cardiovascular status should be monitored continuously in the PACU. Hypotension should be avoided, as it may lead to left ventricular decompensation and acute heart failure.

Blood. The arthritic patient will usually exhibit anemia, most commonly of the hypochromic microcytic variety. In most cases this anemia can be treated by blood transfusion. Postoperative hematocrit and hemoglobin levels should be determined when the patient arrives in the post anesthesia care unit. Blood loss should be extensively

TABLE 36–4. Corrective Surgery for Rheumatoid Arthritis

Operative Site	Common Operative Procedure
Neck	Atlanto-axial arthrodesis
Shoulder	Synovectomy and partial excision of acromion
Elbow	Synovectomy and radial head excision; resection arthroplasty
Wrist	Synovectomy and excision of distal ulna
Hand	Metacarpal phalangeal arthroplasty and flexor and extensor tenosynovectomy
Hip	Cup or total replacement arthroplasty
Knee	Synovectomy (often bilateral), arthroplasty
Foot	Resection arthroplasty (often bilateral)

From Jenkins, L. C., and McGraw, R. W.: Anesthetic management of the patient with rheumatoid arthritis. Can. Anaesth. Soc. J., *16*:408, 1969.

monitored, including observation of stools for blood. The contents recovered from the nasogastric tube (if present) should be checked for blood, as these patients may suffer from a bleeding peptic ulcer secondary to long-term aspirin and steroid therapy.

Fluid Balance. Renal function is usually impaired in the chronic rheumatoid arthritic patient. Therefore, drugs that are primarily excreted by the kidneys should be avoided,

TABLE 36–5. PACU Hazards in Patients with Rheumatoid Arthritis

Area of Concern	Complication
Respiratory system	
Airway	Hypoplastic mandible restriction, cervical spine motion, atlanto–axial subluxation, laryngeal tissue damage
Ventilation	Rheumatoid nodules in lung, chronic diffuse interstitial fibrosis, costovertebral joint disorder which will inhibit ventilation, thoracic vertebrae flexion deformity which will inhibit ventilation, tuberculous lung
Cardiovascular system	Pericardial, myocardial, coronary artery pathology, aortic valve regurgitation, arrhythmias
Hemopoietic, hepatic and renal systems	Anemia, leukopenia, bleeding tendency (decreased platelets), renal amyloidosis
Miscellaneous	Skin fragility; postoperative chest complications, such as atelectasis, hypercarbia, and hypoxia; multiple joint disease

Modified from Jenkins, L. C., and McGraw, R. W.: Anaesthetic management of the patient with rheumatoid arthritis. Can. Anaesth. Soc. J., *16*:408, 1969.

and urinary output should be monitored at regular, perhaps hourly, intervals.

OBESITY

Obesity, the most common nutritional disorder in civilized countries today, presents many difficulties to the post anesthesia care unit nurse. Many definitions of obesity can be found in the literature. The pooled statistics of American Life Insurance Company state that a person is obese if he or she exceeds the expected or ideal weight, corrected by age and sex, by more than 10 percent. *Morbid obesity* is a term that denotes a weight of twice as much as that predicted for age, sex, body build, and height. Morbidly obese patients can be divided into two groups. Obesity with normal levels of arterial carbon dioxide tension is referred to as *simple obesity* and includes 90 to 95 percent of morbidly obese patients. The other group, which represents 5 to 10 percent of obese patients, is referred to as having the *obesity-hypoventilation (pickwickian) syndrome*. This is characterized by extreme obesity and episodic somnolence, and by hypoventilation (increased $Paco_2$) with twitching, plethora, edema, periodic respiration, secondary polycythemia, right ventricular hypertrophy, and right ventricular failure.

The most useful anthropometric index for determining obesity is the *body mass index (BMI)*. This measurement employs the person's weight (in kilograms) divided by height squared (in meters):

$$BMI = \frac{\text{weight (kg)}}{\text{height (m)}^2}$$

The patient with a BMI of 27 (25 to 30 percent overweight), usually presents minimal risks in the perioperative period. A BMI of more than 30 is associated with an increased perioperative mortality.

Physiologic Considerations in Obesity

Respiratory System. Preoperative evaluation of obese patients reveals that 85 percent of them have exertional dyspnea and some degree of orthopnea. Periodic breathing, especially when sleeping, may also be present.

Obese patients tend to develop some degree of thoracic kyphosis and lumbar lordosis owing to a protuberant abdomen. In addition, the layers of fat on the chest and abdomen reduce the bellows action of the thoracic cage. The overall lung-thorax compliance is reduced, leading to an increased elastic resistance of the system. Usually the diaphragm is elevated and the total work of breathing is increased as a result of the deposition of abdominal fat. Because of these factors, the oxygen cost of breathing is three or more times that of normal, even at rest.

The primary respiratory defect of obese patients is a marked reduction in the expiratory reserve volume (ERV). The reason for the decrease in expiratory reserve volume and other lung volumes is that the obese patient is unable to expand his chest in a normal fashion. Therefore, diaphragmatic movement must account for the changes in lung volume to a much greater extent than thoracic expansion. As previously discussed, the diaphragmatic movement is moderately limited owing to the anatomic changes of obesity that account for the decreased lung volumes.

In the obese patient, the functional residual capacity (FRC) may be below the closing capacity in the sitting and supine positions. Therefore, the dependent lung zones may be effectively closed throughout the respiratory cycle (see Chapter 4). Consequently, inspired gas is distributed mainly to the upper or nondependent lung zones. The resulting mismatch of ventilation to perfusion produces systemic arterial hypoxemia (Fig. 36–1).

The hypoventilation and ventilation-perfusion abnormalities that contribute to systemic arterial hypoxemia also contribute to retained carbon dioxide, resulting in hypercarbia, which can be observed in the pickwickian syndrome.

Cardiovascular System. It has been estimated that 30 pounds of fat contain 25 miles of blood vessels, and that the increased

The relationship of body mass to systemic arterial hypoxemia.

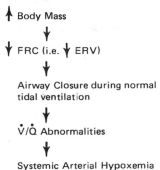

Figure 36–1. The relationship of body mass to systemic arterial hypoxemia. (Adapted from Drain, C., and Vaughan, R.: Anesthetic Considerations of Morbid Obesity. *AANA J.* 47(5):556–565, 1979, p. 558.)

body mass in obesity leads to an increased oxygen consumption and carbon dioxide production. It is not surprising that the cardiac output and the total blood volume are increased in the obese state. This increase in cardiac output is a result of an increase in stroke volume rather than an increase in heart rate, as the latter usually remains normal.

The transverse cardiac diameter has been shown to be greater than normal in approximately two thirds of obese patients. There seems to be a linear relationship between cardiac diameter and body weight.

It has been suggested that obesity predisposes to electrocardiographic changes. The Q-T interval is often prolonged and the QRS voltage is reduced (owing to the increased distance between the heart and the electrodes). Finally, there is an increased likelihood that ventricular arrhythmias can occur in the obese patient.

There is a positive correlation between an increase in body weight and increased arterial pressure. A weight gain of 28 pounds can increase the systolic and diastolic blood pressure by 10 and 7 torr respectively. The increase in blood pressure is probably due to the increased cardiac output.

Chronic heart failure, although not common, does occur in persons with long-standing morbid obesity with or without hypertension. It is usually characterized by high output and biventricular dysfunction with the left ventricle predominating. Clinically, heart failure may be difficult to diagnose because pedal edema may be chronically present.

Cerebral blood flow in obese persons does not differ significantly from that in normal persons. Oxygen uptake of the brain remains normal in the obese person. However, the fraction of the total body oxygen accounted for in the cerebral metabolism is less than normal since the total body oxygen requirement is increased. Although the kidneys of obese subjects weigh more than those of their normal counterparts, renal blood flow is the same or slightly lower than that found in patients of normal weight.

Pregnancy. Problems associated with obesity in pregnancy occur relatively frequently. Studies indicate that patients weighing at least 250 pounds have a 35 percent chance of operative obstetrics. In fact, some form of obstetric complication(s) may be observed in 63 percent of obese patients. There is seven times more toxemia, five times more pyelonephritis, and ten times more diabetes mellitus than in similar groups of nonobese pregnant patients.

Other Disorders. Diabetes mellitus has been associated with obesity. It is the third most prevalent preoperative pathologic condition found in obese patients. Adult diabetics are often obese, and an improved glucose tolerance test follows weight reduction. Other associated problems that may be clinically present include abnormal liver function tests, fatty infiltration of the liver, gallstones, hiatal hernia, and varicose veins.

PACU Care

Respiratory. Significant problems can and do arise in the post anesthesia care unit phase of the perioperative care of the obese patient. In fact, the problems associated with obesity are becoming more apparent to all PACU nurses since the advent of the jejunoileal bypass and gastric stapling procedures for the treatment of morbid obesity. There is a direct correlation between incidence of postoperative pulmonary complications and degree of obesity. The mortality rate after upper abdominal operations in obese patients is two-and-one-half times that of their nonobese counterparts.

Positioning can be a valuable therapeutic tool to improve arterial oxygenation. It has been demonstrated that position significantly affects the Pa_{O_2} for 48 hours postoperatively. The obese patient should be cared for in a semi-Fowler position unless cardiovascular instability exists. *Routine use of the supine position should be avoided*, as the functional residual capacity (FRC) can decrease below the closing capacity, and thus reduce the number of ventilated alveoli, which will ultimately lead to hypoxemia. Moreover, early ambulation in the PACU is of great value in enhancing lung volumes of the obese patient.

In the postoperative period, the position of the operative incision is a factor, because it has been demonstrated that in obese patients with a vertical incision, there exists a more marked postoperative hypoxemia than in obese patients who receive a transverse incision. Therefore, supplemental inspired oxygen may be necessary for up to 3 to 4 days postoperatively in patients with a vertical incision. Serial arterial blood gases can serve as a guide to supplemental oxygen administration. Along with this, when the patient arrives in the post anesthesia care unit and an arterial line is in place, arterial blood gases should be drawn to provide a baseline guide for proper ventilation. If the patient arrives in the PACU with the endotracheal tube in place, the patient should be started on a ventilator. The nurse should then auscultate for bilateral breath sounds to ensure proper placement of the endotracheal tube. Because of the many technical difficulties associated with tracheal intubation of the obese patient, the PACU nurse should constantly monitor the patient for proper placement of the tube. If it becomes displaced, the patient should be ventilated with a bag-valve-mask system, and the anesthesia personnel should be summoned immediately.

Cardiovascular pathophysiology may re-duce cardiac reserve, especially in the older obese patient. A reduction in arterial oxygen tension due to incision site or postoperative position will cause an increase in cardiac output in order to facilitate tissue oxygen delivery. This could lead to cardiac decompensation in an already compromised cardiovascular system. Arterial hypoxemia should be avoided, since many obese patients cannot compensate for the increased cardiac output demand and the concomitant pulmonary vasoconstriction caused by the reduced arterial oxygen tension.

Not only is early postoperative ambulation important in enhancing lung volumes, but it will also help reduce the incidence of venous thrombosis. Indeed, relatively immobile obese persons are particularly susceptible to the development of pulmonary emboli.

Cardiovascular. The obese patient has a higher incidence of hypertension, coronary artery disease, myocardial infarction, and cardiomegaly. Therefore, careful electrocardiographic monitoring should be employed. If an arterial line was not utilized intraoperatively, a blood pressure cuff that covers one-third to one-half the length of the upper arm should be utilized. A baseline blood preasure reading when the patient arrives in the PACU will prove valuable when compared with the intraoperative readings to assess the accuracy of the blood pressure reading.

Fluid Dynamics. Because fatty tissue is 6 to 10 percent water, as compared with lean tissue, which is composed of 70 to 80 percent water, alteration in fluid requirements is likely to occur in the obese patient. In the normal individual, the percentage of body water is 65; in the obese individual the body water is about 40 percent of his total weight. Calculations of fluid requirements must be adjusted to compensate for this reduction in total body water.

Psychologic. Psychologic support of the obese patient should not be overlooked when administering PACU care. Many of these patients have become obese because of repeated episodes of emotional stress.

Body image, along with the ability to interact with others, may be a problem for obese patients; they may appear to be very demanding and aloof from others. It is important for the post anesthesia care unit personnel to establish a positive rapport with the obese patient preoperatively. Along with this, it is important that the PACU staff not inflict any negative feelings about the patient, or about morbid obesity in general, on the obese patient. Hence, the added psychologic support will serve to minimize fear and anxiety and ultimately improve the outcome of the obese patient.

CIGARETTE SMOKING

Cigarette smoking affects the manner in which a patient recovers from an anesthetic. The PACU nurse should be aware of the diverse reactions that smoking can have on the patient who is emerging from an inhalation anesthetic.

Although the literature on the relationship between smoking and its effects on anesthesia is meager, it does indicate an increase in the risk factor when a patient smokes.

Respiratory Effects

A growing body of convincing scientific literature suggests that almost all pulmonary disease is related in some way to the inhalation of infectious or irritant particulate material. Cigarette smoke in its gaseous phase contains nitrogen, oxygen, carbon dioxide, carbon monoxide, hydrogen, argon, methane, hydrogen cyanide, ammonia, nitrogen dioxide, and acetone. In the particulate phase, cigarette smoke contains nicotine, tar, acids, alcohol, phenols, and hydrocarbons. When a smoker inhales nicotine from a cigarette into the lungs he will actually receive 25 to 30 percent of the nicotine contained in the cigarette. Thirty percent is destroyed by combustion, and 40 percent is lost in the side stream. Therefore, if a person inhales the smoke from a cigarette containing 2.5 mg of nicotine, 1 mg of nicotine will actually be absorbed by the

lungs. It was also found that filters made very little difference in this absorption. Contrary to some opinions, smoking cigars and pipes does also present risk for pulmonary disease.

The carbon monoxide combines with the hemoglobin molecule at the same point as does oxygen. It has an affinity for this receptor point that is 210 times greater than that of oxygen. Therefore, the oxygen-carrying capacity of hemoglobin is reduced, and the end result is that less oxygen is given up to the tissues by the hemoglobin. When carbon monoxide combines with hemoglobin, the compound formed is called *carboxyhemoglobin*. The amount of carboxyhemoglobin in the blood is especially important in the patient who has a diseased myocardium, as myocardial oxygenation is limited by the flow of the blood through the coronary arteries. During stress, such as in surgery and anesthesia, the amount of carboxyhemoglobin saturation could lead to severe myocardial hypoxia in heavy-smoking patients with coronary artery disease, because the diseased coronary arteries cannot increase the flow significantly. The only means of preventing hypoxia is to increase the extraction of oxygen from the hemoglobin. Small amounts of carboxyhemoglobin may hinder the uncoupling of the oxygen, resulting in yet more oxygen retention at any given tension. This effect clearly would be greater when the oxygen tension is further reduced by local ischemia and any additional vasoconstriction associated with smoking.

Smoking is an important causative factor in chronic pulmonary disease, especially in the obstructive type. The pulmonary function alterations characteristic of smokers usually include a reduction in vital capacity, an increase in residual volume to total lung capacity, an uneven distribution of inspired gas, a decrease in dynamic compliance, and an increase in nonelastic resistance.

Chronic bronchitis is the disease most often associated with smoking and is seen quite frequently by the PACU nurse. Hypertrophy of bronchial mucous glands, with production of excessive mucus, is the hallmark of this disease. A vicious circle develops as this failure to remove the mucus leads to retention of pathogenic organisms and irritants. The resulting distorted alveolar septa and the increased pressure on the alveoli from chronic bronchitis can lead to emphysema.

Cigarette smoke can cause a progression from hyperplasia to metaplasia to neoplasia in the lungs. Sometimes associated with bronchial carcinoma is the *Eaton-Lambert syndrome*, often referred to as the "myasthenic syndrome," because its symptoms resemble those of myasthenia gravis. This syndrome in some way affects neuromuscular transmission, and patients experience the classic symptoms of muscle weakness. These patients are especially sensitive to the skeletal neuromuscular blocking agents used in clinical anesthesia. If the anesthetist is unaware of this syndrome and administers the normal dosage of skeletal muscle relaxants, the patient will probably be unable to ventilate spontaneously upon emergence from anesthesia even when pharmacologic reversal of the muscle relaxant is attempted. In this situation postoperative mechanical ventilation will be necessary.

Cardiovascular Effects

The correlation between vascular disease and smoking is strong. Smoking may influence thrombosis, and since thrombi and platelets contribute to the development of arteriosclerosis, smoking can help to cause arteriosclerosis and its complications.

Inhalation of nicotine produces a release of catecholamines, activates the carotid and aortic chemoreceptor bodies, and directly stimulates the muscles of the vessel walls. As a result, the immediate effects of smoking even a small number of cigarettes can be fairly marked—producing increases in heart rate, peripheral resistance, cardiac workload, and blood pressure. Each of these actions causes a greater myocardial oxygen demand. Furthermore, as the smoker's hemoglobin can provide less oxygen to the myocardium, it is not surprising that smoking can cause cardiac arrhythmias, either through myocardial anoxia or through epinephrine release.

PACU Care

In a study involving 49 complications out of 785 operations, it was noted that patients who smoked had a significant increase in pulmonary complications[30] as compared with nonsmokers. Another study indicates that patients who smoke more than two packs of cigarettes a day are especially prone to perianesthetic complications.[25] Many of these complications developed when cigarette smokers had a preexisting chronic respiratory disease, usually bronchitis. The major postoperative complications associated with smoking are infection, atelectasis, pleural effusion, pulmonary infarction, and bronchitis.

Complications associated with the chronic cigarette smoker revolve around the inability of the patient to clear secretions. The goal of nursing care in the PACU centers around clearing the tracheobronchial tree. This necessitates frequent suctioning, cascade coughing, and the use of the sustained maximal inspiration (SMI) maneuver. If, upon auscultation, rales and rhonchi are heard, percussion and postural drainage should be initiated.

Because cardiovascular disease is associated with a long history of cigarette smoking, the patient should have continuous electrocardiographic monitoring. Arrhythmias, such as premature venticular contractions (PVCs), should be sought, as they may be the first sign of decreased myocardial oxygenation in the cigarette smoker.

REFERENCES

Chronic Obstructive Pulmonary Disease (COPD)

1. Burrows, B., Knudson, R., Quan, S., et al.: Respiratory Disorders: A Pathophysiologic Approach. 2nd ed. Chicago, Year Bok Medical Publishers, Inc., 1983.
2. Drain, C.: Comparison of two inspiratory maneuvers on increasing lung volumes in postoperative upper abdominal surgical patients. Unpublished Master's Thesis. Tucson, The University of Arizona, 1980.

3. Katz, J., Benumof, J., and Kadis, L.: Anesthesia and Uncommon Diseases: Pathophysiologic and Clinical Correlations. 2nd ed. Philadelphia, W. B. Saunders Co., 1981.

Myasthenia Gravis

4. Katz, J., Benumof, J., and Kadis, L.: Anesthesia and Uncommon Diseases: Pathophysiologic and Clinical Correlations. 2nd ed. Philadelphia, W. B. Saunders Co., 1981.
5. Miller, R.: Anesthesia. 2nd ed. New York, Churchill Livingstone, Inc., 1986.
6. Stoelting, R., and Dierdorf, S.: Anesthesia and Co-Existing Disease. New York, Churchill Livingstone, Inc., 1983.

Diabetes Mellitus

7. Biddle, C., and Hernandez, S.: Perioperative control of diabetes mellitus—revised. AANA J., 51(2):138–141, 1983.
8. Katz, J., Benumof, J., and Kadis, L.: Anesthesia and Uncommon Diseases: Pathophysiologic and Clinical Correlations. 2nd ed. Philadelphia, W. B. Saunders Co., 1981.
9. Lynch, J.: Preoperative and intraoperative insulin needs in diabetic patients. AANA J., 52(3):275–279, 1984.
10. Miller, R.: Anesthesia. 2nd ed. New York, Churchill Livingstone, Inc., 1986.
11. Stoelting, R., and Dierdorf, S.: Anesthesia and Co-Existing Disease. New York, Churchill Livingstone, Inc., 1983.
12. Taitelman, U., Reece, E., and Bessman, A.: Insulin in the management of the diabetic surgical patient. JAMA, 237(7):658, 1977.

Rheumatoid Arthritis

13. Fink, D., and Raymon, R.: Rheumatoid arthritis of the cricoarythenoid joints: an airway hazard. Anesth. Analg., 54(6):742, 1975.
14. Katz, J., Benumof, J., and Kadis, L.: Anesthesia and Uncommon Diseases: Pathophysiologic and Clinical Correlations. 2nd ed. Philadelphia, W. B. Saunders Co., 1981.

Obesity

15. Brown, B. (ed.): Anesthesia and the Obese Patient. Philadelphia, F. A. Davis Co., 1981.
16. Drain, C., and Vaughan, R.: Anesthetic considerations of morbid obesity. AANA J., 47(5):556–565, 1979.
17. Katz, J., Benumof, J., and Kadis, L.: Anesthesia and Uncommon Diseases: Pathophysiologic and Clinical Correlations. 2nd ed. Philadelphia, W. B. Saunders Co., 1981.
18. Paul, D., Holt, J., and Boutrous, A.: Cardiovascular and respiratory changes in response to change of posture in the very obese. Anesthesiology, 45(1):73, 1976.
19. Vaughan, R., et al.: Post operative hypoxemia in obese patients. Ann. Surg., 180(6):877, 1974.

Cigarette Smoking

20. Aronson, R., Weiss, S., Ben, R., and Komaroff, A.: Association between cigarette smoking and acute respiratory tract infections in young adults. JAMA, 248:181–183, 1982.
21. Austin, R.: Cigarette smoking and chronic bronchitis. Br. Med. J., 2(6046):1261, 1976.
22. Ayres, S.: Cigarette smoking and lung diseases: an update. Basics of Respiratory Disease. American Lung Association, 1975.
23. Bayes, J.: Asymptomatic smokers: ASA I or II? Anesthesiology, 56:76, 1982.
24. Berman, L.: Cigarettes, coronary occlusions, and myocardial infarctions. JAMA, 246:871–872, 1981.
25. Biddle, C., and Biddle, W.: A survey of perianesthetic complications in the asymptomatic smoker. AANA J., 51(5):481–484, 1983.
26. Drain, C.: Cigarette smoking—its effects on anesthesia. AANA J., 42(4):323–325, 1974.
27. Erikssen, J., et al.: Chronic effect of smoking on platelet count and platelet adhesiveness in presumably healthy middle-aged men. Thromb. Haemost., 38(3):606–611, 1977.
28. Friedman, F.: Mortality in cigarette smokers and quitters: effects of baseline differences. N. Engl. J. Med., 30:1407–1410, 1981.
29. Schenker, M., Samet, J., and Spiezer, E.: Effect of cigarette tar content and smoking habits on respiratory symptoms in women. Am. Rev. Respir. Dis., 125:684–690, 1982.
30. Wightman, J.: A prospective survey of the incidence of postoperative pulmonary complications. Br. J. Surg., 55:85–91, 1968.

37

Postoperative Care of the Geriatric Patient

Care of the geriatric patient is of particular importance in the post anesthesia care unit (PACU) because of the physiologic changes that usually occur during the later years. These include insufficient oxygenation of the blood, improper elimination of carbon dioxide, fluid and electrolyte imbalance, drug toxicity, nerve palsies, and psychologic changes. It is difficult to define chronologically when old age begins, because some persons age much more quickly than their chronologic age indicates. Legally, however, old age is defined as 65 or older.

AGE-RELATED PROBLEMS

Cardiovascular System

When first admitted to the post anesthesia care unit, the geriatric patient often presents many physiologic and psychologic problems. With advancing age, the cardiovascular system often undergoes some changes. The aged heart has less reserve and less ability to adjust to stress. Coronary sclerosis is common, and there is usually some atrophy of the myocardial fibers. There is a delay in the recovery from excitability in the aged heart muscle, and it is more susceptible to dysrhythmias. Cardiac output in the aged is lower than it is in the

young, and there is less ability to increase it during periods of stress.

The systolic blood pressure is usually higher in the geriatric patient owing to degenerative arterial disease, which decreases elasticity of the large arteries. This disease makes it difficult for the cardiovascular system to react to stress. Hypotension should be avoided because of the danger of thrombosis and the reduced amount of oxygen that can be transported to the vital organs. Hypertension, on the other hand, must be equally avoided. The most immediate problem of hypertension in the aged is damage from a cerebral vascular hemorrhage. Other areas of concern are hypovolemia, increased susceptibility to hemorrhage, and anemia.

Respiratory System

The aging process frequently affects the respiratory system. The thoracic bone structure usually becomes calcified, a condition that decreases the elastic recoil properties of the chest wall, which causes a premature balance in the elastic forces of the lungs and the chest wall. Thus the functional residual capacity (FRC), vital capacity (VC), and total lung capacity (TLC) are decreased (see

Chapter 4). As a person ages, the ratio of residual volume (RV) to total lung capacity progressively rises, making ventilation less and less adequate. Senile emphysema causes the intrapulmonary mixing of gases to become less effective, leading to hypoxemia and hypercarbia. The upper respiratory tract is also affected by advancing age, leading to increased secretions and airway resistance.

In the post anesthesia care unit, the geriatric patient's ventilation should be constantly assessed. The stir-up regimen of reposition, cascade cough, and sustained maximal inspiration (SMI) is mandatory for the geriatric patient (see Chapter 18) to reduce the incidence of postoperative pulmonary complications. Along with this, secretions should be removed by assisting the patient to cough and, if required, by suctioning. Positioning to facilitate good ventilatory excursion may be difficult in the geriatric patient owing to bone deformity or arthritis, or both. Usually, head-up positions will promote proper ventilation.

Neuromuscular System

The weight of the brain decreases with advancing age. Along with this, the loss of neurons caused by the aging process is particularly marked in the cerebral cortex. These atrophic changes interfere with the basic neuronal process and are responsible for the increased susceptibility of the elderly to central nervous system side effects of drugs that are seen clinically in the post anesthesia care unit.

In relation to anesthesia, aging is associated with a progressive decrease in the minimum alveolar concentration (MAC) for general inhalational anesthetic agents (see Chapter 12). Hence, in the post anesthesia care unit, patients of advanced age may experience a prolonged emergence following the administration of an inhalational anesthetic. There seems to be a loss of neurotransmitters and synaptic function, along with a decrease in the number of axons supplying peripheral muscles and in the number of muscles innervated by each axon. Consequently, over time, denervation

and atrophy of the skeletal muscles become apparent, which leads to a reduction in conduction velocity in peripheral nerves. This is why the dose requirement for regional anesthetics progressively declines with advancing age.

Renal System

As in other organ systems, there is a progressive decrease in renal function and mass with advancing age, which includes a decrease in the glomerular filtration rate (GFR) and renal blood flow. Thus, with a reduced cardiac and renal function, the geriatric patient is especially susceptible to fluid overload. Along with this, the mechanisms involved in maintaining the constancy and volume in the extracellular fluid are blunted with progressive age. This reduction in functional adaptive renal mechanisms is responsible in part for the problems in fluid and electrolyte balance seen in geriatric patients. An electrolyte of particular importance in the context of advancing age is *sodium*. The geriatric patient will progressively have a blunted response to sodium deficiency; i.e., patients in this age group lose the ability to conserve sodium in response to acute reduction in sodium intake. The geriatric patient, because of this salt-losing tendency, may experience such symptoms as confusion, loss of thirst, and disorientation in the post anesthesia care unit. This is particularly true when a transurethral resection of the prostate (TURP) is performed or, for that matter, any surgical procedure in which urinary irrigation is utilized. The geriatric patient who has experienced this type of surgical procedure should be monitored in the PACU for a deficiency in this electrolyte.

The first symptoms of sodium deficiency is probably disorientation. Because some patients in the geriatric population may normally be somewhat disoriented, it is important that the PACU nurse differentiate among the possible types of disorientation. Electrolyes should be drawn and analyzed immediately, before any sedation is administered to the patient. Should the level of sodium be below normal, intravenous sodium will resolve the clinical picture of disorientation rather rapidly.

Another electrolyte of concern when caring for the geriatric patient is *potassium*. Advancing age is associated with a progressive decrease in plasma renin concentration. Along with this, there is an equal reduction in the concentration of aldosterone, which acts on the distal tubule to increase sodium reabsorption and to enhance the excretion of potassium, thereby protecting against hyperkalemia. With advancing age, the protective mechanism to prevent hyperkalemia during periods of potassium challenge is lost. Given that the glomerular filtration is reduced in the geriatric patient, when potassium is administered hyperkalemia may result. Therefore, along with monitoring the electrocardiogram for the peaking of T waves, electrolytes should be monitored particularly when a geriatric patient has received potassium salts intravenously in the perioperative period.

Because of the reduction in physiologic function of the renal system associated with advancing age, kidney function should be monitored in the post anesthesia care unit, including fluid and electrolyte balance. The fluid intake and output should be monitored meticulously, as these patients are subject to oliguria and, in some cases, anuria. Also, drugs dependent on renal excretion for their elimination (such as gallamine) will be affected by the decrease in kidney function, leading to a prolonged plasma concentration and, ultimately, to a prolongation of the effect of the drug.

Hepatobiliary System

Advancing age is associated with a progressive reduction in hepatobiliary function. Hepatic blood flow is progressively reduced, and an age-related decrease in the functioning of the hepatic microsomal enzymes has been demonstrated. This ultimately leads to an age-related reduction in the biotransformation actions of the liver, and drugs that are dependent to a major extent on hepatic metabolism will usually have a prolonged effect in the elderly population. Because there is considerable danger of hepatic injury from drugs, hypoxia, and blood transfusions, in the routine PACU care of the geriatric patient, careful attention should be given to appropriate airway care to enhance oxygenation and to ensuring that the appropriate dosage of depressant drugs is given.

Drug Interactions

The physiologic response to a drug occurs in a twofold manner. The first process deals with the drug concentration at the site of

TABLE 37–1. Adverse Effects or Drug Interactions Associated with the Geriatric Patient[3, 4]

Drug	Adverse Effect or Drug Interaction
Antibiotics	Prolongation of muscle relaxants
Antidysrhythmics	Prolongation of muscle relaxants
Benzodiazepines	Decreased metabolism
Diazepam	Increased CNS effects
Chlordiazepoxide	Prolonged drowsiness
Flurazepam	
Digoxin	Decreased renal excretion with increased CNS disorientation, anorexia, nausea, and cardiotoxicity; blood levels 2 to 3 times higher in the elderly with any given dose.
Diuretics	Hypokalemia Hypovolemia
Halothane	Decreased anesthetic requirement
Lithium	Clearance decreased by 65% and effective dose by 30% compared with age 25. Increased side effects of tremor, diarrhea, and edema.
Meperidine	Markedly elevated plasma levels, and decreased red blood cell and plasma binding of drug Increased incidence of nausea, respiratory distress, and hypotension
Methyldopa	Enhanced hypotensive effects
Pancuronium	Decreased clearance from plasma
Propranolol	Plasma level approximately 3 to 4 times higher in the elderly, owing to decreased metabolism Bradycardia, congestive heart failure, bronchospasm, mental confusion, and attenuation of autonomic nervous system activity
Tricyclic antidepressants	Increased anticholinergic effects—confusion, agitation, and disorientation Cardiac conduction disturbances Increased anesthetic requirements
Warfarin	Enhanced sensitivity

action and is termed *pharmacokinetics*. The second process deals with the ability of the drug to react with a specific receptor and to translate that effect on the receptor into a physiologic response, which is called *pharmacodynamics*. Advancing age is associated with progressive alterations in both the pharmacokinetics and the pharmacodynamics of drug therapy. Furthermore, the geriatric patient may experience pharmacologic problems because of the multiple types of drugs being taken and the adverse drug interactions that may occur. Table 37–1 may be utilized to determine the possible adverse effects or drug interactions that may take place in the geriatric patient during the perioperative period.

Psychologic Aspects

The psychologic aspects of PACU care of the geriatric patient center around maintaining the patient's self-esteem. Feelings of uselessness and lack of self-worth promote tension and anxiety, which, in turn, can affect the patient's physiologic status. Geriatric patients are usually set in their ways, and it is important for them to be able to contribute to their own care. Because their hearing and vision may be impaired, these patients tend to isolate themselves and may not be able to understand oral communication very well. Therefore, when conversing with a geriatric patient with possible or proven hearing loss, it is important to speak slowly and distinctly, and in a loud voice.

REFERENCES

1. Del Portzer, M.: Geriatric cardiovascular problems. AANA J., 44(6):609, 1976.
2. Katz, J., Benumof, J., and Kadis, L.: Anesthesia and Uncommon Diseases: Pathophysiologic and Clinical Correlations, 2nd ed. Philadelphia, W. B. Saunders Co., 1981.
3. Krechel, S. (ed.): Anesthesia and the Geriatric Patient. New York, Grune & Stratton, Inc., 1984.
4. Miller, R.: Anesthesia. 2nd ed. New York, Churchill-Livingstone, Inc., 1986.
5. Stoelting, R., and Dierdorf, S.: Anesthesia and Co-Existing Disease. New York, Churchill-Livingstone, Inc., 1983.

CHAPTER

38

Postoperative Care of the Pediatric Patient

Pediatric anesthesia is a popular subspecialty in the practice of anesthesiolgy. For clarification, the newborn is defined as less than 72 hours old, the infant less than 1 month old, and the child less than 13 years old. Infants and children cannot be regarded as just small adults, since their immaturity presents various definite physiologic differences. Some of the main differences lie in the endocrine, cardiovascular, and respiratory systems and in the regulation of body temperature.

Anesthetic management of the pediatric patient has been revised in several areas as comprehension of pediatric physiology and pathophysiology has improved. Because of this greater understanding, pediatric anesthesiology and post anesthesia care have become even more challenging and rewarding.

ANATOMIC AND PHYSIOLOGIC DIFFERENCES

Endocrine System

At birth, the infant has a diminished response to surgical trauma because the cortical cellular organization is not as fully functional as that of the adult adrenal cortex. Some physicians may utilize supplementary cortisone therapy during the postoperative period to improve the response in infants to surgical stress.

Cardiovascular System

Average pulse and blood pressure measurements for newborns, infants, and children are summarized in Tables 38–1 and 38–2. With the advent of more sophisticated blood pressure monitoring devices, measurements in infants can now be taken with

TABLE 38–1. Average Blood Pressure of Children*

Age	Systolic (mm Hg)	Diastolic (mm Hg)
Newborn	75–85	40–50
2 wk–4 yr	85	60
5 yr	87	60
6 yr	90	60
7 yr	92	62
8 yr	95	62
9 yr	98	64
10 yr	100	65
11 yr	105	65
12 yr	108	67
13 yr	110	67
14 yr	112	70
15 yr	115	72
16 yr	118	75

*From Vaughan, V. C., and McKay, R. J. (eds.): Textbook of Pediatrics. 10th ed. Philadelphia, W. B. Saunders Co., 1975.

494

TABLE 38–2. Average Pulse Rate at Different Ages*

Age	Lower Limits of Normal	Average	Upper Limits of Normal
Newborn	70	120	170
1–11 mo	80	120	160
2 yr	80	110	130
4 yr	80	100	120
6 yr	75	100	115
8 yr	70	90	110
10 yr	70	90	110

*From Vaughan, V. C., and McKay, R. J. (eds.): Textbook of Pediatrics. 10th ed. Philadelphia, W. B. Saunders Co., 1975.

great accuracy. It is important to monitor the infant's blood pressure, as shock can develop rapidly; and as Smith points out, "observation of the blood pressure is actually more important in infants and children than in adults."[10] This is because the pediatric patient does not have the physiologic reservoirs (e.g., blood volume) to rely upon in situations in which shock can occur. The author has observed that the pediatric patient will ordinarily demonstrate the usual signs of impending shock or airway obstruction, and yet, if the problem is not rectified rapidly, the pediatric patient's physiologic status will deteriorate two to three times faster than in the adult. Hence, the PACU nurse must always monitor the physiologic parameters of the pediatric patient, and if abnormalities arise, prompt interventions are essential.

The heart rate of the pediatric patient is another parameter that should be monitored constantly in the PACU. After the patient's arrival, when the vital signs are obtained, the PACU values should be compared first with the pre- and intraoperative recordings of vital signs. Changes in the heart rate of the pediatric patient are one of the first clues of impending physiologic dysfunction. In the PACU, the heart rate of infants and children is influenced by physical activity, and by the administration of atropine, glycopyrrolate, and anesthetic agents: Crying, struggling, or pain can increase the heart rate; glycopyrrolate (Robinul), an anticholinergic drug like atropine, may elevate the heart rate mildly, but not as much as atropine does; anesthetic agents

such as halothane, enflurane, and isoflurane will cause a decrease in heart rate.

The hemoglobin and number of blood cells are high at birth. Values then decrease rapidly until age 3 months. The rates then rise slowly to the normal adult value by age 12 years (Fig. 38–1).

Respiratory System

Newborns are usually obligate nose breathers and are prone to airway obstruction. This is because the newborn has small nares, a large tongue, a small mandible, a short neck, and a large amount of upper airway lymphoid tissue. Consequently, when ventilating a newborn by use of a face mask, the nurse should be careful not to apply too much pressure over the soft tissue of the neck, because pressure of this kind can easily obstruct the airway.

The vocal cords of the newborn are situated at about the level of the fourth cervical vertebra, as opposed to the location at the sixth cervical vertebra in the adult. Normally, in the adult, the opening of the vocal cords is the narrowest portion of the trachea and, in the newborn, the narrowest portion of the trachea is the cricoid cartilage (see Chapter 4). The clinical implications of this anatomic feature are that if edema about the cricoid cartilage should occur because of infection or mechanical irritation from an endotracheal tube, significant narrowing of the airway may occur. Also, because the cricoid ring is the narrowest part of the larynx, this limits the size of the endotracheal tube to be used. The endotracheal tube selected should allow a slight leakage around itself when positive pressure is applied by use of an anesthesia bag. Finally, the epiglottis of the newborn is U-shaped and usually long and narrow, as compared with the flatter epiglottis of the adult.

Newborns are diaphragmatic breathers. This is because the ribs are situated horizontally in a cylindrical thorax, which limits thorax expansion. Consequently, the ventilatory effort is due almost entirely to the movement of the diaphragm. Because newborns are diaphragmatic breathers, they are

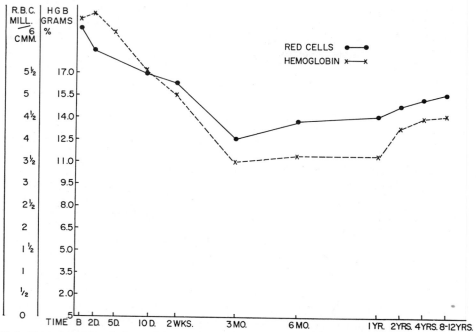

Figure 38–1. Normal variation in hemoglobin and red blood cell count during infancy and childhood. (From Kaplan, S., In Nelson, W. E. [ed.]: Textbook of Pediatrics. 7th ed. Philadelphia, W. B. Saunders Co., 1959.)

very susceptible to ventilatory problems, such as hypoventilation when the excursions of the diaphragm are impeded. Hence, gastric distention due to faulty bag and mask ventilation, improper positioning, or bowel obstruction can certainly produce inadequate ventilation. In addition, the sternum and anterior rib cage are compliant, and the intercostal and accessory muscles of respiration are poorly developed. In the premature infant, the sternum may be retracted deeply with each inspiration, causing impaired ventilation.

As in the adult, the newborn's primary drive to ventilation is carbon dioxide (see Chapter 4). However, the secondary drive in the newborn is different from that of the adult. The newborn under a week of age will respond to a reduction in the partial pressure of oxygen by hyperventilation followed by hypoventilation. This secondary drive response is aggravated by hypothermia, a condition that can occur in the post anesthesia care unit.

The respiratory rate is higher and the tidal volume lower in infants and in chil-

dren. When ventilation equipment, such as a mask, is used, dead space is increased. The Radford nomogram can be used to predict basal tidal volume (Fig. 38–2).

The respiratory control center in the in-

TABLE 38–3. Endotracheal Tube Size in Children

Age or Weight	Endotracheal Tube Size Internal Diameter (mm)	External Diameter (French)	Length (cm)	Suction Catheter (French)
Under 1500 gm	2.5 uncuffed	12	8	6
Newborn– 6 mo	3.0 uncuffed	14	10	6
6–18 mo	3.5 uncuffed	16	12	8
18 mo–3 yr	4.0 uncuffed	18	14	8
3–5 yr	4.5 uncuffed	20	16	8
5–6 yr	5.0 uncuffed	22	16	10
6–8 yr	5.5 cuffed	24	18	10
8–10 yr	6.0 cuffed	26	18	10
10–12 yr	6.5 cuffed	28	20	12
12–14 yr	6.5 cuffed	28	20	12
14–16 yr	♂7.0 cuffed	30	22	12
	♀6.5 cuffed	28		
16–21 yr	♂7.5 cuffed	32	22	12
	♀7.0 cuffed	30		

Note: Endotracheal tube should fit so as to allow full expansion of both lungs on manual inflation but allow a definite leak with pressure of 20 to 25 cm H_2O.

From Smith, R. M.: Anesthesia for Infants and Children. 4th ed., St. Louis, C. V. Mosby Co., 1980.

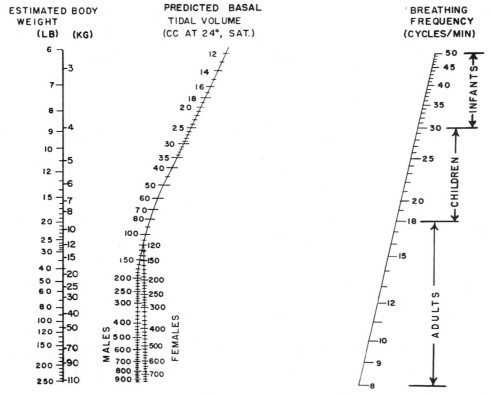

Figure 38–2. Nomogram for predicted basal tidal volume. Corrections to be applied: add 10 percent if subject is awake; add 9 percent for each degree centigrade of fever; add 8 percent for each 1000 meters of altitude above sea level; calculate the required tidal volume. If a tracheostomy is in use, subtract the patient's estimated physiologic dead space (i.e., subtract 1 ml/kg body weight). Add the dead space of the anesthetic apparatus. (From Radford, E. P., Jr., Ferris, B. G., Jr., and Kriete, B. C.: Reprinted by permission from the New England Journal of Medicine, 251:877, 1954.)

fant and child is easily fatigued; therefore, ventilatory reaction to high carbon dioxide tensions or to low percentage of oxygen is not rapid. As a result, the infant may not be able to compensate for rapid changes in arterial blood gases. Along with this, infants and small children may breathe irregularly and be unable to respond to oxygen, owing to their lack of a mature respiratory center; periodic breathing is often seen in this age group.

Endotracheal intubation is becoming more widely accepted in pediatric anesthesia (see Table 38–3 for guide to proper-sized endotracheal tubes). The advantages of this technique are decreased dead space, avoidance of laryngospasm and gastric distention, and prevention of aspiration. However, the incidence of postintubation edema

from trauma and infections may be increased.

The Kidney and Fluid Balance

Fortunately, the kidney of the newborn matures rapidly. By the end of the first month, the kidneys reach about 90 percent maturity. However, at about 5 days of age, renal function is characterized by an obligate salt loss, slow clearance of fluid overload, and an inability to conserve fluid. Consequently, newborns who are 5 days or less in age are intolerant of both dehydration and fluid overload. The blood volume of the newborn varies from 60 to 130 ml/kg, depending on the position of the baby in relation to the placenta and perineum during delivery and whether the cord was

TABLE 38–4. Maintenance Fluids and Normal Urine Output in Pediatric Patients

Age	Body Weight	24-Hour Fluid Requirement	Normal Urine Output (ml/kg/hr)
Premature and full-term newborn less than 5 days	3–3.5 kg	50–70 ml/kg	0.3–0.7
Premature and full-term newborn over 5 days up to 1 month	3.5–4 kg	150 ml/kg	1.0–2.7 (5–7 days)
Over 1 month up to 1 year	4–10 kg	100 ml/kg	3.0 (over 7 days)
1 to 5 years	10–20 kg	1000 ml, plus 50 ml/kg over 10 kg	2.0 (over 2 years)
5 years to adult	20–>70 kg	1500 ml, plus 20 ml/kg over 20 kg	1.0

Adapted from Dripps, R., Eckenhoff, J., and Vandam, L.: Introduction to Anesthesia: The Principles of Safe Practice. 6th ed. Philadelphia, W. B. Saunders Co., 1982.

"milked" toward or away from the newborn before its clamping. The blood volume of the infant is about 80 to 85 ml/kg, as compared with 65 ml/kg in the adult female and 70 ml/kg in the adult male.

Water distribution in the various body compartments is markedly different among the premature newborn, the normal newborn, the child, and the adult. Premature and normal newborns have the most water in their extracellular fluid compartment. This condition will continue until about the second year, when adult proportions of 20 percent extracellular and 40 percent intracellular water are reached. Table 38–4 summarizes the daily maintenance fluids and normal urine output for the pediatric patient.

Important considerations for fluid management of the pediatric patient include monitoring for hyper- or hypovolemia and ensuring proper administration of fluids. Consequently, the monitoring of the pediatric patient should include the following parameters: (1) urine output, specific gravity, and osmolality; (2) temperature; (3) ECG, pulse, and blood pressure; (4) hydration of the mucosa; and (5) blood loss. It is essential to make an accurate assessment of blood loss intraoperatively and postoperatively, because a miscalculation of just a few milliliters can have a serious impact on the total blood volume of the infant. If the pediatric patient loses 10 percent of blood volume, the possibility of blood replacement is usually considered by the physician. In losses of up to 15 to 20 percent of blood volume, replacement is usually instituted. The usual blood replacement is such that for each 1 ml lost, 1 ml of whole blood is administered to the patient.

During the administration of fluids, the PACU nurse should ensure that the indwelling catheter is patent and not infiltrated, and should use a constant infusion pump to facilitate the proper administration of the correct volume and rate of fluids. To prevent inadvertent overhydration, not more than one third of the day's maintenance intravenous fluid volume should be measured into the intravenous bag at any one time.

Infants and newborns expend a great amount of energy maintaining alveolar ventilation, cardiac output, muscular activity, and an appropriate temperature. Because of these high-energy metabolic processes, glycogen and fat stores may be mobilized and depleted rapidly. Consequently, in the PACU, cold, stress, pain, and increased muscle activity compound the need for adequate caloric intake. Therefore, one of the cornerstones of fluid replacement in the PACU is the provision of enough glucose intake to maintain the glycogen and fat stores. One-fourth to one-third strength saline solution in 5 percent dextrose is the most common maintenance fluid used in the PACU care of the pediatric patient.

PEDIATRIC ANESTHESIA TECHNIQUES

Administration of anesthetic drugs to the pediatric patient has progressed from the technique of open drop ether to the nonrebreathing technique. The Bain circuit is sometimes used in pediatric anesthesia, as it offers the advantages of conserving body heat, of not utilizing valves, and of keeping the patient normocarbic (see Chapter 12).

The most popular 100 percent potent inhalation anesthetic agents used for pediatric anesthesia are halothane, isoflurane, and enflurane. All offer rapid induction and rapid emergence. Halothane remains the most popular pediatric inhalational agent; freedom from airway irritation and smooth emergence are especially important characteristics of halothane that make it the anesthetic of choice. The Liverpool technique, which consists of nitrous oxide, oxygen, and curare, can be used for patients under 3 years of age. It also offers the advantage of rapid emergence.

Ketamine, a dissociative anesthetic, is sometimes used in pediatrics as an induction agent or for short procedures that do not require muscle relaxation. Emergence time depends upon route of administration and whether or not the drug was repeated during the operation.

PACU CARE OF THE PEDIATRIC PATIENT

When the pediatric patient arrives in the post anesthesia care unit, vital signs, including core temperature, should be obtained and a warmed and humidified air/oxygen mixture (high flow) administered before the report from the anesthetist is given. The patient should be placed in lateral position; however, following an intraoral surgical procedure, the patient should be placed in prone position to facilitate adequate drainage of secretions or blood. During the report, dressings should be checked for drainage and the intravenous infusion line should be checked for patency and for assurance that the line is adequately secured. Also, children's teeth should be checked routinely on admission to the PACU, especially if loose teeth are present, and again before discharge. Because of the improved anesthesia techniques and rapid-acting anesthetic agents, the pediatric patient will usually arrive in the post anesthesia care unit awake and responsive, and with good muscle tone. These patients usually respond quickly to the stir-up regimen. However, about 10 to 15 percent of pediatric patients recovering from general anesthesia will exhibit hyperactive behavior. They will require constant nursing care to prevent injury to themselves, as they are extremely restless and often scream loudly. This agitation or excitement may be related to drug responses, hypoxemia, pain, or awakening in strange surroundings. Therefore, if a pediatric patient is demonstrating hyperactive behavior, the PACU nurse should assess the patient in the aforementioned areas before providing interventions.

Cardiovascular and Fluid Monitoring

If the pediatric patient is moderately to severely ill, monitors for central venous pressure, electrocardiographic status, urine output, specific gravity, and an arterial line may be used.

The central venous pressure line is usually inserted via the superior vena cava or the external jugular vein. It provides information on blood volume and serves as an avenue for fluid replacement. The arterial line, which is inserted through the umbilical or radial artery, can measure blood pressure and heart rate, and provide for instantaneous blood gas sampling. The electrocardiograph provides information on cardiac rate and rhythm. Blood pressure and pulse should be ascertained and recorded every 5 to 10 minutes, depending on the physical status of the patient. Any deviation in the cardiac or pulmonary physiologic parameters should be reported immediately to the attending physician.

Dressings should be watched for excessive bleeding. Such bleeding should be reported at once to the attending physician, as the infant and small child do not have enough blood volume to compensate for losses.

The urine output and specific gravity will yield information on kidney function and volume expansion.

Respiratory Monitoring

The rate and depth of ventilation should be monitored in the PACU. Respiratory depression occurs with greater frequency if muscle relaxants are used during anesthesia.

Infants and small children usually have a low incidence of postoperative atelectasis, because crying from pain or unhappiness will automatically keep the airway clear. Older children tend to remain in one position and to not move about. They must be encouraged to cough and to perform the sustained maximal inspiration (SMI) maneuver to prevent atelectasis. If the pediatric patient is unable to perform the SMI maneuver, deep breathing should be encouraged.

Temperature Regulation

Newborns, infants, and children are very sensitive to heat loss because they have a relatively large surface area, a relatively small amount of subcutaneous fat, and very poor vasomotor control, and because they seldom shiver. Ordinarily, to maintain a body temperature within normal limits, they metabolize brown fat, cry, and move about vigorously. Thus, newborns, infants, and children respond to a cold environment by increasing their metabolism, which ultimately leads to an increase in oxygen consumption and to the production of organic acids. If a child in this age group arrives in the post anesthesia care unit with inadvertent hypothermia, the nurse should assess the patient for (1) vital signs—core temperature, pulse, and respiratory rate—and (2) the degree of emergence from anesthesia. The patient should be monitored on a continuous EKG, as dysrhythmias and cardiovascular depression are associated with hypothermia. If the patient is experiencing a delayed emergence from anesthesia, the nurse should protect the patient from aspiration of gastric contents and from hypoventilation by positioning (Fig. 38–3) and stimulation. Finally, to avoid excess oxygen demand and acidosis that are associated with hypothermia, newborns and infants should be maintained in a neutral thermal environment in the PACU by the use of incubators, infrared heating, blankets, or elevated room temperature.

A word of warning is needed here. If a water mattress is to be utilized to rewarm the patient, the temperature setting should not be more than 37°C, and four layers of sheets should be used between the mattress and the skin to prevent burns. Whatever rewarming method is used, the temperature of the device should be monitored constantly to prevent overwarming. Records should be kept of core body temperature (rectal, esophageal, or tympanic), room temperature, and device temperature.

Psychosocial Considerations

When the pediatric patient emerges from a general inhalational anesthetic, certain emotional needs should be met by the PACU nurse, so as to facilitate positive outcomes of perioperative experience. Infants can become distressed when physical needs are not met. Taking into consideration the type of surgery and the degree of emergence from anesthesia, the primary care giver should hold or rock the patient if age-appropriate, or do both. This will usually relax the patient, and infants especially enjoy cuddling, rocking, fondling, and hearing the voice of the nurse. Because the infant mimics facial expressions, the nurse should smile and use facial expressions of happiness when caring for the child. Another consideration is that the post anesthesia care unit is a strange environment for the child. Many times dolls, teddy bears, and other familiar objects from home are taken to surgery and will arrive with the patient in the PACU. These special toys should remain with the child, especially during emergence, to help cope with the environmental change.

Children at ages 1 to 3 are at the stage of autonomy versus self-doubt. They may exhibit independence that alternates with sudden dependence and the need for periodic cuddling and reassurance. Negativism may be the child's means of demonstrating con-

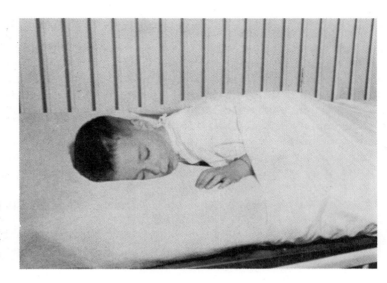

Figure 38–3. After operation the child lies face down with shoulder supported and one arm and leg flexed. (From Smith, R. M.: Anesthesia for Infants and Children. 3rd ed. St. Louis, C. V. Mosby Co., 1968, p. 188.)

trol; thus, "no" may actually mean "yes." Children of this age are prone to temper tantrums, ritualistic behavior, and breath-holding spells. The PACU nurse should be sure to differentiate apnea from breath-holding spells when assessing the respiratory status of the patient. Three-year-olds are certainly special children, loveable but stormy. They are too young to use their own reason and become impatient at times. It is therefore important for the PACU nurse to avoid criticism and provide acceptable behavior alternatives to the patient.

Between the ages of 3 and 6 years the child begins to become independent. However, in the post anesthesia care unit, dependency can occur because of pain, course of disease, or immobilization. Guilt can occur when the child desires to remain dependent. Consequently, the PACU nurse should provide as much opportunity for independence as possible. This can be done by allowing the child to select alternatives in care.

Ages 6 to 12 coincide with school entrance. These children are striving for approval when tasks are completed and usually do not tolerate failure, as it promotes their sense of inferiority and inadequacy. Because children lose control when they are immobilized or ill, the nurse should allow as much individualization and self-care as possible. The nurse should also encourage

self-expression and compliment the child on accomplishments during recovery from anesthesia.

The adolescent years of ages 12 to 18 are a transitory time characterized by vacillations between dependence and independence, idealism and realism, confidence and uncertainty. Privacy is of utmost importance to these patients; therefore, the adolescent's body should be covered as much as possible to prevent exposure and resulting embarrassment.

COMPLICATIONS

Because the pediatric patient does not have the physiologic reserves of the adult patient, when complications occur, serious untoward sequelae can and will take place. Hence, the PACU nurse must monitor for and react to any complication in a timely fashion.

Retrolental Fibroplasia

Retrolental fibroplasia is a neovascularization and scarring of the retina due to elevated inspired oxygen tensions. The risk of this retinal pathology is to neonates, especially premature infants who are born before 36 weeks' gestation. The risk of developing retrolental fibroplasia is negligible beyond 44 weeks after conception. Therefore, the preterm neonate who has a gestation of 36 weeks will remain at risk until about 8 weeks of age. Current recommendations are that the PaO_2 for the premature infant be between 40 and 60 torr and between 60 and 80 for the normal newborn. The FiO_2 should be kept below 0.4. The exact length of time the patient must be exposed to the hyperoxic environment for retrolental fibroplasia to develop is unknown. In susceptible patients who are exposed to a hyperoxic environment, blood gas tension should be measured and an oxygen analyzer used to confirm the oxygen concentration. The key thought when dealing with this situation is that attempts to prevent arterial hyperoxia must be tempered with the realization that unrecognized arterial hypoxemia can result in irreversible brain damage.

Idiopathic Respiratory Distress Syndrome

Infant respiratory distress syndrome (IRDS), also called *hyaline membrane disease*, is a severe disorder of the lungs of the newborn. The incidence of IRDS increases with maternal diabetes, toxemia, hemorrhage, and prenatal asphyxia. The basis of the pathogenesis of IRDS is insufficient surfactant levels. Surfactant can be described as having the following two functions: (1) reducing surface tension so that less pressure is required to hold the alveoli open, and (2) maintaining alveolar stability by adjusting surface tension to changes in alveolar size. Insufficient surfactant levels will increase surface tension at the alveolar air-liquid interface, resulting in alveolar collapse, an inordinate increase in the work of breathing, and impaired gas exchange. This impaired gas exchange will result in hypoxemia and hypercarbia. Along with this, the pulmonary vascular resistance will be increased, resulting in hypoperfusion of the pulmonary and systemic circulations. This hypoperfusion along with hypoxemia will cause tissue hypoxia and metabolic acidosis.

More specifically, low surfactant levels will produce a high surface tension in the alveoli, which, besides causing alveolar collapse, will reverse the gradient for transcapillary fluid movement. Hence, the products derived from the blood, as well as cellular debris, will be pulled into the alveoli. This cellular "junk" will end up lining the alveoli and making up what is referred to as the hyaline membrane. Profound atelectasis results and the lungs become very stiff, which leads to a severely reduced functional residual capacity (FRC), hypoxemia, and, finally, ventilatory failure.

The cardinal signs of IRDS, which appear soon after birth, are tachypnea, grunting respiration, and chest retraction. Treatment for neonates with IRDS includes oxygen therapy, fluid restriction, temperature regulation, chemical monitoring (glucose, bilirubin, and arterial blood gases), and continuous positive airway pressure (CPAP). If, during CPAP, the infant becomes apneic and develops hypercarbia with a respiratory acidosis (pH $\leq$ 7.2), or if the arterial oxygen tension falls below 50 torr, then mechanical ventilation is begun. The mechanical ventilation will probably utilize high positive end-expiratory pressure (high PEEP) to ventilate the exceptionally stiff lungs of these neonates.

Airway Obstruction

In the post anesthesia care unit, each pediatric patient who has been intubated during anesthesia should be monitored for signs of airway obstruction. When laryngeal swelling occurs, the diameter of the airway of the infant or small child can become significantly reduced; in fact, 1 mm of edema in the infant's trachea at the cricoid level will decrease the diameter of the airway by 75 percent! The symptoms of laryngeal obstruction, in order of appearance, are croupy cough, hoarseness, inspiratory stridor, and aphonia. These symptoms are accompanied by increasing restlessness, tachypnea, use of accessory muscles of respiration, retraction of the suprasternal notch and intercostal spaces, and drawing in of the upper abdomen. If these symptoms appear, the PACU nurse should act immediately to relieve the obstruction *and* should send someone to notify the anesthesiologist, as the progression of these symptoms can be rapid.

Treatment of postintubation croup involves use of a high humidity atmosphere that is oxygen-enriched, optimum body hydration, and administration of antibiotics when indicated. Steroids such as dexamethasone (Decadron) are usually prescribed to decrease the laryngeal inflammation. If laryngeal edema is allowed to progress, the patient may require reintubation or a tracheostomy. If tracheostomy is performed, the PACU nurse should observe the patient for pneumothorax, mediastinal emphysema, and bleeding. Auscultation of the chest should be done every 15 minutes for breath sounds to ascertain if the tracheostomy tube is above the bifurcation of the trachea (at the carina). The PACU nurse should also determine during auscultation whether excess secretions are present. If suctioning is required, sterile suction technique should be utilized. Aspiration of secretions should be done by slow suction to prevent injury to the tissue. Before the tracheostomy suctioning is instituted, the procedure should be explained fully to the child in language that can be readily understood.

A 75 percent atmospheric humidity should be provided to the pediatric patient with a tracheostomy. This will help to decrease the viscosity of the sputum. Maintenance of good hydration is also important if an infection is present.

Malignant Hyperthermia

Although malignant hyperthermia (MH) is discussed in detail in Chapter 42, a brief description of the condition is given here, because the incidence of MH is approximately 1 in 14,000 in children, as compared with 1 in 52,000 in adults. This genetically determined condition is triggered by inhalational anesthetic agents, such as halothane and succinylcholine, and by stress. The pathophysiology of the condition centers around the enhanced release and diminished reuptake of calcium in the skeletal muscle. This causes sustained skeletal muscle contraction and, ultimately, profound hyperthermia. The drug dantrolene effectively treats MH by inhibiting further release of calcium in the skeletal muscles. In most cases, the malignant hyperthermia occurs in the operating room; however, a patient could first experience the disorder in the post anesthesia care unit, or the successfully treated MH patient could have an exacerbation of MH in the PACU.

In most cases of MH, the first clinical clue is tachycardia or other dysrhythmias; then tachypnea and a profound increase in tidal volume will be observed in the spontaneous-breathing PACU patient. The temperature will begin to rise, sweating will occur, and the patient's skin will become mottled.

Blood chemistry will reveal an elevated potassium and an initially elevated calcium that will then fall below normal. Arterial blood gases will demonstrate severe metabolic acidosis with an elevated $PaCO_2$ and a decreased pH. The PaO_2 may be normal, depending on the FiO_2.

To facilitate a reversal of this condition, the PACU nurse must understand the pathophysiology of MH and should know exactly where the MH emergency cart (as described in Chapter 42) is located. If a patient appears to be developing MH, SEND FOR HELP! Start ventilating the patient, using high-flow 100 percent oxygen, and check to be sure the IV is patent. Once the appropriate personnel arrive, have one person mix the dantrolene (20 mg/60 ml of sterile water).

A note of warning is needed. Be sure that the sterile water does not contain any preservatives, as much sterile water will be used. The usual dose of dantrolene is 1 to 2 mg/kg over 1 to 2 minutes. This can be repeated up to 10 mg/kg or until the patient's temperature is reduced.

SPECIAL CONSIDERATIONS
Gastrointestinal Surgery

Pediatric patients recovering from gastrointestinal surgery should be observed for prolonged paralytic ileus; if it goes beyond 72 hours, the physician should be notified, because complications such as intestinal obstruction, local abscess, or pneumoperitoneum may be present. During the PACU report on the patient, nursing personnel on the surgical unit should be properly warned about the possibility of prolonged paralytic ileus occurring.

Otolaryngologic Surgery

Pediatric patients who have tonsillectomies and other operations on the pharynx, larynx, and esophagus require intensive PACU care, because the airway can become obstructed postoperatively as a result of surgical manipulation and bleeding. When the patient is admitted to the PACU, the laryngeal and pharyngeal reflexes should be present. The patient should be placed in the tonsillectomy position (Fig. 38–3), prone with the arm and leg flexed and the head turned to the side. This position improves drainage of secretions and blood from the mouth, preventing possible aspiration. The patient should be kept in this position until the gag reflex has returned completely.

REFERENCES

1. Berman, S.: Pediatric Decision Making. Philadelphia, B. C. Decker, Inc., 1985.
2. Dripps, R., Eckenhoff, J., and Vandam, L.: Introduction to Anesthesia: The Principles of Safe Practice. 6th ed. Philadelphia, W. B. Saunders Co., 1982.
3. Frost, E., and Andrews, I.: Recovery Room Care. Int. Anesthesiol. Clin., 21(1):1983.
4. Jolin, R.: Neonatal physiology and anesthesia. AANA J., 51(6):594–603, 1983.
5. Levin, R.: Pediatric Anesthesia Handbook. 3rd ed. New York, Medical Examination Publishing Co., Inc., 1984.
6. Miller, R.: Anesthesia. 2nd ed., New York, Churchill Livingstone, Inc., 1986.
7. Oaks, A.: Critical Care Nursing of Children and Adolescents. Philadelphia, W. B. Saunders Co., 1981.
8. Rackow, H., and Salanitre, E.: Modern concepts in pediatric anesthesiology. Anesthesiology, 30(2):208, 1969.
9. Rando, J.: A review of pediatric fluid therapy. AANA J., 48(5):437–440, 1980.
10. Smith, R.: Anesthesia for Infants and Children. 4th ed. St. Louis, C. V. Mosby Co., 1980.
11. Stoelting, R., and Dierdorf, S.: Anesthesia and Co-Existing Disease. New York, Churchill Livingstone, Inc., 1983.

Postoperative Care of the Pregnant Patient

Karen D. Spadaccia, R.N., B.S.N., C.C.R.N., C.E.N.

The incidence of surgery performed on pregnant women for reasons unrelated to the pregnancy itself has been reported by various statistics to be as high as 40,000 to 50,000 cases per year. The most common conditions requiring surgical intervention are acute appendicitis, ovarian cysts, and breast tumors. However, there are reports of more complicated procedures such as craniotomies, open heart surgery, and aneurysm repairs that have been successful in pregnant patients.

When caring for the pregnant patient postoperatively, one must remember that there are two patients requiring nursing care and assessment: mother and fetus. Nursing care should be directed toward emotional support for the mother, as well as the avoidance of uterine stimulation that could produce preterm labor. Also of prime importance is prevention of respiratory depression in the mother and the maintenance of normal uterine placental blood flow to ensure adequate fetal supply of oxygen and nutrients.

PHYSIOLOGIC CHANGES OF PREGNANCY

Almost every system in the body is affected in some way during pregnancy, either by hormonal changes or because of the increasing size of the uterus. The changes that will impact on post anesthetic nursing care will be discussed (Table 39–1).

Cardiovascular Changes

The cardiovascular system undergoes significant change as pregnancy advances.

TABLE 39–1. Physiologic Changes in Pregnancy

Respiratory System
Anatomic changes
Lung volumes
Ventilation
Acid-base balance
Cardiovascular System
Blood volume and constituents
Hemodynamic changes
Gastrointestinal Tract
Hepatic Function
Renal Function

Blood volume increases along with the number of platelets, fibrinogen levels, and the level of activity of several clotting factors. However, there is a smaller rise in circulating red blood cells. This difference results in a lower hematocrit and hemoglobin level (usually in the low 30s) even though there is an actual increase in red cell mass. This is known as *physiologic anemia of pregnancy.*

Serum cholinesterase activity declines. The implications of these changes for the nurse are the predisposition for thromboembolism and the possibility of prolonged paralysis and apneic period following the administration of succinylcholine.

Hemodynamic Changes. Cardiac output and heart rate increase progressively during pregnancy until, at 30 to 34 weeks' gestation, the cardiac output is 30 to 50 percent above normal, and the heart rate is about 10 beats per min above normal, with EKG changes and heart sounds possibly developing (Table 39–2). Arterial blood pressure decreases slightly because there is a decrease in peripheral vascular resistance in an attempt to compensate for the increased cardiac output.

Perhaps the most significant effect on the cardiovascular system for the nurse to consider in routine post anesthesia management is obstruction of the inferior vena cava and the pelvic veins by the enlarging uterus. This condition, known as *Scott's syndrome,* can develop by the second trimester and causes supine hypotension. It becomes mandatory to avoid the supine position postoperatively, because it can significantly aggravate the obstruction. The

TABLE 39–2. Possible Alterations in Cardiovascular Parameters During Pregnancy*

Heart sounds are louder with the development of a split S_2
Short systolic murmur
More forceful apical impulse
Inverted T waves in leads III V_1 and V_2
Left axis deviation in the second through sixth months
Flattened T waves
Depressed S-T segments

*If findings develop during pregnancy, they usually disappear after delivery.

side-lying position is the one of choice in the PACU.

It is also important to note that collateral circulation for venous return develops through the intervertebral venous plexus and the azygos vein. This condition reduces the volume of the epidural and subarachnoid spaces. Therefore, the amount of drug required during regional anesthesia should be decreased. Keeping this in mind, the PACU nurse should assess the patient upon admission for a high block and monitor dermatome levels frequently thereafter.

Respiratory Changes

The diaphragm elevates and the rib cage flares, so that at term 85 percent of respiratory effort is intercostal and 15 percent is diaphragmatic (normally approximately 70 percent is intercostal and 30 percent is diaphragmatic). There is also a rise in the respiratory rate and in the tidal volume, which causes a significant rise in alveolar ventilation. The functional residual volume and the residual volume of air in the lungs decrease.

There is capillary engorgement of the upper respiratory tract, and pregnant women may complain of nasal stuffiness.

Gastrointestinal Tract Changes

There is a slowing of gastric emptying because the stomach is displaced as the uterus enlarges. Therefore, the PACU nurse must be cognizant of the potential for vomiting and aspiration, particularly in post–general anesthesia patients. Muscle relaxants may have been used, resulting in the patient's normal protective mechanisms being obtunded. Once again, the side-lying position becomes of significant importance.

Hepatic Changes

Liver function results are abnormal but there is no evidence of alteration in function, and blood flow remains constant. Therefore, those anesthetic agents that are metabolized in the liver should have the same duration of effect.

Renal Changes

Early in pregnancy, the kidneys receive an increased blood flow; therefore, glomerular filtration rates and urine formation increase. This is necessary to handle the increased amount of waste products produced. Monitoring of output should reflect this expected increase in volume. Intervention may be required for hypovolemia even though the urine output is within acceptable ranges for a nonpregnant patient.

CARE OF MOTHER AND FETUS IN THE PACU

Studies have not shown one anesthetic technique to be better than another in the gravid patient. As with nonpregnant patients, the choice of technique is determined by:

1. Surgery to be performed
2. ASA classification of patient
3. Anesthetist's preference
4. Patient's preference
5. Underlying disease entities

The care of the patient postoperatively should be the same as for any patient undergoing that procedure or for one recovering from that particular anesthetic. There are, however, additions to the routine nursing care that must be instituted for all pregnant patients.

Positioning

To alleviate compression of the vena cava, the uterus should be displaced to the left, either by positioning the patient on her left side or by tilting the pelvis using a folded sheet or bath towel under the woman's right iliac crest. Slight elevation of the legs and the use of thigh-high elastic stockings should be standard.

Psychologic and Emotional Support

The mother's concern for her unborn child is paramount. Constant reassurance is mandatory. If possible, allow the mother to listen to the fetal heartbeat frequently during the recovery phase. Explain all procedures and why they are being done before carrying them out. If your PACU allows visitors, involvement of the father should also be considered.

Fetal Monitoring

The fetal heart rate must be monitored every 15 minutes if the fetus has reached viability (Table 39–3). If available, an indirect fetal monitoring system should be utilized for constant assessment of fetal stability (Fig. 39–1).

The second type of monitoring required is to observe the patient closely for signs of premature labor. These include spontaneous rupture of membranes, increased fetal heart rate, presenting of vaginal mucus plug, uterine palpitations, uterine contractions, and restlessness of the mother.

Initially, the patient may not feel the contractions or be aware of membrane rupture; therefore, palpation of the abdomen and assessment of vaginal discharge must be performed by the nurse. Should premature labor begin, transfer of the patient to the labor and delivery area as soon as possible is recommended. A tocolytic drug may have to be given to stop labor. These drugs should be administered by personnel familiar with proper protocols for administration and with their side effects.

Pain Management

Since the growth of consumer awareness, the administration of medication during pregnancy has become a controversial issue, and one that must be dealt with on an individual basis. For pain management immediately post anesthesia, when the patient is in a hypersuggestive state, the use of distraction techniques, i.e., guided imagery

TABLE 39–3. Fetal Heart Rates

Normal fetal heart rate	120–160 beats/min
Moderate tachycardia	160–180 beats/min
Marked tachycardia	180 + beats/min
Moderate bradycardia	100–120 beats/min
Marked bradycardia	100 − beats/min

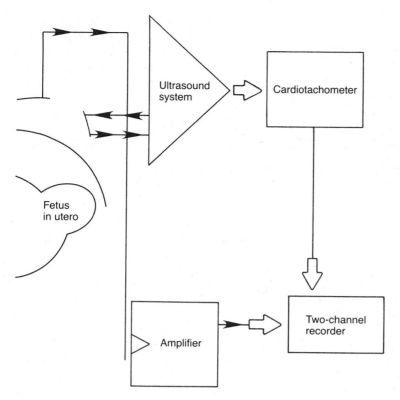

Figure 39–1. Indirect fetal monitoring system. Doppler/ultrasound device transmits a beam to determine fetal heart rate. When striking a moving object within the fetus, such as a mitral valve leaflet, the frequency of the transmitted beam is shifted up or down depending on which way the leaflet is moving. This valve movement is counted and displayed as a heart rate on the recorder.

and breathing exercises, has had favorable results in place of drugs.

If a mild analgesic is required, the drug of choice is acetaminophen (Tylenol) and, for moderate pain management, propoxyphene (Darvon). Both these drugs have been evaluated through prospective studies and have been shown to pose minimal risks to the fetus if used appropriately for short-term pain management. Narcotic analgesia may be warranted for severe pain but must be utilized judiciously, keeping in mind the respiratory depressive effects.

The gravid patient in the PACU is a rare occurrence and one that requires a great deal of knowledge and the ability to provide continual support during this stressful situation. The nurse must be able to provide a quiet, calm, reassuring atmosphere for the patient. The objective of the care delivered is an optimum environment for both mother and fetus.

REFERENCES

1. Kelly, M.: Maternal position and blood pressure during pregnancy and delivery. Am. J. Nurs. *82*:809–812, 1982.
2. Kovaks, R. R.: When your patient is also pregnant. AORN, *36*(4):559–565, 1982.
3. Mersheimer, W. L., and Kazarian, K.: Surgical Disease in Pregnancy. Philadelphia, W. B. Saunders Co., 1974.
4. Niebyl, J.: Drug Use in Pregnancy. Philadelphia, Lea & Febiger, 1982.
5. Shnider, S. M., and Webster, G. M.: Maternal and fetal hazards of surgery during pregnancy. Am. J. Obstet. Gynecol. *92*(7):891–899, 1985.
6. Vestal, K. W., and McKenzie, A. M. (eds.): High Risk Perinatal Nursing. Philadelphia, W. B. Saunders Co., 1983.
7. Ziegal, E. E., and Cranley, M. S.: Obstetric Nursing. 8th ed. New York, Macmillan Publishing Company, 1984.

40

Postoperative Care of the Patient with Sickle Cell Anemia

Sickle cell anemia is an inherited type of hemolytic anemia. It is a chronic disease marked by exacerbations. The clinical manifestations are based entirely on sickling of the red cells and its consequences.

In recent years, more than 100 abnormal hemoglobins have been described in humans. This particular form of hemoglobin, when exposed to low oxygen tensions, causes the red blood cell to distort its shape (sickle) and to cause infarction and other complications. Normal hemoglobin is labeled hemoglobin A, while this sickling hemoglobin is labeled hemoglobin S. Hemoglobin S is thought to have arisen in Arabia in Neolithic times, and from there to have spread eastward and westward; it is found today in parts of India, east and west Africa, the West Indies, and among American blacks.

The common sickle cell disorders are sickle cell trait (SA), homozygous sickle cell disease (SS), sickle cell–hemoglobin C disease, and sickle cell–thalassemia. A combination of thalassemia and sickle cell anemia occurs in sickle cell–beta thalassemia.

Sickle cell trait is found in about 8 to 12 percent of the black population, who are heterozygous for sickling, and represents a combination of sickle hemoglobin (SA) and normal hemoglobin (AA). The red blood cells of such persons contain from 20 to 40 percent hemoglobin S but are not misshapen under normal living conditions. The individual may suffer sickling if exposed to any conditions that cause hypoxia, such as depressed respiratory function from anesthetics in the post anesthesia care unit (PACU).

The most common form of sickle cell disease is the homozygous sickle cell disease (SS). It occurs in about 1 in 400 to 1 in 500 blacks in the United States. These persons have inherited sickling genes from both parents. They usually have 80 to 100 percent hemoglobin S. Sickling is present all the time and minor reductions in oxygen tension can cause a sickle cell crisis. The onset of symptoms occurs around the age of 2, and rarely do these persons live past the age of 40.

Sickle cell–hemoglobin C disease is caused by the presence of the gene for sickle hemoglobin and the gene for hemoglobin C. The course of the disease is usually milder than that of the homozygous sickle cell disease (SS), although the person will experience discomfort and occasional sickle cell crises.

Sickle cell–thalassemia, which occurs in persons who have traits for sickle cell– and beta-thalassemia, has a less severe course and symptoms in comparison with the other forms of these diseases. The sickle cell crises is not seen as commonly in this disease.

PATHOGENESIS

To understand the pathogenesis of this disease, it is helpful to know what happens to the red blood cell when sickling occurs. If oxygen tension is lowered, long crystals called "tactoids" are formed within the red blood cells, owing to rearrangement of the amino acid chains or polymers. The cell membrane becomes distorted by the twisting of the polymers. The result is the sickle cell shape for which the disease is named (Fig. 40–1). The process can be reversed if the oxygen tension is raised.

The actual pathologic action of sickling occurs in the microcirculation. Because of increased viscosity and the distortion of the red blood cells with the formation of tactoids, which prevents the cells from molding to the size and structure of the capillaries, the sickled cells are wedged in the capillary bed, occluding normal flow. As the cells aggregate, a thrombus is formed.

Symptoms depend on whether the thrombus becomes an embolus, and, if so, on where it becomes lodged; infarctive episodes will be caused in that tissue. Areas of infarctive crisis are the spleen, myocardium, kidney, liver, mesentery, bone marrow, and brain.

Oxygen tension causes sickling, but several other precipitating factors are also involved, such as acidosis, hypotension, regional vasodilatation, dehydration, hemoconcentration, stasis of blood, hypothermia, sepsis, decreased cardiac output, and respiratory impairment.

ANEMIA AND ANESTHESIA

It is generally believed that anesthesia is not hazardous to sickle cell trait (SA) patients. Nevertheless, it must be kept in mind that sufficiently adverse hypoxic conditions can precipitate a sickling crisis. Definite hazards arise with anesthesia for the sickle cell disease (SS) and the sickle cell–hemoglobin C disease patients. General anesthesia, because of its ability to cause the intravascular sickling syndrome, has been the object of much research. The most important factor in this syndrome is hypoxemia, which generally occurs during the recovery period rather than intraoperatively. Local anesthesia or nerve blocks are the techniques of choice. Epidural or spinal techniques should be avoided, owing to the

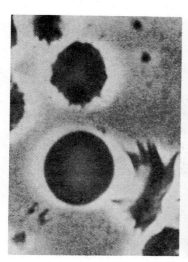
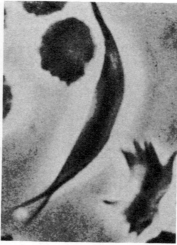

Figure 40–1. Comparison of a normal cell and a sickle cell. (From: Sickle cell anemia. Medical World News, December 3, 1971, p. 38.)

possibility of hypotension with these two methods.

PACU CARE

Prevention of sickle cell crisis is the main objective in the PACU phase. If diagnostic procedures are not available, or if emergency surgery prevents testing for the sickling trait, all black patients should be treated as possible carriers of the trait, since the incidence of this disease is relatively high among blacks.

In the patient with sickle cell disease (SS), the postoperative period is of crucial importance. This is because incisional pain, analgesics, pulmonary infections, and low arterial oxygen partial pressures are all predisposing factors to the formation of sickle cells. Hence, in the PACU, supplemental humidified oxygen, along with appropriate monitoring of intravascular volume and core temperature, is of utmost importance for ensuring the positive outcomes of the patient.

Temperature regulation is important for the patient with sickle cell disease. While cold reduces tactoid formation, it also reduces body metabolism, which may lead to crisis. Hyperthermia causes excess sweating, however, and may lead to dehydration, which can also cause sickling. Temperature monitoring and the use of hypo- hyperthermia blankets can allow maintenance of body temperature in the optimal range of 36° to 37°C.

Cardiac monitoring is important because the frequency of arrhythmias, such as extrasystole or prolonged P-R interval, in sickling patients is high. Vasodilators or vasoconstrictors should be avoided, if possible, since the dilators may cause hypotension and the vasoconstrictors may cause circulatory stasis.

Respiratory rate and volume should be monitored closely, so that hypoxia can be avoided. Arterial blood gas monitoring can aid in assessing respiratory status, and postoperative pain should be managed with drugs that do not depress respiratory function.

Kidney function should be monitored because the renal tubules will become blocked by the hemolyzed red blood cells if crisis occurs, and infarcts may occur in some areas of the kidney. Insertion of a urinary catheter to monitor urinary output at regular intervals will prove useful.

SICKLE CELL CRISIS

The types of crisis seen in sickle cell anemia are vaso-occlusive, aplastic, sequestration, and hemolytic. The *vaso-occlusive crisis* is the most common type and is characterized by tissue ischemia, infarction, and necrosis. The bones, tendons, synovia, spleen, liver, and intestine are common sites of occlusion. Infections, dehydration, high altitudes, extreme physical exertion, and emotional upsets can trigger this type of crisis.

The *aplastic crisis* is most grave and constitutes a medical emergency. It is characterized by a sudden drastic fall in red blood cell production. The patient will initially appear weak and have signs of cardiac decompensation.

The spleen is involved in *sequestration crisis*. A large amount of blood becomes trapped in the spleen, and hypovolemia and shock are the outcome—this constitutes a medical emergency. Clinically, the patient's blood pressure will decrease and the pulse will rise. Palpation and percussion will reveal an enlarged mass in the right upper quadrant of the abdomen.

Bacterial infections, poisons, and medications, such as phenothiazines or sulfonamides, aspirin in large quantities, and quinine, are capable of producing *hemolysis* of the red blood cell. The patient also has an enzyme deficiency (glucose-6-phosphodehydrogenase) in this type of sickle cell anemia.

If crisis occurs, the following modes of treatment are recommended: Keep the patient warm, treat infections, and maintain oxygenation, hydration, and alkalinization. Heparin may be administered to reduce the risks of embolus formation, and magnesium sulfate may also be indicated for its vaso-dilator and anticoagulant properties.

REFERENCES

1. Guyton, A.: Textbook of Medical Physiology. 7th ed. Philadelphia, W. B. Saunders Co., 1986.
2. Katz, J., Benumof, J., and Kadis, L.: Anesthesia and Uncommon Diseases: Pathophysiologic and Clinical Correlations. 2nd ed. Philadelphia, W. B. Saunders Co., 1981.
3. Maduska, A.: Sickling dynamics of red blood cells and other physiologic studies during anesthesia. Anesth. Analg., *54*(3):361–364, 1975.
4. Miller, R.: Anesthesia. 2nd end. New York, Churchill Livingstone, Inc., 1986.
5. Sponner, T., and Dark, M.: The management of sickle cell patients undergoing surgery. Laryngoscope, *86*(4):506–508, 1976.
6. Stoelting, R., and Dierdorf, S.: Anesthesia and Co-Existing Diseases. New York, Churchill Livingstone, Inc., 1983.
7. Vickers, M.: Medicine for Anaesthetists. 2nd ed. St. Louis, C. V. Mosby Co., 1982.

41

Postoperative Care of the Patient with Nausea and Vomiting

One of the most perplexing problems for the PACU nurse is that of the "syndrome" of postoperative nausea and vomiting. Although, through the years, the incidence of nausea and vomiting has decreased, the problem is still perennial in every PACU. The surgeon hopes that nausea and vomiting will be minimal, as disturbances in electrolyte balance and wound healing are associated with such upsets. The PACU nurse also appreciates a decreased incidence of these upsets since, when patients are vomiting, airway management can become most difficult.

MECHANISM OF ACTION

The *vomiting center* is located in the medulla near the dorsal nucleus of the vagus nerve (Fig. 41–1). It can be excited by reflex impulses arising in the pharynx, stomach, or other portions of the gastrointestinal tract. Foreign materials, such as blood and mucus or irritant gases in the stomach or other portions of the gastrointestinal tract, can produce this syndrome. The vomiting center can be excited by impulses received from cerebral centers. Drugs such as anes-

thetic agents and narcotics sensitize the vestibular apparatus, the organ of balance. This explains why two of the principal causative factors of nausea and vomiting are rough handling of the patient during transportation and frequent changes of position in the immediate recovery period.

The vomiting center can be excited by chemical materials carried to it in the blood. Drugs such as apomorphine, morphine, and meperidine (Demerol) arrive this way, exciting the vomiting center directly. This is designated as *central vomiting*. The vomiting center can be excited by interference with its blood supply. Severe cerebral anoxia and increased intracranial pressure are examples of this. Finally, the vomiting center can be excited by dehydration and electrolyte imbalance.

INCIDENCE

Studies indicate that the incidence of nausea and vomiting is higher in women than in men. There is a lower incidence in those patients premedicated with morphine than in those who received meperidine (Demerol). Of great interest is that patients

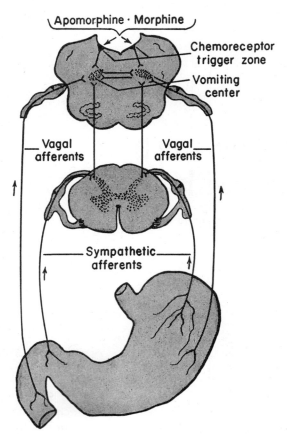

Figure 41–1. The afferent connections of the vomiting center. (From Guyton, A. C.: Textbook of Medical Physiology. 7th ed. Philadelphia, W. B. Saunders Co., 1986, p. 803.)

who received their anesthetic by mask have a higher incidence of nausea and vomiting than patients who received their anesthetic by endotracheal tube. Other possible causes of nausea and vomiting of statistic significance are hypotension during surgery, intra-abdominal surgery, increased duration of surgery, obesity, and a history of motion sickness.

In a study by Andersen and Krohg,[1] postoperative nausea was significantly related to pain. Opiates of sufficient dosage tended to reduce pain and abate nausea, and they seldom provoked nausea. If the dosage of the analgesic is inadequate, the nausea may persist, and further supplemental doses of analgesic may be required. Other techniques for relief of pain that should be

instituted concomitant with the administration of opiate are repositioning the postoperative patient, coughing, deep breathing, and the administration of oxygen.

Patients who received a nitrous-narcotic anesthetic and whose state was reversed postoperatively with an excessive dose of naloxone (Narcan) will usually exhibit nausea and vomiting in the recovery period. Goodman and Gilman[2] state that naloxone (Narcan) itself has no emetic properties. Therefore, the analgesic state should be reestablished to eliminate the vomiting reaction.

PACU CARE

If the patient complains of nausea, he should be encouraged to cough and breathe deeply, and oxygen should be administered if there is any suspicion of hypoxemia. A cold washcloth placed on the patient's forehead and words of encouragement will sometimes extinguish the nausea. It is mandatory for the nurse to remain with the patient, as the patient can go into the vomiting stage at a moment's notice. It must be remembered that the danger of aspiration of vomitus and obstructed airway is always present.

If the nausea persists or is severe, the patient can be given a pharmacologic remedy per a physician's order (Table 41–1).

The nursing care of the patient who is vomiting centers around airway management. The patient should be placed in a head-down position so that the vomitus will drain away from the lungs. Oral suctioning should be instituted if the patient is not able to control his airway completely. Oxygen should be administered when there is any question of compromise of the respiratory status. Rapid assessment of the patient's respiratory status should be made during and after the vomiting episode. This is done by auscultation of the chest bilaterally for adventitious sounds. Any possible aspiration of vomitus should be reported to the physician immediately. If the airway becomes obstructed, place the patient in a head-down position, turn his head to one

TABLE 41–1. Drugs Used to Control Nausea

Drug	Route of Administration	Action	Side Effects
Prochlorperazine (Compazine)	PO, IM, suppository	Antiemetic, tranquilizer	Drowsiness, dizziness, hypotension, extrapyramidal reactions
Trimethobenzamide (Tigan)	PO, suppository, IM	Antiemetic	Drowsiness, Parkinson-like symptoms, hypotension, blurring of vision
Hydroxyzine (Atarax or Vistaril)	PO, IM	Reduces anxiety, antiemetic	Potentiates narcotics and barbiturates, and other CNS depressants; drowsiness, dry mouth
Droperidol (Inapsine)	IM, IV	Antiemetic, tranquilizer	Drowsiness, hypotension, extrapyramidal reactions
Benzquinamide (Emeticon)	IM or IV (slowly)	Antiemetic, antihistaminic, mild anticholinergic, sedative	Drowsiness, headache, hypertension, arrhythmias during IV administration, increased temperature, dry mouth, flushing, blurred vision

side, and try to remove foreign material by suctioning or with the finger. While performing this maneuver, send another person for a physician or anesthetist. A third person should remain to assist the nurse.

REFERENCES

1. Anderson, R., and Krogh, K.: Pain as a major cause of postoperative nausea. Can. Anaesth. Soc. J., 23(4):366, 1976.
2. Goodman, L., and Gilman, A.: The Pharmacological Basis of Therapeutics. 6th ed. New York, Macmillan Publishing Company, 1980.
3. Katz, J., Benumof, J., and Kadis, L.: Anesthesia and Uncommon Diseases: Pathophysiologic and Clinical Correlations. 2nd ed. Philadelphia, W. B. Saunders Co., 1981.
4. Miller, R.: Anesthesia. 2nd ed. New York, Churchill Livingstone, Inc., 1986.
5. Stoelting, R., and Dierdorf, S.: Anesthesia and Co-Existing Disease. New York, Churchill Livingstone, Inc., 1983.

42

Postoperative Care of the Patient with Malignant Hyperthermia

In the past, there have been reports in the medical literature about young, healthy persons who, after exercise in hot weather, developed "heat stroke" that was followed by death. Clinical reports of this syndrome continued to appear, especially of patients in the operating room developing an accelerated temperature during induction of anesthesia, and by the 1950s, more information was secured. Today, because of research, the morbidity and mortality from this syndrome have been reduced. Its cause is a genetically determined condition called *malignant hyperthermia (MH)*. MH is precipitated by certain general inhalational anesthetics, depolarizing skeletal muscle relaxants, amide local anesthetics, and stress. The incidence of malignant hyperthermia ranges from 1 in 14,000 to 1 in 15,000 in children, and 1 in 50,000 in adults. The onset of malignant hyperthermia usually occurs during induction of anesthesia. Once the acute episode is treated in the operating room, the patient may be admitted to the post anesthesia care unit (PACU). There have been reports of malignant hyperthermia recurring in the post anesthesia care unit. Because successful management of

MH depends upon early assessment and prompt intervention, the PACU nurse must be well versed in the pathophysiology and treatment of this syndrome.

IDENTIFICATION OF MH–SUSCEPTIBLE PATIENTS

Genetics

Humans probably inherit susceptibility to malignant hyperthermia by more than one gene or more than one group of possible mutational forms of a gene. The pattern of inheritance may range from recessive to dominant, with graded variations in between. The ease of initiation of an episode of MH seems to depend on the degree of genetic susceptibility and on environmental factors; this explains why some patients who are known to be susceptible show no signs of malignant hyperthermia when exposed to confirmed MH triggering agents. It is also possible that a malignant hyperthermia–susceptible (MHS) patient could be given an anesthetic in the presence of trigger agents; this patient might not experience an acute MH reaction intraoperatively, but it could develop instead in the post anesthesia care unit.

Evaluation of Susceptibility

Identification of patients, before anesthesia, who may be susceptible to MH is of major therapeutic importance. MH–susceptible patients, upon history and physical examination, will usually demonstrate some subclinical muscle weakness or abnormality, such as deficient fine motor control. Many MH–susceptible individuals complain of muscle cramps that occur spontaneously, during an infectious illness, or during or after exercise. When these cramps are present, they may be so severe that they are almost incapacitating. The patient may also describe heat prostration during physical exertion which is associated with environmental heat stress. Along with this, there may be a positive patient history or a positive genealogy going back for two generations; i.e., the patient or immediate relatives may show MH symptoms during an anesthestic experience. Physical examination of the MH–susceptible individual may reveal myopathies such as wasting of the distal ends of the vastus muscles and hypertrophy of the proximal femoral muscles of the thigh. Other myopathies that are associated with MH susceptibility are cryptorchidism, pectus carinatum, kyphosis, lordosis, ptosis, and hypoplastic mandible. Interestingly, electromyographic changes are seen in less than half of MH–susceptible patients. Electrocardiograms (ECG) of MH–susceptible patients may reveal ventricular or atrial hypertrophy, or both, bundle branch block myocardial ischemia, and ventricular dysrhythmias. Measurements of blood CPK (creatine phosphokinase) are usually about 70 percent reliable in estimating susceptibility to MH.

The most definitive test for detecting MH susceptibility is the biopsy of skeletal muscle. Samples are obtained from the quadriceps muscle and are subjected to isometric contracture testing. The skeletal muscle of the MH–susceptible patient will have an increased isometric tension when exposed to caffeine or halothane.

Patients at high risk for development of an acute MH crisis have been classified as follows: (1) patients who have an MH–positive muscle biopsy or who have survived an acute MH crisis; (2) patients who have a first-degree relative known to be MH susceptible or to have had a positive muscle biopsy; (3) patients whose family members have a clinically demonstrated muscle abnormality; and (4) patients who are members of a family whose plasma CPK measurements have been found to be elevated in one or more samples (taken on at least three occasions).

NORMAL SKELETAL MUSCLE PHYSIOLOGY

Although a complete discussion of skeletal muscle contraction can be found in Chapter 14, a brief synopsis will be given here. The events leading to the contraction of a skeletal muscle begin with an electrical impulse that is transmitted down the axon to the motor nerve terminal, where vesicles containing acetylcholine are located. Upon stimulation, the contents of the vesicles are released. This quantum of acetylcholine crosses the myoneural junction and interacts with its receptor on the postsynaptic membrane. This receptor activation causes a transient increase in the permeability for sodium and potassium ions which ultimately creates an electrical action potential (nerve impulse) that is propagated along the muscle membrane. This action potential electrically excites the sarcolemma and releases into the myoplasm calcium ions that are stored in the sarcoplasmic reticulum. These calcium ions then attach to troponin C, an inhibitory muscle protein that, when stimulated by the calcium, permits the actin and myosin protein filaments to interact and cause muscle contraction. The calcium ions in the myoplasm are then taken up by a reuptake mechanism into the sarcoplasmic reticulum. The process by which the electrically excited sarcolemma is coupled to the calcium released from the sarcoplasmic reticulum is known as excitation-contraction (E-C) coupling.

PATHOPHYSIOLOGY OF MALIGNANT HYPERTHERMIA

When a susceptible patient is exposed to a trigger agent, such as halothane, causing MH to occur, the clinical features are produced by an excess of calcium ions in the myoplasm. Although the exact pathophysiology of malignant hyperthermia is not known, it appears that in MH the reuptake of calcium from the myoplasm by the sarcoplasmic reticulum is decreased; it has also been suggested that the E-C coupling mechanism is defective. With an elevated calcium ion concentration in the myoplasm, the skeletal muscle contraction will be intense and prolonged, finally leading to a hypermetabolic state of acid and heat production. More specifically, heat is produced by the accelerated and continued synthesis and use of adenosine triphosphate (ATP) during glycolysis. The metabolic by-product of glycolysis, lactic acid, is transported to the liver, where part of it is oxidized to provide the ATP necessary to help make glucose. This glucose, along with glycogen, is released from the liver and transported back to the metabolically active muscle, where the entire cycle repeats. This revolving process liberates much heat and produces a significant amount of metabolic acid. Respiratory and metabolic acidosis develop because of this hypermetabolic state, and symptoms such as tachycardia, tachypnea, ventricular dysrhythmias, and unstable blood pressure will appear. Because of intense vasoconstriction, the skin is mottled and cyanotic (Table 42–1). Interestingly, elevated body temperature can actually be a late sign of malignant hyperthermia; for this reason, the nurse should not prolong the assessment of the patient on the assumption that the patient's temperature must be significantly elevated before intervention is attempted. Once the patient's temperature begins to rise, it may increase at a rate of 0.5°C every 15 minutes and may approach levels as high as 46°C.

Muscle rigidity will occur in about 75 percent of the patients who experience MH. This is especially true in MH–susceptible patients following the administration of suc-

TABLE 42–1. Signs and Symptoms of Malignant Hyperthermia

Signs (Objective Findings)
*Central venous desaturation**
*Central venous hypercapnia**
*Metabolic acidosis**
*Respiratory acidosis**
Hyperkalemia
Myoglobinemia
Elevated creatine phosphokinase

Symptoms (Subjective Findings)
Tachycardia†
Tachypnea†
Ventricular dysrhythmias
Cyanosis
Skin mottling
Fever—hot, flushed skin
Rigidity
Profuse sweating
Unstable blood pressure

*Primary sign
†Primary symptom

cinylcholine. In fact, the spasm of the masseter muscles following the injection of succinylcholine may be so severe that the nurse cannot open the patient's mouth to insert an airway. It is important to remember that the onset of skeletal muscle rigidity following the administration of succinylcholine could be a sign of the impending development of malignant hyperthermia.

Triggering of Malignant Hyperthermia

Various environmental stimuli and pharmacologic agents can stimulate an acute episode of malignant hyperthermia (Table 42–2). Fatigue, emotional upset, or very hot and humid weather can trigger a waking febrile episode. Patients usually respond to dantrolene, surface cooling, and other symptomatic treatment. The anesthetic agents that trigger MH seem to affect the sarcoplasmic reticulum or the E-C coupling mechanism or both. Because of their wide use, halothane and succinylcholine are the most common trigger agents. Amide local anesthetics, such as lidocaine, are also trigger agents; it has been demonstrated that lidocaine causes the release of calcium ions into the myoplasm in vitro. In MH–susceptible patients or in patients who have had an episode of acute malignant hyperthermia

TABLE 42–2. Environmental Stimuli and Pharmacologic Agents That May Trigger Malignant Hyperthermia (MH)

Environmental Stimuli
Extensive skeletal muscle injury
Emotional crisis
Very hot and humid weather
Strenuous and prolonged exercise

Pharmacologic Agents
Halothane
Enflurane
Isoflurane (?)
Succinylcholine
d-Tubocurarine
Gallamine (?)
Amide local anesthetics—lidocaine, mepivacaine, bupivacaine, etidocaine
Caffeine

in the operating room, all possible trigger agents should be stringently avoided. As another precaution, because emotional upsets will trigger MH, the PACU nurse should provide a stress-free environment for the MHS patient.

Pharmacologic Agents Associated with Malignant Hyperthermia

Dantrolene Sodium (Dantrium). Dantrolene is a muscle relaxant that is chemically and pharmacologically unrelated to other muscle relaxants. It is the only known pharmacologic agent that is effective in the treatment of malignant hyperthermia. The site of action of this drug is distal to the endplate within the muscle fiber. The main pharmacologic action of dantrolene results in a reduction in the release of calcium by the sarcoplasmic reticulum without affecting reuptake. Consequently, the concentration of calcium in the myoplasm is reduced, inhibiting the E-C coupling mechanism and causing muscle contraction to cease. When administered orally, dantrolene has a half-life of 8 hours; when administered intravenously, the half-life is 5 hours. When it is used in the treatment of acute malignant hyperthermia, the intravenous dosage is 1 to 2 mg/kg, which can be repeated every 5 to 10 minutes with a maximum dose of 10 mg/kg. If the acute episode of MH occurs in the operating room and the patient is

treated successfully, dantrolene therapy will be continued into the recovery (PACU) period to prevent recurrence of MH. After the acute period in the post anesthesia care unit has passed, the patient will be given oral dantrolene in four divided doses. Because dantrolene is poorly soluble, it is supplied in vials in the form of a lyophilized powder. To reconstitute a vial of lyophilized powder, 60 ml of sterile water for injection, U.S.P. is added to the vial, and it is shaken until the solution is clear; many compatibility problems arise when dantrolene is mixed with solutions other than sterile water for injection, U.S.P. Also, *the sterile water for injection, U.S.P., that is used to reconstitute the dantrolene should not contain any bacteriostatic agents.* This is because it is not unusual to use over 2000 ml of diluent during the treatment of acute MH in a 70 kg adult.

Procainamide (Procamide, Procapan, Pronestyl). Procainamide once was the main drug in the treatment of malignant hyperthermia. The use of procainamide is controversial, particularly since the recommended initial dose is two to five times its cardiotoxic dose. Some authors suggest that if this drug is used in the treatment of MH, isoproterenol should be administered to maintain cardiac function. The recommended dose of procainamide is 0.5 to 1 mg/kg/min, up to a maximum dose of 15 to 30 mg/kg. The dosage should be lowered when there is a reduction in the heart rate or dysrhythmias. At a lower dose range, procainamide may be useful in the treatment of the dysrhythmias during the acute episode of MH.

PERIOPERATIVE MANAGEMENT OF THE MH–SUSCEPTIBLE PATIENT

Preoperatively, the MH–susceptible patient may be given oral dantrolene in four divided doses of 4 to 7 mg/kg/day for 1 to 3 days prior to the administration of the anesthetic. The patient is usually well premedicated; however, anticholinergics, such as atropine, should be avoided because they interfere with the normal heat loss mechanisms and, in the case of atropine, can cause

TABLE 42–3. Drugs That Are Considered Safe to Administer to a Malignant Hyperthermia– Susceptible Patient

Nitrous oxide
Diazepam
Droperidol
Pancuronium
Thiopental
Ketamine
Fentanyl
Morphine
Ester local anesthetics—procaine, tetracaine,
    2-chloroprocaine

tachycardia which could cause confusion in diagnosis of acute MH. Also, phenothiazines should be avoided in the perioperative period, as they may cause a release of calcium from the sarcoplasmic reticulum. Intraoperative anesthesia requires the use of agents that will not trigger an episode of malignant hyperthermia (Table 42–3). Although regional anesthesia avoids the use of the general inhalational anesthetic agents and skeletal muscle relaxants, elevated temperatures in MH–susceptible patients have been reported with its use. If local anesthetic agents are to be utilized, amides such as lidocaine and mepivacaine should be avoided.

Intraoperative monitoring of the MH–susceptible patient includes electrocardiogram, temperature, arterial blood gas including acid-base determinations, and precordial stethoscope. These monitoring parameters should be continued into the PACU period (Table 42–4). Because some MH–susceptible patients have had malignant hyperthermia triggered in the postop-

TABLE 42–4. Suggested Components of Monitoring of the Patient with Acute Malignant Hyperthermia

Continuous electrocardiogram (consider 12-lead ECG
    and EEG after acute phase)
Core and axillary temperature
Urine output
Arterial pressure line
Pulse and blood pressure
Central venous pressure*
Swan-Ganz catheters*

*Should be considered; however, do not delay treatment if the insertion of these monitors is physically or technically difficult.

erative period, they should be followed for a minimum of 24 hours postoperatively and should not be subjected to anxiety or stress. These patients should be reassured that doctors and nurses have very reliable instruments to monitor for malignant hyperthermia, and that prompt and effective treatment will be provided if it develops.

TREATMENT OF ACUTE MALIGNANT HYPERTHERMIA IN THE POST ANESTHESIA CARE UNIT

The cornerstone of the successful treatment of MH is early detection (see Table 42–1). Table 42–5 lists the suggested equipment and drugs to be used in the treatment of acute malignant hyperthermia that should be kept in the post anesthesia care

TABLE 42–5. Suggested Equipment and Drugs to be Used in the Treatment of Malignant Hyperthermia

Equipment Needed in the Treatment of Acute Malignant Hyperthermia
Intravenous lines with assorted cannula gauges
Central venous pressure sets (2)
Sterile venous and arterial strain gauge
Swan-Ganz catheter
Laboratory test tubes for blood chemistry analysis
Crystalloid solution (ten 1000 ml bottles)—
    labeled **FOR HYPERTHERMIA ONLY** and stored in
    the PACU refrigerator
Bucket of cracked ice—labeled **FOR HYPERTHERMIA
                    ONLY** and stored in freezer of
                    the PACU refrigerator
Cooling blanket
Fan

Drugs Needed in the Treatment of Acute Malignant Hyperthermia
Sodium bicarbonate (12 ampules of 8.4% strength)
Mannitol (4 ampules—12.4 gm/50 ml)
Furosemide (4 vials)
Calcium gluconate (2 ampules—100 mg/10 ml)
Potassium chloride (2 ampules)
Glucose (2 bottles of 50% strength)
Iced IV saline (ten 1000 ml bottles in refrigerator)
Procainamide (2000 mg)
Regular insulin (1 ampule of 100 units)
Dantrolene (Dantrium intravenous)—36 vials of
    lyophilized powder with at least 2200 ml of sterile
    water for injection, U.S.P. (without a bacteriostatic
    agent) to reconstitute the dantrolene

Note: All the above equipment and drugs should be stored in a box or cart in the PACU. The box or cart should be labeled **HYPERTHERMIA**.

unit. If the assessment indicates that the patient is developing acute malignant hyperthermia, the following steps should be taken[4]:

1. Discontinue the use of any trigger agent (see Table 42–3) and SEND FOR HELP!

2. Rapidly ventilate the patient with large tidal volumes, using a bag-valve-mask system and oxygen (total oxygen flow should exceed 15 L/min). Oral endotracheal intubation should be performed if the patient's airway is compromised.

3. Insert arterial and central venous lines and send venous and arterial blood samples to the laboratory for immediate results on electrolytes and arterial blood gas analysis.

4. Start reconstituting the dantrolene as soon as possible.

5. Administer the intravenous dantrolene—1 to 2 mg/kg over 1 to 2 minutes, up to 10 mg/kg or until the patient's temperature starts to decrease.

6. *Cool the patient.* Cover all exposed surfaces with towels soaked in water. Cover the wet towels with ice. Use cooling blankets and fans if possible. Use cold gastric lavage and hydrate with iced intravenous fluids. To avoid hypothermia, discontinue all the cooling interventions when body temperature decreases to 38°C.

7. Administer sodium bicarbonate intravenously at a dosage of 1 to 2 mEq/kg. When results of the arterial blood gas analysis are available, correct the base deficit using sodium bicarbonate according to the following formula[5]:

base deficit =
0.3 × weight (kg) × base excess (mEq/L)

If $Paco_2$ is elevated, increase the tidal ventilation of the patient. Do not administer sodium bicarbonate to correct respiratory acidosis, as the $Paco_2$ will only increase, which may lead to ventricular fibrillation.

8. Constantly monitor the patient's core temperature, blood pressure, pulse, cardiac rhythm, and pupil size and reactivity and watch for cyanosis (see Table 42–4).

9. The hyperkalemia can be treated with IV insulin and glucose (0.25 to 0.5 units/kg of insulin to 0.25 to 0.5 gm/kg of glucose).

10. If possible, catheterize the bladder and monitor urinary output and appearance. To secure a high urinary output, furosemide (1 mg/kg) or mannitol (1 gm/kg) may be given.

11. *Do NOT treat dysrhythmias with LIDOCAINE* because it is a trigger agent. Do not give intravenous calcium because it may also cause dysrhythmias.

12. Hypotension can be treated by the infusion of cold crystalloid solution.

13. Continue to send arterial and venous blood samples to the laboratory for prompt determination of arterial blood gases and electrolytes.

14. Look for such hopeful prognostic signs as a lessening coma, hyperactive tendon reflexes, and a stabilization of the temperature. Once the temperature returns to normal, continue constant observation of the patient.

COMPLICATIONS FOLLOWING ACUTE MALIGNANT HYPERTHERMIA

Renal failure can occur because of myoglobinuria or hypotension. Consumption coagulopathies, such as disseminated intravascular coagulation (DIC), have been reported along with acute heart failure and pulmonary edema. Brain deterioration can occur in patients who are not promptly diagnosed and treated for MH.

REFERENCES

1. Britt, B.: Malignant Hyperthermia. Int. Anesthesiol. Clin. *17*(4):1–182, 1979.
2. Gronert, G.: Malignant hyperthermia. Anesthesiology, *53*:395–423, 1980.
3. Katz, J., Benumof, J., and Kadis, L.: Anesthesia and Uncommon Diseases: Pathophysiologic and Clinical Correlations. 2nd ed. Philadelphia, W. B. Saunders Co., 1981.
4. Miller, R.: Anesthesia. 2nd ed. New York, Churchill Livingstone, Inc., 1986.
5. Stoelting, R., and Dierdorf, S.: Anesthesia and Co-Existing Disease. New York, Churchill Livingstone, Inc., 1983.
6. Yarborough, J.: Malignant hyperthermia. AANA J., *52*(1):58–64, 1984.

43

Postoperative Care of the Patient Suffering From Shock

Shock may be considered a severe pathophysiologic syndrome associated with abnormal cellular metabolism, which in most cases is due to poor tissue perfusion. Shock may also be due to other factors, such as sepsis. Shock can be divided into three stages: a nonprogressive or compensated stage, a progressive stage, and an irreversible stage. In the nonprogressive stage, the tissue perfusion is decreased but not enough to cause the vicious circle of cardiovascular deterioration. When the patient enters the progressive stage, cardiac deterioration has reached the point at which, if shock is not treated, death will ensue. The hallmark of the irreversible stage is that all forms of treatment prove inadequate to save the life of the patient.

TYPES OF SHOCK

The types of shock are hypovolemic or hemorrhagic shock, neurogenic shock, anaphylactic shock, septic shock, and cardiogenic shock (See Table 43–1).

Hypovolemic Shock

Hypovolemic shock is the most common type of shock encountered in the PACU. A diminished blood volume will lead to a decreased systemic filling pressure, which will have as a consequence decreased return. The cardiac output falls and shock ensues.

A patient can lose approximately 10 percent of his blood volume without any appreciable loss in arterial pressure or cardiac output. As the person approaches 15 to 18 percent blood loss, the arterial pressure and cardiac output begin to fall. Both fall to zero when the blood loss is 35 to 45 percent of the total blood volume (Fig. 43–1).

As blood volume is lost, sympathetic reflexes become activated and cause peripheral vasoconstriction and reflex tachycardia, blood flow is allowed to decrease, and cardiac depression, vasomotor failure, and vascular failure ensue.

Treatment. Treatment for hypovolemic shock involves improving the blood volume status by the administration of blood products appropriate to the patient's condition.

Neurogenic Shock

Neurogenic shock results from loss of vasomotor tone without any loss of blood volume. Some of the causes of neurogenic shock are deep general anesthesia, spinal

TABLE 43–1. Types of Shock

Type	Definition	Causes	Symptoms
Hypovolemic shock	Caused by a decrease in the intravascular volume relative to the vascular capacity, and is generally associated with a blood volume deficit	Hemorrhage Excessive vomiting Excessive diarrhea Severe dehydration	Hypotension Tachycardia Cool, clammy skin Low central venous pressure Decreased urine output
Neurogenic shock	Caused by damage to or pharmacologic blockage of the sympathetic nervous system, producing vasodilatation of the arterioles in the affected portion of the body and increased vascular capacity	Deep general anesthesia High spinal anesthesia Disease or damage of the spinal cord Brain damage	Hypotension (high spinal anesthesia and spinal cord damage) Bradycardia (high spinal anesthesia and spinal cord damage) Hypertension (early) then hypotension (late) in the patient with brain damage Tachycardia (early) then bradycardia (late) in the patient with brain damage
Septic shock	Associated with severe sepsis. It can be divided into *hyperdynamic*, associated with impaired cell metabolism with normal or increased cardiac output, or *hypodynamic*, which has relative or absolute hypovolemia due to increased capillary leakage and low cardiac output	The effects of various noxious chemicals and vasoactive substances liberated from damaged, ischemic, or infected tissues	High fever Marked vasodilatation Sludging of the blood Hypotension Tachycardia
Cardiogenic shock	Caused by impaired function of the heart as a pump	Acute myocardial infarction Pulmonary embolus Tamponade	Hypotension Bradycardia or tachycardia Increased central venous pressure
Anaphylactic shock	An exaggerated hypersensitivity reaction to a drug or other substance	Administration or contact with some type of antigen	Bronchospasm Hypotension Arrhythmia Cardiac arrest

anesthesia, and spinal cord disease or damage. In the PACU, this type of shock may be seen after spinal anesthetics that reach above the fourth thoracic dermatome.

Treatment. Treatment of neurogenic shock uses the Trendelenburg position and the administration of oxygen. If blood pressure does not improve, alpha adrenergic vasopressors can be utilized to cause peripheral vasoconstriction to get more blood to the heart to improve the cardiac output. Administration of fluids will also contribute to the restoration of normal hemodynamics in these patients.

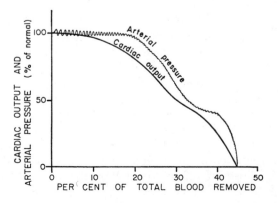

Figure 43–1. Effect of hemorrhage on cardiac output and arterial pressure. (From Guyton, A. C.: Textbook of Medical Physiology. 5th ed. Philadelphia, W. B. Saunders Co., 1976, p. 358.)

Anaphylactic Shock

Anaphylaxis is an exagerated hypersensitivity reaction to a drug or other substance. The theoretic basis for anaphylaxis is that when a person is exposed to a specific antigen, antigen-specific immunoglobuin E (IgE) antibodies are formed that interact only with that particular antigen. Subsequent exposure causes a series of intramembrane and intracellular events that culminate in the release of histamine and of the slow-acting substance of anaphylaxis (SRS-A) from the cell. These mediators, in turn, may directly elicit local and systemic pharmacologic effects, may cause the release of other mediators, or may activate reflexes that ultimately produce the clinical picture of anaphylaxis. Histamine is believed to be the major mediator of anaphylaxis. It is found in mast cells and in basophils. It can cause bronchial constriction, increased capillary constriction, and vasodilation.

The onset of anaphylaxis following the administration of the antigen is usually seen within 30 minutes. This time can be delayed up to an hour or more depending on how rapidly the antigen is taken up by the circulation. The symptoms of anaphylaxis include conjunctivitis, vasomotor rhinitis, pilomotor erection, pruritic urticaria, angioedema, various gastrointestinal disturbances, laryngeal edema, bronchospasm, hypotension, arrhythmias, cardiac arrest, coma, and death. These symptoms are highly variable and unpredictable. Fatal anaphylaxis may be limited to one symptom or a wide spectrum of symptoms. Because of the high degree of variability of responses, any systemic manifestation must be considered as the beginning of a severe anaphylactic reaction and be treated vigorously.

Treatment. Five classes of drugs can be utilized in the treatment of an anaphylactic reaction. These are adrenergic agonists, methylxanthines, antihistamines, anticholinergics, and corticosteroids. The first line of treatment is epinephrine, usually in a dose of 0.3 ml of 1:1000 IM or IV. The rationale for the selection of epinephrine is that it produces both alpha and beta effects. It also reverses rhinitis, urticaria, bronchoconstriction, and hypotension during anaphylaxis.

The methylxanthines are utilized when bronchial relaxation and an increase in cardiac output are desired. Aminophylline is the drug of choice in this group. Anticholinergics such as atropine, scopolamine, or glycopyrrolate (Robinul) can be utilized to help relax the bronchiolar smooth muscle and block further cholinergic stimuli. Antihistamines such as diphenhydramine (Benadryl) help block the actions of histamines. Corticosteroids can be utilized, as evidence suggests that they have some potential benefits, especially when the anaphylactic reaction is not improved by other forms of treatment and persistent bronchospasm or hypotension is present.

The anaphylactic reaction is a medical emergency. It is important for the PACU nurse to recognize and respond when a patient exhibits any one of the symptoms of anaphylaxis. The drugs mentioned should be available in the unit at all times. Oxygen should be administered immediately to the patient, as the pathophysiology of this reaction appears to affect the pulmonary structures to a high degree. The blood pressure and pulse should be continuously monitored. The respirations should also be monitored for rate, depth, and rhythm. The larynx should be observed for edema, which is characterized by "crowing" respirations. A physician should be called immediately to institute further treatment of the patient if this occurs.

Septic Shock

Septic shock results from a widely disseminated infection in the body. Some causes of septic shock are peritonitis, generalized infection resulting from a localized infection, and a generalized gangrenous infection caused by gas gangrene bacilli.

The early clinical features of septic shock include high fever, marked vasodilation, and sludging of the blood. As the septic shock progresses, its end stages resemble those of hypovolemic shock.

Septic shock can be divided into two types, *hyperdynamic* and *hypodynamic*. The hyperdynamic type is associated with a normal or increased cardiac output. It is associated with impaired cell metabolism, which prevents the tissues from properly utilizing nutrients such as glucose and oxygen. Increased arteriovenous shunting or improper distribution of blood will aggravate this tendency.

Hypodynamic septic shock is associated with a low cardiac output. These patients have a relative or absolute hypovolemia, which is due to an increased capillary leak throughout the body, particularly in the inflamed or infected area.

Treatment. Once septic shock has occurred, the patient must be given *definitive therapy*, such as early surgical débridement or drainage of the wound and appropriate antibiotics. Other recommended measures, including fluid replacement, steroid administration, pulmonary therapy, and the use of vasoactive drugs, represent *adjunctive therapy*, which will be useful when preparing the patient for surgical intervention or to support the patient until the infectious process is controlled.

Cardiogenic Shock

Cardiogenic shock is caused by an impaired function of the heart as a pump. The heart begins to fail, usually owing to an acute myocardial infarction or rupture of the ventricular septum, or to the development of significant mitral incompetence. With this type of cardiogenic shock the patient will exhibit such problems as peripheral vascular resistance, increased pulse rate, and cool, clammy skin. Up to 10 to 15 percent of these patients may exhibit symptoms of significant hypotension and bradycardia, and they may not have cold, clammy skin.

Because of the increased peripheral vascular resistance, the central venous pressure usually rises. Because the heart is unable to pump blood in significant amounts to all parts of the body, the urine output falls, as does the arterial oxygen content (PaO_2), and the arterial carbon dioxide ($PaCO_2$) rises. The arterial blood lactate rises, leading to metabolic acidosis.

Treatment. It is suggested that cardiogenic shock treatment can be divided into three main categories: (1) medical treatment, (2) circulatory assists, and (3) surgery. Medical treatment is centered around a pharmacologic reversal of the causative factors of the cardiogenic shock. Oxen should be administered, as should bicarbonate after a base deficit has been determined. The drugs used in treatment should contribute to increasing the performance of the heart without increasing the myocardial oxygen demand and returning the peripheral vascular resistance to a more normal level. Drugs such as dopamine may prove effective for this condition because of its positive inotropic effect and minimal effect on peripheral vascular resistance. It also increases renal and mesenteric blood flow. Hypovolemia and electrolyte imbalance should also be corrected.

Circulatory assists use the balloon counter pulsator, which helps mechanically to decrease the work of the heart and increase coronary perfusion. Surgical correction of cardiogenic shock can help a small number of patients, depending on whether or not the medical facility has the capability to perform open heart surgery. Other factors involved are the selection of the patient and timing of surgery.

REFERENCES

1. Alspach, J., and Williams, S.: AACN: Core Curriculum for Critical Care Nursing. 3rd ed. Philadelphia, W. B. Saunders Co., 1985.
2. Dripps, R., Eckenhoff, J., and Vandam, L.: Introduction to Anesthesia: Principles of Safe Practice. 6th ed. Philadelphia, W. B. Saunders Co., 1982.
3. Guyton, A.: Textbook of Medical Physiology. 7th ed. Philadelphia, W. B. Saunders Co., 1986.
4. Miller, R.: Anesthesia. 2nd ed. New York, Churchill Livingstone, Inc., 1986.
5. Stoelting, R., and Dierdorf, S.: Anesthesia and Co-Existing Disease. New York, Churchill Livingstone, Inc., 1983.
6. Wilson, R. (ed.): Principles and Techniques of Critical Care. Volume I. Kalamazoo, Mich., The Upjohn Co., 1976.

44

Cardiopulmonary Resuscitation in the Post Anesthesia Care Unit

In the last decade, many advances have been made in cardiopulmonary resuscitation. The morbidity and mortality rates have been substantially reduced after cardiac arrest because of these new techniques. In the post anesthesia care unit (PACU) there is a high probability that the nurse will be confronted with a patient who requires cardiopulmonary resuscitation. It is, therefore, of utmost importance that the PACU nurse be completely familiar with all facets of cardiopulmonary resuscitation, and that essential equipment be readily available (Table 44–1).

PATHOPHYSIOLOGY OF DEATH

When the blood flow ceases, generalized tissue anoxia takes place. In the brain, the anoxia causes a reversible loss of function. Owing to this anoxia, the patient will lose consciousness and, if ventilation is not restored, will become completely apneic because the control center for respiration is blocked. At this point, the patient is clinically dead and, if cardiopulmonary resuscitation is not instituted within three to six

minutes, irreversible brain damage will occur and the patient will be biologically dead. It is critical that the PACU nurse recognize and react quickly and efficiently in this medical emergency.

INDICATIONS FOR RESUSCITATION

The precipitating factors in cardiac arrest are hypoxia, anesthetic agents, and hypotension. All of these factors occur in the post anesthesia care unit.

Hypoxia is difficult to recognize. It is suspected when the patient has tachycardia, and is restless, sweating, and cyanotic. Absence of cyanosis is not proof of adequate oxygenation, since anemia or cutaneous vasodilation may give a pink color in spite of profound hypoxia, of which cyanosis is a late sign. Hypercarbia should be considered if the patient becomes progressively somnolent. Another symptom to be considered is loss of muscle tone, although a brief tonic seizure can occur in the first few seconds after cardiac arrest, and the pupils will begin to dilate bilaterally and symmetrically immediately after the arrest. Dilation of the

TABLE 44–1. Essential Equipment and Drugs for Cardiopulmonary Resuscitation

Respiratory Management
Oxygen supply (two E cylinders) with reducing valves capable of delivering 15 L/min with masks and reservoir bag
Oropharyngeal airways (Guidel type—pediatric; small, medium, and large)
Laryngoscope with blades (curved and straight, for adult, child, and infant) and extra batteries and bulbs
Assorted adult-sized (cuffed) and child-sized (uncuffed) endotracheal tubes with stylet and 15 mm/22 mm adapters
Syringe (10 ml) with clamp for inflating endotracheal tube cuff
Bag-valve-mask unit, with provision for 100 percent oxygen ventilation
Suction (preferably portable), with catheters, sizes 6–18 French
Yankauer suction tips
Tracheotomy set and tubes

Circulatory Management
Portable defibrillator-monitor with ECG electrode-defibrillator paddles or portable DC defibrillator and portable ECG
    monitor
Portable electrocardiogram machine, direct-writing, with connection to monitor
Venous infusion sets (micro and regular)
Indwelling venous catheters, catheter outside needle (sizes 14–22), catheter inside needle (sizes 14–22), central
    venous pressure catheters
Intravenous solutions (5 percent dextrose in water and lactated Ringer's solution)
Cutdown set
Sterile gloves
Urinary catheters
Assorted syringes and needles, stopcocks, venous extension tubing
Intracardiac needles
Tourniquets, adhesive tape, alcohol sponges
Thoracotomy tray
Essential drugs as listed in Table 44–5
Useful drugs
    Aminophylline
    Dexamethasone (Decadron)
    Dextrose 50 percent (Ion-trate Dextrose 50 percent)
    Digoxin (Lanoxin)
    Diphenhydramine hydrochloride (Benadryl)
    Ethacrynic acid
    Furosemide (Lasix)
    Isoproterenol hydrochloride (Isuprel)
    Lanatoside C (Cedilanid)
    Levarterenol bitartrate (Levophed)
    Metaraminol bitartrate (Aramine)
    Methylprednisolone sodium succinate (Solu-Medrol)
    Morphine
    Naloxone (Narcan)
    Nitroglycerine
    Pancuronium bromide (Pavulon)
    Phenylephrine hydrochloride (Neo-Synephrine)
    Potassium chloride
    Procainamide (Pronestyl)
    Propranolol hydrochloride (Inderal)
    Quinidine
    Sodium Nitroprusside (Nipride)
    Succinylcholine chloride (Anectine)
    Tubocurarine chloride
    Verapamil

pupils will be complete within two minutes after arrest.

Assessment of these patients is for airway obstruction and apnea. The nurse should look for movements of the chest and abdomen and listen and feel for the movement of air in the lungs. In complete obstruction no respiratory movements will be seen and the breath sounds will be absent. If a partial obstruction exists, there may be a crowing sound, which usually indicates laryngospasm; gurgling, which usually indicates foreign matter; or wheezing, which indicates bronchial obstruction.

Rapid assessment of the heart by auscultation may reveal cardiac standstill or bradycardia. If a stethoscope is not available, the carotid pulse can be checked. The carotid artery is large and lies just anterior to the sternocleidomastoid muscle in the neck. Use of the carotid pulse also reduces time in assessing the patient, as the nurse can check the airway, pupils, chest, and pulse simultaneously. If the patient is connected to an electrocardiograph, the following dysrhythmias may be observable:

1. Ventricular asystole
2. Bradycardia
3. Premature ventricular contractions, greater than 6 per minute, multifocal, or R on T phenomena
4. Ventricular tachycardia
5. Ventricular fibrillation
6. Atrioventricular blocks of all degrees
7. Atrial fibrillation and flutter

In essence, the indications for cardiopulmonary resuscitation are either respiratory arrest or cardiac arrest or both. Nursing assessment should be conducted in seconds, and cardiopulmonary resuscitation should be instituted rapidly.

As cardiopulmonary resuscitation is begun, another nurse should be called. Optimally, there should be two attendants, one to assist in the administration of resuscitation and the other to summon emergency aid.

STEPS IN CARDIOPULMONARY RESUSCITATION

The A-B-C steps in cardiopulmonary resuscitation are *airway, breathing* and *circulation.*

Airway

Some patients may arrive in the post anesthesia care unit still experiencing the depressant effects of the anesthetic. In some of these patients, the obtunded patient's tongue and epiglottis may fall back to the posterior pharyngeal wall, which will occlude the airway. When this happens, the nurse should place the patient in a supine position, with the head tilted backward and the neck hyperextended. The nurse should then lift the angle of the lower jaw upward using moderate pressure (Fig. 44–1). Many times this maneuver will be all that is required for spontaneous respirations to occur. If spontaneous respirations do not occur, the oral cavity should be inspected for foreign material and the mouth suctioned if necessary. If large particles are present, turn the head to the side, place the patient in a

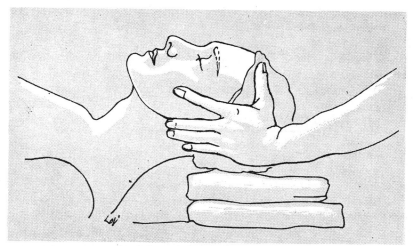

Figure 44–1. Technique of lifting jaw with fingers behind the mandible to overcome soft tissue obstruction of the upper airway. (From Dripps, R., Eckenhoff, J., and Vandam, L.: Introduction to Anesthesia: The Principles of Safe Practice. 6th ed. Philadelphia, W. B. Saunders Co., 1982, p. 111.)

head-down position, and remove the particles manually.

Breathing

If spontaneous ventilation does not occur, positive pressure breathing must be instituted. If possible, an Ambu bag, or some other type of bag-valve-mask unit, connected to an oxygen source should be utilized (Table 44–2). The nurse should be positioned at the patient's head, not at his or her side. The mask should be fitted over the mouth and nose with the neck hyperextended. The lower jaw should be lifted up at its angle with the other fingers of the hand holding the mask. The thumb of that hand should be placed at the top of the mask, pushing down to provide compression over the bridge of the nose to reduce air leaks (Fig. 44–2).

The patient should be ventilated four times. While the PACU nurse is ventilating the patient, an assistant should assess the adequacy of the positive pressure breathing by auscultation of the chest. If an assistant is not present, the nurse should check to see if the chest rises and falls or if air escapes during expiration. These are considered rough estimates of ventilation, and may not be completely accurate about its adequacy. If breath sounds are not heard during auscultation or if the rough estimates are inconclusive, an oropharyngeal airway should be inserted (Fig. 44–3) and ventilation continued. The assessment of

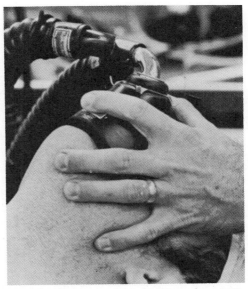

Figure 44–2. Holding the mask with one hand. (From Dorsch, J., and Dorsch, S.: Understanding Anesthesia Equipment. Baltimore, Williams & Wilkins, 1975, p. 225.)

adequacy of ventilation should then be repeated. The patient should be hyperventilated with large tidal volumes so that the excess carbon dioxide can be removed. The flow of oxygen to the bag should be about 15 L per min.

If a bag-valve-mask system is not available, mouth-to-mouth ventilation should be instituted until appropriate support materials and personnel become available. The technique involves hyperextending the neck and lifting up on the jaw with one hand and holding the nose shut with the other (Fig. 44–4). An airtight seal is formed with the nurse's mouth over the patient's mouth. The patient is ventilated 15 to 20 times per minute. The patient is observed to see if the chest rises and falls or if air escapes on expiration. For infants and small children, the nurse can cover the mouth and nose simultaneously to provide a good seal. The infant has a very pliable neck, so that forceful flexing of the head may in itself cause obstruction; therefore, the nurse must not exaggerate the flexed position in infants.

If the PACU nurse is unable to ventilate the patient, endotracheal intubation should

TABLE 44–2. Criteria for Bag-Valve-Mask Unit

Self-refilling, but without sponge rubber inside (because of the difficulty in cleaning and disinfecting, and in eliminating ethylene oxide, and because of fragmentation)
Nonjam valve system at 15 L/min oxygen inlet flow
Transparent, plastic face mask with an air-filled or contoured, resilient cuff
Standard 15 mm/22 mm fittings
No popoff valve, except in pediatric models
System for delivery of high concentrations of oxygen through an ancillary oxygen outlet at the back of the bag or by an oxygen reservoir
True nonrebreathing valve
Oropharyngeal airway
Satisfactory practice on mannequins
Available in adult and pediatric sizes

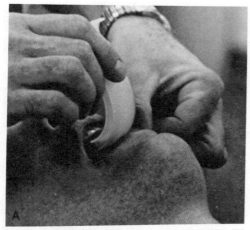

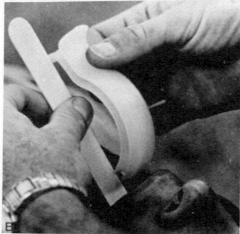

Figure 44–3. Insertion of oral airway: *A*, airway is turned 180 degrees from final resting position; *B*, airway is inserted with the use of tongue blade to displace the tongue forward. (From Dorsch, J. and Dorsch, S.: Understanding Anesthesia Equipment. Baltimore, Williams & Wilkins, 1975, p. 228.)

be performed. Other indications for endotracheal intubation are inability of the patient to protect his airway, prolonged mechanical ventilation, cardiac arrest, and respiratory arrest. Because of the delays, difficulties, and complications in placing an endotracheal tube, only the PACU nurses or physicians who have intubation experience should perform this maneuver in an emergency situation.

INTUBATION OF THE TRACHEA

The PACU nurse should be familiar with the technique of tracheal intubation and be capable of performing intubation quickly and efficiently, knowing that the conditions under which intubation is performed in the post anesthesia care unit are less than ideal. The patient's position in the bed, excess upper airway secretions, and intact reflexes increase the degree of difficulty in performing this maneuver in the PACU. Although the technique for intubation will be presented in this text, the PACU nurse is strongly encouraged to perform it on a mannequin, and then to do it in the operating room under the supervision of an anesthesiologist or nurse anesthetist. The PACU nurse should continue to perform intubation on a monthly basis in the operating room under the same supervision in order to remain adept at this skill.

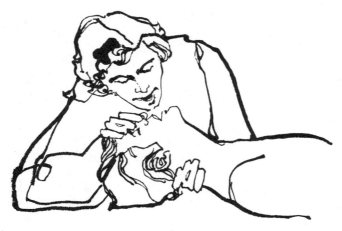

Figure 44–4. Mouth-to-mouth resuscitation. (Reprinted with permission © American Heart Association.)

Equipment for Tracheal Intubation

Adult and pediatric intubation trays should be kept in the post anesthesia care unit at all times. For a list of the suggested items to be kept on the intubation trays, see Table 44–3. Table 44–4 gives the recommended sizes for endotracheal tubes. Because of their importance, the laryngoscope and tracheal tubes will be discussed in detail.

Laryngoscope. The *laryngoscope* is used to visualize the larynx and the anatomic structures in close proximity to the larynx (Fig. 44–5). The laryngoscope has two parts: the *handle* and the *blade*. The *handle*, which is available in several sizes, is used to hold the laryngoscope and to house the batteries that provide the electrical source for the light on the side of the blade. The *blade* consists of three parts: the spatula, the flange, and the tip. The *spatula* can be straight or curved and is the long, main shaft of the blade. It serves to compress and move the soft tissue of the lower jaw to facilitate direct vision of the larynx. The

TABLE 44–4. Recommended Sizes for Endotracheal Tubes*

Age	Endotracheal Tube (internal diameter in mm)
Newborn	3.0
6 months	3.5
18 months	4.0
3 years	4.5
5 years	5.0
6 years	5.5
8 years	6.0
12 years	6.5
16 years	7.0
Adult (female)	8.0–8.5
Adult (male)	8.5–9.0

*One size larger and one size smaller should be allowed for individual variations.

Reprinted with permission © American Heart Association.

flange, which is on the side of the spatula, serves to deflect tissue that could obstruct the direct vision of the larynx. The *tip*, at the distal end of the spatula, is either curved or straight and serves to either directly or indirectly elevate the epiglottis. The blade is attached to the handle at a connection called the hook-on fitting. The PACU nurse is strongly encouraged to practice connecting the blade to the handle.

TABLE 44–3. Suggested Equipment for the Post Anesthesia Care Unit Pediatric and Adult Endotracheal Trays

Pediatric Endotracheal Equipment
Small laryngoscope handle
#2 Macintosh curved blade
#1 Miller straight blade
Pediatric oral airways
Assorted pediatric masks
    Child's anatomic masks
    Rendell-Baker-Soucek masks
Assorted tracheal tubes
    Reverse angle endotracheal (RAE) tubes
    Cole tubes
    Reinforced latex tube with stylet
    Plastic thin-walled tube

Adult Endotracheal Equipment
Laryngoscope handle
Laryngoscope blades
    #2 and 4 Miller
    #3 Macintosh
Stylet
Sterile gauze with topical water-soluble anesthetic
    lubricant
Sizes 6 mm through 9 mm cuffed tracheal tubes
10 ml syringe to inflate the cuff
Small hemostat
Tongue blades for airway insertion
Assorted-sized oropharyngeal airways.

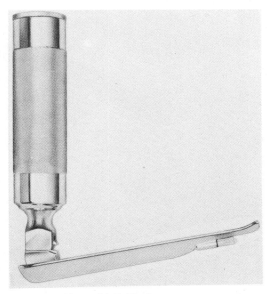

Figure 44–5. The laryngoscope.

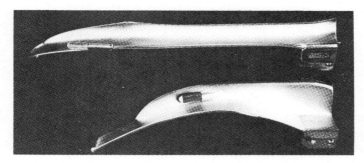

Figure 44–6. The most frequently used laryngoscope blades: the Miller (top) and the Macintosh blade (bottom). (From Miller, R. [ed.]: Anesthesia. New York, Churchill Livingstone, Inc., 1981, p. 237.)

The Macintosh and the Miller are the most popular blades in use today. The Macintosh is a curved blade with the flange on the left side to aid in moving the tongue so as to enhance visual exposure of the larynx. The Macintosh blade (Fig. 44–6) comes in four sizes: (#1) infant, (#2) child, (#3) medium adult, and (#4) large adult. For most adults, the number 3 medium adult is the blade of choice. The Miller blade (Fig. 44–6) is a straight spatula with a curved tip. This blade has five sizes: (#0) premature infant, (#1) infant, (#2) child, (#3) medium adult, and (#4) large adult. The Miller numbers 0 and 1 are the blades of choice for premature and full-term infants, whose anatomical structures are more receptive to the use of a straight blade. Many anesthesia workers use the number 2 Miller to intubate adults. The PACU nurse is encouraged to utilize both the straight and the curved blades and to then decide on blade preference. In most cases, the curved blade is easier to use than the straight blade; however, the exposure of the larynx is not as good as with the straight blade.

Tracheal Tube. The *tracheal tube* is also called the *endotracheal tube, intratracheal tube,* or *catheter* (Fig. 44–7). It is usually made

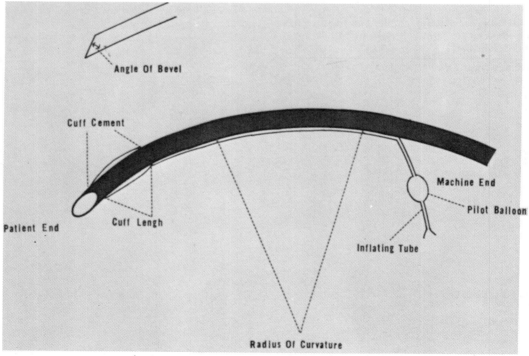

Figure 44–7. The curved tracheal tube. (From Dorsch, J. and Dorsch, S.: Understanding Anesthesia Equipment. Baltimore, Williams & Wilkins, 1975, p. 249.)

from natural or synthetic rubber or plastic. The *proximal end*, or *machine end*, protrudes from the patient's mouth and receives the adaptor. The distal end, or *patient end*, has a slanted portion called the *bevel*. An uncuffed tracheal tube should be used on patients who are 8 years old or younger. Endotracheal tubes are numbered according to their outside diameter. Near the distal end of the tracheal tube is a *cuff*. Also leading away from the cuff is an inflating tube that has a *pilot balloon* at its proximal end to indicate whether the cuff is inflated. Above the pilot balloon is a plug or one-way valve for the inflation syringe.

The cuff is an inflatable sleeve that provides a leak-resistant fit between the tube and the trachea when inflated. It also prevents aspiration and allows positive pressure ventilation of the lungs. There are different types of cuffs: the slip-on and the permanently attached. Concerning inflation volume, there are *high* or *low residual volume* cuffs, referring to the amount of air that can be withdrawn from the cuff after it has been inflated and allowed to deflate spontaneously with the tube patent and open to the air. Local tracheal complications are associated with the cuff, especially after longer periods of intubation. Excessive cuff pressure is the primary factor causing ulceration, necrosis, and tracheal stenosis. This is because high cuff pressure will reduce the blood supply in the tracheal mucosa. For long-term ventilation the cuffs should be long, with a large residual volume and a diameter larger than that of the trachea.

In an emergency, the nurse should choose one size down from that recommended for the patient. When making this choice, many clinicians look at the little finger of the patient, as small-sized little fingers seem to indicate that the patient will have an opening at the vocal cords that is smaller than normal. Also, a stylet made of malleable metal or plastic should be inserted inside the endotrachal tube to improve its curvature. *The stylet must be covered with a water-soluble lubricant to ease its withdrawal from the tube after placement.* The end of the stylet should be about 3 cm from the distal

end of the tracheal tube and should not protrude beyond it.

Technique of Oral Endotracheal Intubation

The essential steps in the technique of oral endotracheal intubation are: positioning the patient, positioning the head, inserting the blade of the laryngoscope, raising the epiglottis, visualizing the vocal cords, placing the tracheal tube, and assessing the patient. The methods for accomplishing these steps are as follows:

Positioning the Patient. Move the patient up so that his head is at the top of the bed. Raise the head of the bed (or the entire bed, if possible) so that the patient's face is approximately at the level of the standing PACU nurse's xiphoid process.

Positioning the Head. Place a firm 4-inch pillow or ring under the head. Flex the patient's head at the neck. This position is called the sniffing position (Fig. 44–8), because of the flexion of the head at the neck and extension of the head. Place right hand on the patient's forehead to extend the head.

Inserting the Blade. With the fingers of the right hand, open the jaw wide, making sure that the lips are spread away from the teeth. With the laryngoscope in the left hand, insert the moistened or lubricated blade between the teeth at the right side of the patient's mouth. Advance the blade slowly inward, past the tonsillar pillars and toward the midline of the oral cavity, sweeping the tongue toward the left side of the mouth. A major key to a successful intubation is moving the tongue to the left, out of the visual path to the vocal cords. At this point, the right hand can be placed under the patient's occiput to extend the head. The epiglottis should now be visualized; it is a red, leaf-shaped structure that will appear behind the tip of the blade as the laryngoscope is advanced down the oral cavity.

Raising the Epiglottis and Visualizing the Vocal Cords. With the epiglottis under direct vision, slip a straight blade just beneath the tip of the epiglottis and gently lift the blade

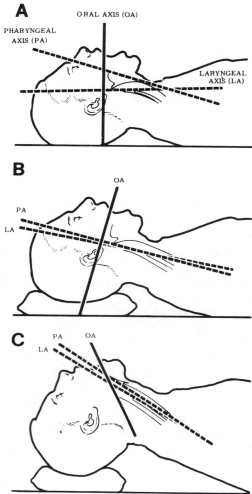

Figure 44–8. Positioning for endotracheal intubation: *A*, patient in supine position—with the alignment of the oral, pharyngeal, and laryngeal axes; *B*, placement of pad or ring under the patient's occiput (sniffing position) will align the pharyngeal and laryngeal axes; *C*, extending the patient's head at the atlanto-occipital joint will now align all three axes, which provides the shortest distance and most nearly straight line from the mouth to the larynx. (From Miller, R. [ed.]: Anesthesia. New York, Churchill Livingstone, Inc., 1981, p. 234.)

forward and upward at a 45-degree angle, holding the wrist rigid (Fig. 44–9). If a curved blade, such as the Macintosh, is used, slip the tip of the blade between the epiglottis and the base of the tongue (Fig. 44–9). With the left hand, lift forward and upward at a 45-degree angle on the handle. The epiglottis will fold onto the blade and the vocal cords should then be visible.

Whether using a curved or straight blade, do not use the handle as a lever with the upper teeth acting as a fulcrum, as the tip of the blade will push the larynx up and out of sight, chipping or breaking the teeth.

At this point, if the vocal cords cannot be seen, have an assistant apply gentle external downward pressure on the larynx (the Sellick maneuver) and the vocal cords should come into view. If the blade is passed too far, it will enter the esophagus. If this happens, withdraw the blade, ventilate the patient with 100 percent oxygen and perform the procedure again. While ventilating the patient, think about what went wrong, and design an alternative strategy.

Placing the Tracheal Tube. The tracheal tube, with a stylet appropriately placed to maintain a curve and the cuff deflated, is placed in the right hand by an assistant. While visualizing the vocal cords, pass the tracheal tube with the right hand to the right of the tongue and the blade through the vocal cords until the cuff disappears behind the vocal cords or until the tip of the tracheal tube protrudes 2 to 3 cm into the trachea.

Assessing the Patient. Once the tracheal tube is in place, while holding on to the tube with the right hand, remove the blade with the left hand. Place the laryngoscope on the patient's bed or on a table, remove the stylet, connect the patient to a bag-valve or anesthesia bag system with a high flow oxygen source, and inflate the cuff. Continue to hold the tracheal tube with the right hand, and ventilate the patient while an assistant auscultates the chest for breath sounds. If no breath sounds are heard, deflate the cuff, remove the tracheal tube, and ventilate the patient with a mask using 100 percent oxygen. While ventilating the patient, consider why the attempt was unsuccessful, review the procedure again, and reintubate. If breath sounds are heard on only one side of the chest, withdraw the tube at 1 cm intervals until the breath sounds are bilateral. Adjust the volume of air until there is minimal or no air leakage around the cuff. The cuff leak is assessed by placing the bell of the stethoscope over

A   **B**

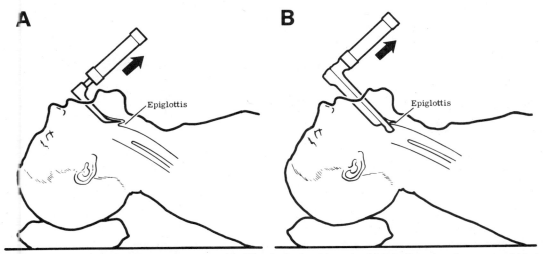

Epiglottis   Epiglottis

Figure 44–9. Proper positioning of laryngoscope blade to facilitate endotracheal intubation: *A*, using a curved blade (i.e., Macintosh), the tip is placed into the space between the base of the tongue and the pharyngeal surface of the epiglottis which is called the vallecula; *B*, using a straight blade (i.e., Miller), the tip is placed on the laryngeal surface of the epiglottis. Regardless of the type of blade used, once the blade is in position, the forward and upward movement on the handle (as denoted by the arrows) will exert pressure on the long axis of the blade, which will serve to elevate the epiglottis and expose the vocal cords. (From Miller, R. [ed.]: Anesthesia. New York, Churchill Livingstone, Inc., 1981, p. 238.)

the larynx. Once tube placement and cuff pressure are correct, secure the tube with adhesive tape.

Ventilation of the Patient. The adult patient should be ventilated approximately 14 to 18 times per minute at a tidal volume of 8 to 10 ml per kg. Infants should be ventilated at approximately 26 to 30 times per minute at a volume large enough to raise their chest on inspiration. However, when time permits, a tidal volume of 7 ml per kg should be used. Children should be ventilated at a rate of 18 to 24 breaths per minute. The tidal volume to be delivered can be determined in the same manner for infants.

Circulation

Assessment should be done to see if a carotid pulse is present or, if a stethoscope is available, whether an apical heart sound is present. In infants and small children, the hand can be placed over the precordium to feel the apical beat. Absence or questionable presence of the pulse is the indication for instituting external cardiac compression.

External Cardiac Compression

External cardiac compression (Fig. 44–10) should be performed with the patient in horizontal position on a firm surface, and the lower extremities elevated to promote venous return. Stand at the patient's side and place the heel of one hand over the lower half of the sternum, about 1.5 to 2 inches above the tip of the xiphoid process. Place the other hand on top of the first one. Keeping the arms straight and the shoulders over the patient's sternum, depress the lower sternum a minimum of 1.5 to 2 inches. The sternum should be held down for half a second, then released rapidly. Pressure is reapplied every second or at a slightly faster rate. Rates slower than 60 per minute do not provide sufficient blood flow. In children, the sternum is compressed with one hand only; in infants, it is compressed with the tips of two fingers. In infants and children a rate of 100 to 120 compressions per minute is recommended.

The compressions must be regular, smooth, and uninterrupted. If the external cardiac compression is done correctly, the systolic blood pressure will approach 100 mm Hg, the diastolic pressure will be zero, and the mean pressure will be 40 mm Hg. The amount of circulation is only 20 to 40 percent of normal, so the rhythmic compressions should not be interrupted for more than a few seconds.

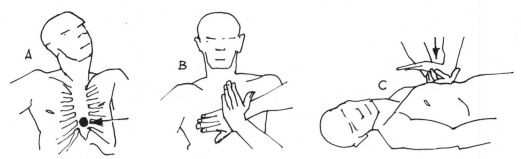

Figure 44–10. External cardiac compression. *A,* Point of lower hand placement at the sternum. *B,* Two hand placement with heel of one hand on top of the other with fingers straight. *C,* Sternal compression, about 4 to 5 cm toward spine. (From Dripps, R., Eckenhoff, J. and Vandam, L. *Introduction to Anesthesia: The Principles of Safe Practice.* 6th ed. Philadelphia: W. B. Saunders Company, 1982, page 404, Figure 35–3).

External cardiac compression must be combined with ventilation of the lungs. If only one nurse is administering the cardiopulmonary resuscitation, a ratio of 2 ventilations to every 15 sternal compressions at one-second intervals should be utilized. The patient's head should be hyperextended while ventilating. A rolled towel or blanket placed under the shoulders will maintain this position. Both the ventilation and the compressions should be performed at the patient's side to decrease the time interval in going from one maneuver to the other (Fig. 44–11).

If two persons are administering cardiopulmonary resuscitation, the ratio of ventilation to compression should be 1 to 5. One person compresses the sternum at one-second intervals and the second person interposes one deep lung inflation after every fifth sternal compression. If ventilation of the lung is difficult in the nonintubated

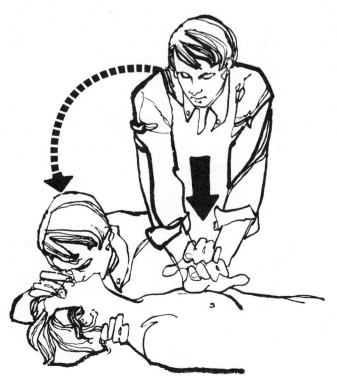

Figure 44–11. One-person cardiopulmonary resuscitation includes 15 chest compressions (rate of 80 per minute) and two quick lung inflations. (Reprinted with permission © American Heart Association.)

patient, use the 2 to 15 ratio even when two persons are conducting the resuscitation

Sternal compressions should be interrupted every two minutes to check for return of spontaneous pulses. If there is no return, continue the sternal compressions; if spontaneous ventilation occurs, ventilate the lungs when the patient inspires to assist ventilation. Once the patient's spontaneous ventilation is determined to be adequate, the positive pressure ventilation can be discontinued, although the nurse should continue to administer oxygen to the patient.

MEDICAL THERAPY

Other resuscitative efforts to be instituted by another nurse, when possible, include starting an intravenous solution of 5 percent dextrose in Ringer's lactate with a 16- or 18-gauge needle. The patient should be connected to an electrocardiograph and monitored on lead 2. The cardiac arrest cart should be brought to the patient's bedside and medications prepared for administration. The essential and useful drugs should be readily available (Table 44–5).

Atropine Sulfate

Atropine sulfate, an anticholinergic agent, will reduce vagal tone, enhance atrioventricular conduction, and accelerate the

TABLE 44–5. Drugs for Cardiopulmonary Resuscitation

Essential
Sodium bicarbonate
Epinephrine
Atropine sulfate
Lidocaine
Calcium chloride
Dopamine (Intropin)
Dobutamine
Useful
Vasoactive drugs
Bretylium tosylate (Bretylol)
Levarterenol
Metaraminol
Isoproterenol
Procainamide (Pronestyl)
Propranolol
Corticosteroids
   Methylprednisolone sodium succinate
   Dexamethasone phosphate

cardiac rate. It is especially useful in preventing cardiac arrest in patients with profound bradycardia due to myocardial infarction, especially when hypotension is present. The initial dose of this drug is 0.5 mg intravenously, and it may be repeated until the pulse rate is higher than 60. The total dose should not exceed 2 mg except in cases of third degree atrioventricular block, when larger doses of this drug may be required.

Sodium Bicarbonate

Sodium bicarbonate is used to combat acidosis. The initial dose of this drug is 1 mEq per kg of body weight intravenously. When blood gas determinations are not accessible, half the initial dose can be administered at 10-minute intervals. Once effective spontaneous respirations are restored, administration of the sodium bicarbonate should be discontinued. This drug and epinephrine should not be administered intravenously in the same infusion, since the sodium bicarbonate can inactivate the epinephrine.

Bretylium Tosylate

Bretylium (Bretylol) has postganglionic adrenergic-blocking properties, antidysrhythmic actions, and a positive inotropic effect. Use of bretylium should be considered when ventricular fibrillation and ventricular tachycardia are refractory to therapy with lidocaine or procainamide, and to repeated countershocks. If the patient is experiencing ventricular fibrillation, 5 mg per kg of undiluted bretylium should be given rapidly. After injection, electrical defibrillation should be administered to the patient, as bretylium's ability to terminate ventricular fibrillation resides in its synergistic actions with D.C. countershock. If the ventricular fibrillation continues after the initial dose of bretylium and D.C. countershock, the dose can be increased to 10 mg per kg and repeated as necessary. The dosage of bretylium for refractory or recurrent ventricular tachycardia is 5 to 10 mg per kg. The bretylium is injected intravenously over a period of 10 minutes.

Calcium Chloride

Calcium chloride will increase the myocardial contractility, prolong systole, and enhance ventricular excitability. It is useful in cardiovascular collapse and may enhance electrical defibrillation. The usual dose of this drug is 2.5 to 5 ml of a 10 percent solution. It should be injected intravenously at 10-minute intervals. It should not be administered together with sodium bicarbonate, as a precipitate will form. Calcium chloride should be administered continuously to a patient on digitalis therapy or to patients who have atrioventricular block.

Corticosteroids

Corticosteroids are indicated in the treatment of cardiogenic shock or lung shock, which may be a complication of cardiac arrest. The dosage forms are 5 mg per kg of methylprednisolone sodium succinate or 1 mg per kg of dexamethasone phosphate. Table 44–6 describes drugs commonly utilized for infants and children.

Dobutamine

Dobutamine is a synthetic derivative of isoproterenol that acts directly on the β_1 receptors in the heart. Its principal action is to increase myocardial contractility without greatly changing peripheral resistance or heart rate. Dobutamine is useful in the treatment of congestive heart failure and for the patient who is emerging from cardiopulmonary bypass surgery. The dosage for dobutamine via continuous intravenous infusion is 2.0 to 10 μg per kg per min. This direct-acting β_1-adrenergic receptor–stimulating agent can cause tachycardia, dysrhythmias, nausea, headache, angina, palpitations, and dyspnea, especially when blood levels are in excess of 20 μg per kg per min.

Dopamine

Dopamine (Intropin) is a naturally occurring biochemical catecholamine precursor of norepinephrine. Dopamine exerts a positive inotropic effect (change in contractile force) and a minimal chronotropic effect (change in contractile rate) on the heart. Therefore,

TABLE 44–6. Commonly Used Drugs for Infants and Children

Drug	Suggested Dose	Remarks
Epinephrine	Intracardiac: 0.3 to 2 ml diluted 1:10,000 (0.1 ml/kg)	
Calcium chloride (10%)	IV: maximum dose of 1 ml/5 kg; intracardiac: 1 ml/5 kg diluted 1:1 with saline	Use caution in digitalized children
Sodium bicarbonate	IV: 1 ml (0.9 mEq)/kg diluted 1:1 with sterile water	Repeat dosage after pH obtained and base deficit calculated
Levarterenol bitartrate (Levophed)	Infants–IV: 1 mg in 500 ml of 5% D/W Children–IV: 2 mg/500 ml of 5% D/W	Titrate to desired effect. Not to be used in endotoxic shock or renal shutdown
Metaraminol bitartrate (Aramine)	IV: 25 mg/100 ml 5% D/W	Titrate to desired effect
Mephentermine sulfate (Wyamine)	IV: 0.05 mg	
Lidocaine (Xylocaine)	Infants–IV: 0.5 mg/kg Children–IV: 5 mg and repeat until desired effect obtained IV drip: 6 mg/kg/4 hr (100 mg in 500 ml of 5% D/W)	Not to exceed 100 mg/hr
Isoproterenol hydrochloride (Isuprel)	IV drip: 1–5 mg/500 ml of 5% D/W	Titrate to desired effect

the contractility of the heart is increased without changing the afterload (total peripheral resistance), which will lead to an increase in cardiac output. The increase is in the systolic and pulse pressures, with virtually no effect on diastolic pressure. Dopamine is not associated with tachyarrhythmias and produces less of an increase in myocardial oxygen consumption than does isoproterenol. Blood flow to peripheral vascular beds may decrease, while mesenteric flow increases. One of the major reasons for the increased use of dopamine clinically is its action on the renal vasculature, i.e., that of dilatation. This action is secondary to the inotropic effect and decreased peripheral resistance produced by dopamine. Therefore, the glomerular filtration rate is increased with the renal blood flow and sodium excretion.

The usual dose of dopamine is 0.4 to 1.6 mg per minute until adequate blood pressure is attained. The dopamine infusion is made by adding 200 mg dopamine to 250 ml of 5 percent dextrose and water. The resulting solution will be 0.8 mg per ml. The dopamine should not be given through an infusion with sodium bicarbonate, as the dopamine is inactivated in an alkaline solution.

In the intubated patient in whom an intravenous route cannot be established, epinephrine or lidocaine can be instilled into the trachea via the endotracheal tube to produce the pharmacologic effects. The epinephrine can be diluted with sterile distilled water as a 1 to 2 mg per 10 ml solution. Lidocaine is diluted with sterile distilled water to a 50 to 100 ml solution.

The intramuscular route can be utilized only when adequate spontaneous circulation is present. Atropine sulfate in a dose of 2 mg or lidocaine in a dose of 300 mg will be effective if given by this route.

Epinephrine

Epinephrine increases myocardial contractility, elevates perfusion pressure, and, in some instances, restores myocardial contractility. The dosage is 0.5 mg, which is diluted in 10 ml, or 5 ml of a 1:10,000 solution. It should be administered intravenously every 5 minutes during the resuscitative effort. Intracardiac injection of this drug should be done by a physician trained in this technique.

Isoproterenol

In patients who have complete heart block in which profound bradycardia is present, isoproterenol (Isuprel) is an effective immediate treatment. It is also effective in profound bradycardia that does not respond to atropine sulfate. The dose of this drug is 2 to 20 μg per minute. This solution

can be made by adding 1 mg isoproterenol to a 500 ml solution of 5 percent dextrose in water. This will yield a concentration of 2 μg per ml.

Levarterenol Bitartrate

Vasoactive drugs may be effective in the resuscitation period. If the patient has peripheral vascular collapse, with hypotension and absence of peripheral vasoconstriction, levarterenol bitartrate (Levophed) in a dose of 16 mg per ml or metaraminol bitartrate (Aramine) in a dose of 0.4 mg per ml of dextrose and water can be titrated intravenously to support the blood pressure.

Before levarterenol bitartrate is administered, it should be ascertained that the intravenous cannula is correctly positioned inside the vein. Any extravasation of this drug will produce tissue necrosis. Metaraminol can also be administered intravenously in a 2 to 5 mg bolus.

Lidocaine

Lidocaine, also a local anesthetic agent, is useful as an antiarrhythmic agent. It is administered slowly intravenously at a dose rate of 50 to 100 mg and can be repeated as necessary. Lidocaine can be administered in a continuous infusion at 1 to 3 mg per minute, usually not exceeding 4 mg per minute.

Intravenous Nitroglycerin

Nitroglycerin dilates the large coronary arteries, increases coronary collateral blood flow, and can improve perfusion of ischemic myocardium. This drug relaxes all smooth muscle, particularly vascular smooth muscle. The ventricular systolic and diastolic volumes fall, resulting in a reduced myocardial wall tension, which leads to a decreased myocardial oxygen demand. Intravenous nitroglycerin is indicated for unstable angina pectoris, acute myocardial infarction, and congestive heart failure. This drug should be administered via an automated infusion pump. The dose is about 10 to 20 μg per min. The dosage, which can be increased by 5 to 10 μg per min every 5 to 10 minutes, is usually titrated to achieve the desired clinical effect.

Sodium Nitroprusside

Sodium nitroprusside (Nipride) is a rapid-acting, potent peripheral vasodilator. Because it will cause an immediate reduction of peripheral arterial resistance, sodium nitroprusside is especially useful in the treatment of hypertensive crisis. It is also useful in the treatment of patients with left ventricular failure and pulmonary edema. For dosage and precautions associated with sodium nitroprusside, the reader is encouraged to review Chapter 5.

Procainamide

Procainamide (Pronestyl) may be useful in suppressing premature ventricular complexes and recurrent ventricular tachycardia that do not resolve after treatment with lidocaine. If ventricular ectopy has not been resolved by at least 225 mg of lidocaine administered by intermittent bolus injection and intravenous lidocaine infusion of 4 mg per min after each bolus, procainamide should be administered. The intravenous dosage of procainamide is 100 mg every 5 minutes (20 mg per min). The bolus administration of procainamide should be stopped when the dysrhythmia is suppressed, or the QRS complex is widened by 50 percent, or hypotension occurs, or the total dose of the procainamide reaches 1 gm. The maintenance rate of procainamide is 4 mg per min, and the therapeutic blood level for this drug is 4 to 8 µg per ml.

Intravenous procainamide should be administered cautiously in the PACU, especially to those patients suffering from acute myocardial infarction. Severe hypotension can result from rapid injection. Hence, arterial blood pressure and ECG monitoring are essential during the administration of the drug. The warning signs of impending hypotension are a widening of the QRS complex and a lengthening of the PR or the QT interval.

Propranolol

In patients with ventricular fibrillation who do not respond well to lidocaine, the beta blocker propranolol (Inderal) may be administered. The usual dose is 1 mg slowly infused intravenously. The dose can be repeated up to a total dose of 3 mg and should be given when the patient is being monitored by electrocardiograph. Because this drug is a beta-blocking drug, it should be used with extreme caution in patients who have pulmonary disease or cardiac failure.

Verapamil

Verapamil, a slow channel blocker, is primarily useful in emergency cardiac situations as an antidysrhythmic agent. More specifically, the drug is highly effective in the treatment of paroxysmal supraventricular tachycardia (PSVT). The dosage of verapamil is 0.075 to 0.15 mg per kg, which is administered via intravenous bolus over a one-minute period. Not over 10 mg of the drug should be administered at any one time. After 30 minutes, if the initial response is not adequate, a dose of 0.15 mg per kg can be repeated. Again, this dose should not be over 10 mg, and the total cumulative dose of verapamil within the 30-minute period should not be greater than 15 mg.

ELECTRICAL CARDIOVERSION

Cardioversion depolarizes all cardiac cells, restoring synchrony and allowing the predominant pacemaker to regain control of the rhythm. Direct current countershocks should be administered as soon as possible if the heart is known to be in ventricular fibrillation. It is also indicated in ventricular tachycardia and ventricular asystole (Table 44–7).

TABLE 44–7. Recommended Energies for Countershock

Arrhythmia	Amount of Shock (watt-seconds or joules)
Atrial tachycardia	50
Atrial flutter	50
Atrial fibrillation	200
Ventricular tachycardia	200
Ventricular flutter	200
Ventricular fibrillation	200 (advance quickly to 400 if unsuccessful)

The electrode position should be kept standard, one electrode just to the right of the upper sternum below the clavicle and the other electrode just to the left of the cardiac apex or left nipple. Standard electrode paste or 4 × 4 gauze pads saturated with normal saline will provide conduction of the electrical impulse.

REFERENCES

1. Dripps, R., Eckenhoff, J., and Vandam, L.: Introduction to Anesthesia: The Principles of Safe Practice. 6th ed. Philadelphia, W. B. Saunders Co., 1982.
2. Luce, J., Cary, J., Roso, B., et al.: New developments in cardiopulmonary resuscitation. JAMA, 244:1366, 1980.
3. McIntyre, K., and Lewis, A.: Textbook of Advanced Cardiac Life Support. New York, American Heart Association, 1981.
4. Morrow, D., and Luther, R.: Anaphylaxis: etiology and guidelines for management. Anesth. Analg., 55(4):493, 1976.
5. Standards for cardiopulmonary resuscitation and emergency cardiac care. JAMA, 244(5):453–509, 1980.
6. Wood, M., and Wood, A.: Drugs and Anesthesia: Pharmacology for Anesthesiologists. Baltimore, Williams & Wilkins, 1982.

Index

543

Post anesthesia care unit (PACU)
    (*Continued*)
    size of, 3–5, *4*
    staff orientation to, 11–13, 12t, 13t
    staffing of, 5, 9–11, 11t, 15
    visitors to, 15–16
    warming lights for, 259
Postanesthesia care, 243–260, *250*, 251t,
    253, *254*
Postanesthesia recovery score (PARS),
    17, 17t
Postoperative care, sustained-maximal
    inspiration and, 61
Post-tetanic facilitation, during neuro-
    muscular blockade, 207
Potassium, deficiency of, and muscle re-
    laxants, 203–204
    in geriatric patients, 491
    drug interactions with, 223t
    loss of, after anesthesia, 178
Precapillary sphincter, 72
Prednisolone, drug interactions with,
    224t
Prefrontal area, of brain, *114*
Pregnancy, changes in, cardiovascular,
    505–506, 506t
    gastrointestinal, 506
    hemodynamic, 506
    hepatic, 506
    physiologic, 505–507, 505t
    renal, 506
    respiratory, 506
    ectopic, definition of, 435, *436*
        postoperative care for, 438–439
    postoperative care during, 507
    surgery during, incidence of, 505
Pregnant patients, fetal monitoring of,
    507, 507t, *508*
    pain management of, 507–508
    position of, 507
    postoperative care for, 507–508
    psychologic support of, 507
Preload, definition of, 65
Premotor cortex, 114–115, *114*
Pressure-volume (P-V) curve, *36*, 36–37,
    37
    anesthesia effect on, 39–40, *40*
Prilocaine, relative potency of, 212t
PRL. See *Prolactin*.
Procainamide, drug interactions with, 222
    for CPR, 540
Procaine, drug interactions with, 223t
    for local anesthesia, 213t
    relative potency of, 212t
Prochlorperazine, for nausea, 515t
Procidentia, definition of, 437
Projection fibers, of brain, 112
Prolactin (PRL), 143
Pronestyl. See *Procainamide*.
Propanidid, anesthetic effects of, 192
    metabolism of, 192
    side effects of, 192
Propranolol, drug interactions with,
    222
    for CPR, 540
Proprioception, definition of, 110
Prostaglandins, in hypoxemia, 42
Prostate, surgery for, 429–431
    approaches to, 429–430

Prostatectomy, definition of, 421
    drainage after, 430, *430*
Prostigmin. See *Neostigmine*.
Protein synthesis, in liver, 101
Pseudocholinesterase, and ACh, 196
    deficiency of, 201
Psychedelics, complications of, postop-
    erative, 476
Psychosocial assessment, postoperative,
    240–241
Pterygium, definition of, 287
PTH. See *Parathormone*.
Ptosis, definition of, 287
    myasthenia gravis and, 479
Pudendal nerve, 139
Pulmonary artery pressure, hemody-
    namic monitoring of, 338
Pulmonary capillaries, fluid movement
    from, 42–43, *43*
Pulmonary capillary wedge pressure,
    hemodynamic monitoring of, 338
Pulmonary circulation, 41–42
    gas exchange in, 41–42
    interstitial fibrosis and, 41
    neuroendothelial bodies in, 41
    nutrition and, 42
    systemic and, 41
Pulmonary edema, 43
    crackles in, 43
    treatment for, 43–44
Pulmonary forces, balance of, 39–40, *40*
Pulmonary function, abnormal, 58–60
    age and, 59–60
    normal, *60*, 60–61, *61*
    obesity and, 59
    postoperative risks to, 58–59
    postoperative sighless breathing and,
        60
    tests of, 58–59
Pulmonary hysteresis, 36–38, *37*
Pulmonary stretch receptors, 57
Pulmonary vascular resistance, hemody-
    namic monitoring of, 344
Pulse, character of, 233
    deficit of, 65
    irregularities in, 233
    postoperative, 232
        pressure of, 233–234
    radial, obliteration of, 218
    variations of, pediatric, 494–495, 495t
Pupils, activity of, cranial injury and,
    382–383
Purkinje fibers, 69
P-V curve. See *Pressure-volume curve*.
Pyelitis, definition of, 84
Pyeloplasty, definition of, 420
Pyelostomy, definition of, 420
Pyelotomy, definition of, 420
Pyloric obstruction, gastroenterostomy
    for, *407*
Pyloric stenosis, surgery for, 414
Pyloromyotomy, definition of, 409
Pyloroplasty, definition of, 409
Pyramidal signs, definition of, 366
Pyramidal tracts, of brain, 113
Pyramids, renal, 85, *85*
Pyridostigmine, and neuromuscular
    transmission, 200
    dosage of, 200